Nurse's HomeCare Handbook

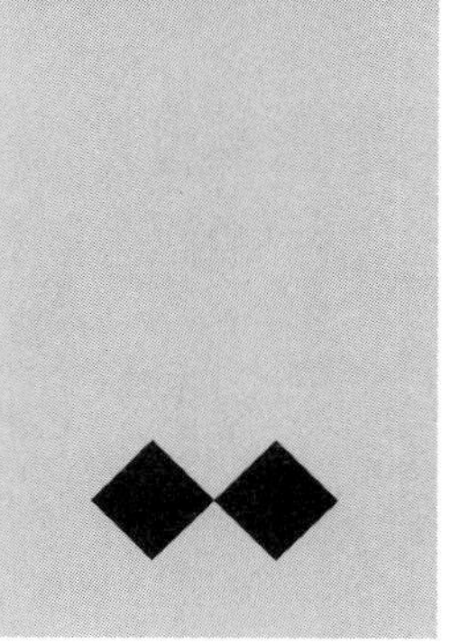

Nurse's HomeCare Handbook

SPRINGHOUSE CORPORATION

Springhouse, Pennsylvania

STAFF

Senior Publisher
Matthew Cahill

Editorial Director
Donna O. Carpenter

Clinical Director
Judith Schilling McCann, RN, MSN

Art Director
John Hubbard

Managing Editor
H. Nancy Holmes

Clinical Consultant
Collette Bishop Hendler, RN, CCRN

Clinical Editors
Maryann Foley, RN, BSN; Carla M. Roy, RN, BSN, CCRN; Beverly Ann Tscheschlog, RN

Editorial Project Manager
Catherine E. Harold

Editors
Jane V. Cray, Kathryn Goldberg, Howard Kaplan, Doris Weinstock, Patricia A. Wittig

Copy Editors
Cynthia C. Breuninger (manager), Karen C. Comerford, Mary T. Durkin, Stacey A. Follin, Brenna H. Mayer

Designers
Arlene Putterman (associate art director), Susan Hopkins Rodzewich (project designer), BJ Crim, Jacalyn Bove Facciolo, Donald Knauss, Amy Litz, Jeffrey Sklarow

Manufacturing
Deborah Meiris (director), Patricia K. Dorshaw (manager), Otto Mezei

Production Coordinator
Stephen P. Hungerford, Jr.

Editorial Assistant
Beverly Lane

Indexer
Barbara Hodgson

The clinical procedures described and recommended in this publication are based on research and consultation with medical and nursing authorities. To the best of our knowledge, these procedures reflect currently accepted clinical practice; nevertheless, they can't be considered absolute and universal recommendations. For individual application, recommendations must be considered in light of the patient's clinical condition and, before administration of new or infrequently used drugs, in light of the latest package-insert information. The authors and the publisher disclaim responsibility for any adverse effects resulting directly or indirectly from the suggested procedures, from any undetected errors, or from the reader's misunderstanding of the text.

Printed in the United States of America.

NHCH-01398

A member of the Reed Elsevier plc group

Library of Congress Cataloging-in-Publication Data
Nurse's HomeCare Handbook.
p. cm.
Includes index.
1. Home nursing I. Springhouse Corporation
[DNLM: 1. Home Care Services—United States—handbooks. WY49 N9735 1998]
RT120.H65N87 1998
610.73—dc21
DNLM/DLC 97-50211
ISBN 0-87434-894-3 (alk. paper) CIP

CONTENTS

CONTRIBUTORS AND CONSULTANTS

Mary Bannan, RN, BSN
Staff Nurse
Western Medical Services
Media, Pa.

Marcie Barnette, RN, MSN, FNP
Director of Organization Improvement
Visiting Nurse Association of Washington, D.C.

Janice Gasho Brennan, RN, MSN, MSOM, CCRN
Regional Coordinator for Quality Assurance and Clinical Outcomes
Allegheny University Hospital Home Care Services
Philadelphia

Barbara M. Braithwaite, RN, MSN, CS
Clinical Nursing Instructor
Burlington County College
Pemberton, N.J.

Karen T. Bruchak, RN, MSN, MBA
Assistant Administrator, Cancer Clinical Programs
University of Pennsylvania Cancer Center
Philadelphia

Heidi Brush, RN,C, BSN
Nursing Supervisor, Home Care Department
Doylestown (Pa.) Hospital

Marsha L. Cornell, RN, MSN
Assistant Professor
Armstrong State College
Savannah, Ga.

Kathleen M. Cummings, RN, BSN, CRNH
Vice-President, Clinical Services
Kansas City (Mo.) Hospice

Cindy Dillon, RN, MS
Disease Management Program Development, Home Care
Children's Hospital of Philadelphia

Joann K. Erb, RN, MSN
Course Coordinator, Advanced Medical-Surgical Nursing
Abington Memorial Hospital School of Nursing
Willow Grove, Pa.

Claire J. Fisher, RN, ARNP, CNM
Certified Nurse-Midwife
Lahey-Hitchcock Clinic
Manchester, N.H.

Latrell P. Fowler, RN, PhD
Assistant Professor
Medical University of South Carolina
Florence

Terry L. Gampher, RN, BSN
Nursing Supervisor
Visiting Nurse Association of Greater Kansas City (Mo.)

Ginny Wacker Guido, RN, MSN, JD
Professor and Chair, Department of Nursing
Eastern New Mexico University
Portales

Judy Willis Hileman, RN, PhD, ARNP
Assistant Professor and Coordinator of Distance Education
School of Nursing
University of Missouri at Kansas City

Patricia P. Hrebicik, RN
Home Health Aide Supervisor
LifeQuest Home Care
Quakertown, Pa.

Cynthia Lange Ingham, RN, BSN
Public Health Nursing Specialist
Vermont Department of Health
Burlington

Susan Jeffries, RN, MSN
Case Manager, Research
University of Pittsburgh Medical Center

Susan K. Markel, RN, BSN, MS, CNSN, CRNI
Senior Director, Clinical Development
Option Care, Inc.
Bannockburn, Ill.

Dawna Martich, RN, MSN
Clinical Director
Medi Home Health Agency
Upper St. Clair, Pa.

Lyn L. McNair, RN,C, IBCLC
Maternal-Infant Home Care Coordinator
Doylestown (Pa.) Hospital

Carol F. Metcalf, RN, BSN, PhD
Professor
Truckee Meadows Community College
Reno, Nev.

Ruth D. Mitchell, RN, MS
Director, Community Nursing Organization
Visiting Nurse Service of New York
Long Island City

Janet Byram Newsom, RN, MSN, CDE, CETN, CNS
Clinical Nurse Specialist and Independent Consultant
Marshall, Tex.

Lori Martin Plank, RN, MSN, MSPH, CS, FNP, GNP
Coordinator, Adult Nurse Practitioner Program
Gwynedd Mercy College
Gwynedd Valley, Pa.

Rosilyn Reiss, RN
Visiting Nurse
Visiting Nurse/Home Care Department
Doylestown (Pa.) Hospital

JoAnne Resnic, RN, BSN
Case Management Coordinator
Paidos Health Management Services, Inc.
Paoli, Pa.

Christine E. Shebest, RN
Clinical Supervisor
Visiting Nurse/Home Care Department
Doylestown (Pa.) Hospital

Larry E. Simmons, RN, MSN
HIV Clinical Nurse Specialist
Visiting Nurse Association of Greater Kansas City (Mo.)

Laureen M. Tavolaro-Ryley, RN,C, MSN
Geropsychiatric Clinical Nurse Specialist
Benjamin Rush Geropsychiatric Associates
Pennsylvania Hospital
Philadelphia

Pamela Wendt, RN, BSN
Vice President, Clinical Services
Nursefinders, Inc.
Arlington, Tex.

Janet H. Wright, RN, MSN
Assistant Professor
Armstrong Atlantic State University
Savannah, Ga.

Joan Zieja, RN, MPH
Assistant Professor of Nursing
Holy Family College
Philadelphia

FOREWORD

Home care has a long and rich tradition in the nursing profession and continues to be one of the most challenging specialty areas of nursing practice. Changing sociocultural patterns and population trends, political and legislative influences, health care system reorganization, and restructured reimbursement patterns have dramatically influenced home care. Cost containment measures have resulted in shorter hospital stays as well as different types of alignments, partnerships, and negotiated contracts for home health care and durable medical equipment.

These changing trends not only influence how home care services are organized, delivered, and paid for, but they also affect nursing roles in caring for vulnerable populations at every stage of life. Although home care nurses have long functioned in an independent and flexible manner, they carry increasing responsibility for managing the complex health and illness needs of patients and their families — persons with differing health beliefs, values, cultural norms, and communication levels. Effective communication and negotiation skills are essential to interaction with patients and families, doctors, care providers, case managers, discharge planners, and paraprofessionals in maintaining continuity of care.

High levels of technology, ranging from intermittent infusion devices to ventilator care, require home care nurses to have in-depth assessment and teaching skills as well as the ability to support families in integrating technological devices into their home life. Each of these areas raises ethical and legal concerns regarding patient and family involvement in planning for level-of-care and end-of-life decisions as well as nursing responsibilities in providing a safe living environment and adhering to standards of practice. Clearly, the multiple care demands of home nursing require a high degree of knowledge and skill to meet the needs of patients and families who encounter illnesses or other life changes that necessitate care and support in their home environment.

Planning and delivering high-quality home care in changing systems requires ready access to current information through a versatile, practical guide such as the *Nurse's Home-Care Handbook.* The purpose of this comprehensive reference is to enable home care nurses to respond in a knowledgeable and timely way to these professional and clinical challenges. This highly informative handbook provides current information on a wide range of topics, including in-depth assessment of various population groups, safe performance of common procedures, managing technology in the home, handling difficult patients or unsafe situations, avoiding legal hazards, and improving decision-making and management skills. Each entry is clearly and concisely written and highlighted with charts, illustrations, and explanatory tables.

Throughout the book, special graphic symbols draw the reader's attention to important information. The "Critical Decisions" logo identifies flowcharts that illustrate the process of critical thinking and evaluation skills that nurses use in decision making. The "Emergency Interventions" logo highlights the actions a nurse would take when encountering emergencies in the home, and the "Teaching Points" logo points to specific teaching information the nurse would include in an individual teaching plan.

Carefully selected and reviewed, the entries in *Nurse's HomeCare Handbook* provide an authoritative and convenient reference that addresses basic and complex issues facing both experienced home care nurses and nursing students seeking to improve their skills. It is sure to become one of the most frequently used references for home care nurses, nurse case managers, home care administrators, and others seeking to provide effective patient- and family-centered home care services.

Patricia Ann Roth, RN, EdD
Professor of Nursing
Coordinator, Case Management Program
University of San Diego

Nurse's HomeCare Handbook

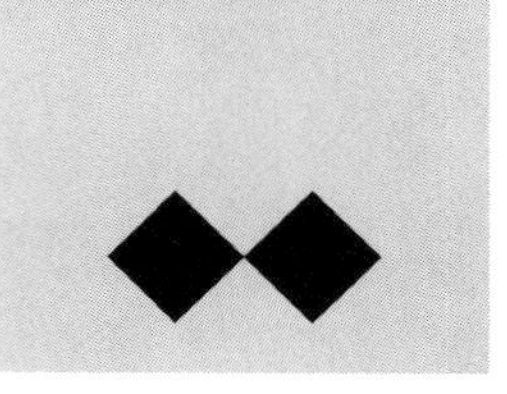

CHAPTER 1

Home care as a specialty

Like all nursing specialties, home health nursing offers a wealth of challenges and rewards. Unlike many other specialties, however, the challenges and rewards of home health nursing involve a broad set of nursing skills that extend well beyond the bounds of clinical expertise.

As a home health nurse, you must be ready to tackle issues as diverse as the patients and families in your charge. In addition to providing expert care, for example, you'll also need to balance your patient's need for care with funds available to pay for it. You'll need to understand the workings of insurance companies, equipment suppliers, and government agencies. You'll need to know how to ensure reimbursement. You'll need to be able and willing to coordinate the services of multiple health care providers, all to the patient's benefit. And you'll need to be prepared to teach, motivate, and counsel patients and their families through possibly confusing, frightening events with compassion and professionalism.

In this chapter, you'll find an introduction to some of the concepts unique to home health nursing. Grasping these concepts — and those presented in later chapters — will help you build a foundation for success in this rapidly growing, highly rewarding specialty.

◆ COLLABORATING WITH THE PATIENT

One of the most obvious distinguishing features of home health nursing is the environment in which it takes place: the patient's home. Here, in the home, you have the opportunity to create a sense of intimacy rarely found in other settings. At the same time, however, you wield considerably less control than you would in other settings. In fact, it's useful to remember that you are, in effect, a guest in your patient's home.

In an acute care setting, you can alter your patient's diet, activity, medications, treatment regimens, visitors, and sleep schedules as you deem necessary to meet his clinical needs. In his home, you must recognize and accept his autonomy.

That means you'll need to develop collaborative ways to accomplish your plan of care. Think of yourself as an enabler, a motivator, and a source of information and encouragement, in addition to being a provider of care. Use your awareness of the patient's autonomy to help build a mutually respectful therapeutic relationship — a relationship in which your patient and his family help set goals and participate in nursing care decisions.

By recognizing the unique influence of the home environment, you can interact with the patient and his family in a manner that increases their independence and their ability to take responsibility for themselves. You can help them build on their own strengths in their own environment. In doing so, you'll help them become your long-term partners in maximizing the patient's health.

◆ INCREASED RESPONSIBILITY

Typically, nurses who work in acute care settings have a circumscribed set of clinical duties and ready backup in case a problem arises. When each shift ends, a new nurse comes in to take over. In contrast, the home health nurse must manage a considerably bigger picture with considerably more independence. Even experienced nurses who switch to home health may at first feel intimidated by the sudden sense of independence — even isolation.

As a home health nurse, you're responsible for all your patient's health needs: assessment, teaching, direct care, case management, coordination, and psychosocial support. It all falls to you. And it isn't limited by the hours in a shift. Consequently, you can't adopt a task-oriented mindset. Instead, you must always keep the patient's big picture in mind.

Astute assessment

Astute assessment skills are a crucial element in managing the patient's care. Over time, you'll develop a keen eye for worsening problems, potential dangers, and the need for assistance.

In the meantime, hone your assessment skills to suit each patient's condition. For example, if you're accustomed to visiting new mothers 1 or 2 weeks postpartum and your new patient was discharged just 12 hours after delivery, you'll need to make sure you obtain appropriate knowledge for assessing this differing clinical situation.

Accurate information

In general, to be successful in seeing and responding to your patient's big picture, you'll need an extensive generalist's knowledge base and the ability to find specific information quickly, as you need it. Fortunately, with rapid technological advancements over the past decade, you have access to more resources — and more convenient resources — than ever.

For example, many medical and drug references are available on handheld computers. Billing and communication can take place online. And cellular phones, pagers, and laptop computers can keep you in touch with crucial resources almost whenever you need them.

Of course, there are still plenty of resources available in traditional formats too, including drug and laboratory handbooks, clinical procedure manuals, and patient education handouts. Many such references are made to fit into a pocket or a small bag.

Some sources of clinical information are right in the patient's community. For example, the patient's pharmacist can confirm which medications he takes and can answer questions about a drug's adverse effects or interactions. The discharge planner at the acute care facility from which the patient was discharged can provide valuable information as well. If the patient has sought help from community social service organizations or other professional services, those professionals may be helpful as well.

Whichever types of resources you prefer, the point is the same. You are responsible for the accuracy of your patients' care. So it's imperative that you cultivate your knowledge base and your ability to find accurate information as you need it.

When help is needed

Another important issue in managing home care is recognizing when you — or your patient — needs help beyond what you can provide. At the least inkling of uncertainty, it's your responsibility to find someone with the appropriate expertise to serve your patient.

That may mean bringing another clinician along on your next visit or holding a telephone conference about the patient. Or you may want to phone another professional from your patient's home. In any case, you'll need to make appropriate decisions to seek additional help as soon as your patient needs it.

Emergency response

If your patient develops an emergent problem, you'll need to make sure he receives care in an appropriate time frame and from the most appropriate professionals. In acute care settings, an emergency typically receives an almost immediate response. At home, there's a considerable risk that it won't.

Plus, what constitutes an emergency typically differs between the home setting and an acute care setting. For example, patients are more likely to fall at home and less likely to have someone nearby who's qualified to assess the results of the fall. Even an unexpected change in a patient's condition may warrant an emergency response — whether or not a patient's caregivers realize it.

You'll need to instruct patients and their families carefully about situations that could signal an emergency. They need clear knowledge about how and when to call you. And you need clear knowledge about how to judge — possibly at a distance — situations that may need an emergency response.

Finally, patients in an acute care setting receive emergency treatment almost without regard to the cost of that treatment. In the home setting, you don't have that luxury. So, when making a decision about the most appropriate emergency care, you'll also need to figure in the availability of funds to pay for that care.

Counseling and teaching

Contrary to acute care settings, patient teaching in home health nursing is typically a crucial element of ongoing nursing care. Starting with your first visit, you'll need to assess — and continually reassess — the teaching needs of your patient and his family.

For example, one of your first teaching assignments will likely involve home safety. Few laypeople know the steps they should take to ensure a safe home environment. Other teaching assignments typically involve the patient's caregivers, who may be called on to provide care that professionals administer in an acute care setting.

Remember that patients and families in acute care settings typically receive teaching that pertains only to the crisis that created a need for acute care. They may be largely unprepared to carry through with the patient's overall needs after discharge.

In the home setting, your teaching can be less crisis-oriented and more health-oriented. By providing generous counseling and teaching, you can — and must — help your patient and his family maximize health, independence, and quality of life.

◆ THE KEY TO SUCCESS

The most successful and satisfied nurses in home health care are those who possess the coping skills and per-

Profile of a home health nurse

The successful home health nurse needs to have the personal and professional traits listed below:
- ◆ self-direction and autonomy
- ◆ strong generalized and specialized clinical skills
- ◆ willingness to assume responsibility for the patient and his plan of care
- ◆ desire to develop new nursing and administrative skills
- ◆ service-driven, patient-oriented interpersonal skills
- ◆ acceptance of the need to balance clinical goals with the patient's reality
- ◆ acceptance of each person's lifestyle and its effect on health
- ◆ sense of humor to help patient and colleagues get through rough times.

sonality traits that are particularly helpful in the home environment. These include the ability to be flexible, to problem-solve, to comfort, and to interact openly with people of various cultures, languages, and lifestyles. (See *Profile of a home health nurse.*) In addition, successful home health nurses learn to balance potentially conflicting priorities.

Maintaining balance

Besides developing helpful personal qualities, you'll also need to balance many contrasting factors when caring for patients in their homes. For example, you'll have to balance the need to create a trusting, intimate care environment with the need to maintain your professional composure and distance.

Although a home visit is not a social occasion, a certain amount of socialization is necessary to establish rapport. You'll need to set boundaries on your disclosure of personal information to maximize the therapeutic aspect of your work.

You'll also need to balance your desire to care for your patient personally with the need to empower him and his family by letting them learn to deliver care. When you needlessly limit the patient's or his family's efforts, you may devalue them and make them feel inadequate. Obviously, this feeling will only hamper their ability to maximize the patient's health and independence.

So, although delivering care personally may make you feel effective and needed, it may run counter to your real goal of helping your patient. Instead, you'll need to shift the balance toward the patient and family. And you'll need to learn how to derive your sense of personal accomplishment from your patient's success rather than from your indispensability.

Another important example is the need to balance your senses of realism and altruism. Most of the patients you see as a home health nurse will have extensive, sometimes longstanding problems that may or may not relate specifically to their need for home nursing. Always remember that you won't be able to solve all patient and family problems, just those responsive to nursing interventions.

Above all, it's important to reflect on your actions and attitudes as they relate to your patients' dignity and autonomy. You can't succeed by imposing your needs and goals on your patients. Instead, you'll need to strike a fine balance that provides them with what they need to develop their own goals and satisfy their own needs to the extent that they're able.

Cultural considerations

Each day, you'll probably visit the homes of patients who differ strikingly from you in their cultural, religious, and socioeconomic traits. Yet you'll need to merge into their lives without disruption or conflict. How can you accomplish this?

In general, you can do so by maintaining a sense of openness and sensitivity. Do your best to avoid stereotypical attitudes and preconceived notions. It's incumbent upon you to be attuned to basic cultural values and beliefs and to ascertain the extent to which they influence each patient.

For example, when you stand in the doorway of a new patient's home, begin to acquaint yourself with the cultural, religious, and economic influences visible in the environment. Scan the room for religious items and symbols, reading material, television or radio programs in progress, furnishings, pictures, and foods. Pay attention to the patient's and family's education levels, communication styles, time and personal space issues, family rituals, and specific health and nutritional practices and beliefs.

Take in what you can about your patient, but remember not to supplement your findings with assumptions. The more you can assess and accept each patient's unique set of beliefs, values, and circumstances, the more you'll be able to promote his physical and psychological health.

◆ THE TEAM APPROACH

In virtually all avenues of health care today, patients receive care from teams of professionals. As a home health nurse, you typically will be charged with coordinating your patients' multidisciplinary health team.

This is a job of crucial importance. Without collaboration and coordination, there can be no continuity of care and little chance of accomplishing a multifaceted plan of care.

In addition to his doctor, the patient's team may include professionals from a number of diverse specialties, including a physical therapist or assistant, speech therapist, occupational therapist, social worker, home health aide, respiratory therapist, nutritionist, dietitian, and others. (See *The home health team*, pages 6 and 7.)

You also may work with a number of community and family members and with subcontractors who also provide patient services. You'll need strong interpersonal skills to solicit information, answer questions, organize services, direct care, and teach. (See chapter 2 for more information on interpersonal skills.)

One of the keys to success in coordinating your patient's care is to start right away. As soon as multidisciplinary care begins, start coordinating the included activities. Don't wait for the patient to develop a problem.

Coordinating a patient's care may involve a number of time-consuming tasks, such as arranging joint visits to the patient's home, scheduling conference calls, and orchestrating meetings. Remember, however, that these tasks are imperative to achieving coordinated, efficient care. They're well worth the effort.

Also keep in mind that in home health care, the responsibilities and functions of each member of the health care team are dictated by Medicare, state licensing boards, state home health regulations, and accrediting bodies. You'll need to become familiar with their requirements so you can follow them faithfully when coordinating your patient's care.

The home health team

Your patient's multidisciplinary team may include some or all of these members.

Physical therapist

Physical therapists evaluate neuromuscular and functional ability and use such treatments as therapeutic exercise; massage; transcutaneous electrical nerve stimulation; water, heat, ultraviolet, and ultrasound therapy; postural drainage; and pulmonary exercises. They must possess at least a bachelor's degree and be licensed by the state in which they practice.

Occupational therapist

Occupational therapists help patients develop and maintain the ability to perform activities of daily living. Specific interventions include performing exercises to increase upper body strength and mobility, making and fitting splints, adjusting and using upper extremity prostheses, teaching feeding techniques, and identifying special devices to promote independence. Occupational therapists must possess at least a bachelor's degree and be registered by the National Occupational Therapists Association.

Speech-language pathologist

Also called speech therapists, these professionals help patients who have communication, hearing, or swallowing problems. They also teach other providers and family members how to help patients develop communication skills. Typical interventions include language boards, computers, sign language, exercises, and games. Speech therapists must possess a master's degree and be certified by the American Speech, Hearing, and Language Association.

Social worker

Social workers help patients and families deal with social, emotional, and environmental issues. Some social workers focus on psychotherapy; others focus on community programs and systems. The social worker chosen should specialize in the patient's or family's problem area. Social workers must possess a master's degree in social work and be certified by the Association of Certified Social Workers.

Home health aide

Duties of the home health aide may include light housekeeping, cooking, shopping, and laundry. Under supervision, they provide some direct care, such as overseeing exercises, monitoring temperature, and providing skin and indwelling urinary catheter care. Home health aides must pass a course that meets Medicare and state standards. They must work under the supervision of a nurse or physical therapist unless hired by the family directly.

Personal care assistant

Also called homemakers, personal care assistants tend to patients' personal needs. States that reimburse for these services

The home health team *(continued)*

under Medicaid mandate the specific training, supervision requirements, and activities allowed. Personal care services aren't reimbursable by Medicare.

Physical therapy assistant
Assistants may provide some types of physical therapy under direct supervision by a licensed physical therapist. They must graduate from a 2-year college program, be approved by the American Physical Therapy Association, be licensed by the state, and have at least 2 years of experience.

Social work assistant
Under the supervision of a social worker, social work assistants help identify and apply appropriate resources. They must possess a bachelor's degree but need no training in psychotherapy or mental status evaluation.

Additional personnel
This category may include such professional team members as a respiratory therapist, nutritionist, or dietitian. It also may include escorts for nurses going into high-crime areas, translators (for written communication), and interpreters (for verbal communication).

In general, it's up to you to provide full documentation of your patient's care. Ensure that your documentation is fastidious and accurate and that it fully reflects discussions among the members of your patient's care team. (See chapter 15 for more information on documentation.) Include all discussions of the patient's plan of care, progress toward goals, problems, and discharge plans. Also document all conferences, phone conversations, and other contacts with team members. Besides ensuring coordinated care, doing so will also ensure compliance with Medicare requirements.

◆ WHAT AGENCIES OFFER

As a home health nurse, you may tend to think of yourself as working for your patients. In many ways, you are. However, your paycheck probably will come from some type of home health agency. (See *Types of home health agencies*, page 8.) In general, home health agencies provide a range of patient care services, including professional services, paraprofessional services, and equipment and supplies. Examples of professional services include:

- nursing
- physical therapy
- social work
- speech and language therapy
- occupational therapy
- diet or nutrition therapy
- respiratory therapy.

Examples of paraprofessional services include:

- home health aide services
- homemaker services
- home attendant or personal care services
- escort or transportation services.

A long and changing list of equipment and supplies is available to home care patients, including:

- commodes

Types of home health agencies

According to the National Association for Home Care, there are more than 15,000 home care agencies in the United States. About two-thirds participate in Medicare. Typically, they fit into one of the following categories.

Visiting nurse association (VNA)
A freestanding, voluntary, nonprofit organization governed by a board of directors and usually financed by tax-deductible contributions and earnings.

Public (official) agency
An agency operated by a state, county, city, or other unit of local government. Public agencies are primarily responsible for preventing disease and for community health education. They often provide direct patient services as well.

Private nonprofit agency
A freestanding, nonprofit agency that's privately developed, governed, and owned.

Private for-profit agency
A freestanding, for-profit home health agency. May be organizationally linked to a VNA or a private, nonprofit agency and may be housed under the same roof.

Combination agency
A combined government and voluntary agency. Sometimes combination agencies are considered VNAs.

Hospital-based agency
An operating unit or department of a hospital. (Agencies that have working arrangements with hospitals or are owned by hospitals but operated as separate entities are classified as freestanding agencies under one of the categories above.)

Rehabilitation facility–based agency
A home health arm of a freestanding rehabilitation facility.

Skilled nursing facility
A home health arm of a freestanding skilled nursing facility.

- wheelchairs
- oxygen equipment
- hospital beds
- walkers
- catheters
- dressing supplies
- respirators
- needleless insulin injectors.

Keep in mind that home health agencies provide equipment and supplies based on their ability to receive reimbursement for them. Consequently, you'll need to remember the definitions for both categories of items.

Medical supplies typically are defined as items essential for diagnosing or treating a patient's illness or injury. Durable medical equipment (DME) is defined as medically necessary equipment that can be used over and over again, such as wheelchairs and hospital beds. It must serve a primarily medical purpose, can't be useful for those who are not sick or injured, and must be appropriate for home use.

As a home health nurse, you need to be familiar with the types of equipment and supplies that are and aren't reimbursable by various payers. You also need to verify coverage before obtaining special equipment. Because regulations in this area tend to change regularly, check with your local supplier of medical equipment and supplies for the most recent reimbursement guidelines.

Many home health agencies offer additional services as well as those listed above, including infusion therapy, long-term care planning, mental health programs, community nursing, health education programs, elder-care consultations, and others. Additional services are limited only by the creativity of those involved and the needs of the individual agency's local patients.

Footing the bill

No matter what type of agency you work for, you almost certainly will hold at least partial responsibility for ensuring that funds are available to pay for your patients' care. This is a major difference between home health nursing and virtually every other nursing specialty.

Funds to pay for your patients' care may come from several sources, including Medicare, Medicaid, private health insurance, out-of-pocket payments, and long-term care insurance.

Medicare

Signed into law in 1965, Medicare includes provisions for home health care that enable elderly and disabled citizens to receive nursing and other health services at home. In addition, the legislation specifies regulations and standards for all home health agencies that participate in the Medicare program. Typically, Medicare covers services ordered by a doctor that relate to an acute medical condition.

Medicaid

A federal- and state-funded program, Medicaid provides health care for indigent persons. It's funded by general tax revenues rather than by mandatory contributions (such as Medicare and Social Security). Consequently, states can structure their own Medicaid eligibility benefits as long as they adhere to certain minimum benefit levels. Home health care is an optional benefit, but most states cover at least some home health services.

Medicaid services often are very different from those covered by Medicare. In fact, in some states, Medicaid covers custodial and comfort measures, such as homemaker services.

Private health insurance

Some commercial insurance policies cover home health care. The benefits vary from policy to policy; usually, they're limited to services that substitute for more costly inpatient or outpatient care after surgery or prolonged hospitalization.

Out-of-pocket payments

Often viewed as the last resort in paying for health care services, private funds or out-of-pocket payments come directly from the patient or his family. Private funds are best used to supplement services not covered by another payer or when other payer sources are exhausted.

Long-term care insurance

Sold as a supplement to Medicare and private insurance, a long-term care policy usually covers nursing home and home health care.

Certification

When choosing the agency for which you'll work, consider whether or not it's been certified. About two-thirds of home health agencies are certified to receive payment for their services from federal and third-party sources (such as commercial insurance and managed care organizations).

Keep in mind that certified agencies may occupy a more secure position in the changing health care industry. As more and more government services become privatized, governing bodies, such as cities and counties, have discovered that an official agency with Medicare certification is a desirable commodity. In some cases, doing business with such an agency can help to lower government spending.

To become Medicare certified, a home health agency must meet Medicare standards and be approved by the federal Health Care Financing Administration (HCFA). Certified agencies also must comply with local and state home health agency licensing requirements. In some states, agencies are tightly regulated; in others, they're largely unregulated.

Certified agencies must offer at least the following services:

- part-time or intermittent nursing care by or under the supervision of a registered professional nurse
- physical, occupational, or speech-language therapy
- medical social services
- part-time or intermittent services by certified home health aides
- medical supplies and durable medical equipment.

Home health agencies, home care aide organizations, and hospices may choose not to seek Medicare certification for a number of reasons. For example, some agencies don't provide the kinds of services that Medicare covers. Others may prefer to avoid Medicare's regulatory demands. Noncertified home health agencies must arrange alternate funding sources, such as third-party payers, managed care organizations, and private funds.

Accreditation

Another factor to weigh when choosing an employer is an agency's accreditation status. Accreditation is a voluntary process in which one of several independent organizations lends its stamp of approval to an agency and the services it provides. The two organizations best known for accrediting home health agencies are the Joint Commission on Accreditation of Healthcare Organizations (JCAHO) and the Community Health Accreditation Program (CHAP).

In its mission to improve the quality of health care delivery, JCAHO sets widely accepted standards for and accredits most types of health care organizations. Some payers now require JCAHO accreditation for subcontractors.

CHAP, a subsidiary of the National League for Nursing, surveys a variety of community health organizations. Its mission resembles that of JCAHO: to improve the quality of health care.

The newest credentialing body for home health agencies is the National Committee for Quality Assurance (NCQA). This private, nonprofit organization evaluates and provides information about the quality of managed health care. It has two purposes: accrediting managed care companies and measuring patient care outcomes. In the future, NCQA may be used to compare home health agencies within specified regions.

NCQA standards originated with the Health Plan Employer Data and Information Set (HEDIS), which was developed by a coalition of health maintenance organizations (HMOs). Some states use HEDIS to compare hospitals within regions. HCFA is aggressively urging states to use HEDIS for comparing the performance of Medicaid HMOs, for making purchase decisions, and for holding plans accountable.

◆ RULES OF REIMBURSEMENT

To function with expertise as a home health nurse, especially in a certified agency, you'll need to understand the rules on which payers base reimbursement for services. Typically, they consider the acuity of the patient's condition, his need for skilled services, and the opinion of a doctor.

To receive reimbursement from Medicare for home health care, the patient must be homebound, and he must require skilled nursing or physical therapy on an intermittent basis. Because interpretations of skilled therapies can be subjective, you'll want to carefully identify and document each patient's need for care available only from a skilled professional.

For example, when deciding whether a service qualifies as skilled care, ask yourself questions like these: Is the service complex, requiring the knowledge and skill of a registered nurse? Does the patient's condition warrant skilled intervention? Can this service be performed by a nonmedical person? Does the teaching required by a patient involve knowledge and demonstrations that must come from a registered nurse?

If a patient's services qualify for reimbursement from Medicare, it typically comes through what Medicare calls a fiscal intermediary — an agency, usually an insurer, designated by HCFA to act as a reimbursing agent. Some agencies hire a "surveyor" to interpret the applicable rules of reimbursement, and then shape their operations to conform with the surveyor's interpretation. The fiscal intermediary for your agency will monitor your documentation and nursing notes from time to time to verify the need for reimbursement.

Keep in mind that reimbursement can be denied even after services are provided. Obviously, it's important to provide adequate documentation to prove that services qualify for reimbursement. It's also important to avoid multiple denials of reimbursement; they could affect your agency's reimbursement status.

◆ FUTURE TRENDS

Unquestionably, the delivery of health care in the United States has changed dramatically over the past decade or so. The changes result primarily from wild increases in health care expenditures. For example, in 1960, the United States spent $27.1 billion on health care, or 5.3% of the gross domestic product. By 1991, total health care expenditures had risen to $751.8 billion, a figure that equaled 13.2% of the gross domestic product ($2,686 per person).

Because home health is considerably less expensive than care delivered in an acute setting, most experts suspect that the demand for home health care will continue to rise. Indeed, Medicare's home health expenditures more than tripled between 1990 and 1994, from $3.9 billion to nearly $14 billion.

Despite this good news for the future of home health, you almost certainly will be forced to adapt to continued cost-cutting measures, such as capitation or fixed reimbursement rates per visit.

Managed care

The most important development in the bid to cut health care costs has been the growth of managed health care plans. (See *Common managed health care plans.*) Home health agencies may subcontract with or be owned by managed care organizations that offer any or all of these plan types.

Usually, when your patient belongs to a managed care plan (especially an HMO), you'll be authorized to provide a certain number of home visits. Unauthorized visits won't be reimbursed. If you feel that your patient requires more home care than the authorized number of visits, you'll need to contact the managed care organization, explain the patient's status, and urge the organization to authorize additional visits.

If you're accustomed to collaborating with a professional health care team to determine how many home visits your patient needs, this authorization process can become frustrating. You may feel that your professional judgment is being questioned and infringed upon.

However, it's important to recognize that more people than ever are enrolled in managed health care plans. Many states require Medicaid beneficiaries to enroll in managed care plans. And many organizations offer managed care plans to Medicare beneficiaries. Although the percentage of Medicare recipients in managed care is still low, it's growing rapidly. Why? Because managed care plans offer more covered benefits than Medicare for the same monthly cost.

Thus, the nurses most successful in home care will be those who develop skills in negotiating with managed care plans to the benefit of the agency and the patient. As more and more people join managed care plans and the number of covered home visits declines, it becomes even more important to evaluate and teach patients carefully and thoroughly and to help identify alternative sources of care whenever possible. Keep in mind that many HMOs would consider covering even nonmedical services if those services were less costly and still effective.

Competition

Like all industries seeking to cut costs, the health care industry has undergone and will continue to undergo mergers, buyouts, consolidations, and realignments. Home health agencies are no exception. That's why it's important to take note of the industry trends in your area. Home health agencies, like other organizations, are restructuring to help increase market influence and gain economies of scale.

This increased competition, while unnerving to most employees, can actually benefit your patients. Why? Because patient satisfaction must remain a primary goal for every agency. Keep in mind that many people who need home care will need it again in the future. Those who are satisfied with their first round of care are almost certain to call the same agency for continued care.

Increased competition has also altered the routes by which patients come to home care agencies. These days, patients may enter the home care system — or be removed from it — through facilities as diverse as subacute facilities, assisted living facilities, limited extended care facilities, and outpatient treatment facilities. Subacute and assisted living facilities probably exert the largest influence.

Subacute facilities

Subacute facilities are a subsector of the skilled nursing facility industry. They're designed to better serve

Medicare patients discharged from acute care settings. These patients are too sick to be treated at home but don't need all the services available in hospitals. After leaving this type of facility, patients commonly need home care as well.

Assisted living facilities

These facilities offer housing, support services, personalized assistance, and health care to patients who need help with activities of daily living. They seek to foster the patient's dignity and independence. They commonly involve the patient's family, neighbors, and friends.

Assisted living facilities provide services and a home setting at a lower cost than many home health agencies and intermediate care nursing homes. Many have their own certified home health agency or a contracted agency. Reimbursement is primarily by private pay.

Technology

Possibly the least understood factor affecting the future of health care is technology. However, even though no one knows exactly how rapidly evolving technology will affect home care, it almost certainly will. In fact, its influence has already begun.

Plummeting computer prices combined with rapid increases in computing power are allowing development of systems that extend beyond the bounds of individual facilities, agencies, and professional offices. Improved data management promises to decrease duplicated data-collection efforts. It also may decrease the time nurses spend trying to find such crucial patient data as history, nursing problems, and treatment.

In addition to advances in computing, technology continues to increase the availability of devices for home use. A variety of miniaturized equipment is suitable for use by home health nurses. For example, noninvasive monitors are available to assess blood oxygen levels, electrocardiogram machines have shrunk to the size of a box of chocolates, and hand-

Common managed health care plans

As more and more of your patients enter managed health care plans, it's ever more important for you to understand their basic features. Here's a brief description of some of the most common managed care plans.

HMOs
In a health maintenance organization (HMO), each member has a primary care doctor who delivers or coordinates all of the member's care. Self-referred care is not covered.

Point-of-service plan
Each member has a primary care doctor through whom the member obtains care at the lowest out-of-pocket cost. Self-referred care is covered at a restricted benefit level.

Preferred provider organization
Members receive the highest benefit levels when they seek care from doctors contracted with the plan.

Physician-hospital organization
This is basically a preferred provider organization that includes contracted doctors and hospitals in a specific service area.

held blood sample analyzers give readings within 2 minutes.

Improved telecommunications also holds the possibility of revolutionizing some aspects of home health care. For example, through telephones equipped with special video capability, it's possible to gather some types of data without actually visiting the patient's home. You can check vital signs, schedule daily events, teach patients, and remotely manage the patient's plan of care. Some systems even allow you to manipulate the video camera to get a closer look at a wound, watch an aide demonstrating patient care, or accomplish a myriad of other changing needs.

Clearly, to ensure future success as a home health nurse, you'll need to be willing to learn high-tech skills as they evolve. As more homes become equipped with personal computers, technological possibilities will broaden for home health providers, and the home health nurse's role will become more expansive and valuable.

◆ SPECIFIC POPULATIONS

Within the home health care specialty, you may have opportunities to specialize still further. Common home health specialties include maternal and infant care, pediatric care, mental health and psychiatric care, and hospice care. In each case, you'll need skills and education appropriate to serve your specific population.

Maternal and infant care

Home health care is available to mothers and infants from a variety of sources. For example, each state has programs for mothers and infants. Your agency may subcontract with towns, cities, or counties to provide government-mandated services, such as primary preventive care for mothers and infants. Most managed care plans cover both prenatal care and postpartum assessment and teaching.

No matter which type of organization funds your visits, you'll want to start prenatal care as early as possible in the patient's pregnancy. Depending on the patient's needs, you should consider including a wide array of teaching topics during pregnancy and after delivery. (See *Topics for new mothers*.)

During postpartum home visits, you'll evaluate the mother and infant, teach the new mother, and make referrals as needed.

Pediatric care

Especially for medically fragile children and those with flare-ups of chronic diseases, visits from a home health nurse can keep life as normal as possible while also reducing the overall cost of care. Pediatric home health care is covered by private insurers, HMOs, and Medicaid.

Typically, children are considered for home care based on such factors as:

◆ the potential risks and benefits of home care
◆ the child's needs and medical stability
◆ the availability of family members who are willing to learn proper care and provide it at home
◆ an appropriate home setting
◆ medical, social, and educational support in the community.

Especially in pediatric care situations, you'll need to take special steps to avoid creating conflicts with the parents' role expectations, boundaries, and general home care habits. You can help reduce potential conflicts by discussing house rules as well as the family and nurse relationship.

Remember that even though the child is your patient, one of your primary responsibilities will be teach-

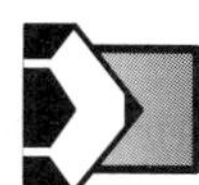

TEACHING POINTS

Topics for new mothers

Even if your pregnant patient already has other children, you should review teaching topics such as those listed here.

During pregnancy

◆ Benefits of prenatal care
◆ Importance of taking personal responsibility for self and developing fetus
◆ Physiologic changes that occur during pregnancy
◆ Milestones of fetal growth and development
◆ Principles of health and nutrition
◆ Benefits of exercise
◆ Dangers of using drugs, alcohol, or tobacco during pregnancy
◆ Coping with domestic violence during pregnancy
◆ Planning the delivery process
◆ Stages of labor
◆ Breast-feeding techniques and problem solving
◆ Future birth control
◆ Preparation for parenthood
◆ Other sources of prenatal care, including community childbirth classes, self-help groups, governmental programs, family planning services, and school-based clinics

After delivery

◆ Caring for an infant
◆ Normal variations in infants
◆ Milestones of growth and development
◆ Follow-up health care for mother and infant
◆ Immunization schedule for an infant
◆ Physiologic changes after delivery
◆ Breast- and bottle-feeding techniques
◆ Exercises to regain muscle tone
◆ How to recognize postpartum depression
◆ Family planning
◆ How to balance home, work, and family
◆ How to find child care, if needed

ing parents and other family members. In addition to teaching specifically about the child's disorder, be sure to reinforce general child-care principles, such as immunization schedules and measures that promote the child's growth and development.

Finally, make sure you're familiar with child protection laws in your state. As a home health nurse, you'll be on the front line in detecting possible abuse and neglect. It's crucial that you understand the legally mandated reporting responsibilities in your state and that you're prepared to identify and report child neglect and abuse.

Mental health and psychiatric care

Every year, about 15 out of 100 people require mental health care. Of those, about 1.5% may need home care. Because of this limited population, only a small number of home health agencies provide mental health and psychiatric home care.

To obtain Medicare reimbursement for these services, you'll need to meet specific educational and practice regulations. Also, the patient must have a psychiatric diagnosis and meet Medicare's homebound and skilled care requirements. In some cases, mental (or behavioral) home health care may include patients with closed-head injuries, patients who undergo alcohol detoxification at home, and patients who need continuity of care at home.

Hospice care

Since it was formalized in 1974, hospice care has grown steadily as an option for patients in the terminal stage of illness. This type of care seeks to make the dying process as dignified, comfortable, and emotionally, spiritually, and socially supportive as possible.

Hospice care can be financed through Medicare, most state Medicaid programs, many private insurance plans, HMOs, individuals, and charity. Hospices may be for profit or nonprofit. Nearly all emphasize care in the patient's home. Most also offer a broad array of services from an interdisciplinary team in various inpatient and outpatient settings.

Hospice benefits vary depending on the financing body. For example, the Medicare hospice benefit covers:

- nursing care
- doctors' services from the hospice program
- medical appliances and supplies
- drugs to manage symptoms and relieve pain
- short-term inpatient and respite care
- homemaker and home health aide services
- social work
- counseling
- spiritual care
- volunteer assistance
- physical therapy, occupational therapy, and speech-language therapy
- pathology services
- bereavement services.

To receive reimbursement from Medicare, the hospice must be certified by HCFA. Reimbursement comes as a capped per diem rate based on four possible payment categories: routine home care, continuous home care, respite care in an approved facility (5-day maximum per episode), and general care in an acute facility for pain- or symptom-control that can't take place at home.

No matter what kind of nursing care you administer in the home setting, it's important to remember that the patient in need of home health care is your biggest, but not your only, concern. To be successful as a home health nurse, you also need to concern yourself with the patient's doctor, who brings referrals to your employer; with payers, who may demand deep discounts on referred services while still expecting high patient satisfaction; and with the future of your agency or its corporate parent.

Clearly, home health nursing encompasses a much broader level of skill and awareness than many other nursing specialties. In the remaining chapters of this book, you'll learn much more about the skills and strategies that build a foundation for success in home health nursing. Armed with knowledge, experience, and dedication, you'll be well prepared to take part in the rewarding field of home health nursing.

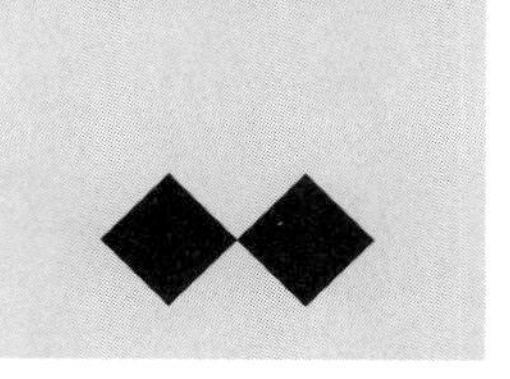

CHAPTER 2

Bolstering management skills

To be successful as a home health nurse, you'll need to develop and use a wide range of practical management skills. Not only do you need such skills when dealing with patients, but you also need them so you can interact with administrators and deftly coordinate teams of professionals and other providers.

High on the list of management skills helpful to home health nurses are the abilities to communicate well, resolve conflict, handle change, and carry out day-to-day agency business. Like all nurses, you'll also need to be well-equipped to assess varying situations, set systematic goals, and develop strategies to meet those goals. You'll need to organize, prioritize, and be able to motivate and reward people of widely differing personality types and professions.

In short, to be successful in today's home health environment, you must excel at managing yourself, your patients, your colleagues, and your employer's business — all with little or no supervision. This chapter outlines the important elements in ensuring your management success.

◆ COMMUNICATING EFFECTIVELY

In one way or another — in words or writing, body language or silence, whether we realize it or not — humans communicate virtually all the time. Often, we communicate almost without thinking.

As a home health nurse, however, you must communicate consciously, on purpose, with skill and understanding. Your ability to communicate clearly is one of your most important assets. It strengthens your nurse-patient relationships, improves teamwork and clinical accuracy, and creates trust between you and your colleagues.

The first step in honing your communication skills is to realize that communication is a process. It contains specific steps that can be learned, used, and improved.

The communication process

In a general sense, communication refers to sending and receiving messages. It's an interactive process that requires a sender and a receiver working together to share information. Good communication minimizes the amount of confusion and misunderstanding created by the interaction.

The overall process of communication breaks down into several discrete steps that involve identifying an idea to be communicated, encoding it into a message before sending it, and decoding the message after receiving it. (See *Communication in action,* page 18.)

An equally important portion of the communication loop is the final one: feedback from the receiver to the

Communication in action

Successful communication doesn't happen by accident. In fact, it requires both the sender and receiver to complete several important steps.

First, the sender identifies an idea to be communicated. Then the sender must encode that idea into a format understandable to the receiver. Finally, the sender must deliver the resulting message.

The receiver must decode the message out of its format and back into an idea. Then the receiver interprets the idea using his or her own knowledge, experience, and intelligence.

Feedback from the receiver to the sender helps verify that the message arrived correctly.

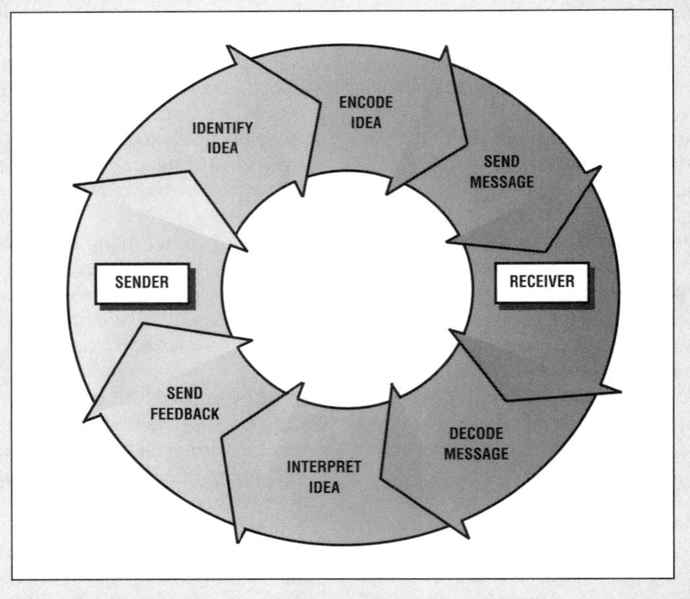

sender. This final step reflects back to the sender how the receiver interpreted the decoded message. It provides the sender with confirmation that the message was received as sent, or it gives the sender a clue that the message may have been misunderstood. In that case, the sender can clarify the message and send it again.

Ideally, it's helpful to give and receive prompt feedback in a mutually understood language — either verbal or written. In practice, however, you may need to decipher a receiver's feedback from an incidental response, such as a facial expression, body language, voice tone, and so on. Sometimes you may be forced to interpret your receiver's response by observing the actions that take place after the communication ends.

Obviously, the most precise and successful communication involves an ongoing comparison of messages sent and received. However, particularly when communicating with those who differ widely in language, training, experience, or knowledge, you'll find many parts of the process in which the message may become distorted or the interaction may break down.

Roadblocks to communication

Even in carefully constructed communication, understanding can be hampered by a variety of personal and situational roadblocks. For example, your message may be blocked by "noise."

In this case, noise doesn't mean actual, audible sounds that interfere with hearing, although obviously that kind of noise can impair communication as well. Rather, noise refers to any factor that distracts the receiver or blurs the message.

For example, cultural differences may distort a message. Feeling threatened or fearful may prevent the receiver from taking in parts of a message. And unusual clothing, scents, facial expressions, or movements may reduce the receiver's ability to concentrate.

Another inevitable roadblock to communication comes from the uniqueness of each person. No two people are exactly alike; no two have had the same education, life experiences, or cultural background. These differences between people give each one of us a unique frame of reference that may cause us to encode or decode messages differently than others would.

As a home health nurse, it's especially important that you recognize the influence of another roadblock — crisis — on communication. Typically, crisis creates a high level of stress, anxiety, confusion, and eventual fatigue. All of these conditions make it difficult for a sender to create clear messages and for a receiver to interpret messages, retain information, and formulate questions.

Being aware of the most common roadblocks to communication can help you frame your message as clearly as possible, ask for feedback to help assess a receiver's comprehension, and follow up with additional information, as needed.

The flow of communication

Another concept important to maintaining clear communication is recognizing the influence of power or position. Communications experts have outlined several patterns by which communication tends to flow, along with the potential pitfalls of each pattern.

In a nutshell, communication can flow vertically, horizontally, or in clusters. These directional flows tend to align with the relative power and influence of the sender and receiver. (See *How messages flow*, page 20.) Usually, however, the most satisfying form of communication is a fourth style, interpersonal communication, which operates independently of levels of power and influence.

Vertical communication. Communication flows vertically — downward or upward — when the sender and receiver possess different levels of power or authority. When the sender has more power or authority than the receiver, communication is said to be downward. When the sender has less power or authority, the communication is said to be upward.

For example, if you're explaining the need for lifestyle alterations to your hypertensive patient, you're engaging in downward communication.

How messages flow

Depending on the message to be delivered and the people delivering it, communication can flow vertically, horizontally, in clusters, or interpersonally, as described here.

Vertical communication

In this communication pattern, messages can originate at the top of a hierarchy and move down (downward communication) or can originate lower in the hierarchy and move up (upward communication). In downward communication, people lower in the hierarchy may receive only partial information and may not be included in discussion or mutual decision making.

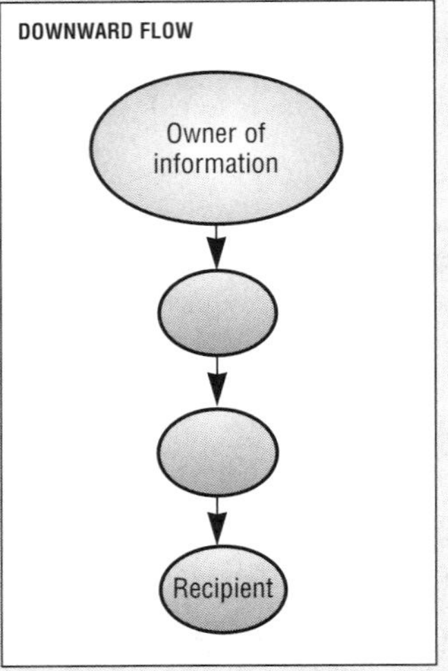

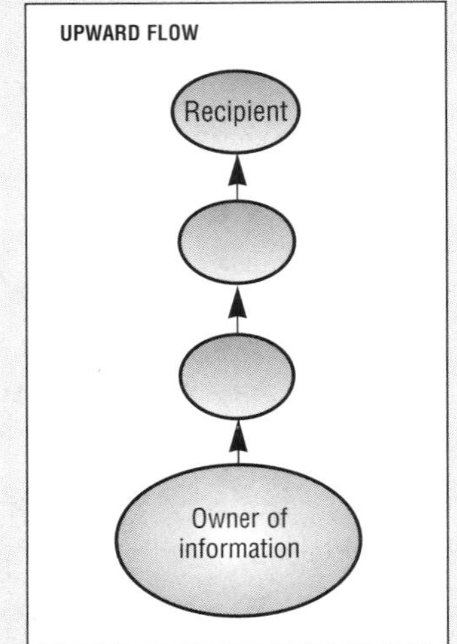

Horizontal communication

In this pattern, information passes laterally among people who have similar levels of power and authority in the hierarchy. Because of this pattern's "whisper down the lane" quality, messages may lose details, goals may lose clarity, and information may lack consistency or continuity.

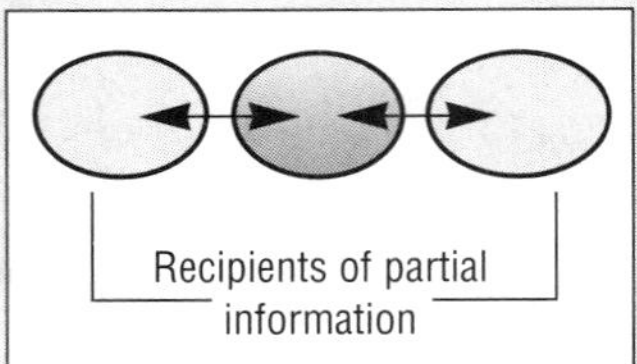

How messages flow *(continued)*

Clustered communication
In this pattern, information flows among individuals in small, separate clusters, but there is little or no communication between clusters. Information, knowledge, and details are not shared beyond the individuals in the cluster.

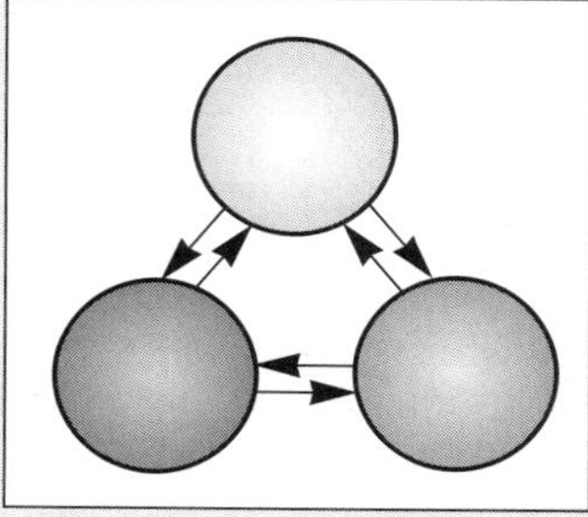

Interpersonal communication
In this pattern, information moves freely among people regardless of their status in the hierarchy. No one person owns the information, and it isn't passed up, down, or over to people. All are recipients and owners of the knowledge, which creates the potential to produce better, more comprehensive decisions.

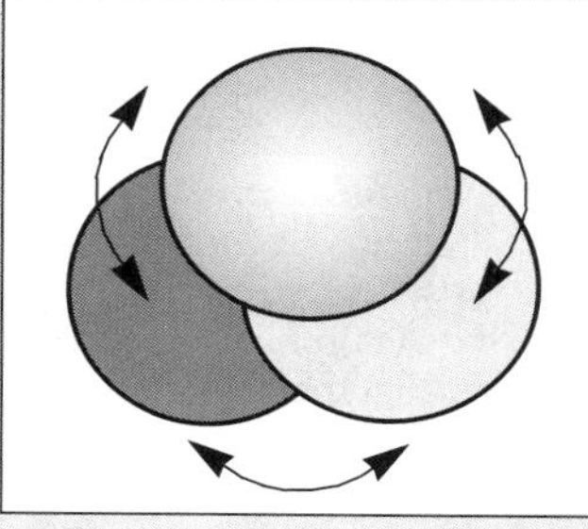

Clearly, as a health care provider, you have more power and authority on health matters than your patient does. In general, downward messages include instructions, explanations, procedures, feedback, and motivational messages.

On the other hand, if a patient is explaining to you why she didn't follow your instructions completely, she's engaging in upward communication. Upward communication allows the "superior" to know the "subordinate," to correct misinterpretations, to identify initial signs of trouble, and to consider the subordinate's views.

Both types of vertical communication create potential pitfalls and problems. In downward communication, for example, many senders tend to rely too much on written rather than verbal messages (using both provides a good balance). Also, senders in downward communication may tend to overload receivers with messages or may fail to time the messages appropriately.

Upward communication, although helpful in building morale and forming strong organizations, typically doesn't happen as fully as it should. For this type of communication to be effective, all participants must trust that upward messages will be heard, considered, and responded to in an appropriate manner and time frame.

Horizontal communication. This pattern of communication includes both direct and diagonal messages. Direct horizontal messages flow between colleagues with similar levels of power and authority but differing areas of responsibility. Consulting with your patient's physical therapist, for example, creates horizontal communication.

Diagonal communication is similar to direct horizontal communication, but it involves participants of somewhat different status levels. Consulting with your patient's home health aide, for example, may be a diagonal type of communication.

In general, horizontal communication tends to flow more quickly and more accurately than vertical communication because the similar status levels create less noise and distraction. Horizontal communication tends to involve such tasks as coordination of activities, problem solving, sharing of information, and conflict resolution. Problems in this type of communication commonly stem from rivalry, competition, mistrust, and lack of motivation.

Clustered communication. Particularly during periods of rapid change or in organizations that limit the flow of communication, informal communication networks usually develop. Commonly known as the grapevine, this powerful, clustered communication pathway cuts across all levels of a hierarchy and all formal avenues of communication.

The grapevine is usually fast and accurate. However, it tends to thrive in an atmosphere of mistrust, anxiety, and ambiguity. Consequently, if you find that communication on your teams and in your organization is circumventing established routes, you'll want to make a special effort to communicate openly with everyone involved. Encourage all team members to do the same. And be sure to directly confront any misinformation being spread via the grapevine.

Interpersonal communication. In this pattern of communication, ideas flow freely among people rather than being passed formally from a person who knows (or owns) information to a person who doesn't. Communication is one of the major building blocks with which interpersonal relationships are constructed. The therapeutic interpersonal relationship also provides the foundation on which you can build success as a home health nurse.

Developing interpersonal relationships

In your professional life, you'll want to create and nurture a network of supportive interpersonal relationships among patients, peers, other professionals, and ancillary personnel. The qualities of a healthy interpersonal, or dyadic, relationship bring benefits to both people involved. (See *Elements of a healthy relationship*.) Plus, positive interpersonal relationships increase job satisfaction and improve information flow.

As you interact in your interpersonal relationships, remember that the climate in which communication occurs may be more important than the specific message being communicated. Defensive or hostile environments restrict communication. Supportive environments can encourage communication of even the most difficult and frightening messages.

When interacting with patients and the people on your care teams, try to minimize qualities that make for a hostile environment. For example, try to avoid too much emphasis on evaluation. Try not to be too controlling or dogmatic. Avoid communicating a lack of concern for others or a sense of your own superiority.

Instead, to help create a warm, open, relaxed atmosphere among your patients and your team, do your best to be nonjudgmental. Take a team approach to solving problems rather than seeking someone to blame for them. Communicate equality and empathy. Stay open to change. Be willing to take spontaneous steps.

Most likely, you already know the benefits of creating a supportive climate for patient and colleague interactions. To make the most of that climate, you'll also want to hone certain skills that keep communication precise and pleasant.

Elements of a healthy relationship

Healthy interpersonal relationships offer a number of benefits to both participants, especially when they:

- meet person-to-person on a regular basis
- empathize and communicate understanding to each other
- regard each other warmly, positively, and unconditionally
- perceive mutual acceptance and empathy for each other
- create an open and supportive climate
- exhibit trusting behavior.

Building communication skills

You can make your efforts at communication more effective by developing a number of practical skills.

First, don't base decisions on partial information. Instead, make a point of asking questions to gain as much information as possible. Investigate the thoughts and feelings of all involved. Not only will you make everyone feel heard, but you'll also be better able to explain the reasons behind your eventual decision — to yourself and those around you.

Also, be sure to consider the personal impact that a problem or situation has on the people it affects. Be sensitive to the significance of a situation by observing, listening, asking questions, and clarifying messages.

Next, never make assumptions. It only takes a few extra thoughts and sentences to ensure that you've communicated the whole picture. Doing so will help avoid the inevitable misunderstandings created by messages that are abbreviated by assumptions.

Do what you can to transform implicit ideas to explicit ones. Clarify perceptions and encourage feedback. Make sure the lines of communication are open by offering your perceptions, then asking for others' reactions to them.

Avoid speaking in generalities. Instead, try to obtain specific details and facts to clarify the situation. Then learn to speak only for yourself, no one else.

Don't assume that your opinion or interpretation of a situation is the same as everyone else's — or more correct than someone else's. Try to avoid the tendency to turn differences of opinion into issues of right and wrong. Remember that you can't begin to know how another person feels about a situation — or why. All you can do is accept another person's opinion as valid, even if you disagree with it.

To help develop morale and a sense of shared caring, use "we" statements rather than "you" statements when appropriate. This habit helps prevent patients and team members from seeing themselves as separate or secondary. It opens the door to everyone's ideas and opinions, which helps everyone feel a part of the health care process.

Work to routinely clarify your expectations by providing as much pertinent information as possible. By clarifying expectations, you create a climate of trust. You prevent your patients or colleagues — indeed, yourself — from being unpleasantly surprised, and you avoid the anger and defensiveness that mark relationships based on dominance or power, in which you have a monopoly on needed information.

In general, try to communicate as clearly as possible by repeatedly using the same language or symbols when communicating a concept. Always find a way to communicate in a language understandable to your receiver, and avoid using jargon or technical terms that your listener may not understand. That goes for team members as well as patients.

Of crucial importance in communicating well is the ability to change your mind. Don't stubbornly cling to your own opinions, because doing so will prevent you from really hearing someone else's. Instead, listen to the thoughts and opinions of others. Then alter your own as you recognize the need to do so.

Finally, improve your communication skills by asking for frequent feedback. Using verbal and nonverbal clues, assess the extent to which your receiver understood your message, and clarify it as needed. Also use that clarification process to help yourself communicate more accurately to other people on different occasions.

Don't forget that another person's frame of reference may be dramatically different from yours based on educational, experiential, or cultural differences. By following these principles for improving your communication skills, you can build a bridge over these differences and help ensure quality communication.

Screening tests

Another tool that may help you communicate better is an awareness of your personality type and those of your patients and team members. Sociologists and psychologists have developed a number of assessment tests and screening tools that identify personal preferences in gathering information, perceiving the world, and dealing with others.

These tests provide a nonjudgmental assessment that can help you encode messages in a manner most effective for the receiver to comprehend. They can also help you identify personal strengths and weaknesses as well as sources of friction in a nonthreatening manner.

One of the most popular of these screening tools is the Myers-Briggs Type Indicator (MBTI). It helps point out differences among people through four pairs of personality characteristics that you can use to understand more about how each person makes decisions, processes information, and interacts with the world. (See *MBTI personality types*.)

The personality characteristics used in the MBTI reflect opposing tendencies in four major areas. When using the MBTI as a tool to better understand yourself, your patients, and your colleagues, remember that the eight characteristics aren't exclusive. Don't think of them as rigid pigeonholes. Instead, think of them as tendencies. A person's individual decisions or actions may reflect any of the eight characteristics. But taken as a group, each person's decisions and actions tend to reflect a preference

MBTI personality types

The Myers-Briggs Type Indicator (MBTI) personality screening tool gives you insights into how your patients and team members think, process information, and interact with the environment. In the four categories shown below, every person tends to identify with one of the paired characteristics more than the other.

The first pair suggests overall personality type: either introverted or extroverted. This difference offers insight into a person's attitudes toward others and typical methods of social interaction.

The second pair reflects a method of perceiving the environment: by sensing or by intuition. The sensing person tends to rely more on information gathered through the senses. The intuitive person tends to rely more on hunches and instincts.

The third pair reflects the process used to make decisions or judgments: by thinking or by feeling. The thinking person prefers to use logic in decision making. The feeling person is more likely to base decisions on how they'll affect others.

The last pair reveals how a person handles change and the flow of information: by judging or by perceiving. The judging person prefers planning, organization, and deadlines. The perceiving person tends to prefer a more flexible, open-ended approach that responds readily to new information.

Introverted
- Turns inward
- Gains energy from introspection and reflection
- Processes information by withdrawing, limiting emotions, and conserving personal energy
- Drained by group interactions

Extroverted
- Turns outward
- Gains energy from the environment and from other people
- Enjoys talking, sharing ideas, and offering opinions
- Has trouble listening to others and pausing to think about options

Sensing
- Uses senses to gather information
- Focuses on the present
- Is comfortable with the unknown
- Prefers logic and details
- Has a practical nature

Intuitive
- Uses instincts to gather information
- Focuses on future possibilities
- Is effective in creating ideas but may miss details
- Becomes easily bored with routines
- May prefer hunches over facts

(continued)

MBTI personality types *(continued)*

Thinking	Feeling
◆ Makes decisions based on logic ◆ Is analytical, objective, and critical ◆ Prefers rules and values justice ◆ May be impersonal and stubborn once a decision is made	◆ Makes decisions based on personal values and the effect on others ◆ Is warm and compassionate ◆ Values harmony and friendship ◆ May have trouble maintaining subordinates' performance or criticizing it
Judging	**Perceiving**
◆ Desires organization and closure ◆ Prefers to plan ahead and make decisions ◆ Tends to control or regulate work ◆ Values punctuality and responds to deadlines ◆ Is good at making decisions but may be perceived as inflexible	◆ Is open and receptive to new information and ideas ◆ Is adaptable to change but tends to resist deadlines and keeping plans ◆ May procrastinate ◆ Values spontaneity and flexibility ◆ May have trouble starting projects without an immediate deadline

for just four characteristics over the other four. Keep in mind that a person's preferences may change over time as he or she develops or focuses on different skills.

To use the MBTI effectively, you'll need special training in administering and interpreting it. Proper use of this test will most likely improve your understanding of yourself as well as your colleagues and patients. This understanding can help you communicate as effectively as possible on a consistent basis.

◆ RESOLVING CONFLICT

Even when you do your best to communicate with clarity and understanding, conflicts are sure to arise. They're an inevitable result of the differences between people. It's natural for these differences to lead to disagreements and differing opinions. Conflicts may involve you personally, or they may arise between family members, including the patient, or between team members. In any case, it's your job to help resolve them.

Many conflicts arise because an initial minor disagreement leads to the realization that two people have a string of disagreements or a group of related problems that stem from the first — a situation called the iceberg phenomenon. Conflict also may arise when expectations rise. No matter how conflict arises, however, it typically takes on emotional and moral overtones if people feel that they must defend their beliefs.

Although conflict can be disconcerting and uncomfortable, it does not have to cause long-term damage. In fact, how you handle conflict with your patients or among your team members can make the difference between creating a negative, damaging experience and a positive, constructive experience.

Managing conflict well requires that you analyze situations effectively and use creative problem-solving skills. Doing so can actually allow conflict to help unify a diverse group. Even parties who agree to disagree may come to see the process as a positive one. Here are some points to keep in mind.

Defining conflict

Conflict can be intrapersonal, interpersonal, or intergroup. Like communication, conflict can also be vertical or horizontal.

Intrapersonal conflict occurs when a person feels internal tension. It involves a personal struggle with opposing values or desires. Commonly, intrapersonal conflict relates to personal definitions of right and wrong, role clarification, unrealized goals, or unmet needs.

Interpersonal conflict involves two people. It can occur at any time but occurs most often when one or both parties are fatigued or stressed.

Intergroup conflict involves two groups of people. They may be small groups, such as a few family members disagreeing with other family members, or they may be large groups, such as those who favor abortion and those who don't. When intergroup conflict arises, each group increases cohesion within itself. Its members become more task-oriented, leadership becomes more autocratic, and the group becomes more structured.

Dangers of interpersonal and intergroup conflict include development of adversarial relationships, stereotyping, scapegoating, and decreased communication. However, when handled astutely, conflict also has the potential to foster problem solving, provide intellectual stimulation, and facilitate personal development.

Management strategies

When most people think of conflict resolution, they think of methods to end a dispute and move on in harmony. In some ways, that concept is correct and necessary. In a larger sense, however, it's important to understand and accept that conflict always exists in one form or another. It may rise and fall in intensity. It may involve large and small issues but it always exists. Accepting this fact will render you much more able to manage conflict over time, rather than becoming frustrated and defeated by it.

A number of ideas and strategies are available to help you manage conflict. For one, it's useful to remember that conflict commonly progresses in stages. (See *The stages of conflict*, page 28.) Accurately assessing the stage of a conflict can help you develop appropriate interventions.

For another, remember that people or groups tend to play out certain roles when they enter a conflict. Determining the role adopted by a participant in a conflict also can help you determine appropriate interventions. Watch specifically for three roles that may surface during a conflict: the aggressor, the victim, and the instigator. The aggressor attacks others. The victim enjoys suffering and indignation. The instigator relishes the role of provoker and observer of others' conflict.

The stages of conflict

When trying to manage conflict, remember that most conflicts progress in relatively predictable stages. They're outlined here in general terms.

Latent conflict
During this first stage, conditions come together to set the stage for an outright conflict. For example, two people may have differing goals, personalities, values, interests, roles, or tasks to perform. There may be a conflicting need for resources or conflicting sets of regulations. In this stage, although conditions are ripe for conflict, it has not yet begun.

Perceived conflict
As involved parties realize that differences exist between them, such as those listed above, they become intellectually aware of a conflict. This perception is based on logic, not emotion at this stage. Some conflicts can be resolved at this stage by using logic and reason.

Felt conflict
After the involved parties realize they have a conflict, emotions begin to rise. The extent and direction of these emotions will vary with the people involved, their cultural backgrounds, their personal experiences, and their thoughts about their opponents. In fact, these emotions may play a significant part in how the rest of the conflict develops and plays out. Remember that it's possible to perceive conflict and not develop feelings about it; it's also possible to feel conflict and not be able to perceive the cause.

Manifest conflict
In this stage, the conflicting parties take action. They may withdraw and avoid the problem. They may argue. They may compete for dominance. Or they may discuss the conflict and try to resolve it. Studies suggest that men are more likely to address conflict, while women are more likely to try to avoid it. In your role as team leader, be careful to investigate and resolve buried conflicts among (primarily female) nurses. By doing so, you can help keep unspoken conflicts from damaging your team's effectiveness.

Aftermath conflict
Depending on how a conflict was managed, anger and damaging emotions may be left over. In fact, if a conflict isn't handled appropriately, the aftermath stage can be more damaging to the group than the conflict itself.

To manage a conflict that involves these roles, you'll need to equalize the power bases between aggressors and victims and actively control instigators.

Ultimately, your success in managing conflict stems largely from the role *you* adopt in the process. In general, people tend to adopt one of five management styles when it comes to managing conflict: avoidance, accommodation, confrontation, compromise, or collaboration. Some lead to success. Others are doomed to failure.

Avoidance

If an issue has only minor importance or if resolving it seems to demand a higher cost than the reward it promises, you may think it's easier to sidestep the problem, ignore it, or avoid it. For a time, this response may seem to work. In many cases, however, it only delays an inevitable and larger conflict.

Accommodation

In the accommodation role, you allow the other party to win by sacrificing your own position. This tactic typically applies to political situations or conflicts in which the issue is important to only one of the two parties. Although it creates a win-lose situation, this method of conflict management may promote team harmony if the "loser" can still function as part of the team.

Confrontation

Confrontation is a highly assertive style of conflict management in which one of the disagreeing parties pursues his or her own goals or needs without agreement from other affected parties. Naturally, this style tends to create anger and frustration rather than mitigating them. Confrontation is a win-lose style that may provide a quick solution to a problem. But it's usually an unpopular solution.

Compromise

Compromise, also called negotiation, typically produces a lose-lose situation in which both parties must give up something to reach a rapid solution. This strategy is commonly used when the conflicting parties have similar levels of power or authority. Although many people think of compromise as a primary tool of conflict management, it tends to create resentment and a negative view of the process on both sides of the table. Plus, it may provide only a temporary solution to the problem.

To help avoid the pitfalls of compromise, learn to recognize some of the most common negotiation tactics before you respond to them. For example, a person in conflict with you may ridicule you in an attempt to undermine you psychologically. The person may bring up unrelated issues (the smoke-screen tactic) in an attempt to draw your attention away from the real issues. The person may try to use your vulnerabilities to force concessions. Seduction, flattery, and gifts can divert your attention from the real issues, as can flaunting gender differences or using illness or helplessness tactics. The person may try to make you feel guilty or try to convince you that a certain solution is in your best interest. Finally, the person may refuse to negotiate at all, thereby winning despite your objections.

Collaboration

In most cases, collaboration offers the best avenue for resolving a conflict amicably and permanently. This style fosters a win-win situation and promotes assertive yet cooperative communication and teamwork. Each party must agree on the same goals and develop a solution to meet them. This style promotes creativity and the sharing of views and ideas, and it improves the performance of both parties. Because of the higher level of creativity and sharing, collaboration typically requires more time to come to a solution than the other techniques.

Ensuring success

Last but not least, to succeed in conflict management, you must be willing and able to communicate openly with the people involved. You must develop and use skills in team building and assertive communication and, to maintain the respect of all involved, you must be fair. To accomplish these goals for your care teams and your patients' families, try to:

- be descriptive rather than judgmental
- be clear and specific rather than vague and general
- give feedback when it can be heard, understood, and implemented
- give feedback when its accuracy can be checked by others
- focus on behaviors, not attitudes
- avoid bringing up past issues or stirring up past grievances
- use assertive messages when conveying criticism or feelings
- focus on one individual at a time, not the whole group
- listen attentively.

In addition to communicating openly yourself, you'll also need to encourage others to be open, honest, and fair. Remember that many intelligent people have not learned these skills. For example, encourage eye contact. Urge people to share their feelings and emotions, and then require all participants to treat those feelings with respect. Give feedback about verbal and nonverbal messages that could color the interpretation of messages. Specifically, call attention to differences between a person's verbal and nonverbal cues. Above all, reinforce all positive interactions to help continue the group's growth. Finally, when the group seems to have achieved a resolution to a conflict, test the participants for consensus.

To fully discharge your personal and professional responsibilities, you'll need to be able to manage conflicts using all the skills and ideas listed here. The rewards of doing so will quickly become apparent, not only to your patients and colleagues, but to you as well.

◆ IMPLEMENTING CHANGE

In your role as a home health nurse and a team leader, you'll often be attempting to effect change in a patient's or family's health care behaviors. This is a difficult job, requiring tenacity and encouragement from you and your care team. Although many people resist change, you can help the process by understanding how change occurs and how to make it permanent.

The first step is to understand change itself. By definition, change is a repatterning of behavior or a substituting of one behavior for another. In a general sense, it's a three-step process that involves unfreezing the status quo, making the change, and then refreezing. Unfreezing results from a motivation to change. During the change, driving forces increase enough in intensity to overcome resisting forces. Refreezing is the stabilization of that change. By working closely with patients and their families, you can help them make changes that will maximize the patient's health and well-being.

Assisting the change agent

When it comes to health care behaviors, change rarely happens spontaneously. Instead, members of the health care team must shepherd the patient through it. This process involves several crucial steps, including articulating the behavior that needs to change, assessing the patient's motivation and capacity to change, specifying change objectives, facilitating the change, maintaining the change, and terminating the helping role.

The person responsible for making a change is called the change agent. In home health care, it's important for you to recognize that the patient is the change agent, not you or your team members. To the extent that a patient's behavior reflects family functioning, the patient's family members may be change agents as well.

It's your role and the role of your team to help the change agent accomplish his goals. Your home health patient probably has already had an interaction with the health care system that made him aware of a need to change something about his behavior. Hopefully, that awareness will be enough to provide a degree of motivation. Your reinforcement and explanation of the need to change can help as well.

As a home health nurse, your primary role usually will be to help the patient develop strategies to make a change he already knows he needs to make. Use your powers of observation and your clinical and personal experience to help the patient solve problems and navigate roadblocks. Help him to realize that he'll obtain a greater reward by making the change than by preserving the status quo.

As you see the patient begin to change, recognize that the process may pass through a number of stages. (See *The stages of change,* pages 32 and 33.) Make sure that all team members are working together to encourage the patient's progress. Throughout the change, continue to gather data, monitor the patient's progress, and communicate the need to keep going. Try to help the patient develop specific goals and strategies to implement the change. Then evaluate his progress and emotional state, and adjust the goals as needed. Reward and praise his efforts throughout the process.

If the patient's family must make changes as well, concentrate on motivating and educating the most receptive members. Help all family members see the benefits of making the change. If you have time, phase the change in gradually. Use informal conversations to help reinforce aspects of the change and increase the family's receptiveness to it. If possible, cultivate an ally in the family, who can encourage other members (and the patient) to change. Provide extra reinforcement to early or tentative changes. Also try to create support systems among family members.

Organizational change

In an organization such as a home health agency, anyone can be a change agent. Usually, the most successful changes stem from the actions of an "intrapreneurial" change agent — someone inside the organization who can help build trustworthy networks, identify marketing advantages, and foster professional development, personal satisfaction, and recognition for employees of the organization.

If you're a change agent in your organization, you must demonstrate leadership while continuing to complete your usual functions. You'll need to develop strategies and tactics that accomplish the change while consuming the least possible amount of your organization's time and resources. You may need to enlist help from within the organization (a facilitative strategy), perhaps in the form of a committee. You'll need to gather all pertinent facts and opinions (an informational strategy) to prove the need for the change and plan an appropriate process. You may also need to convince some people in the organization that the change is

The stages of change

Like grief, change usually requires a complex adjustment that takes place in stages. Recognizing the stages involved, such as those listed below, can help you encourage your patients to make the changes they need.

Equilibrium
A patient who is satisfied with the status quo is in equilibrium. He feels little reason to change and, in fact, prefers not to change. If he begins to feel pressure to change, as when a doctor recommends lifestyle changes, he becomes uneasy and insecure.

Denial
As the prospect of change becomes inevitable and equilibrium disintegrates, the patient may feel that his energy has been drained. He may feel incapable of resisting change, yet unable to make the change. He may experience changes in his health, emotional state, and thinking patterns. To help him through this stage, employ active listening and show personal concern.

Anger
Usually, anger develops next. The patient may look to someone else to make the change, or he may balk at doing it himself. He may say he can't do it or won't do it. He may resent needing to do it. At this stage, you'll need to use your problem-solving skills, legitimize your patient's feelings, and help him manage his anger effectively.

Bargaining
If your patient begins to use "if only" statements, he has entered the bargaining stage. Although he may seem logical and rational, he's not using his energy to make the change, but rather to look for ways to avoid making it. To help him, start identifying his needs and using your conflict management and negotiation skills.

Chaos
When facing the need for a change that won't go away, the patient may begin to feel insecure, powerless, and disoriented. His energy diffuses. He may feel a loss of identity and direction. To help him, reinforce his feelings as a recognized stage of change, and reassure him that these feelings will pass.

Depression
Eventually, the patient will probably begin to feel depressed. He'll talk about the "good old days" and may engage in self-pity. Be aware that this depression may be preparatory or reactive. If it's preparatory, the patient is grieving over his old life in preparation for making the change. If it's reactive, he's still resisting the change. Continue to provide information and support even during reactive depression. Be patient, but don't downplay the need for change as a way to make the patient feel better.

The stages of change *(continued)*

Resignation
Eventually, the patient will become resigned to the need for change. He'll stop resisting. In this stage, he's passive, not enthusiastic. In fact, you may still see remnants of anger and depression. At this stage, allow the patient to progress at his own pace. Don't try to prod him into hurrying the process.

Openness
As the patient becomes more comfortable thinking about making a change, he'll begin to grow into it. He may not be able to self-start, but he'll be open to recommendations and assistance. He'll be working *with* you, not against you. He still may not seem enthusiastic about the change, however. Not until the patient reaches this stage is he really open to learning about the change he needs to make. Be sure to provide him with plenty of information when he's open to it.

Reemergence
Once the patient lets go of the old and begins to invest in the new, he's in the reemergence phase. Now he'll begin to work on the change for himself instead of simply being willing to work with you. He'll establish new roles and a new identity that incorporates the change. He'll be reenergized.

really necessary (an attitudinal strategy).

By learning to facilitate change, both in your organization and in the homes of your patients, you'll be instrumental in permanently improving personal and professional lives, including your own.

◆ UNDERSTANDING THE BUDGET

In home health nursing, you'll probably have more fiscal responsibility than nurses in many other specialties. Even if you aren't charged with administrative duties, you still should make it your business to understand fiscal matters, including budgets, and your agency's goals to the extent that you know them. Doing so could mean the difference between your agency's success and failure in an increasingly competitive health care market.

One of the primary financial tools in any agency is the budget. A budget is a plan that compares revenues with expenses. It's a formal, proactive document typically created at the beginning of a project or the fiscal year to help predict profitability and provide guidelines for spending. Budgeting can help you set goals, improve organizational communication, and coordinate group efforts. A budget may also be used as a motivational tool by measuring productivity and performance in the agency.

Most agencies use several types of budgets, including a master budget, a long-range budget, an operating budget, a capital budget, a cash bud-

Types of budgets

Most home health care agencies use a variety of budgets, including those described below. Learn about your agency's budgets because they will undoubtedly affect your daily practice.

◆ Master budget — a set of all budgets in the organization

◆ Long-range budget — a plan for revenues and expenses over an extended period of time, usually more than 1 year

◆ Operating budget — a plan that compares revenues received and expenses incurred in operating the organization

◆ Capital budget — a plan for items that will provide long-term service, such as building renovations, new computers, or medical equipment

◆ Cash budget — a plan that compares cash income and expenses, usually for a month-long period

◆ Special budget — a plan to analyze a specific program or product line

get, and one or more special budgets. (See *Types of budgets*.) Although you may not participate in much of the budgeting process, the results of the process will almost certainly influence your day-to-day practice.

In most agencies, the operating budget is the one with which you're most likely to be involved. Understanding it requires that you grasp two major concepts: revenue and expenses.

Revenue

Revenue refers to gross income. It's analogous to your salary before taxes are removed and before you spend any of it. In home care, revenue includes reimbursements provided by various insurers and fees collected from private-pay patients. In assembling an accurate operating budget, the administrator must have a good idea of the mix between reimbursed services and private-pay services.

Throughout the year, the agency's managers will perform a case mix analysis to classify the types of services the agency provided, the number of visits provided, and the reimbursement rates of the various payers. This assessment can help administrators keep track of past and predicted income.

Expenses

Expenses — or costs — are the other main component of the operating budget. Costs may be either fixed or variable. Fixed costs don't change with the volume of services provided. They include managers' salaries and overhead. Variable costs change with the volume of services provided. They include hourly wages and patient care supplies.

Costs also may be classified as direct or indirect. Direct costs are related to the service provided, such as wages, travel expenses, and care supplies. Indirect expenses include building overhead, marketing, accounting, and legal services.

Staff salaries represent the largest expense in an operating budget. Consequently, one of the most important steps in creating an accurate operating budget is to predict the need for staff. The cost of home services hinges on the number of visits the agency can provide each day. This prediction is based on the agency's history, goals, and available staff and on a careful analysis of the environment, including health care legislation and competing agencies.

The first step in identifying staffing requirements is to predict the average number of visits a nurse can provide in a day. This number can be calculated from agency figures, area norms, or equations devised by such organizations as the National League for Nursing. Factors to consider include the geographic distance between patients and the types of services provided. For example, a typical medical patient may require about 45 minutes of nursing care per visit. However, a typical maternal-infant visit may take 2 hours. Consequently, the maternal-infant visiting nurse will average fewer daily visits.

When it comes to full-time staff, the manager will also have to account for paid time that's not spent visiting patients. There's a formula for predicting the number of full-time staff positions needed to provide one full-time equivalent, known as an FTE. Once you consider sick time, vacation time, inservice time, conference time, holidays, office duties, and personal time, you find that it takes 1.2 to 1.5 full-time staff nurses to provide one FTE.

When an administrator compares the cost of providing service (expenses) with the income obtained from various payers (revenue), the resulting figure should be a positive number. Otherwise, the agency will lose money. If the figure is a negative number (or too small a number), the administrator will need to find high-cost, low-income services to delete. Another alternative is to improve the bottom line by increasing volume while keeping fixed costs the same. Many agencies negotiate contracts with high-volume payers, such as managed care organizations, to help accomplish that goal.

At times it's useful to consider the relative loss incurred by home care. If the loss is less than that incurred by other facilities in the same health care organization, then using home care services despite the loss may provide the best "big picture" patient management.

Even if you aren't responsible for making these fiscal decisions, understanding basic budgeting concepts can help you support your agency's goals. This knowledge also can provide guidelines for team members and help develop a team that can build decisions on a sound fiscal foundation.

◆ ENSURING REIMBURSEMENT

Although you may not have direct budgeting responsibilities, you *are* responsible for managing reimbursement for your services and those of your care teams. You are responsible not only to your agency, but to your patients as well.

Why? Because, as your patients' advocate, you have the responsibility not only to provide the care they need, but also to advocate for them and their families by making the most of funds available for their care.

Obviously, your agency's future depends on a steady stream of reimbursements or private payments. Particularly for reimbursements, your agency depends almost entirely on your documentation to prove that services you delivered should indeed be reimbursed.

You'll find detailed documentation guidelines in chapter 15. In general terms, however, your documentation must accurately reflect your patient's environment and health status, the nursing interventions provided, and the patient's response to those interventions. You'll also need associated

Requirements for Medicare reimbursement

Use this list to help make sure that your patient meets the criteria for reimbursement of home care services by Medicare.

◆ Your agency must be certified to receive Medicare funds.

◆ The patient is over age 65, is permanently disabled, or has end-stage renal disease.

◆ The patient has no other primary source of medical insurance.

◆ The patient has a doctor who manages his home care.

◆ The doctor must see the patient periodically.

◆ The patient has a plan of care that's been prepared and signed by his attending doctor. It must be on the proper form (HCFA form 485). It must be updated at least every 62 days.

◆ The plan of care must specify the type, frequency, and duration of services the patient needs as well as the discipline that will provide them.

◆ The patient is homebound. In other words, he has a physical or mental impairment that makes it unsafe for him to leave his home without supervision. (Document his homebound status clearly and repeatedly throughout his home care.)

◆ The patient needs part-time, intermittent skilled nursing, physical therapy, or another service that qualifies for Medicare's home care benefit. In Medicare terms, part-time means up to 8 hours a day, 35 hours a week. Intermittent means that visits occur at least once every 60 days. If the patient needs visits 5 to 7 days a week, your documentation must specify an end date.

documentation about the abilities and involvement of caregivers, your case coordination, and plans for future care.

In all likelihood, you'll need to be most concerned about meeting documentation requirements established by Medicare — the most common source of reimbursement. It's also important to learn all you can about managing your interactions with managed health care organizations.

Medicare

In chapter 1, you learned about the basics of reimbursement and the major sources of funds available to pay for home care. If your agency is certified to receive Medicare funds, you'll also need to know the specific rules governing Medicare reimbursement. (See *Requirements for Medicare reimbursement*.)

Medicare covers six types of home health services: skilled nursing, home health aide, physical therapy, occupational therapy, speech therapy, and medical social work.

As you know, skilled nursing refers to a variety of tasks in the home, including observation and assessment, wound care, administration of injectable medications, and patient teaching. This care must be provided on an intermittent and part-time basis. Skilled nursing visits are deemed part-time if each visit lasts less than 1 hour and intermittent if they occur at least once every 60 days.

Remember that rehabilitative services can only be provided if the patient demonstrates the potential to respond to those services. Meeting these requirements requires detailed and explicit documentation by the visiting nurse. It also requires careful record keeping and file management. You'll need to clearly document the reason for your patient's homebound status. Provide an accurate picture of his health status and level of independence. Also note the types of assistance your patient needs or devices he uses for mobility. Finally, document the distance the patient can ambulate and whether doing so worsens his symptoms.

Describe your patient teaching, including materials provided to the patient and the patient's responses. When documenting wound care, include the types and amounts of dressings used, along with measurements of the wound and its progress in healing.

The plan of care must be clear, complete, and free from errors. Orders for care by the various health disciplines must meet the criteria for allowable services in the home. Nursing care must be skilled, and all outcomes must be measurable. Appropriate forms must be signed and submitted in a timely manner for reimbursement to occur.

Be aware that the Health Care Financing Administration (HCFA), which funds Medicare, may review your documentation. If its agents deem your care ineligible for reimbursement, HCFA will deny your request for funds. If HCFA determines that you should have known that a service wouldn't be covered, it bestows what's called a technical denial.

For any denial of reimbursement, your agency will most likely appeal the decision. Clear, detailed documentation is all the more important if this situation arises.

Other payers

Although Medicare is the major payer when it comes to home care, you'll also need to know how to interact with other payers — especially managed care organizations.

To ensure reimbursement from a managed care organization, you'll need to make sure that the patient is eligible for coverage under the plan, the services you provide are covered under the plan, and the services have been deemed medically necessary, usually by the patient's personal doctor. Managed care organizations also concentrate heavily on measurements of quality and outcomes.

When caring for a managed care patient, remember that the plan's home care standards may differ widely from those of Medicare. For example, the patient may not need to meet the same homebound criteria, and you may be able to alter care schedules to meet the patient's unique needs.

To ensure quality home care for patients covered by managed care plans, you'll need to communicate regularly with representatives of the managed care organization. Consult with the plan's case manager to make sure that the goals you create for your patient are both medically appropriate and covered. Then you'll have to communicate the goals clearly, so the patient comprehends the expectations for care.

For instance, the managed care plan's case manager may expect the patient or a caregiver to start providing the patient's wound care within 2 weeks, while the patient may expect that you'll be providing it. If you determine that the case manager's expectations can't be met, then you'll need to talk further.

In fact, it's prudent to talk with the plan's case manager frequently and in detail. When explaining your patient's need for continued or additional care, do it in terms important to the case manager. Remember that managed care organizations seek to provide high quality care at the lowest possible cost. As you can imagine, sometimes these goals conflict. It may well be up to you to convince the case manager that providing additional care now will save money later.

Finally, if you believe that limitations imposed by a managed care plan may harm your patient, then you'll need to appeal the plan's decisions up the hierarchy. In fact, you may need to talk directly with the case manager's supervisor or the organization's medical director. Be prepared to provide persuasive reasons why your patient needs additional care.

Obviously, providing care to patients covered by managed care plans will require clear thinking, effective communication skills, and persistence to ensure that your patients receive all the care they need, when they need it.

At times, you may have to handle difficult conflicts between the patient's needs and the payer's requirements. If the organization denies care you think your patient needs, provide information to help patients and their families understand the limits of coverage; then do your best to offer alternatives. Above all, be sure to consider all sources of support, not just the most obvious ones. Try to view the patient's environment and funding sources as broadly as possible. And don't assume that family funds won't be available if third-party funds dry up.

In fact, a surprising number of patients and families don't understand that they can purchase home health care directly and that doing so may allow the patient to remain safely and comfortably at home. In a matter-of-fact way, do your best to outline all options to the patient and family; then let them decide their best course of action.

Whether you're a new nurse or you've been practicing for years, working in home health care requires you to continually exercise a host of management skills. To manage people effectively, you'll need to use skills in communication, relationship-building, conflict resolution, and change management. To manage agency requirements, you'll need to understand the influence of budgets and the requirements of a number of payers. But remember that making these management skills an integral part of your daily practice will help not only your patients and your agency, but you as well, in all aspects of your professional and personal life.

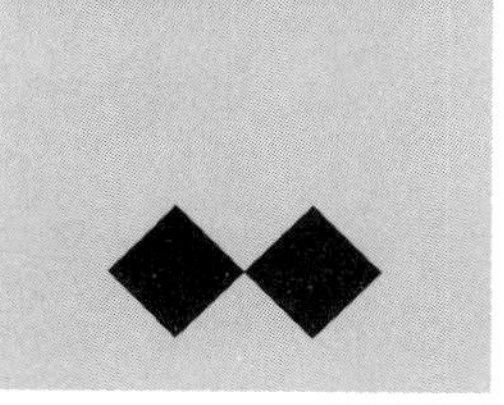

CHAPTER 3

Avoiding legal hazards

Patients today are more knowledgeable and involved in their health care decisions than ever before. They readily seek second opinions, ask probing questions, and demand answers to sometimes complex and difficult clinical problems. Occasionally, they also seek legal advice when treatments or medical professionals fail to meet their expectations.

Clearly, the threat of litigation can add anxiety to your professional life, but it doesn't need to hamper your ability to practice with confidence. Even in the home health arena, where you're faced with increased autonomy and decreased control over your patients and their environment, you can avoid most legal hazards.

How? By knowing your patients' rights and working to uphold them. In this chapter, you'll find up-to-date advice on such legal issues as patient rights, patient self-determination, responding to abuse, working with incompetent or noncompliant patients or caregivers, and handling the threat of litigation.

◆ UNDERSTANDING PATIENTS' RIGHTS

The concept of patients' rights has been evolving since the mid-1960s — a time of broad advances in civil rights for many segments of the population. (See *A timeline of patient rights,* pages 40 and 41.) At that time, President John F. Kennedy determined that patients in the health care system had four basic rights:

- ◆ the right to safety
- ◆ the right to be informed
- ◆ the right to choose
- ◆ the right to be heard.

In the years since then, a number of events — legislative, judicial, and medical — have advanced the rights of patients in America's health care system. (See *A patient's bill of rights*, page 42.)

In theory, patient rights are clearly defined. In practice, however, you'll have to take extra steps to make sure you understand them and uphold them. They include such important concepts as confidentiality, the right to privacy, informed consent, and what to do when a patient refuses therapy or wishes to stop therapy.

Confidentiality and the right to privacy

Although the United States Constitution doesn't formally sanction a right to privacy, the earliest articles proposing such a basic right were published in 1890. Since that time, a series of Supreme Court decisions (*Roe v. Wade*, 1973; *Griswald v. Connecticut*, 1965; *Eisenstadt v. Baird*, 1972; and *In re Quinlan*, 1976) have carved out such rights.

Today, the concept of privacy includes several issues. It concerns a patient's right to information about

A timeline of patient rights

The concept of patient rights has been evolving since the 1960s. Some of the landmark decisions are described below.

1959

◆ National League for Nursing issues first patient bill of rights, a model for today's document.

1973

◆ American Hospital Association issues *A Patient's Bill of Rights.*
◆ Hospitals recognize patient rights.
◆ States begin to legally recognize patient rights.
◆ First in a series of federal bills is passed ensuring rights for disabled persons.

1976

◆ New Jersey Supreme Court gives Karen Quinlan's parents the right to remove life-sustaining equipment from a child in a persistent vegetative state.

1980

◆ Federal Mental Health Systems Act is enacted to ensure rights for patients receiving mental health services.

1987

◆ Omnibus Reconciliation Act provides for the rights of patients receiving long-term care.

his health status, freedom from unwanted intrusion by health care workers, and freedom from disclosure of private facts by health care personnel. Because home health nurses see patients in their private environments, this nursing specialty probably faces the greatest risk for invasion of privacy.

Nursing implications

How can you uphold your patients' rights to privacy? In general, by maintaining the confidentiality of his health-related information and providing sufficient information for patients and their families to make realistic, competent decisions about health care. For example, you'll want to:

◆ help your patient understand his illness, the goals of his planned treatments, and his ultimate prognosis
◆ develop plans of care that incorporate the patient's goals and wishes
◆ make sure that the nursing diagnoses you select meet your patient's goals and expectations.

1990

◆ Supreme Court paves the way for the Patient Self-Determination Act by ruling that states can block removal of feeding tubes when no clear evidence exists of the patient's opposition to life-sustaining treatment.

◆ Hospice Association of America issues bill of rights for patients receiving hospice care.

◆ Americans with Disabilities Act ensures rights for disabled persons in workplaces and public facilities.

1991

◆ Patient Self-Determination Act requires Medicare- and Medicaid-funded health care providers to ask patients about advance directives and provide forms to patients who want them.

1997

◆ Federal law mandates that a note documenting whether or not the patient has an advance directive be placed prominently in the patient's chart.

◆ Advance Planning and Compassionate Care Act is introduced in congress. It strengthens advance directives and the existing federal law, the Patient Self-Determination Act.

By involving the patient in decision making about his care, interventions, risks, and outcomes, you not only keep the patient informed about his care but also reduce the chance that he or his family will seek legal assistance should the ultimate outcome be less than expected.

Ensuring open communication and patient decision-making power is generally considered part of the nurse's role as patient advocate. Courts have consistently held that nurses possess a vital and legally enforceable role as patient advocate. Giving patients adequate information, in terms they can comprehend, from which they can make sound decisions about their health care, ensures that you are serving as your patient's advocate.

For legal reasons as well as professional ones, be sure to openly discuss your patient's ability to follow your health care instructions. If necessary, give repeated instructions and ask for multiple return demonstrations over a specified time frame so you can be sure that the patient or his family

A patient's bill of rights

The American Hospital Association has issued a document outlining the rights of patients in the American health care system. Even though much of the document pertains to hospital care, it offers guidance for home health nurses as well. Here's a list of its main points.

Every patient has the right to:

- ◆ considerate and respectful care
- ◆ up-to-date, understandable information about his diagnosis, treatment, and prognosis
- ◆ privacy
- ◆ confidentiality
- ◆ a reasonable response to a request for care or transfer
- ◆ continuity of care.

Every patient also has the right to:

- ◆ give consent for care or refuse care
- ◆ complete advance directives, including a living will, a natural death document, and durable power of attorney for health care
- ◆ review his own medical records and obtain a copy of them, except where restricted by law
- ◆ know about potential business conflicts of interest among health care providers
- ◆ agree or refuse to participate in research studies without fear of receiving inadequate care
- ◆ know about hospital policies and practices that relate to patient care.

members can fulfill his health care needs.

Also be sure to carefully document your teaching and return demonstrations. Doing so further attests to your evaluation that a patient can be self-sufficient in a variety of ways, including correctly taking ordered medications, correctly performing needed treatments (ranging from simple dressing changes to self-suctioning by ventilator-dependent patients), and adhering to exercise regimens, diet modifications, and smoking cessation.

If a patient or his family can't follow instructions or adequately perform specific tasks, you'll need to find alternate ways to make sure his health care needs are met. Such alternate means could include scheduling more frequent visits, using home health aides or other ancillary personnel, or exploring the benefits of moving the patient to long-term care or an assisted-living facility.

Finally, keep in mind that your patient has the right to see or obtain a copy of his health records. When it comes to other, unrelated people, however, it's up to you to keep his health records private. Reveal information about his health only with his consent or when required by law.

Informed consent

In general, barring an emergency or unexpected need, your right to treat a patient is based upon a contractual relationship that requires the consent of both parties. Consent is the voluntary authorization by a patient or the patient's legal representative to do something to the patient.

Consent becomes important from a legal perspective because patients can sue for battery (touching of their person without permission to do so) if they didn't consent to a procedure or treatment before you carry it out.

This means that a patient can bring a lawsuit against you and be awarded damages even if he was helped by the procedure or treatment. Thus, consent concerns your right to treat a person, not the manner in which the treatment was delivered or the result of that treatment. You can deliver safe, competent care and still be sued for lack of consent.

The right to give consent and the right to refuse consent are based on a long-recognized common-law right of persons to be free from harmful or offensive touching of their bodies. In a landmark case early this century, the court declared that "every human being of adult years has a right to determine what shall be done with his own body, and a surgeon who performs an operation without his patient's consent commits an assault for which he is liable in damages" (*Schloendorff v. Society of New York Hospitals*, 1914).

Technically, consent is an easy yes or no. In reality, however, the key to consent is the patient's level of understanding. Remember that the law concerning consent in health care requires that the patient give an *informed* consent. That means you're responsible to give the patient as many material facts as he needs to reasonably understand his situation and make informed choice among his options.

What are the material facts you'll need to provide? Certainly, they differ for each patient. In general, however, make sure you outline all the patient's available alternatives and the risks and dangers of each one. Failure to disclose all the needed facts in language the patient can understand doesn't negate the patient's consent, but it does leave you open to potential litigation if the patient later says he didn't understand you. (See *Elements of informed consent,* page 44.)

In summary, if you fail to obtain consent, you can be sued for battery. If you fail to obtain informed consent, you can be sued for negligence and malpractice.

The right to informed consent did not become a judicial issue until 1957. In a landmark decision, the California courts found a doctor negligent for failing to explain the potential risks of a vascular procedure to a patient subsequently paralyzed by the procedure (*Salgo v. Leland Stanford, Jr., University Board of Trustees*, 1957).

Some courts have extended the right to informed consent to what may be termed *informed refusal*. That means you may be held liable if you fail to tell patients the risks of refusing a treatment or therapy. *Truman v. Thomas* (1980) was one of the first cases to recognize this important corollary to informed consent. In that case, the court awarded damages against a doctor for failure to inform a patient of the potential risks of not having a recommended Papanicolaou test.

Types of consent

Consent can be conferred in several ways. *Expressed consent* is given through direct words, either oral or written. For example, you tell the patient that you're going to give him an injection and the patient says, "Okay, but can you use my left arm instead of my right?" As a rule, expressed consent is the type usually sought and received by health care providers.

Implied consent is inferred by the patient's conduct or assumed in an emergency. Implied consent has its foundation in the classic case of *O'Brien v. Cunard Steamship Company* (1899). In that case, a ship's female passenger joined a line of people receiving vaccinations. She neither questioned nor refused the

Elements of informed consent

To be informed, the patient must receive, in terms he can comprehend, the following information:

◆ a brief but complete explanation of the treatment or procedure to be performed

◆ the name and qualifications of the person who will perform the treatment or procedure and, if others will assist, their names and qualifications

◆ an explanation of any serious harm that may occur during the treatment or procedure, including death if it's a realistic outcome, as well as pain and discomforting adverse effects during and after the procedure

◆ a description of any alternatives to the recommended treatment or procedure, including the risk of doing nothing at all

◆ an explanation of the risks incurred by refusing the recommended treatment or procedure

◆ assurance that he can refuse the recommended treatment or procedure without having other types of care or support discontinued

◆ the fact that he can still refuse even after the treatment or procedure begins; for example, the entire course of radiation treatment need not be completed if the patient denies consent for further therapy.

injection. In fact, she willingly held out her arm for the vaccination. Later she unsuccessfully brought suit for battery.

Suppose your patient simply holds out his arm when you say you need to give him an injection. You can infer from the patient's conduct that he both understood and consented to the injection. Health care practitioners commonly obtain implied consent for minor procedures and routine care.

Implied consent is presumed in emergency situations or for minors whose parent or guardian can't be contacted. However, remember the requirements of this situation: the patient must be unable to make his wishes known, and a delay in treatment would result in permanent harm. The treatment given must be that which a reasonable patient would allow. Another important requirement in emergency consent is that the health care provider must have no reason to believe the patient would deny care if he were able. So, for example, the provider can't wait until after the patient loses consciousness to order treatment that the patient has previously refused such as a blood transfusion.

Unless state law requires a written document, the law views oral and written consent as equally valid. As a precaution, however, it's best to remember that oral consent is much more difficult to prove should consent, or the lack of it, become a legal issue. As a convenience and to prevent such court issues, most facilities require written consent. In the home setting, it's wise to obtain written consent as well.

Standards of disclosure

How do you know how much information a patient needs before he can give informed consent? State courts have created standards of disclosure that offer some guidelines. These tests or standards of disclosure have evolved to assure that patients are informed in their decisions and to allow a means of determining the adequacy of the disclosure. (See *Defining standards of disclosure.*)

Most states use a medical community standard, sometimes referred to as the *reasonable medical practitioner standard.* This standard has evolved from the landmark *Karp v. Cooley* (1974) decision and is based on a model of medical paternalism. The standard requires that the health care provider "disclose facts which a reasonable medical practitioner in a similar community and of the same school of medical thought would have disclosed regarding the proposed treatment."

This standard is fluid and changing. It's based on prevailing medical thought and the local community. It must be established in court through expert medical witness testimony. Usually, this standard requires that you tell the patient inherent risks (including serious injuries), but not necessarily unexpected risks that could occur after the treatment or procedure begins. Courts favor more rather than less facts for full disclosure.

The second and third tests involve a reasonable patient standard. The *objective patient standard* is based on disclosure of risks and benefits based on what a prudent person in the given patient's position would consider material. Thus, this standard is also known as the prudent patient standard or material risk standard. Material facts are those that may make a significant difference to the reasonable and prudent patient. The court in *Korman v. Mallin* (1993) found that the "determination of materiality is a two-step process: (1) defining the existence and nature of the risk and the likelihood of occurrence; and (2) whether the probability of that type of harm is a risk which the reasonable person would consider."

The third test is the *subjective patient standard*, which requires the full disclosure that a particular patient, rather than a reasonable patient, would have wanted. The judge and jury must determine what risks were or were not material to that particu-

Defining standards of disclosure

Arguments for standards of full disclosure center on four key points:

◆ The patient assumes all the risk because it's his body and life that are ultimately affected.

◆ Informed consent mandates increased communication between the patient and the health care provider. With increased communication, the health care provider is less apt to violate the informed consent standards and is more likely to fully answer the patient's questions.

◆ Informed consent creates better health awareness by the consumer and ultimately encourages better health care practices.

◆ Informed consent raises the quality of health care because the provider must explain all risks and benefits of the proposed procedure and must outline alternatives, thus highlighting the best type and quality of care needed.

lar patient's decision with respect to the treatment accepted or refused. No expert testimony is required on the scope of disclosure, although expert testimony may be required to establish risks and alternatives to therapy. Only a handful of states have adopted this standard.

Some states have tried to bypass these three tests of disclosure by creating statutes to define what must be disclosed to a patient before therapy or surgery. These medical disclosure laws mandate that certain risks and consequences be printed on the face of the consent form in language that the patient can be reasonably expected to understand.

Some states haven't adopted a single standard for disclosure, but rely on individual case-by-case analysis. Others restrict informed consent to certain types of procedures, such as operative or surgical procedures.

Obtaining informed consent

By law, doctors carry the burden of responsibility for obtaining informed consent. In practice, however, they commonly delegate that responsibility to nurses even though a nurse's failure to obtain informed consent would extend back to the doctor who delegated the task. Agencies and health care facilities have no responsibility for obtaining informed consent unless:

1. the doctor or independent practitioner is an employee or agent of the agency; or

2. the agency knew or should have known about the lack of informed consent and took no action. Court cases and individual state statutes have repeatedly upheld this last principle.

The practical principle to remember is that, especially in home health care, obtaining informed consent will commonly fall to you. You must obtain it for all procedures and treatments, not just medical procedures. You'll typically rely on oral expressed consent or implied consent easily inferred by the patient's actions. If the patient can't communicate, permission may be derived from the patient's admission to the hospital or obtained from his legal representative.

To keep your patient's consent truly informed, you'll need to continually assess his competence and communicate openly with him. Clearly explain each procedure, its risks, the alternatives, and the risks of not undergoing it. Respect your patient's right to refuse a procedure if he doesn't want it, and make sure you know your state's laws on the patient's right to refuse life-sustaining treatment. Depending on where you work, you could face charges for honoring or failing to honor this request.

Remember that informed consent is a fluid and changeable concept. For example, if a patient wants to revoke his consent, he can. If you realize that an informed consent, even a written one, doesn't meet the standards of true informed consent, you'll have to start again. Usually, this happens when the patient doesn't understand an explanation of a procedure, but you don't detect the misunderstanding until later.

Remember that you, the attending doctor, and your health care agency all face liability if you have reason to suspect that standards of informed consent haven't been met. If that happens, you must speak up. Contact your supervisor and the responsible doctor. Both parties need to know about the patient's change of mind or lack of comprehension.

Likewise, if a reluctant patient asks for more information about a procedure recommended by his doctor, don't try to talk him through his reluctance. Instead, contact the doctor.

Who must consent

Equally important to the need for the patient to have all material facts on which to base an informed choice is the fact that the correct person must consent to the procedure or treatment. Informed consent becomes a moot point if you obtain the wrong signature.

Adulthood. Most states recognize their residents as adults once they reach age 18, although some actions, such as marriage, may classify a person as an adult before he reaches legal age. According to state law, the basic rule is that if the patient is an adult, only he can give or refuse consent.

For persons under age 18, a parent, guardian, or other approved adult must give informed consent for medical procedures or treatments. If the minor's parents are currently married to each other or have joint custody of the minor, state law usually allows either parent to give valid informed consent. If a divorce has resulted in sole custody or total abrogation of parental rights, then the parent with custody is considered the party to either give or deny consent.

State law also determines who may give consent in the absence of a parent. If the state has a family consent doctrine, the approved adult could be a grandparent, a brother or sister, or an aunt or uncle. These issues are state-specific, so you may find exceptions to these general rules. For example, a Georgia court ruled that a do-not-resuscitate order could not be enforced without the signature of both parents.

In some cases, you may be able to forego consent by a minor's parent or guardian, for example, when:

- ◆ the emergency doctrine applies.
- ◆ the child is an emancipated or a mature minor.
- ◆ you have a valid court order to proceed with the therapy.
- ◆ the law recognizes the minor as having the ability to consent to the therapy.

Emancipated minors are persons under the state's legal age who are no longer under their parent's control and regulation and who are managing their own financial affairs. Emancipated minors can give or refuse valid consent for proposed therapies. Examples of emancipated minors include married minors, underage parents, and minors in the armed services. In selected states, college students may be viewed as emancipated.

Mature minors, a concept recognized by a handful of states, may also consent to medical care. This concept originates in family law and involves the child's right to decide which parent will have custody of him after a divorce. The mature minor is a person between ages 14 and 17 who can understand the nature and consequences of the proposed treatment and is making decisions on a daily basis.

Obtaining valid informed consent when minors declare themselves to be emancipated or mature can be a problem. The best course of action is to postpone elective procedures or treatment until it can be determined whether the minor can give valid consent under state law. If a true emergency exists, you should document the existence of the emergency and proceed under an emergency consent doctrine.

The law also recognizes the right of minors to consent for selected therapies without informing their parents of the treatment. This exception is allowed to encourage minors to seek and receive necessary treatment without fear of reprisal from their parents. Instances for which minors may give consent include:

◆ diagnosis and treatment of infectious, contagious, or communicable diseases
◆ diagnosis and treatment of substance dependence, substance addiction, or any condition directly related to the substance dependence
◆ obtaining birth control devices
◆ treatment during a pregnancy, as long as the treatment pertains to the pregnancy.

Competence. In addition to being legally able, the person giving or refusing consent must be mentally able in the eyes of the state. Legally, competence means that:
◆ the court has not declared the person incompetent; and
◆ the person is generally able to understand the consequences of his actions.

Usually, legal competence results from assessment by a doctor or other health care professional — not necessarily a psychiatric specialist. You may be charged with performing this assessment at the time you request informed consent. Keep in mind that it's prudent to request confirmation from another health professional if you suspect:
◆ underlying mental retardation
◆ a mental disorder
◆ a disease that affects the patient's mental functioning.

In the case of the elderly patient, especially if he has periods of confusion combined with periods of competence, it's best to document how you assessed the patient for competence at the time of consent or its refusal. A simple entry clarifying the patient's competence may well prevent a future lawsuit or the threat of one.

Courts generally have upheld a strong presumption of continued competence. Such cases involved persons whose minds sometimes wandered, those who were disoriented at times and, in one case, a person who was confined to a mental institution. In each case, the court sought evidence to show that the person was capable of understanding the alternatives to the procedure as proposed and could fully appreciate the consequences of refusing consent to the procedure (*In re Milton*, 1987).

Guardianship. If an adult patient isn't competent to give informed consent, you'll need to obtain consent from a legal guardian. This person may be appointed by the patient or the court. A guardian appointed by the patient must possess a valid, written power of attorney.

If the patient did not appoint a representative while he was still competent, the court will do so. First, the court must declare the adult incompetent. Then it will appoint a guardian, either temporarily or permanently. If the court has reason to believe the adult is only temporarily incapacitated, it will appoint a guardian until the adult is able to once again manage his personal affairs.

Three types of guardians may be appointed. (See *Types of guardians.*) Usually, the court selects a guardian from the patient's family because courts typically feel that a family member will have the patient's best interest at heart. Family members are also most likely to know the patient's desires. If the spouse of the incompetent adult is also elderly and ill or has periods of confusion, an adult child may be appointed guardian.

In some states, even if the patient hasn't been deemed incompetent by a court, the family may be asked to make decisions for a temporarily incompetent patient. For example, an illness or traumatic event may render the patient incapable of making decisions and giving consent, and it's

Types of guardians

The court may appoint one of three types of guardians, as listed below. However, because the language and requirements for guardianship vary from state to state, be sure to verify that your state's requirements have been met before you accept someone's guardianship papers as valid.

Guardianship of property
This appointment allows the guardian to make decisions about financial matters. It gives no authority to make medical decisions for an incompetent patient.

Guardianship of person
This appointment allows the guardian to make medical decisions for the incompetent patient. It gives no authority to make financial decisions.

Plenary guardianship
This appointment allows the guardian to make all types of decisions about the incompetent patient's medical and financial needs.

common for a doctor to ask the family about medical matters for an unconscious patient. The order of preference in cases involving adult patients is usually:

1. spouse
2. adult child or grandchild
3. parent
4. adult brother or sister
5. adult niece or nephew.

Be sure to validate state laws and judicial decisions because family consent may not be valid in some states. In those states, consent is obtained by a court-appointed representative or through a valid durable power of attorney for health care document. (See *Durable power of attorney for health care*, page 50.) Lack of valid consent may become a court battle, especially if the practitioner acts on family consent and there is disagreement among family members as to the course of action to take.

Remember that guardians and representatives have a narrower range of permissible choices than they would if deciding for themselves, and some states insist that the patient's known choices be considered first. Any expressed wishes concerning therapy or refusal of therapy made while the patient was still fully competent should be evaluated and followed if at all possible.

The right of refusal
Remember that a patient has the right to refuse medical care at any time, even after he has given consent. The right hinges on the common-law right of freedom from bodily invasion and on the constitutional rights of privacy and religious freedom. The patient or guardian need only notify the health care provider that he no longer wishes to continue therapy. In limited circumstances, if the danger of stopping therapy poses too great a harm for the patient, the law may allow its continuance. For example, immediately after surgery, the patient can't refuse procedures intended to ensure a safe transition out of anesthesia.

(Text continues on page 52.)

Durable power of attorney for health care

The form and content of a durable power of attorney for health care can vary from state to state. The following is an example of a typical format. Review any document you receive to ensure that it meets your state's requirements.

Durable power of attorney for health care designation of health care agent

I, ________________________, appoint ________________________
(NAME)

____
(ADDRESS) (PHONE)

my agent to make any and all health care decisions for me except to the extent I state otherwise in this document. This durable power of attorney for health care takes effect if I become unable to make my own health care decisions and this fact is certified in writing by my doctor.

LIMITATIONS ON THE DECISION-MAKING AUTHORITY OF MY AGENT ARE AS FOLLOWS:

____

____

DESIGNATION OF ALTERNATE AGENT

(You are not required to designate an alternate agent but you may do so. An alternate agent may make the same health care decisions as the designated agent if the designated agent is unable or unwilling to act as your agent. If the agent designated is your spouse, the designation is automatically revoked by law if your marriage is dissolved.)

If the person designated as my agent is unable or unwilling to make health care decisions for me, I designate the following persons to serve as my agent to make health care decisions for me as authorized by this document, who serve in the following order:

A. First alternate agent

Name: ____
Address: ____
Phone: ____

B. Second alternate agent

Name: ____
Address: ____
Phone: ____

The original of this document is kept at ________________________
The following individuals or institutions have signed copies:
Name: ____
Address: ____
Name: ____
Address: ____

DURATION

I understand that this power of attorney exists indefinitely from the date I execute this document unless I establish a shorter time or revoke the power of attorney. If I am unable to make health care decisions for myself when this power of attorney expires, the authority I have granted my agent continues to exist until the time I become able to make health care decisions for myself.

This power of attorney ends on the following date:

PRIOR DESIGNATIONS REVOKED

I revoke any prior durable power of attorney for health care.

ACKNOWLEDGMENT OF DISCLOSURE STATEMENT

I have been provided with a disclosure statement explaining the effect of this document. I have read and understand the information contained in the disclosure statement.

(YOU MUST DATE AND SIGN THIS POWER OF ATTORNEY)

I sign my name to this durable power of attorney for health care

on this ______ of ________________, ______ at ______________

(DAY) (MONTH) (YEAR)

______________________________ ______________________________

SIGNATURE PRINTED NAME

STATEMENT OF WITNESSES

I declare under penalty of perjury that the principal has identified himself or herself to me, that the principal signed or acknowledged this durable power of attorney in my presence, that I believe the principal to be of sound mind, that the principal has affirmed that the principal requested that I serve as witness to the principal's execution of this document, that I am not the person appointed as agent by this document, and that I am not a provider of health or residential care, an employee of a provider of health or residential care, the operator of a community care facility, or an employee of an operator of a health care facility.

I declare that I am not related to the principal by blood, marriage, or adoption and that to the best of my knowledge I am not entitled to any part of the estate of the principal on the death of the principal under a will or by operation of law.

WITNESS'S SIGNATURE: ______________________________

PRINTED NAME: ______________________________

DATE: ______________________________

ADDRESS: ______________________________

If a patient or guardian refuses treatment, be sure to carefully explain (and document that you explained) the potential consequences of refusal, such as further deterioration of the patient's physical condition or the hastening of death. In some cases, if the patient refuses treatment that would aid diagnosis or reduce injury or illness, his third-party reimbursement may be denied.

Exceptions to informed consent

The courts recognize four exceptions to the need for informed consent in circumstances in which consent is usually required. These include:

- emergency situations
- therapeutic privilege
- patient waiver
- prior patient knowledge.

From a practitioner standpoint, consent is still needed to prevent charges of a battery, but the informed consent requirements are eased.

Emergencies. In an emergency, where the patient can't give consent and delaying care will do harm, you can proceed on his implied consent. Some courts have recognized that if there's time to give information, a limited disclosure may be valid. If no time exists or the patient cannot understand your disclosure because of physical disability, then you need not try to give him information or later ask the patient or his guardian to sign an informed consent form. Emergency consent negates the need for a completed informed consent form. The patient's doctor simply needs to document the reason for proceeding under an emergency consent doctrine.

Therapeutic privilege. Therapeutic privilege has its origin in the common-law defense of necessity. It allows primary health care providers to withhold information that they believe would be detrimental to the patient's health. However, this belief must involve more than fear that giving the information would lead to the patient's refusal.

In using this exception, you must be able to show and document that full disclosure of material facts would likely hinder or complicate the patient's treatment, cause him serious mental harm, or upset him so much that he could no longer make rational decisions.

Therapeutic privilege isn't favored by the courts and comes into play only when the patient is severely emotionally disturbed and his current medical status presents an imminent danger to his life. Some courts have held that a relative must concur with the patient's decision to consent and that the relative must be given full disclosure, whereas other courts have held that no relative needs to give concurrent consent. Once the risk to the patient has abated, the doctor must fully disclose information previously withheld from the patient.

Patient waiver. The patient may waive his right to full disclosure and still consent to a treatment or procedure. However, to be valid, the waiver must be initiated by the patient himself. If a health care provider suggests that the patient consider a waiver, the resulting document isn't valid.

Prior knowledge. If the patient already heard a full explanation of a procedure or treatment that he needs again, there is no liability for failing to disclose complete information a second time. Likewise, there is no liability for failing to disclose information that's considered common knowledge.

◆ UNDERSTANDING PATIENT SELF-DETERMINATION

A person's right to decide what will or will not happen to his body has its origins in constitutional (legal) rights and autonomy (ethical) rights. Usually, the right of self-determination arises with issues surrounding death and dying. However, it applies to all aspects of consent and its refusal. In particular, you should be familiar with the concepts of advance directives, removal of life-sustaining treatment, refusal of heroic resuscitation, and a patient's right to die.

Advance directives

To help patients make their wishes known if the time comes when they can't speak for themselves, nearly all states have adopted advance directives. Advance directives can take many forms. Many states recognize more than one, so patients have choices that best suit their individual needs and circumstances.

Living wills

Living wills began in the 1960s and gained popularity in the wake of highly publicized court cases involving patients in persistent vegetative states. In a living will, a competent person outlines, for medical personnel and family members, his wishes regarding treatment decisions should he become unable to communicate. (See *Living will,* page 54.) A living will isn't necessary for a patient who's competent and able to make his wishes known. However, when a previously competent person becomes seriously ill and incompetent, a living will can provide important information.

Historically, the language of a living will is broad and vague. It gives the health care provider little direction concerning the circumstances and actual time the declarant wishes the living will to be honored. Typically, living wills are not legally enforceable: The medical practitioner may choose to abide by the patient's wishes or to ignore them as he sees fit. In addition, the living will does not protect the practitioner from criminal or civil liability, so many doctors have been afraid to proceed under a living will's direction for fear that family members or the state might file wrongful death charges.

Natural Death Act

To protect practitioners from potential civil and criminal lawsuits and to ensure that the patient's wishes are followed when he is no longer able to make his wishes known, the Natural Death Act was enacted. This act created legally recognized living wills that serve the same function as living wills, but with statutory enforcement. Virtually all states have enacted some form of natural death legislation. Recognizing that a doctor may be unwilling to follow the directive, several of these laws require a reasonable effort on the part of the doctor to transfer the patient to a doctor who will abide by the patient's wishes.

Statutory provisions for Natural Death Acts vary greatly from state to state. Generally, a person over age 18 may sign a natural death document. The person must be of sound mind and capable of understanding the purpose of the document. The Natural Death Act document is usually a declaration that withholds or withdraws life-sustaining treatment from the patient should he enter a terminal state. The document must be in written form, signed by the patient, and witnessed by two people, each of whom is age 18 or older.

Living will

The format and content of a living will can vary; the example below is one possible form. Remember that a living will carries no legal enforcement. This document can only provide guidance about a person's wishes should heroic measures be required to sustain the person's life.

Living will

To my family, my doctor, my lawyer,
my clergyman, to any medical facility
in whose care I happen to be, to any
individual who may become responsible
for my health, welfare, or affairs:

Death is as much a reality as birth, growth, maturity, and old age — it is the certainty of life. If the time comes when I, ______________, can no longer take part in decisions for my own future, let this statement stand as an expression of my wishes, while I am still of sound mind.

If the situation should arise in which there is no reasonable expectation of my recovery from physical or mental disability, I request that I be allowed to die and not be kept alive by artificial means or "heroic measures." I do not fear death itself as much as the indignities of deterioration, dependence, and hopeless pain. I, therefore, ask that medication be mercifully administered to me to alleviate suffering even though this may hasten the moment of death.

This request is made after careful consideration. I hope you who care for me will feel morally bound to follow its mandate. I recognize that this appears to place a heavy responsibility upon you, but it is with the intention of relieving you of such responsibility and of placing it upon myself in accordance with my strong convictions, that this statement is made.

____
SIGNATURE

____
DATE

____
WITNESS

____
WITNESS

Some states also specify that the witnesses to the Natural Death Act document not be:

◆ related to the patient by blood or marriage
◆ entitled to a portion of the patient's estate by will or intestacy
◆ financially responsible for the patient's medical care

◆ the attending doctor, his employee, or an employee of the facility in which the declarant is a patient

◆ the person who, at the request of the patient, signed the declaration because the patient couldn't.

The form of the Natural Death Act also varies from state to state. Some states provide no suggestion as to the contents of the document. Others have a mandatory form that must be completed by the declarant. Still others suggest a form but allow additional directions to be added if they're not inconsistent with the statutory requirements. For states that have no set form, private organizations have suggested formats for these special directives. (See *Natural Death Act,* pages 56 and 57.)

Once signed and witnessed, most natural death documents are effective until revoked, although some states require that they be reexecuted every 5 years or another stated time frame. In most states, natural death provisions cannot be activated if the patient is pregnant. To maintain the highest validity, the declarant should review, date, and sign the natural death document every year or so. This assures family members and health care providers that the directions contained in the Natural Death Act reflect the patient's current wishes. In most states, the Natural Death Act may be revoked by physical destruction or defacement of the document, by a written revocation, or by an oral statement indicating that the person wishes to revoke the previously executed document.

Once a valid Natural Death Act document exists, it's effective only when the person is diagnosed with a terminal condition or enters a vegetative state — where the use of life-support systems would merely prolong the dying process. Most states require that two doctors certify in writing whether a procedure or treatment would prevent or prolong the natural death of a patient who has no chance of recovery. Medications and procedures used merely to prevent the patient's suffering and to provide comfort are excluded from this definition.

Today, many states also allow an oral invocation of a natural death document or allow another person to invoke one for the patient.

Durable power of attorney for health care

Sometimes known as the medical durable power of attorney, the durable power of attorney for health care allows a competent patient to appoint a surrogate or proxy to make health care decisions in the event that he becomes incompetent.

Under most durable power of attorney for health care statutes, the power of attorney includes the right to ask questions, to select and remove doctors from the patient's care, to assess risks and complications, and to select treatments and procedures from a variety of therapeutic options. The power also includes the right to refuse care or life-sustaining procedures. Health care providers are protected from liability if they abide, in good faith, by the agent's decisions.

Agents further have the authority to enforce a patient's treatment plans by filing lawsuits or legal actions against health care providers or family members. Agents have the right to forego treatment, change treatment plans, or consent to additional treatment. In short, they have the full authority to act as the principal would have acted.

Most patients are cautioned to appoint persons as agents who understand what the patient would want and are capable of making those hard

(Text continues on page 58.)

Natural Death Act

Unlike a living will, a Natural Death Act allows some level of legal enforcement for a patient's end-of-life wishes. The format and content of Natural Death Act documents vary from state to state, so make sure you know what's legal in your state. The example below is a format used in Texas.

Natural Death Act

Directive to Doctors
For persons 18 years of age and over

Directive made this ______________ ______________ ______________
(DAY) (MONTH) (YEAR)

I, ______________________________, being of sound mind, willfully and voluntarily make known my desire that my life shall not be artificially prolonged under the circumstances set forth below, and do hereby declare:

1. If at any time I should have an incurable condition caused by injury, disease, or illness certified to be a terminal condition by two doctors, and where the application of life-sustaining procedures would serve only to artificially prolong the moment of my death, and where my attending doctor determines that my death is imminent whether or not life-sustaining procedures are utilized, I direct that such procedures be withheld or withdrawn and that I be permitted to die naturally.

2. In the absence of my ability to give directions regarding the use of such life-sustaining procedures, it is my intention that this directive shall be honored by my family and doctors as the final expression of my legal right to refuse medical or surgical treatment and accept the consequences of such refusal.

3. If I have been diagnosed as pregnant and that diagnosis is known to my doctor, this directive shall have no force or effect during the course of my pregnancy.

4. This directive shall be in effect until it is revoked.

5. I understand the full import of this directive, and I am emotionally and mentally competent to make this directive.

6. I understand that I may revoke this directive at any time.

Natural Death Act *(continued)*

7. I understand that Texas law allows me to designate another person to make a treatment decision for me if I should become comatose, incompetent, or otherwise mentally or physically incapable of communication. I hereby designate ______________________, (PRINT OR TYPE NAME)

who resides at ______________________________________

to make such a treatment decision for me if I should become incapable of communicating with my doctor.

If the person I have named above is unable to act on my behalf, I authorize the following person to do so:

Name:______________________________________

Address:____________________________________

I have discussed my wishes with these persons and trust their judgment.

8. I understand that if I become incapable of communication, my doctor will comply with this directive unless I have designated another person to make a treatment decision for me, or unless my doctor believes this directive no longer reflects my wishes.

Signed:_____________________________________

City, county, and state of residence: ______________________

____

Two witnesses must sign the directive in the spaces provided below.

The declarant has been personally known to me and I believe him/her to be of sound mind. I am not related to the declarant by blood or marriage, nor would I be entitled to any portion of the declarant's estate on his/her decease, nor am I the attending doctor of declarant or an employee of the attending doctor or a health facility in which declarant is a patient, or a patient in the health care facility in which the declarant is a patient, or any person who has a claim against any portion of the estate of the declarant upon his/her decease.

Witness: ____________________________________

Witness: ____________________________________

decisions. Friends, relatives, or spouses may be appointed as agents. Most states allow the patient or potential patient to appoint subsequent agents. In the event the first named person cannot serve or is unwilling to serve in this capacity, then a second or third person has the principal's authority. Without this latter provision, a patient's wishes still might not be honored.

When patients present a durable power of attorney for health care document to you or another health care provider, a legal counsel, risk manager, or similar person for the institution or agency should verify that the document meets state requirements. Competent patients may be required to re-sign the document if there is a deficiency in the original form or if the form doesn't fulfill state requirements.

Some states allow for a directive that lists a variety of treatments and lets patients decide what they would want, depending on the patient's condition at the time. For example, the patient can select life-sustaining therapy if the condition is not terminal or can disallow life-sustaining therapy if the condition is terminal and irreversible. Generally known as a medical or doctor's directive, this document has comparable legal worth to the living will.

Uniform Rights of the Terminally Ill Act

Adopted in 1989, the Uniform Rights of the Terminally Ill Act is narrow in scope and addresses treatment that merely prolongs life for patients who have incurable, irreversible conditions, who will die soon, and who can't participate in treatment decisions. The act's sole purpose is to provide alternative ways to implement legally a terminally ill patient's desires regarding life-sustaining procedures.

Many provisions of this act look identical to some states' Natural Death Act provisions. For example, the qualified patient must be diagnosed as terminal, meaning that life-sustaining procedures would only prolong the dying process.

Doctors unwilling to comply with patient requests not to begin or continue life-support procedures should take all necessary steps to transfer the patient to a doctor who will comply with the provisions of the declaration. Patients diagnosed as being in a persistent vegetative state are not qualified.

Patient Self-Determination Act

The Patient Self-Determination Act became law as part of the Omnibus Budget Reconciliation Act in 1991. It requires health care providers to question patients about the existence of advance directives, and to provide such directives to patients who want them.

This act doesn't confer any new rights on patients in the health care system. Nor does it change any state laws. It simply ensures that they'll know about their existing rights. It may have provided incentive for more states to pass durable powers of attorney for health care statutes, but it does not mandate such passage. The legislation specifically states that providers may not discriminate against a patient based on the absence or presence of an advance directive.

While the act does not legislate communication or conversation, it does encourage communication and conversation about existing directives at a time when the patient is competent to understand and to execute advance directives. Ideally, this increased communication should be between the patient and the primary health care provider.

Written information described in the act is to be provided to adult patients at the following times:

◆ for a hospital admission, at the time of the patient's admission as an inpatient.

◆ for a skilled nursing facility, at the time of the patient's admission as a resident.

◆ for a home health agency, before the patient comes under the agency's care.

◆ for a hospice program, at the time the patient first begins receiving hospice care.

◆ for an eligible managed care program, at the time the patient enrolls with the organization.

Removal of life-sustaining treatment

For years, legal experts have concluded that competent adults have the right to refuse medical treatment, even if the refusal is certain to cause death (this view is consistent with the decriminalization of suicide by most states). But it was not until 1984 and 1986 that appellate courts directly confronted cases in which a clearly competent patient refused necessary life-sustaining treatment.

One case concerned the right of a competent adult with a serious illness that was probably incurable but not necessarily terminal, over the objections of his doctors and the hospital, to have life-support equipment disconnected despite the fact that withdrawal of such devices would hasten his death. The severely emphysemic patient entered the hospital for depression. While hospitalized, doctors saw a tumor on his X-ray films. During a subsequent biopsy, his lung collapsed.

Despite aggressive therapy, a tracheostomy was performed and the patient became ventilator dependent. Although he died during the course of his legal appeal, the California appellate court held that the "right of a competent adult to refuse medical treatment is a constitutionally guaranteed right which must not be abridged" (*Bartling v. Superior Court*, 1984). In *Bouvia v. Superior Court* (1986), the court addressed much the same issue, with much the same conclusion.

Even for an incompetent patient, the court has allowed a family member to make a decision to withdraw life support in consultation with the acute care facility's ethics committee (*In re Quinlan*, 1976). It should be clear, however, that the court system gave Karen Quinlan's father the right to make the ultimate decision, but did not influence his decision.

In another case, however, the court refused to allow family members to make decisions about life-sustaining treatments, saying instead that the decision to discontinue therapy "must reside with the judicial process and the judicial process alone" (*Superintendent of Belchertown State School v. Saikewicz*, 1977).

Yet another case allowed removal of life-sustaining treatment from a patient in a permanent coma who had previously, while competent, said that he didn't want such treatment *(Eichner v. Dillon*, 1980).

The final decision concerning the incompetent patient's right to die seems to have been settled in 1990. In *Cruzan v. Director, Missouri Department of Health* (1990), the court made explicit that right-to-die issues will be decided on a state-to-state basis and that there will be little, if any, U.S. constitutional limits on what states may do. Following the *Cruzan* decision, cases have given more latitude to family members, and courts have struggled to find instances where patients had made some expression, however fleeting, about their desires for sustaining life with artificial or life-support measures.

Clearly, when it comes to removal of life-sustaining treatments from patients with incurable, possibly terminal illness, the waters are murky, especially when the patient is incompetent. These are not decisions to be made independently or without legal consultation.

DNR directives

Some health care facilities have initiated do-not-resuscitate (DNR) directives that patients may execute upon admission. According to the patient's request, the doctor will then follow agency policy in attaching such orders to the patient record. Most agencies require documentation that the patient's decision was made after consultation with the doctor about the diagnosis and prognosis. The order is then reevaluated according to institution policy.

At least one state — New York — has enacted a DNR statute that establishes the hierarchy of surrogates who may request DNR status for incompetent patients. It also requires all health care facilities to ask patients about their desires concerning resuscitation when they're admitted. The act stemmed from worries about the overuse of cardiopulmonary resuscitation.

Hospice care

Some terminally ill patients sidestep the need for natural death documents and living wills by entering hospice care. In many cases, hospice takes place in the patient's home. This philosophy of care allows patients to receive required nursing and medical care and to be kept comfortable, without the fear of being resuscitated or placed on life support when death is imminent.

Congress recognized the need for such terminal care apart from the hospital setting and authorized Medicare reimbursement for hospice care (Public Law 97-248, 1982).

Assisted suicide

Although suicide has been decriminalized in all states, most still prohibit assisted suicide. Some states treat assisted suicide harshly; others prohibit health care providers only from *causing* a suicide, not *assisting* with it. Washington, Oregon, and California have all tried to enact legislation allowing assisted suicide. Michigan has passed laws specifically to stop Dr. Jack Kevorkian from assisting patients with their suicide. Many legal experts predict that the Supreme Court will be the judiciary body to finally attempt to come to terms with this issue.

The Oregon Death with Dignity Act, passed by the voters in November 1994, allows a doctor to write a lethal drug prescription for a competent, terminally ill adult who is a resident of the state (Measure 16). Other provisions that must be met before the prescription is written include these:

◆ Both the attending doctor and a consulting doctor must certify that the patient has no more than 6 months to live.

◆ The patient must make both an oral and a written request for the prescription, followed by a second oral request 15 days or more after the first requests.

◆ The attending doctor must refer the patient for counseling if a psychological illness or depression is suspected.

◆ The doctor must wait at least 48 hours after the third request before prescribing the medication.

Nursing implications

As a home health nurse, you must understand as much as possible about your patients' rights to direct their own care, refuse treatments, withdraw treatments, or avoid heroic resuscitation. Clearly, however, these are complex concepts with personal, professional, and legal ramifications.

When it comes to advance directives, the rules are fairly clear, and you can do a number of things to educate yourself about them. (See *How to handle advance directives,* page 62.) Commonly, the bigger problem is figuring out how to talk with patients about their wishes, especially the exact circumstances under which they want to invoke the document. For example, if your patient has a relatively minor illness, you may find yourself hesitant to question him about an advance directive, even though it's better to have the patient clarify his intentions and requests before something happens.

Remember, in most states family members cannot override the patient's written requests unless they can prove the advance document is invalid, so the only way your patient can be relatively assured that health care professionals will follow his wishes is to make those wishes formal.

The nurse's role in assisted suicide is still developing. The American Nurses Association (ANA) opposes nurse participation either in assisted or active euthanasia because it violates the ethical traditions embodied in the *ANA Code for Nurses*. However, the Michigan Nurses Association supports legalization of assisted suicide for "competent persons whose suffering cannot be relieved or satisfactorily reduced with alternative strategies" (Michigan Nurses Association, 1994).

If a patient asks you directly to help him commit suicide, for now, you must refuse no matter what your personal convictions are on the matter. But you can still help the patient by looking beyond the request itself to what else the patient may be saying. He may be expressing a need for greater pain control or for someone to talk with him about his fears of a terrible death. Do whatever you can to help the patient be comfortable — physically and mentally — and make sure that his advance directives are in place.

Many patients also benefit from talking with a member of the clergy, a social worker, or a mental health professional. Your role is primarily that of advocating for the patient and providing empathetic, caring support. The same is true of family members; allow them to voice their thoughts and feelings and reassure them that you and other health care professionals will intervene in an appropriate manner to prevent their loved one from unneeded pain and suffering.

◆ DEALING WITH ABUSE

One of the most difficult issues for many health care professionals is abuse: the emotional impact of detecting it or suspecting it, the personal and professional uncertainty about when to report it, and the struggle to understand it.

Studies suggest that understanding comes at least in part from looking at an abuser's background. People who abuse others come from all socioeconomic levels and all ethnic groups. No specific psychiatric diagnosis encompasses the abuser's personality and behavior. Many abusers have a history of being abused as children or of witnessing the abuse of siblings or parents. In most cases, abusers lack self-esteem and the security of feeling loved by others.

How to handle advance directives

To handle advance directives safely and correctly, follow these guidelines.

◆ Review your state's statutes regarding durable powers of attorney for health care, natural death documents, and living wills.

◆ Ask your agency's attorney to hold an in-service so all visiting nurses can become fully aware of any statutory requirements and the means by which advance directives are enforced.

◆ Review your agency's policy and procedure manual for any guidelines about advance directives. If no policies exist, ask your agency's administrators for guidance.

◆ Follow all agency policies carefully.

◆ If a patient or family member tells you the patient has signed an advance directive, make sure the agency and the patient's doctor know about it right away.

◆ Document the existence of the advance directive in the patient's medical record; ask for a copy.

◆ Ask your agency's attorney to review the document before you put it in the patient's record.

◆ Make sure that subsequent health care providers know the document exists and that it's been validated.

◆ If the patient revokes the document, verbally or in writing, make a note in your documentation and notify the agency and the attending doctor right away — even if you're not sure of the patient's competence.

◆ Avoid acting as a witness to a living will or natural death document. Because you provide some of the patient's care, acting as a witness may invalidate the document. Usually a friend or someone unrelated to the patient must serve as witness.

◆ Read the patient's living will or natural death document carefully to determine the scope of its provisions. It's much easier to clarify the document while the patient is still competent than to wait until the document takes effect.

◆ If the patient clarifies the document's coverage, document that clarification in your notes. Also alert the attending doctor.

◆ Most states allow you or another person to write and sign an advance directive as a competent patient's proxy. Just make sure the patient is of sound mind — for example, not influenced by drugs that could affect reasoning — because competency may become an important issue in the execution of such a directive.

◆ Document in the record why someone else had to write an advance directive or sign it instead of the patient (partial paralysis, perhaps, or another medical reason that a competent patient would be unable to sign).

◆ If the advance directive goes into effect, help family members in this time of crisis by being available and by answering as many of their questions as possible. Remember that they may need time to accept the consequences of the patient's directive, especially if they're called upon to concur with it or demand its implementation.

Especially in times of crisis, abusers resort to the behavior they learned in childhood. They abuse as they were abused in an attempt to restore their self-esteem and feelings of control. Many abusers have unrealistic expectations of those they abuse. When others fail to live up to those expectations, the abuser feels the need to control, mortify, reject, and physically injure the person at whom the abuse is aimed.

In your role as a home health nurse, remember that abuse has a broad definition. It encompasses physical, mental, and sexual assaults as well as physical, emotional, and medical neglect. Most states mandate that you report, in good faith, suspected abuse of children and elderly people. The "in good faith" provision affords you some protection and latitude because it doesn't require you to have conclusive evidence of abuse, just evidence that a reasonable person would consider suspicious.

Child abuse

Children who are most at risk for abuse include those under age 3 (who represent about half of serious injuries) and those living in households where the parents are remarried or not married. Also, children with behavioral problems, disabilities, or congenital malformations are more likely to suffer abuse. In many cases, the abuser is a boyfriend or husband of the natural mother, but not the children's biological father.

The first statutory laws calling for mandatory reporting of child abuse were passed in the late 1960s and early 1970s. Unfortunately, these laws differed and had no uniform interpretation. To remedy that issue, Congress passed the Child Abusive Prevention and Treatment Act of 1973. This act requires states to meet certain uniform standards to be eligible for federal assistance in setting up programs to identify, prevent, and treat the problem caused by child abuse. The act also established a national center for child abuse and child neglect.

Most child abuse laws have two common characteristics: the empowerment of social welfare or law enforcement bureaus to receive and investigate reports of abuse and immunity from liability for defamation and invasion of privacy to any person who reports an incident of actual or suspected abuse.

Nursing implications

If you suspect or know about child abuse in a patient's home, you'll want to report it to your supervisor or your agency's administrators and to your patient's doctor. Your agency probably has policies and procedures for you to follow in such instances. Be sure to document in your notes that you reported possible abuse and to whom you reported it. Also explain why you came to suspect abuse.

If you fail to report suspected abuse, you can be the target of civil and criminal charges. This is particularly true if further abuse or neglect occurs because of the nondisclosure. The landmark case in this area is *Landeros v. Flood* (1976), in which a doctor was held liable for failure to report suspected child abuse on the grounds of medical malpractice.

In this case, an 11-month-old infant was brought into the emergency department with a leg fracture. The fracture was a type for which a reasonable and careful doctor would have initiated an investigation into possible child abuse. Instead, the child was treated and released to her parents. Shortly afterward, the child was again seen for severe and permanent injuries from continuing abuse. After state authorities took the child from her parents, this lawsuit was brought against the doctor and the acute care facility.

In its findings, the court held that a hospital whose agents or employees knew of or should have suspected that a child requiring care was a victim of abuse could be held liable for the child's subsequent injuries if it failed to report the suspected abuse in the first place. The legal and moral lesson is that it's better to report suspected abuse and be wrong than to avoid reporting it and be wrong.

Also bear in mind that a court could order you to disclose confidential information in a case of child custody and child neglect. In *In re Doe Children* (1978), the court ordered the medical record to be submitted in a child custody case. The court stated that the children's welfare outweighed the parents' right to keep the medical records confidential.

Elder abuse

Estimates put elder abuse in the United States at 700,000 to 1.5 million cases annually. About 1 in 20 older Americans suffer physical abuse, and they tend to suffer it from a wider range of people than children do. The elderly risk abuse from professionals, family members, and caregivers. Those in nursing homes or living with younger family members are most at risk.

Elders are unlikely to report abuse, usually because they or their spouses fear retaliation from their caregivers, they're ashamed of the problem, or they have limited alternatives for living arrangements. Health professionals do not report the abuse because of ignorance of the problem or of their legal responsibilities to report suspected cases, lack of knowledge about or failure to adequately assess at-risk situations, and concerns that an alternative living arrangement may be less tolerable than the current one.

Elder abuse occurs in all socioeconomic groups and at all educational levels. The most common elder abuse is by the patient's spouse, followed by the patient's children or other caregivers. Recent studies indicate that abusers may be either men or women, with men being slightly more abusive.

The most important factor in elder abuse is the elderly person's loss of physical or financial independence. Confusion, incontinence, frailty, and physical and mental disabilities demand enormous amounts of energy, time, and patience from caregivers. Often, caregivers don't feel that they have the time and energy needed to properly care for an elderly relative because of other family duties and work demands. Sometimes called the "sandwich generation," many middle-aged adults today find themselves caring for two generations, their parents and their children.

Nursing implications

You must look for elder abuse in all settings. Watch for unexplained bruises and injuries. Watch especially for fingerprint bruises on the upper arms, inner thighs, and other areas of the body that aren't readily visible. Elders tend to bruise more easily than younger people, but explanations that don't sound realistic — as well as repeated bruises and other physical signs — should alert you to possible elder abuse. (See *Warning signs of elder abuse*.)

Also assess for possible neglect. Listen for subjective statements from your patient that could raise a red flag in your mind. For example, take note if your patient says he's unattended for long periods of time, forced to stay in his bedroom or the bathroom alone, or concerned that family caregivers may be using his personal funds inappropriately.

The legal responsibility of reporting elder abuse varies from state to state. For example, most definitions of elder abuse don't include financial exploitation. Some definitions don't include neglect. The authority to whom you report possible elder abuse also varies from state to state; usually it's to the state adult protective services or social service agency. As with child abuse, you must report all suspected cases of elder abuse in good faith to the correct agency. In your report, include the reasons for your suspicion, the name and address of the patient, and the caregiver's name (if you know it).

In addition, be sure to follow your agency's reporting policy. And document your suspicion and the reasons for it in your patient's record.

Keep in mind that the abused elder may see you as a threat rather than an advocate if you report possible abuse. You'll need all your powers of empathy and communication to navigate this emotionally charged course in your patient's best interest.

Family violence

You also may discover possible abuse among patients and families that don't include children or elders. Instances of family violence are increasing and patients, particularly women, may seek your advice about what to do. Your agency should have a policy and procedure for such cases, and you should advise such patients about local services, such as safe shelters, legal assistance, and reporting to law enforcement agencies. Because this is a population not seen as vulnerable by the law, there are no state-mandated reporting requirements similar to those for children and elders. After advising a patient of her rights, be sure to document her questions and any advice you gave her in her record.

Warning signs of elder abuse

Because older people are unlikely to report abuse or neglect, you need to watch for signs, such as the following:

- repeated bruises that resemble fingerprints and that appear inside the upper arms and inside the thighs
- strong body odor
- clothing that's consistently soiled and in poor repair
- long, dirty fingernails
- appearance of being undernourished.

◆ WORKING WITH INCOMPETENT CAREGIVERS

In an acute care setting, it's rare to come across a caregiver who's incompetent. In the home setting, on the other hand, it's rather common. Why? Because much of the time, the homebound patient's primary caregivers are family members, friends, neighbors, and possibly paid but unprofessional helpers.

An incompetent caregiver is one who can't adequately perform the care the patient needs. Teaching does not help incompetent caregivers because they're truly unable to perform the task, either because they don't have the manual dexterity or aren't available to perform the needed care. If the latter issue best describes the reason for incompetence, ask the patient whether a caregiver will be in the home during the day and discuss other alternatives. For example, an adult day care center may be available for the times that caregivers must be at work.

Nursing implications

If a caregiver lacks the mental and physical aptitude to give safe and necessary care, then you'll need to pursue alternative caregivers, alternative settings for the patients, or additional services through your agency. Explore all avenues, including adding a second person to help the primary caregiver and to remind him of what needs to be done and why. Document the issue, reasons why you suspect that home care isn't meeting acceptable standards, and how you plan to improve the situation as quickly and completely as possible. Follow your agency's policies and procedures in such instances, and make sure other agency employees do as well.

Early identification and documentation of an incompetent caregiver may prevent a malpractice suit against you and your agency because your notes will show that you identified the problem and did everything you could to solve it in a timely manner as your patient's advocate. If a patient persists in his reliance on an incompetent caregiver and fails to use alternative sources for competent nursing care, he shares responsibility for the outcome — a situation known as comparative or contributory negligence. Courts will hold the patient accountable for his failure to follow recommendations concerning his health care.

◆ HANDLING NONCOMPLIANCE

Noncompliance by patients and caregivers is another area of concern. In too many cases, the overall outcome for patient care is hampered by the patient's failure to follow instructions, take medications as ordered, and refrain from activities as requested.

Nursing implications

When assessing a potentially noncompliant patient, listen carefully for indications of noncompliance. For example:

- ◆ Does the patient talk about someone who had the same condition he does, for whom the treatment made no difference?
- ◆ Does the patient say he knows everything he needs to know about his condition, even if you know he doesn't?
- ◆ Does the patient listen and take an active part in the teaching materials and ask pertinent questions?
- ◆ Does the patient deny that he needs to change unhealthy lifestyles?

A patient who talks about other people who weren't helped by treatment may really be telling you that he's already made a decision not to comply with prescribed treatments. If you think this may be the case, ask the patient how and when he'll comply with the care he needs. This gives you an opportunity to modify your teaching plan and address your patient's concerns and misconceptions.

To help your patient comply, make sure you teach and demonstrate information that's relevant to the patient at the given moment. Unless you help the patient understand the relevance of what you're teaching, he may remain noncompliant. Teaching in smaller amounts and addressing specific concerns at each visit may be helpful as well.

Patients need to know what to expect as they begin new medications or treatments. They may have problems adjusting to different doses of medications or problems with selecting foods that they're not accustomed to eating. Explain that such problems are to be expected. Patients may be better able to comply with nursing and medical treatments when they know what to expect and when they know that you'll be asking questions about such problems when you visit.

Be sure to carefully document any statements your patient makes about noncompliance. If he tells you that he doesn't want to follow his plan of care, make note of it. If he tells you why, make note of that as well. Also note how you responded to these problems and what you did to help improve compliance. Inform the patient and family about the consequences of noncompliance, and then document that you did so. And, as time goes by, be sure to document any follow-up issues that relate to compliance. If necessary, have a second person validate the patient's noncompliance.

Remember that your documentation can prove the difference between your negligence and the patient's noncompliance. Also be sure to check your agency's policy about dealing with noncompliant patients.

If you think you may be dealing with a noncompliant caregiver, listen to his conversation. He may communicate a lack of understanding about the patient's condition or the need for special care. He may say he feels burdened by the patient's care. If noncompliance is the issue, start with more education. Make sure he knows what he's supposed to do. If that does not solve the problem, investigate other problems. For example, if his failure to provide special foods or equipment has a financial basis, talk about possible sources of state and local funds.

Again, carefully and promptly documenting the response to noncompliance is vital. Should the noncompliance cause the patient's condition to deteriorate rapidly or cause the patient undue distress and suffering, explore alternative care settings and follow your agency's policy carefully.

◆ RESPONDING TO THREATENED LAWSUITS

Patients or family members may either threaten a lawsuit or actually file one in any health care setting. Home care is no exception. A variety of cases have been initiated by home health care patients, ranging from breach of contract to malpractice to criminal charges. Most have been filed as civil suits, meaning that they involved issues between private citizens. A contract lawsuit is one such example. A contract lawsuit concerns an agreement made between persons, and the adherence of both sides of the contract to their agreement. Typically, a contract lawsuit involves the patient or family and the overall home health agency.

Lawsuits filed against individual nurses usually involve patient rights or possible malpractice or negligence. Cases filed in this category have centered primarily upon the professional nurse's failure to adequately supervise, educate, and delegate care to ancillary home health workers.

Loton v. Massachusetts Paramedical, Inc. (1989) concerned the negligent training and supervision of such a home health worker. In this case, the patient was left unattended in a shower by a personal care worker. The worker left the patient's apartment and went to another area of the building to do the patient's laundry. While the patient was unattended, the temperature of the water rose, eventually to scalding, and the patient fell while trying to readjust the water temperature.

Because of her underlying disability, the patient couldn't move away from the scalding water. When the home health worker returned, she tried unsuccessfully to contact her supervisor, applied ice to the burned area, waited an unspecified period of time, and eventually called an ambulance. The patient sustained third-degree burns over most of her body, which required numerous skin grafts.

The patient sued the agency, alleging that the agency was negligent in failing to properly educate its workers and to train them in the appropriate response to an emergency. The patient received a $1 million award from the agency.

Criminal actions may also be seen in home health nursing. Criminal actions are those that arise because of conduct offensive or harmful to society as a whole. They're enforced by local or state law enforcement officers. Punishment for such actions may include jail time or fines.

In cases of serious neglect, a patient may file a civil lawsuit and law enforcement authorities may bring criminal charges against the agency and its workers. In *Caretenders v. Commonwealth* (1991), a patient receiving home health care services was admitted to the hospital with numerous pressure sores, many of them extending to the bone. The patient was unwashed and had a necrotic odor to her. An indictment was brought against the agency, the administrator of one of its offices, a visiting nurse employed by the company, and a licensed practical nurse who worked in the agency's nursing and supportive care program.

All were charged with knowingly and willfully neglecting the patient, causing serious mental and physical injury. Following a jury trial, the agency was convicted of a class A misdemeanor and fined. A subsequent civil lawsuit was then filed against the same defendants for monetary damages due the patient for their malpractice and negligence.

Some patients or family members are more likely to bring suit than other patients. Because the psychological make-up of these persons breeds resentment and dissatisfaction in all phases of their lives, they are more likely to find fault with health care providers and file lawsuits. Suit-prone people tend to be immature, overly dependent, hostile, and uncooperative. They commonly fail to follow a prescribed plan of care. Unable to be self-critical, they shift blame to others as a way of coping with their own inadequacies. Suit-prone people project their fears, insecurity, and anxieties onto health care providers, overreacting to any perceived slight in an exaggerated way.

There's also a concept known as the suit-prone nurse, a nurse whose personality and mannerisms are more likely to trigger lawsuits. (See *The suit-prone nurse.*) This nurse requires counseling and education to change her behavior and develop more positive interactions with patients and family members, not only to improve the care she delivers but also to lessen the likelihood of future lawsuits.

Nursing implications

Even if you develop good relationships with patients and provide them with quality nursing care, you still run a small risk of being sued — or being threatened with a suit. If you hear such a threat, investigate right away to find out the nature of the problem. In all likelihood, the patient or family has a problem that isn't being addressed or an expectation that's incorrect. Find out whether the person thinks the patient is receiving inadequate care. Does the person think the patient's failure to get better stems from the quality or quantity of care delivered? Does the person believe he's getting less than the truth from you, the doctor, or other agency staff?

Communication through thoughtful and objective questions may be all you need to prevent further misunderstanding. Perhaps the patient needs to be reassessed and the initial plan of care revised. Perhaps a care conference would better determine realistic nursing needs and interventions. Sometimes the reassignment of another nurse will prevent legal action. Again, careful documentation of steps undertaken and discussions conducted may help you and your agency if the patient or family members actually do file suit.

Even under threat of lawsuit, you are still your patient's advocate. You must do everything within your power to meet the needs of the patient and his family. And you must document that you've done so.

If you recognize that you're dealing with a suit-prone patient or family member, try to compensate for the person's shortcomings. Interact on a more personal level. Express satisfaction with the patient's progress and cooperation. Show empathy and concern if the patient has a setback. And keep repeating needed information so the patient and family won't feel uncertain or fearful of the unknown. An atmosphere of attentiveness, caring, and patience helps prevent suit-prone people from actually filing suit.

Especially if you recognize a patient or family member as suit-prone, make sure your documentation includes all the steps you took to offset the person's unhappiness. Recount the positive comments you made, the exact teaching you provided, and any statements the patient or family members made about noncompliance, whether oral or demonstrated.

Explain how you ensured that the patient received all the care he needed, whether you gave it directly, delegated it to a qualified colleague, or taught a family member how to provide it. Remember, objective and complete charting can assist the judge and jury in finding that the patient received competent, quality nursing care.

Above all else, remain calm and do all that can be done to diffuse the situation. Also be sure to let your patient's attending doctor, your agency's risk manager, your direct supervisor, and other appropriate agency staff know that a lawsuit may be filed. In documenting the incident, include what the patient or family member said, the behavior and demeanor of the person threatening the lawsuit, and whom you notified about it. Such documentation further assures a judge that the threat was taken seri-

The suit-prone nurse

Are you or a colleague at increased risk for being sued? Here's a brief personality sketch of the type of nurse most likely to be sued:

- has difficulty establishing close relationships with others
- is insecure and readily shifts blame to others
- tends to be insensitive to patients' complaints or fails to take them seriously
- tends to be aloof and more concerned with the mechanics of nursing than with ensuring meaningful interactions with patients
- inappropriately delegates responsibility to others to avoid personal contact with patients.

ously and that appropriate actions were taken.

Some lawsuits may be preventable if the agency creates realistic policies and procedures and ensures that all nurses employed by the agency carefully adhere to them. For example, your agency should have written standing orders giving direction on the appropriate way to deal with emergencies or unexpected patient needs when an attending doctor is not available. Standing orders should be reviewed and updated on a regular basis and signed by a doctor before being implemented.

Likewise, you should understand the provisions of contracts made with patients who receive your agency's care. Contracts include both written and oral agreements made between the agency and the potential patient. Services offered in an agency's brochure and other advertisements about the agency may be construed as part of the contract.

The contract should specify the following: provider's and patient's respective roles and responsibilities; the duration, type, frequency, and limitations of services; discharge planning; cost and payment schedules; and provisions for obtaining informed consent from the patient or the patient's surrogate for specific interventions.

Many patients threaten lawsuits because of perceived abandonment by the agency. If a patient will be discharged from the agency, make sure you give the patient or family member reasonable notice and adequate health care services up to the actual date of discharge. Keep in mind, however, that the agency isn't obligated to give services without compensation, nor is it obliged to continue caring for patients who threaten the safety of its staff.

To help prevent potential lawsuits, remember and adopt the following principles:

- ◆ Patients and families who are treated honestly, openly, and respectfully and are apprised of all facets of treatment and prognosis are not likely to sue.
- ◆ Communications made in a caring and professional manner tend to protect you against suits.
- ◆ Stay within your area of individual competence, and adhere to all standards of care. Upgrade your technical skills on a regular basis, attend pertinent continuing education classes and in-service programs, and undertake only those actual skills you can competently perform.
- ◆ Make sure you understand basic legal concepts, such as those outlined in this chapter, and incorporate them into your everyday clinical practice.

Even with the best care, no one can guarantee a certain set of results when it comes to patients who are ill or injured. However, by following the principles you've learned in this chapter, you can maximize your patients' satisfaction.

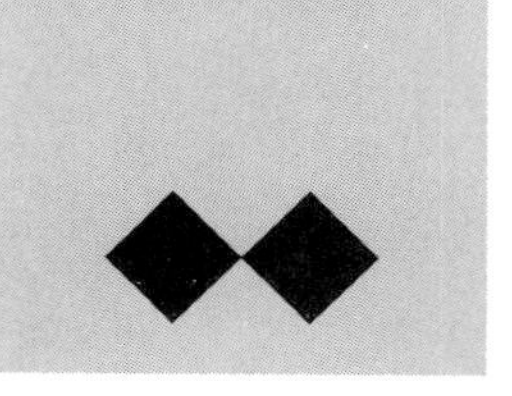

CHAPTER 4

Promoting safety

No matter where you choose to practice nursing, your ultimate goal will be the same: to provide the most accurate, efficient nursing care you can. To meet this goal in the home environment, you'll need more than good nursing skills. You'll also need to take special steps to keep yourself and your patients safe from a variety of potentially harmful influences.

In the home environment, safety is a more complex issue than it is in a controlled setting. There's more for you to think about and watch out for, and there may be more dangers facing you personally. Even in safe homes, you'll need to maintain a level of watchfulness that's typically unnecessary in dedicated health care settings.

This chapter outlines some important concepts you can use to help keep yourself and your patients safe. It includes tips for traveling safely to and from a patient's home, detecting and defusing potential hazards in the home, avoiding dangers related to equipment and restraints, reducing the risk of infection, and making safe use of transportation and emergency services.

By meeting these safety issues head-on, you'll be better able to handle them deftly and get on with the important business of caring for your patients.

◆ KEEPING YOURSELF SAFE

As you know, your job as a home health nurse may take you to a wide variety of homes in neighborhoods that differ markedly in their socioeconomic character. In all the neighborhoods you visit, you must be concerned about *your* safety in addition to that of your patients.

Usually, your agency will provide some of what you need to keep yourself safe. In the final analysis, however, on-the-spot decisions will fall to you. By developing an awareness of safety concerns, plus tools for coping with threats to your safety, you'll be well equipped to discharge your nursing duties with minimal interference from threatening factors.

Agency actions

Although agency administrators obviously won't accompany you on home visits, they will provide support and backup services to help prepare and protect you. For example, before you visit a patient's home, agency personnel will assess the level of risk incurred by providing care in that neighborhood. They may look at reports completed by nurses previously assigned to that neighborhood. They may hire a safety consultant to evaluate and assign risk levels to the communities in your service area. They may also work with the community relations officer of your police district to assess the risk level of various neighborhoods in your area.

Your agency will most likely work to establish close ties with law enforcement officers in your high-risk service areas. Besides helping to assess risk levels, local police departments can help your agency create realistic policies and guidelines for reporting criminal activity, especially when it occurs inside a patient's home. Open communication with local police will help your agency guide you in how and when to report potential problems in a patient's home.

If your patient lives in a high-risk area, the agency will most likely ask an escort or guard to accompany you on your visit. Clearly, even an escort can't guarantee your safety. However, especially if he knows the community, an escort can help avoid trouble areas, provide visible backup to make you appear less vulnerable and, at times, foresee dangerous situations.

In all likelihood, your agency also will have a way to provide immediate backup if you find yourself in a dangerous situation. (If it doesn't have a policy that guarantees this service, consider switching to another agency.) Many home health agencies also provide training in personal safety awareness, drug awareness, and proactive safety measures. Your agency also may provide you with basic safety equipment. (See *Elements of a safety tool kit*.)

Elements of a safety tool kit

Your agency may supply you with safety tools such as the ones listed here. If not, consider obtaining them on your own to help ensure your safety. They include:

- a hand-held alarm that emits a loud noise when activated
- a cellular phone
- a large and powerful flashlight to help identify house numbers and street names in the dark
- a smaller flashlight to help you assess the patient's home and navigate dark halls or stairs
- capsicum (pepper) spray, if you're willing to use it and your agency and local authorities allow it.

By taking these and other concrete steps, agency administrators demonstrate that they have your safety in mind. In addition, they should be willing and ready to stop sending you into any area where you feel threatened or uneasy. In the long run, you'll be better able to promote your own safety if you know your agency stands behind you.

Personal actions

Although your agency can do much to promote your safety, don't forget that you're the one standing on the front line. Ultimately, it's up to you to cultivate an awareness of your surroundings. In a potentially threatening situation, it's up to you to handle yourself appropriately.

Even if you know the neighborhood you visit and consider it to be relatively safe, you still need to understand and follow the three guidelines listed below; they're crucial to maintaining your safety.

◆ *Be prepared.* By knowing the kinds of hazards you may face, you can prepare yourself to minimize or avoid them. Before you find yourself in need of it, make a plan that you can follow in case you need to defend yourself or make a quick exit.

◆ *Be alert.* Rather than worrying needlessly about all the dangers that could befall you, watch for real problems. Excessive worrying can actually put you in greater danger by taking your mind off what's happening right in front of you. Being alert means watching your environment for anything unusual, and responding appropriately.

◆ *Be able to think and act without panic.* In many threatening situations, your best defense is a cool head. Remember that you've made a plan for handling hazards; follow it.

Any home care situation can be dangerous. Whether the hazards you face stem from weapons, drugs, violence, or foreseeable and preventable accidents, you must be aware of potential dangers, take simple precautions to minimize risk, and have a plan for coping with situations that may arise. In addition, keep these specific suggestions in mind.

Dress for success

Believe it or not, what you wear can influence your level of safety when providing home care. Of course, if your agency requires you to wear a uniform and identification tag, do so. If your agency doesn't require a uniform, you'll need to put some thought into your working clothes.

In general, your clothes shouldn't restrict your movements. For example, they shouldn't prevent you from walking briskly. They should allow you to bend, stoop, and stretch without exposing you unduly. On your feet, wear comfortable shoes with nonskid soles that allow you to move quickly and safely in an emergency. Avoid wearing earrings or other accessories that can be grasped and pulled by another person.

Most safety experts advise against carrying a wallet or purse on home visits. Instead, place your agency identification and driver's license in a secure pocket. Some consultants suggest carrying a small amount of money, such as a ten-dollar bill, in an easily accessible pocket. You could use it in an emergency situation or as a distraction for a would-be attacker.

Planning ahead

Before embarking on a series of home visits, make sure you have accurate addresses and directions to your patients' homes. Find out about the neighborhoods you'll be visiting. If possible, question a colleague who's already been to those neighborhoods. That way, you can find out whether drug houses, gang hangouts, or other potentially dangerous areas are located near your destinations.

Before you leave, plan the safest route to your patients' homes, even if that route isn't the most direct one. Make a note of the locations of police stations, public telephones, and other public buildings. Also, be sure to leave a copy of your daily itinerary with your agency. If you'll be visiting high-risk areas, you may want to set up a series of check-in calls so your agency can follow you throughout the day. Never enter a home that's not listed on the posted schedule.

Next, assess your car for road readiness; check the fuel level, tire pressure, windshield wipers, lights, battery, and so on. Carry an extra set of keys. Also, make note of the weather conditions and possible changes in the forecast.

If you want to carry a purse, lock it out of sight in the car's trunk before you arrive at your destination. Don't leave personal items or nursing items visible in the car.

Part of your preparation will be to determine the best time of day to visit each patient. Certainly, clinical considerations may dictate the time of your visit. Also check to see if your patient has a preference. And you may want to consider a few other issues as well. For example, if you'll be visiting a home located near a bar or liquor store, you may want your visit to take place before it opens. Also, remember that Friday afternoons may be more dangerous than other weekdays because of increased alcohol consumption. Finally, be aware that crime may increase on days when Social Security and welfare checks arrive.

Visiting a home

Once you've identified the house or building you'll be visiting, you'll have to find a safe place to park your car. In most cases, you'll want to choose a location as close as possible to the patient's home. However, sometimes a busier, better-lit spot a short distance away may be a better choice. Don't park in a place where you could get wedged beside a van or other large vehicle.

As you move toward your parking place, observe the neighborhood carefully. Assess the approach to your patient's home. If the mood of the neighborhood seems disturbing, or if you see groups of people standing around on the street, drive to a safe, well-lit place and call your supervisor. Perhaps an escort could come to your aid, or a family member could serve as an escort from an acceptable parking place into the patient's home.

If the patient lives in an apartment building, continue to be vigilant even after you get inside. Observe the entrance for suspicious people or activity. Quickly check the building's physical condition for immediate hazards, such as obstacles or poor lighting. Evaluate the stairs or elevator for potential hazards. Depending on what you encounter, you may want to wait for an empty elevator rather than ride with a group of unknown passengers. If the elevator isn't working, ask a family member to escort you from the entrance up to the apartment. In general, try to avoid using the stairs in a large building.

When you enter your patient's home, check with the patient or caregiver to see how many people and animals are present. Try to ascertain where they are and what they're doing. If you detect a potentially hazardous situation, respond appropriately. For example, if you observe people drinking, consider asking them to refrain until you leave.

If you observe illegal drug use, you'll need to follow your agency's policy when responding. Many agencies suggest that you ask participants to stop taking drugs while you're in the home. If they refuse, arrange a different time to visit and then leave. Tell your supervisor what happened as soon as possible.

During your visit, continue to be aware of safety issues related to household hazards, people and animals in the home, medical equipment, and the mechanics of giving care. You'll read about many such hazards later in the chapter. If you feel threatened for any reason when you're in a patient's home, try to be proactive in preventing an incident.

When leaving your patient's home, check the route to your car while still at the patient's door. Have your car keys out and ready. Use extra caution if you see unusual activity, unusual numbers of people congregating, or unusual police activity. You may want to ask a family member to escort you to your car. When approaching the car, quickly observe the area around and under it to check for threatening people or objects, such as broken glass or sharp metal.

Dealing with a hostile dog

When delivering home care, try to avoid interacting with dogs, even those that seem friendly. If you find yourself threatened by a dog despite your precautions, you may be able to thwart a confrontation by following these suggestions:

- Keep the dog in sight, but don't make eye contact with him. Look down or to the side.
- Slowly back toward an exit or a safe area.
- Talk to the dog in a calm, firm voice. Try giving a command, such as "sit" or "stay." If that doesn't work, try talking to him in a soothing, reassuring voice.
- Think about what you could use as a distracting object: a clipboard, perhaps, or a box of tissues. If the dog moves toward you, drop the object in front of him. It may distract him long enough for you to escape.
- If you have a sweater or jacket, wrap it around your forearm. Then, if the dog lunges at you, raise your arm and push it to the back of his mouth. Then, without pulling back, deliver a sharp blow to his nose with your other hand.

Clearly, the secret to handling a hostile dog lies in your ability to keep your head. By watching the dog carefully and responding appropriately, you'll probably be able to escape a potentially dangerous situation.

If you had any problems getting to a patient's home or carrying out your duties while there, document and report them immediately. Doing so will help prevent another staff member from encountering the same or worse problems. Your agency probably has a policy for reporting such incidents in the patient's record and for reporting them to the authorities, particularly if they involve weapons or violence.

Special situations

Certain situation may create added safety concerns — for example, if your patient has an unruly or threatening pet, has one or more children in the home, or lives in an environment marked by violence. If you encounter such situations, being prepared can help you handle them competently.

Animals

If your patient has a dog, even if it seems to be a friendly dog, the safest course of action is to ask the patient to put the animal in another room during your visit. Why? Because even a normally calm dog may grow worried and protective during unfamiliar nursing procedures.

Remember that some procedures may make a dog think you're fighting with or harming its owner, such as administering wound care, giving injections, and performing passive range-of-motion exercises. In general, it's better to avoid these possibly provocative situations by removing the dog from the room.

If you find yourself in a room with a threatening dog, take action to avoid being bitten. (See *Dealing with a hostile dog.*) If you can't avoid the dog and it bites you, you'll need to get immediate treatment for the wound.

Start by washing it thoroughly at the patient's house. Then go to the nearest treatment facility.

After a dog bite, the health department will want to test the offending animal for rabies. Try to describe the dog in detail. If health department personnel can't find it, you'll probably have to undergo rabies prophylaxis.

Remember that rabies is a serious illness that's increasing in frequency. Any time you see an animal acting in an unusual manner, whether it's wild or domesticated, assume that it might have rabies and stay well out of its way. This is especially true if you see a nocturnal animal, such as a raccoon, moving about during the day. If you see an animal that's obviously sick or injured, report it to local animal control authorities as soon as possible.

Cats can be hazardous as well because a scratch from even a healthy cat may carry an increased risk of infection. Even if a patient's cat appears calm and relaxed, don't try to touch or pet it. The best course of action is simply to leave cats and other small pets alone. If you sustain a cat scratch or other injury, wash it carefully at the patient's house, and seek medical attention when you leave.

If you feel that a patient's pet poses a safety hazard, be sure to report it to your agency. That way, other professionals who visit the patient's house will be prepared to ask the patient to remove or contain the pet during home visits.

Personal threats

Even a seemingly safe home can be the setting for a confrontation with a threatening patient or family member. The confrontation may stem from an alcohol- or drug-induced state, a mental or physical illness, or a criminal intention. It may also represent the family's reaction to stress and anger.

No matter what creates a personal threat, it's still frightening and potentially dangerous. That's why your first goal should be to avoid a dangerous situation before it starts. If you can't do that, take steps to minimize the danger and thwart the threat. Look at the overall situation when deciding how to handle a threat: who else is present, whether help is available, the physical strength of the person involved, and the environment itself.

Dealing with hostility. First, quickly assess the possible reason for the personal threat you've encountered. Remember that behavioral changes can accompany a variety of physical and mental illnesses. Are you aware of a disorder that could be affecting the person's behavior or attitude toward you?

Next, determine the level of threat involved. If you're facing low-level hostility, you may be able to calm the person through a simple verbal intervention. Say something like "You seem upset. Can we sit down and talk about your concerns?" This kind of response shows that you care about the person's feelings.

Another course of action would be to say something like "What can we do to increase your comfort with this situation?" This kind of response shows that you care and allows the hostile person to cooperate in reducing the threat and calming the situation. It allows the person to spend energy finding a solution rather than continuing the cycle of hostility.

Also important in your response to a threat is your visible demeanor. Find a way to look calm and confident, no matter how uneasy you may feel. Maintain eye contact and speak clearly and calmly. Be assertive but not aggressive. Express caring for the threatening person. Watch your body language as well. Maintain a relaxed stance. Don't block the door and don't be obvious in your search for a possible escape route.

If a patient or family member seems protective and hostile about having a stranger in the home or perceives your assessment questions to be too intrusive, avoid the tendency to give lengthy explanations of your actions or justifications for your presence. Extended explanations may not address the person's concerns and, in fact, may seem like you're trying to overwhelm him.

You can help to ease this kind of hostility by mentioning the patient's doctor or referral source by name when you first meet the patient or family. Also briefly explain the purpose of your visit and of your assessment questions or procedures. These steps may be enough to allow the visit to proceed smoothly. If not, you may need to defer assessment of all conditions not directly related to the need for home care.

If you think the hostility may stem from fear, try to draw the person out. Find out if he had a frightening encounter with a stranger in the house. Help him express his concerns by asking a sincere question, such as "What would help you feel safer in receiving home health care?"

Handling mental illness. If the threatening person may have a mental illness, the evaluation process is especially important. Watch for signs that the person is losing control; remember that verbal interventions are most effective early in the course of the conflict.

As in other threatening situations, ask the person about his concerns, and ask what he needs to feel better. Suggest that the person come to a quiet place and sit down to talk. Say something like "You seem to have concerns about this. Will you share them with me?" Along with a confident attitude, project an expectation that the threatening person will remain in control. You may even want to say something, such as "I expect you to stay in control of yourself while we talk about this."

Even if you can convince the mentally ill person to talk with you about his concerns, remember that safety is still paramount. Maintain a clear route to the door. Increase your personal space slightly. Avoid having your conversation in the kitchen, where potential weapons may be readily available.

If the person is delusional and believes that *he* is being threatened, respond with a soothing tone and express understanding for his feelings. Say something like "What you're feeling must be very frightening. Even though I'm not seeing or hearing what you are, I understand that it's distressing for you."

Do what you can to try to increase the delusional person's feelings of safety. Tell him that he'll be safe in talking with you, and allow about four times the personal space you usually do. If the person is angry, don't try to touch him. If you do, you'll only increase his agitation while placing yourself in danger of being grabbed or struck.

Defusing dementia. Most patients with dementia, such as that caused by Alzheimer's disease, don't know why they're angry and agitated. In fact, trying to get them to explain their behavior may only increase their anxiety and agitation.

Although violence usually isn't a hallmark of dementia, it can occur from time to time. As with any threatening situation, your best option is to head it off before it develops. For the patient with dementia, this usually means anticipating needs and avoiding unfamiliar situations. A family member who knows the patient's routine can help to determine the best time for your visit, when the patient isn't too tired or hungry.

Ask the familiar family member to introduce you to the patient and explain the reason for your visit. In interviewing the patient, watch how your assessment questions affect him. If impaired memory makes him unable to answer your questions, he may become frustrated and angry. If a loss of language skills makes it difficult for him to communicate, he'll probably grow even more frustrated.

If you see a patient becoming more and more frustrated, respond. First, stop making demands on him. Invite him to sit quietly or walk with you. Be careful not to startle or repel the patient by touching him. Try changing the conversation to one that's not threatening. For example, if you say something about an object easily visible in the room, the patient may be able to focus on it and talk about it without stress.

No matter how you try to defuse the situation, if the patient has an unmet need, he may remain agitated and angry. So you'll need to try to determine the nature of that need — usually a challenging task. Be sure to consider both physical and emotional problems. For example, pain, constipation, or hunger can lead to agitation. An older man with an enlarged prostate may be retaining urine and thus be continually uncomfortable.

Emotional needs can lead to agitation in many ways. For example, if a female patient with dementia insists that she needs to pick up her children after school, she may not be comforted when you tell her that her children are grown and gone. Perhaps the underlying problem is that the patient feels unneeded. Maybe she'd feel more comforted by hearing about her importance to her children and by being invited to do a task.

Clearly, personal threats can arise for a myriad of reasons. By being prepared to assess and respond to potential threats calmly, with a cool head, you'll be well equipped not only to maintain your own safety but to respond appropriately to the needs of your patients and their families.

Weapons

Weapons — especially firearms — present a real and frightening danger for nurses in many home environments, from the inner city, to the suburbs, to rural areas. That's why it's important to know whether firearms are present in the home and what to do about it if they are. (See *Responding to a gun.*) Your agency probably has a policy addressing these issues.

Above all, don't allow your patient or his family to keep a loaded firearm in the same room where you're delivering care. If a patient refuses to remove a loaded gun from the room, preferably to a locked location, don't continue your visit. Instead, leave. Make it clear why you're leaving. Then call your supervisor and the patient's doctor and let them know about the firearm danger. Your agency may have an incident report in which you should document the problem.

If the patient is willing to remove the gun to a safer location, you'll need to establish a verbal or written agreement that he'll continue to store the gun elsewhere when you or your team members visit.

In addition to considering your own safety in the presence of a loaded gun, you must also consider the safety of your patient and his family. If you become aware of a gun, assess the patient's home situation. Does the gun pose a threat to children in the home?

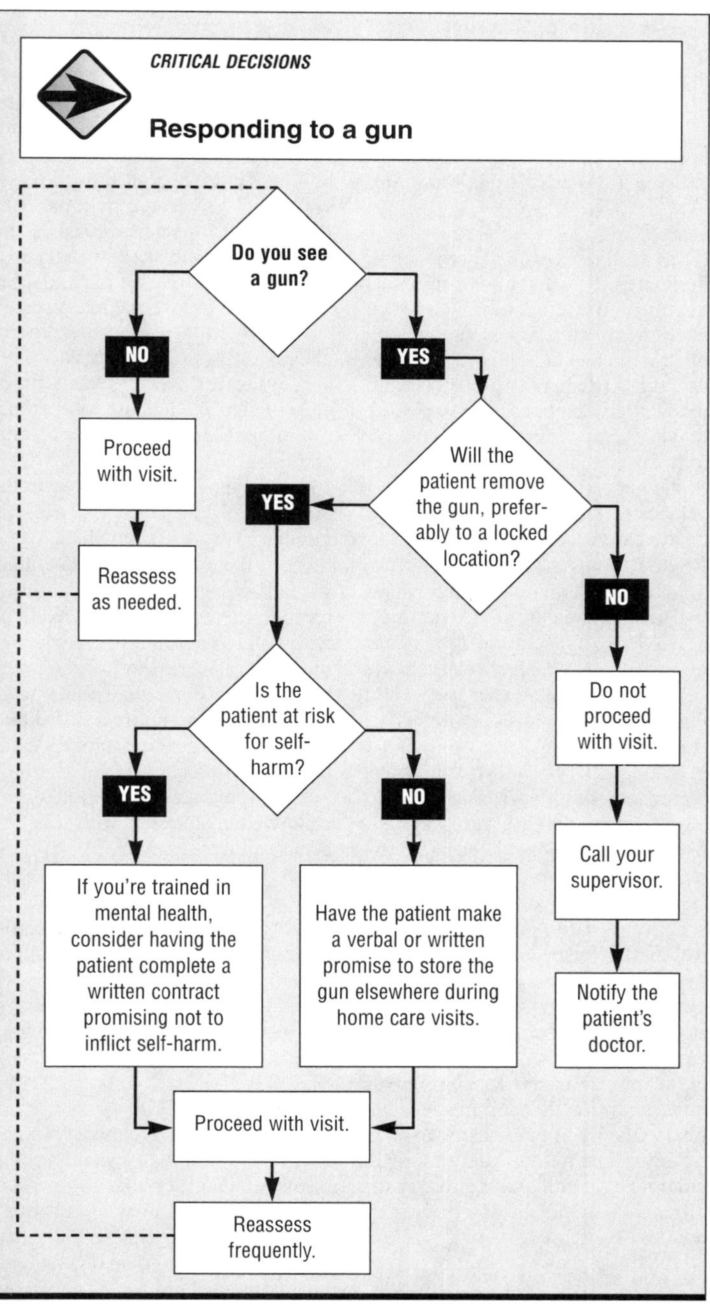
CRITICAL DECISIONS
Responding to a gun
Do you see a gun?
NO
Proceed with visit.
Reassess as needed.
YES
Will the patient remove the gun, preferably to a locked location?
YES
Is the patient at risk for self-harm?
YES
If you're trained in mental health, consider having the patient complete a written contract promising not to inflict self-harm.
NO
Have the patient make a verbal or written promise to store the gun elsewhere during home care visits.
Proceed with visit.
Reassess frequently.
NO
Do not proceed with visit.
Call your supervisor.
Notify the patient's doctor.

Does anyone in the home have a mental illness? Do any family members have a history of violence? If you feel that a gun creates an unacceptable risk for someone in your patient's home, talk with your supervisor about which actions are most appropriate.

Latex allergy

Of all the hazards you may encounter in a patient's home, one of the most deadly can stem from your own equipment: latex gloves, tubing, and other implements. With the increased use of latex in barrier protection and medical equipment, more and more nurses are becoming hypersensitive to it. In fact, although less than 1% of the general public has allergic reactions to latex, more than 10% of health care professionals do.

Sensitivity reactions range from mild contact dermatitis to hives, rhinitis, bronchospasm, and even anaphylaxis. The reaction may increase in severity with each exposure to the substance. If you've ever had a mild reaction to latex gloves or another latex product, you'll need to make a plan for quick action if you find yourself reacting more severely.

For example, carry a supply of nonlatex gloves to avoid unnecessary exposure. Your agency is required to supply these for you if you're hypersensitive to latex. Also wear a medical-alert bracelet. You may also want to ask your personal doctor for autoinjectable epinephrine so you can stop an anaphylactic reaction if you feel it starting. As you know, however, anaphylactic shock can progress quickly. If you develop hives or begin to wheeze after exposure to latex or any other potent allergen, seek emergency medical attention by dialing 911 or the local emergency medical system.

◆ ASSESSING HOME HAZARDS

A big part of your job as a home health nurse is helping to make your patients and their families safe in their homes. To do so, you'll need to assess the risks created by a patient's illness or treatment as well as the existing household risks that could pose a danger to the patient or hinder his treatment or recovery. Finally, you'll need to identify risks caused by inadequate resources, such as limited space; lack of privacy, fresh air, or clean water; inadequate food preparation; and less-than-ideal personal and household hygiene.

If your patient has children in the home, you'll need to be especially vigilant to avoid creating hazards for them or the patient. Remember that, if the patient is the only caregiver present, the children will need to be with you in the room while you provide nursing care. Pay special attention to used sharps and waste materials that could be infectious. Make sure children don't have access to the patient's medications or any hazardous implements. Also make sure children don't interfere with your procedures, the operation of potentially dangerous medical equipment, or the patient's mobility or safety.

After carefully assessing the risks to your patient's safety in his home environment, you can usually do much to reduce risks and maximize the resources available to help your patient recover and live in safety.

Initial assessment

Keep in mind that the most common accidents in the home involve fires, burns, electricity, falls, and poisoning. Plus, certain areas of the house, such as the kitchen and the stairs, may be more dangerous than others. Even normal household habits can prove dangerous to a patient with impaired mobility, vision, or neurologic function.

That's why you'll want to start assessing household safety as soon as you enter a patient's dwelling. Start with an informal observation of the environment. Look at the neighborhood, noting the air quality, noise level, and population density and profile. Remember that these factors will probably vary with the time of day and day of the week. Also look at the exterior of the patient's building. Make particular note of structural problems that could pose a risk to the patient, such as a sagging porch roof, broken or missing steps, or falling plaster.

Inside the home, observe the condition of the walls, ceilings, and floors. Look at the kitchen and bathroom, and check the electricity. Note the presence of clutter or trash in the home because it could create a serious fire hazard.

In addition to your informal observations, you'll also probably need to record your environmental findings in a formal assessment document provided by your agency. Usually, the form will provide space to describe the general state of the patient's home, the availability of water and electricity, and the risk of falls or accidents.

In certain situations, you may need to complete a more in-depth environmental assessment. For example, if you're caring for a child who lives in a home with lead-based paint, you'll need to make specific observations about the extent of this hazard.

To help keep your patients and their families as safe as possible in their homes, perform a systematic assessment of the household hazards listed below. Many household hazards are simple to fix; they just need someone like you to identify them and take action to reverse them.

Fire hazards

Because cigarettes are a common cause of household fires, start your assessment of fire hazards by asking if anyone in the family smokes. Keep in mind that a cigarette dropped onto a sofa, a bed, or an upholstered chair may smolder for hours before suddenly reaching a flashpoint and turning into a major blaze. Do your best to help patients and their families reduce the risks of smoking in the home. (See *Fire safety checklist,* page 82.)

Also check for other fire risks. For example, make sure small stoves and space heaters are placed where they can't be knocked over and well away from furnishings and flammable materials, such as curtains and rugs. Space heaters that use kerosene, gas, or propane should be installed and operated properly. Fuel should be stored according to local fire regulations. Wood- and coal-burning stoves should be installed by qualified persons according to local building codes.

Check to make sure that electrical cords are placed out of the flow of traffic and not under furniture and carpets. Cords should be in good condition, not frayed or cracked. Extension cords should have an amp or wattage rating appropriate for their use. Make sure that electrical outlets and switches have cover plates and that no wiring is exposed. Also make a point of touching the cover plates to make sure they aren't overly warm to the touch. If they are, the wiring is probably unsafe.

Ensure that smoke detectors are in place on every floor of the home. Experts suggest placing them near bedrooms, either on the ceiling or on the wall, 6″ to 12″ (15 to 30 cm) below

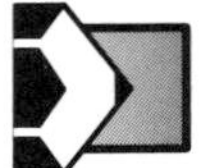

TEACHING POINTS

Fire safety checklist

When teaching fire safety to patients and their families, be sure to include these points:

◆ Use ashtrays for cigarettes and ashes only, not for trash.

◆ Make sure cigarettes are completely out before emptying ashtrays.

◆ Keep matches and lighters away from small children.

◆ Never smoke in bed or in an easy chair.

◆ Avoid overloading electrical circuits.

◆ Don't circumvent the grounding feature in three-prong plugs.

◆ Don't use electrical appliances that have frayed, cracked, or damaged cords or plugs.

◆ If there are young children in the house, place safety covers over unused electrical outlets.

◆ Use light bulbs of the appropriate size and type for lamps or fixtures.

◆ Check smoke detectors monthly to make sure they're functioning properly.

the ceiling. The location should be relatively easy to reach with a step stool so that the patient or a helper can check the batteries and replace them as needed.

Many fire departments suggest changing smoke detector batteries twice a year, using the change to and from daylight savings time as a convenient memory trigger. If you hear a smoke detector in the patient's home or in a common area making the characteristic beeping sound that warns of a low battery, arrange to have the battery replaced or notify the landlord or building management company.

Caution patients and families not to disable a smoke detector to keep it from beeping. If the detector has been mounted too close to smoke and fumes from the kitchen, suggest that your patient remount the device in a location that the manufacturer has recommended or find ways to reduce smoke and fumes emanating from the kitchen. Cleaning the oven or improving the ventilation may solve the problem.

Mobility hazards

To assess your patient's risk of falling, look for cluttered walkways, loose rugs, unsafe steps, unsafe bathrooms, and dangerous obstacles. If necessary, remove unsafe rugs and mats, tack them down, or place nonskid material under them. Make sure uncovered floors aren't slippery, a particular risk in the kitchen and bathroom. Urge the patient's caregivers not to use cleaners that leave surfaces slippery.

Next, look at the patient's stairways. Make sure they're well-lit and have light switches at the top and bottom. Night lights should be plugged into nearby outlets. Handrails should be available and sturdy. They should run continuously from the top to the bottom of the stairs. Fixtures holding the handrails to the walls should be strong enough to withstand a heavy weight. If the patient is frail, suggest installing handrails on both sides of the stairs to increase safety.

The steps themselves should provide secure footing. Make sure that the treads are in good condition, that carpeting isn't loose or frayed, and that no nails or tacks stick up from the stairs or their coverings. Also make sure the patient can easily see the stair edges. Dark or deep pile carpeting can make edges especially hard to see. Warn patients and their families against storing anything on the stairs, even briefly.

Check the rise of outdoor stairs to make sure the patient can readily climb from step to step. If there's a variation in the height of individual stairs, mark them clearly so the patient can see the edges. Even on uniform outside stairs, you may want to suggest that a family member cover them with rough textured paint or adhesive strips to increase safety. Advise them to consider painting the edges white for greater visibility at night.

Finally, make sure that all passages and walkways are well-lit and free from furniture, boxes, or other items that could cause the patient to stumble or fall. Urge the patient to install light bulbs with the maximum wattage recommended for the fixtures in use.

Although mobility hazards can affect any patient, they're especially dangerous for elderly patients or those with problems of gait or mentation. For example, certain types of cerebrovascular accidents and dementias can give the patient a false sense about his ability to walk. Also, patients recovering from surgery or recent injury may be unaccustomed to the temporary limitations on their mobility. Plus, many medications cause dizziness and orthostatic hypotension, which can increase the risk of a fall.

For all these patients, you'll want to make a special effort to identify and remove physical hazards from the environment, provide mobility aids and gait training, ask family members to help the patient move from room to room, and have the patient's doctor or pharmacist evaluate all medications for their potential to contribute to falls.

Food, plant, and product hazards

Foods that are handled or stored improperly can create a serious health threat. Groups especially vulnerable to the effects of food poisoning include the very young, the frail elderly, pregnant women, and immunosuppressed patients. Fortunately, following a few simple rules can increase the safety of all foods in the home. Do your best to help patients and caregivers understand the simple precautions that reduce the risk of food poisoning. (See *Food safety checklist,* page 84.)

During your household assessment, scan indoor and outdoor areas for toxic plants. Make sure that families with young children know about plants that, if ingested, could harm a child. They include such common indoor plants as dieffenbachia, philodendron, and asparagus fern. The degree of harm caused by ingesting these plants depends on the age and general health of the child involved, his degree of sensitivity, and the toxicity of the individual plant. Also warn parents about harmful outdoor plants (such as tulips and firethorn) that produce flowers or berries that could be attractive to children.

Even common food plants can have poisonous parts or can be poisonous if eaten raw or prepared improperly. For example, potatoes that have turned green from exposure to light are toxic and shouldn't be eaten. All parts of the rhubarb plant are poisonous except the well-cooked stem. And many wild mushrooms contain powerful toxins. A good rule of thumb is to recommend that patients and their families avoid eating anything

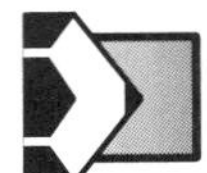

TEACHING POINTS

Food safety checklist

When teaching food safety to patients and their families, be sure to include these instructions:

◆ Wash your hands before handling any food items.

◆ Wash your hands before and after handling poultry, other meats, and food waste.

◆ Wash your hands after using the bathroom or blowing your nose.

◆ Don't defrost foods at room temperature. Instead, defrost them in the refrigerator, run them under cool water, or use a defrost setting on a microwave oven.

◆ Reserve one cutting board only for raw meats. Use a different cutting board for other types of food.

◆ After preparing food, clean your food preparation areas thoroughly.

◆ Discard any food item that smells or looks spoiled.

◆ Discard food cans that are bulging or rusting.

◆ Discard foods that have passed the "sell by" date listed on the label.

◆ Discard food if it has been stored too long at temperatures between 45° and 140° F (7° to 60° C), especially meats and mayonnaise-based items.

◆ Cook foods thoroughly (to above 140° F), especially meats.

◆ Avoid recipes that include raw eggs (such as salad dressings).

◆ Store foods below 45° F. Place a thermometer in the refrigerator to monitor its temperature.

◆ Store cooked foods on the top shelves of the refrigerator and raw foods on the bottom shelves, so juices from uncooked foods won't be able to contaminate cooked foods.

◆ Never return foods (such as mayonnaise) from a serving dish to the original container because you could contaminate the entire container.

◆ Don't store acidic drinks in chipped or damaged galvanized containers because the drink could absorb zinc and cause zinc poisoning.

◆ Don't store acidic foods or beverages in leaded crystal containers because the acid could cause lead to leach into the food or beverage.

◆ Change dishtowels and dishcloths daily; launder them if they've been used to mop up spills or wipe a counter.

that they can't positively identify as a safe food.

Many products used commonly around the home are poisonous when ingested. That's why you should check to see where the patient stores cleaners, antiseptics, and any other product labeled "Keep away from children." Even "safe" products can do damage when used improperly. Consider vitamin and mineral supplements, for example. If ingested in large quantities, the iron they contain can build to toxic levels. Mouthwash can also be toxic in large quantities because many mouthwashes contain large amounts of alcohol.

If you're caring for a patient with dementia who has small children in the home, it's even more important that you assess for food, plant, and product dangers and that you minimize those dangers when you find them. Remember that simply placing dangerous compounds on a high shelf may not ensure safety. Instead, find a way to secure these products behind locks or child-safe devices.

Medication hazards

For a nurse, it's almost second nature to assess for medication hazards, especially interactions and adverse effects. Keep in mind, however, that some medication hazards are more common in the home environment, such as problems with storage and labeling.

Most people tend to store medicines in the bathroom, even though the increased heat and moisture in a bathroom make it a poor storage choice. Check to make sure your patient's medications are stored in a safe location that's not too hot or moist and that's inaccessible to children. Most children have easy access to the bathroom and, because they're curious and agile, may be able to reach medications and undo childproof caps. If an older patient has requested nonchildproof caps, safe storage of medications is doubly important.

Also make sure your patient's medications are in their original containers with legible labels. Urge the patient to discard outdated medications by flushing them down the toilet. Also be sure to teach the patient basic safety information for taking medications properly. (See *Medication safety checklist,* page 86.)

Finally, find out if your patient tends to awaken during the night to take a medication. Many people don't bother to turn on a light in such situations, which heightens the risk of taking the wrong medication. Instead, urge the patient to turn on the light, use a night light, or keep the needed medication by itself in a very specific location. Check the placement of the bathroom light switch.

Kitchen hazards

The kitchen can be one of the most dangerous rooms in the house. Fire and electrical hazards stem not only from stoves, toasters, and other small appliances, but from the close proximity of water and electricity. Accidental burns and fires as well as falls are potential dangers. Don't make the mistake of thinking of burns only in relation to open flames. Other sources of heat also cause serious burns. In fact, the kitchen holds the greatest risk of burns for both adults and children.

When assessing a patient's kitchen, make sure that ventilation systems and range exhausts are working properly, to avoid buildup of indoor air pollutants. Make sure that appliance cords and extension cords are well away from the sink and stove. Also, suggest that the patient have ground fault interrupters installed. These shock-protection devices detect electrical faults and shut off the electricity before a serious injury or death can occur.

Make sure the kitchen is well-lit, especially over the stove, sink, and counter areas, to help avoid burns and cuts. If an older patient complains of glare from the lights, suggest that he use frosted bulbs, indirect lighting, shades or globes on light fixtures, and blinds or curtains on windows.

If the patient is capable of reaching for items on high shelves, make sure he uses a step stool to do so rather than climbing onto a more precari-

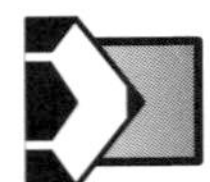

TEACHING POINTS

Medication safety checklist

When teaching medication safety to patients and their families, be sure to include these instructions:

◆ Make sure you know the name of each of your medications, how much you should take, when you should take it, and what side effects you might experience. If you can't remember all this information, write it down and keep it in your wallet.

◆ Every time you visit the doctor, either take all your medications (prescription and nonprescription) with you or take a list with you.

◆ Be sure to take all your medications just as the doctor prescribed them. Don't change the doses or the timing without checking with your doctor.

◆ Make a daily schedule for taking your medications so you're less likely to forget. Use a timer or watch alarm to remind you, if necessary. After taking a medication, mark it on a calendar or schedule sheet to remind yourself that you took it.

◆ Some people like to use a special box with day and time compartments to keep track of which medications to take at which times. If you want to use such a box, check with your pharmacist to make sure your medications aren't sensitive to light, the plastic container, or other medications.

◆ Don't give your medications to someone else to take, and don't take any medications besides your own.

◆ Store your medications in a safe place. If small children live in your home or visit you often, store medications in a locked cabinet. If your bathroom gets warm and steamy, don't store medications there.

◆ Don't keep sleep aids near the bed because doing so raises the risk that you could forget and take two doses at night.

◆ If you keep a steroid inhaler and a bronchodilator by the bed, make sure you don't confuse them during the night. Consider keeping the bronchodilator on top of the night table and the steroid in the drawer.

◆ Don't drink alcohol with any medication.

◆ Tell your doctor if you experience a reaction to a medication.

◆ Read all the information that comes with your medications. If you don't receive package insert information with a new prescription, ask your pharmacist for it.

◆ If you have trouble seeing small print, ask the pharmacist to use large-print labels on your medication containers.

◆ Use only one pharmacy for all your prescriptions.

◆ If you have questions about any of your medications, write them down and take your list of questions to your next doctor's appointment.

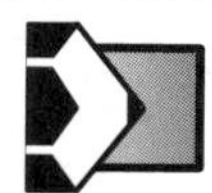

TEACHING POINTS

Kitchen safety checklist

When teaching kitchen safety to patients and their families, be sure to include these instructions:

◆ Never leave pots or pans unattended on a hot stove.

◆ Avoid wearing long or loose sleeves while cooking, or use elastic bands to hold your sleeves back while you cook.

◆ Don't allow the handles of pots or pans to extend past the front edge of the stove, both to prevent children from pulling hot food onto themselves and to prevent you from knocking into the pots.

◆ Make sure insulated pot handles aren't above an open flame.

◆ Make sure you cover noninsulated pot handles before picking them up.

◆ Take care when emptying boiling water into the sink or strainer to avoid splash and steam burns. Use both hands on the pot's handle.

◆ Use back burners before front burners.

◆ Don't allow children to use the stove or oven without supervision.

◆ Secure loose curtains and towels so they can't blow into an open flame or onto a hot burner.

◆ Keep the cords of toasters and coffee pots away from the stove and the edges of counters.

◆ Make sure your utensils are free from grease.

◆ Keep exhaust fans clean.

◆ Keep baking soda nearby to help put out grease fires. Don't store it at the back of the stove, however, because you won't be able to reach through a fire to get it.

◆ Don't spray oven cleaners at or on a pilot light.

◆ Store matches in a secure container away from the stove and inaccessible to small children.

◆ Adjust the hot water heater so tap water doesn't get hot enough to cause burns.

◆ Place hot serving dishes away from children at the table. Leave a pot holder on or near a hot dish.

ous surface, such as a box or chair. The step stool should have a handrail to increase stability when the patient stands on the top step. Make sure the stool's screws and braces are tight and sturdy. In addition to the general items outlined above, remind the patient to follow specific safety precautions when working in the kitchen. (See *Kitchen safety checklist*.)

Bathroom hazards

Because many accidents take place in the bathroom, take special care to assess this room and the activities your patient pursues there. The bathroom is an area of high risk for falls, burns, accidental ingestion of poisons, and potentially serious accidents related to the close proximity of water and electricity.

During your assessment, make sure the bathtub and shower have nonskid mats, abrasive strips, or another nonslip surface. If the patient is frail or unsteady or can't rise from a low sitting position, suggest using a bath stool or shower chair that has nonskid feet.

Also suggest the installation of grab bars beside the toilet and in the tub or shower. Make sure the bars are strong enough to hold a person's weight and firmly attached to the studs behind the surface of the wall. Bars are also available to attach to the sides of the bathtub. If you find this type of bar in use, check to see that it's fastened correctly and securely to the tub.

Although grab bars and bath stools are important aids in preventing falls, remind patients and family members that they can't guarantee safety. You'll need to teach each patient how to use these aids and emphasize the importance of continuing to take steps against falls in the tub or shower, even with bars in place. If, in your judgment, the patient continues to face a high risk of falling in the bath despite safety devices, make arrangements for someone to assist him at bathtime.

To prevent burns, urge the patient's family to set the hot water heater at 120° F (48.8° C) or lower. If they can't adjust the water heater, suggest that they use a thermometer to check the water temperature before starting the bath. For small children and frail elderly patients, bath water shouldn't exceed 110° F (43.3° C). In contrast, water supplied to many bathrooms reaches 140° F (60° C)— a significant burn risk.

If babies or children live in the house, tub safety becomes an even bigger concern. Teach patients and their families that a child can drown in a very small amount of water, even water in the bottom of a cleaning bucket. Urge patients and families never to leave a child alone around water, including during playtime in the tub. In addition to nonskid flooring in the tub, also suggest that families install a cushioned guard over the faucet. The guard will not only keep the child from bumping into the hard faucet, it also will prevent contact with potentially hot metal.

Remember that toileting can increase a patient's risk of falling even outside the bathroom. This is especially true of patients who have trouble transferring or walking when trying to get to the bathroom for toileting. And patients starting a new diuretic may find themselves rushing to the toilet without taking sufficient care. They also may have a heightened risk of falling because of the new illness or recent surgery that led to the need for home care. Keep in mind that many patients overestimate their abilities by basing their expectations on what they could do before their current illness or injury.

For the safety of all family members, suggest that they leave small electrical bathroom appliances unplugged when not in use. Also recommend ground fault interrupters to protect against electrocution.

Bedroom hazards

In the patient's bedroom, check for mobility hazards, such as loose rugs and runners. Even oversized bedding and bedspreads can raise the patient's risk of falling. Try to arrange the room so there's a telephone next to the bed and a light switch nearby. If possible, program emergency numbers into the bedside phone. Install a night light, if necessary. And check the condition of electrical and telephone cords.

Warn the patient and all family members against smoking in bed. Also warn against placing heaters, hot plates, and electric teapots or coffeepots near the bedding. Electric blankets should be used according to the manufacturer's instructions. Usually, that means not tucking them under the mattress or covering them with a bedspread. Covering an electric blanket could make it too hot and increase the risk of fire. Also warn the patient not to fall asleep with a heating pad turned on. Burns can develop over time, even at low settings.

Storage hazards

Household storage areas, including the basement, garage, and workshop, pose particular health hazards that can be reduced by your actions. For example, make sure all work areas have sufficient lighting. Check to see that the patient can reach a light switch without having to walk through a darkened area first. In any dark area, a flashlight should be readily available.

If you find a fuse box in one of these areas, check to see that the fuses are the correct size for the circuit. Make sure appliances and power tools can be plugged into appropriate grounded outlets. Suggest that patients and their families replace old tools that have neither a three-prong plug nor double insulation. Power tools also should have guards in place to protect the operator from moving parts.

Check to see that flammable and volatile liquids are stored in appropriate containers with tight caps to keep toxic fumes from escaping. Remind patients and their families that gasoline fumes can travel a significant distance, then explode when they come in contact with a gas water heater. Gasoline and other flammable substances shouldn't be stored near sources of heat or flame, such as heaters, furnaces, water heaters, stoves, and other gas appliances.

Because improper disposal of toxic materials can contaminate the environment, refer your patient to the local health or fire department for disposal instructions. Many such departments have special pickup or drop-off sites for volatile and hazardous wastes.

Environmental hazards

Certain environmental hazards can pose safety concerns in your patients' homes. They include lead, asbestos, and insect and rodent infestations.

Lead poisoning

Although paint, gasoline, and food cans no longer contain lead, lead poisoning continues to be a major hazard for children in some neighborhoods. The hazard is greatest in neglected older homes that contain significant amounts of lead-based interior paint.

Lead is toxic to humans of all ages, but it's most hazardous to children under age 6. That's primarily because a developing neurologic system is particularly vulnerable to lead poisoning. It's also because typical play activities may expose children to an elevated level of lead-contaminated dust and soil.

We've known for many years that a high level of lead in blood is associated with permanent neurologic damage. Recently, however, researchers have determined that even low lead levels can reduce a child's intelligence and attention span and create reading difficulties, learning disabilities, and behavior problems.

Children usually develop lead poisoning by ingesting lead-laden surface dust. This dust may not even be visible because of its small particle size, but it clings to children's hands and toys and cribs, then enters their bodies through their mouths. The dust falls from chipping, peeling lead-based paint and from paint disturbed by repainting or remodeling projects.

Contaminated soil provides another pathway for ingestion of lead. Usually, the soil has been contaminated

When to screen for lead contamination

Plan to assess lead levels if you note any of the following risk factors:

◆ Interior paint was applied before 1978 (especially before 1950).

◆ Interior paint is visibly deteriorating.

◆ Small children live in the home.

◆ A pregnant woman lives in the home.

◆ Someone in the family tends to eat nonfood items.

◆ Soil outdoors could be contaminated by paint or gasoline.

◆ A family member works in an old, possibly contaminated building.

by leaded gasoline, deteriorating exterior paint or, possibly, industrial sources of lead.

Assessing the danger. In the United States, the federal government requires that certified contractors assess the hazards of lead in private homes. However, you may want to perform a general screening assessment to help gauge the risk of lead contamination in a patient's home.

Your decision to screen for lead will be based primarily on the presence of observable risk factors for lead contamination. (See *When to screen for lead contamination*.) For example, the risk of lead contamination is greater in homes painted before 1978 (when lead-based residential paints were banned in the United States), and not upgraded since then. It's greatest in homes painted before 1950, when paint contained even higher levels of lead.

It's especially important to assess lead levels if a pregnant woman or small children live in an older home. The pregnant woman is at risk for two reasons: First, lead endangers the growing fetus and, second, chelation treatments used to remove lead from the body can damage the fetus.

Try to find out whether children (or adults) in the home tend to eat nonfood items. This condition, called pica, could raise the risk of lead ingestion. Also try to find out if any family members have high-risk occupations. For example, a family member who works in remodeling older buildings may inadvertently bring home enough lead-contaminated dust to harm a small child.

Cleaning up. If your screening assessment leads you to suspect that your patient and his family may be exposed to lead, contact your local health department and request a complete assessment. Health department officials can help homeowners figure out how to safely remove lead-based paints from their home, and they can help residents of rental properties convince landlords to follow recommended maintenance practices.

These maintenance practices include safely removing lead-based paints, taking precautions to prevent the spread of lead-laden dust, and performing specialized cleaning once the paint has been removed. Although you can't take charge of renovating a patient's home, you can remind patients of the hazards of confirmed lead contamination and help convince them to take action.

Asbestos exposure

When you examine a patient's home for hazards, make note of any insulation materials that look crusted, old, and friable. They might contain asbestos, another toxic chemical that can directly affect your patients' and their families' health. At one time, asbestos was considered an ideal building material. Consequently, builders used it in many ways in many areas of the home, including in wall and floor tiles, ceilings, and trim, in addition to using it as insulation.

Now we know, however, that even short-term exposure to asbestos dust can raise a person's risk of lung disease and cancer. The risk is greatest in older buildings, where asbestos-containing materials may deteriorate and shed asbestos-filled dust. In the closed environment of a home, levels of free asbestos can become dangerously high. Even asbestos removal, if done improperly, can raise asbestos levels in the home.

If you care for a patient who lives in a home that's more than 10 years old and you see disintegrating insulation materials that you suspect could contain asbestos, contact the local public utility company.

Insects and rodents

While assessing your patient's home, watch for obvious signs of insect or rodent infestation. You may actually see insects, usually roaches, in a patient's home. To detect rodents, look for droppings or holes in the house's structure.

The reason it's important to assess for insects and rodents in your patients' homes is that they can spread disease. Roaches have been linked to asthmatic conditions, and other insects, such as fleas, ticks, mites, and lice, may increase disease transmission as well. Rodents have been linked to leptospirosis and *Hantavirus* through their urine and feces.

If you know or suspect that a patient's home is infested with insects or rodents, do what you can to help the patient remove them. Provide treatment, as ordered, for conditions resulting from their presence. Until they're exterminated, carry as little as possible into the home with you, place your bag in a clean area, and inspect it discreetly but carefully for insects before you leave. Remember that your equipment and supply bag could carry insects or insect eggs to another patient's home or to your own home.

Ensuring home safety

Clearly, home safety is a wide-ranging topic that deserves your serious and continued attention. However, your patients must work with you to ensure the safety of their homes when you aren't there.

In addition to the teaching you and your team members provide about home safety, suggest that patients or their families write to the U.S. Consumer Product Safety Commission, Washington, D.C. 20207, to obtain a home safety checklist called *Safety for Older Consumers*. Although it's directed at older people, the checklist applies to any home. It's an easy-to-use, illustrated booklet that allows the homeowner to systematically check all areas of the home for hazards. Nurses can obtain copies of this publication to photocopy and distribute to patients by calling (800) 638-2772, extension 300.

◆ USING EQUIPMENT SAFELY

As you know, hospital-based nurses have only limited responsibility for medical equipment used in the facility. If a piece of equipment malfunctions, the nurse simply takes it out of service and finds a replacement that works. Hospital staff members rely on trained technicians to inspect and maintain the equipment, and they assume that if a piece of equipment doesn't meet rigorous safety requirements, it isn't placed on the floor for use.

The home setting is a different world— one that presents many challenges and inconsistencies. The equipment in the home varies widely in age and condition. Nevertheless, it's your responsibility to make sure each patient's medical equipment is safe and works properly.

In fact, if your agency supplies medical devices (apnea monitors, ventilators, infusion pumps, and so on) to your patients, the agency has a legal responsibility to track information about those devices and the patients who receive them. If you encounter a problem with an agency-supplied device, it's your responsibility to report the problem to the appropriate person in your agency, especially if the device causes a serious injury. Follow your agency's reporting policy.

If one or more vendors supply medical equipment to your patients through your agency, your administrators probably have a series of specific criteria that those vendors must meet. Typically, the criteria include performance history, quality control, liability coverage, routine maintenance, and employee training.

Assessing equipment

No matter who supplies your patients' medical equipment, you'll face many challenges in making sure it's safe and effective. For example, many homes have outdated wiring and an unreliable power supply. Also, many patients are forced to rely on antiquated or used equipment that was given or loaned to them. Finally, unlike what happens in a more controlled environment, the patient and family members must operate home-based equipment when you and your team members aren't there.

When evaluating a medical device in the home, consider its safety and its appropriateness for its intended use. Observe the device's general appearance. It should be reasonably clean and be placed in a clear, safe area. If it has a flat top, it shouldn't be used as a utility table or a resting place for food or drinks.

Check the electrical connection to be sure it's in good condition. Make sure the patient hasn't circumvented the grounding feature or forced the plug into an unsuitable socket. The wire shouldn't be frayed or worn, especially around the plug.

Once you're convinced that a piece of equipment is safe, make sure it works properly. Of course, you must be fully competent to use all the equipment your patients may need. In fact, your agency probably has a system in place to evaluate your ability to operate various types of medical equipment.

Teaching safe use

Many of your patients, especially elderly ones, may not completely understand why they need a certain piece of medical equipment. They may not know how to use it properly or the consequences of using it improperly. It's your job to teach them. (See *Equipment safety checklist.*)

Because you're not with a patient at all hours, you need to be confident that the patient or a caregiver can operate needed medical equipment accurately, Your instruction should be precise and complete, yet simple enough for a layperson to understand. Describe backup systems if a power failure could endanger the patient. Document that a patient or his family understood your instructions and gave you an accurate return demonstration.

Even if the patient or a family member knows how to use the medical equipment, your teaching still may not be complete. Check to see if different family members will be operating the equipment at different times, and be sure to teach everyone. Then repeatedly evaluate the patient's and family's ability to use the equipment properly.

Sometimes, a patient or caregiver will tell you that a hospital nurse or equipment supplier explained the equipment before discharge. However, you should still review the instructions and make sure that they can use the equipment properly.

Keep in mind that many types of medical equipment — ventilators, infusion pumps, apnea monitors, electrocardiogram monitors, dialysis machines, and others — are highly susceptible to electromagnetic interference. To prevent such interference, tell the patient and family members not to use pagers, cellular phones, cordless phones, microwave ovens, or radio transmitters around the medical equipment. Remember not to use your own phone or pager around the patient as well.

In addition, even mechanical devices can interfere with medical equipment. Urge patients and their families to call the equipment supplier if they think something is hindering or altering its function.

In all cases, someone should be available 24 hours a day to help patients who have equipment problems. Plus, a backup device should be readily available in case the primary equipment fails. Be sure to review the backup plan periodically with the patient or family. Before you complete your visits, make sure the patient and family know how to contact the supplier, how to ensure reimbursement once the nursing visits stop, and who will take responsibility for the long-term operation of the equipment.

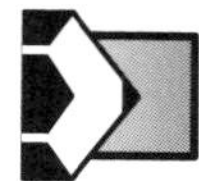

TEACHING POINTS

Equipment safety checklist

Be sure to cover these issues when teaching a patient how to use equipment safely:

- operating instructions
- required maintenance or cleaning
- how to troubleshoot simple problems
- what to do if the equipment isn't working properly
- signs and symptoms that could suggest the equipment isn't accomplishing its therapeutic goal (such as circumoral cyanosis in a patient on oxygen).

Oxygen instructions

One of the most common types of medical equipment used in the home, oxygen delivery is also one of the most hazardous. Therefore, give patients and their families very careful instructions for using oxygen in the home.

Oxygen delivery systems present two possible sets of problems: those related to the equipment and those related to the amount of oxygen the patient receives. (See *Recognizing the risks of oxygen,* page 94.) You'll want to address both potential hazards in your teaching.

Equipment warnings

These days, many patients on home oxygen use a liquid system or a con-

Recognizing the risks of oxygen

Equipment risks	Medication risks
◆ If the tank punctures or a valve breaks off, it could become a projectile. ◆ Using oxygen near an open flame increases the risk of combustion. ◆ If oxygen and oil mingle, an explosion could occur.	◆ Too little oxygen can result in pale or blue-tinged skin, breathing difficulty, restlessness, and decreased mental status. ◆ Too much oxygen reduces respiratory drive in patients with chronic respiratory disease.

centrator as their main method of delivery. However even these patients should have a traditional oxygen tank as a backup in case the power fails or the patient wants to go outdoors. Consequently, all oxygen-dependent patients need warnings and instructions about using oxygen safely.

After showing the patient and family how to operate the liquid system or concentrator, emphasize that they'll need to know how to switch to a traditional oxygen tank as well. Show them how to make the switch and return to the main delivery system.

Stress to the patient and family that the gas in an oxygen tank is stored at extremely high pressures. Tell them that if the tank is punctured or the valve breaks off, the pressure exiting the tank would be strong enough to turn the tank into a missile. Consequently, oxygen tanks should be stored upright and in a safe place where they can't be knocked over.

The small tanks typically found in home use usually come in a carrier equipped with wheels so the patient can walk with the tank. If the patient must be moved in a wheelchair or stretcher, make sure it has a device especially intended to hold the oxygen cylinder. Never place an oxygen cylinder in the patient's lap or between his legs.

Remember that oxygen cylinders must be hydrostatically pressure-tested every 5 to 10 years to make sure they can still withstand the gas pressure. The test date should be stamped on the cylinder. On the type of cylinder that can be tested every 10 years, a star will appear after the date stamp.

Fire and explosion warnings

Most people know that oxygen supports combustion. However, few know, in practical terms, what that means. Tell patients that oxygen will not start a fire but will feed a fire, raising the risk that a spark or cigarette will turn into a large blaze.

For that reason, urge patients and their families never to smoke around oxygen delivery equipment and never to use such equipment around an open flame. Oxygen can make a gas burner flare up, possibly setting afire nearby curtains, towels, or clothing. It can also cause a smoldering cigarette to flare up, possibly causing a devastating burn of the respiratory tract. Remind patients that oxygen will saturate their clothing, towels, and sheets, increasing the risk that a nearby fire could turn disastrous.

Although oxygen tanks won't spontaneously explode, as many patients fear they will, a pressurized oxygen tank could explode if it comes in contact with oil. Consequently, never lubricate an oxygen gauge with a petroleum-based product, and never use petroleum-based adhesive tape to label an oxygen cylinder. Be sure to give patients these warnings as well.

Medication warnings

In addition to warnings about the hazards of oxygen delivery equipment, you'll also need to assess for medication hazards, which arise when the patient receives either too much or too little oxygen.

As you know, signs of adequate oxygenation include pink skin, easy breathing, and unchanged mental status and activity level. If the patient is receiving too little oxygen, you'll begin to notice declining skin color, circumoral cyanosis, difficulty breathing, restlessness, and diminished mental status.

If you detect these signs, check the nasal prongs for patency. Dried secretions commonly block one or both prongs of the cannula. Keep an extra nasal cannula readily available in case you can't clear a blocked prong. Next, check all connections to make sure they aren't leaking, and make sure the flow meter is set at the correct level. If the patient uses an oxygen tank, check the remaining pressure. If the patient uses a liquid system, check the scale at the bottom of the tank. Finally, if the patient uses an oxygen concentrator, make sure the air filter is being washed according to the schedule recommended by the manufacturer.

If you're confident that the patient is receiving the prescribed amount of oxygen but he still shows signs of hypoxia, report the problem to his doctor. If he is in distress, you may need to seek emergency care.

The danger of receiving too much oxygen is highest among patients who have chronic respiratory disease because a chronically high level of carbon dioxide could gradually shift the patient's respiratory drive. Rather than using a high carbon dioxide level as a stimulus to breathe, the patient's body uses a low oxygen level — called a hypoxic drive — as a stimulus to breathe. Therefore, if you give the patient oxygen at too high a flow rate, you could actually diminish his drive to breathe. Usually, such a patient will receive oxygen at a low flow rate to help preserve his hypoxic drive to breathe.

◆ PREVENTING INFECTION

Infection control procedures are common practice for nurses and other health care professionals. However, they may not be such common practice among patients and families in the home care setting. That's why it's important to review your own practices and to teach patients and families what they need to know to avoid disease transmission both inside and outside their home. (See *Elements of infection control,* page 96.)

Obviously, teaching sound infection control techniques to your patients and their families has great potential to promote health and prevent disease for patients, household members, and even the general public. Give patients and their families general instructions for maintaining hygiene and taking precautions against the spread of disease-causing organisms. Also offer specific instructions if the patient or a family member has a particular infectious condition, especially AIDS. (See *Infection control checklist,* page 97.)

Elements of infection control

To help protect yourself from infection and reduce the risk of transmitting infection to patients and their families, be sure to follow standard precautions, as outlined by the Centers for Disease Control and Prevention. Here are some principles to keep in mind:

◆ Wash your hands thoroughly before and after each home visit.
◆ Carry antimicrobial cleaning wipes or "waterless soap" with you in case you can't wash your hands.
◆ Handle all bodily substances as if they are infectious, regardless of the patient's diagnosis. Use barrier protections, such as gloves, gowns, face masks, and eye shields, as needed.
◆ Don't recap used needles unless you use a mechanical device to do so.
◆ Dispose of all sharps (disposable syringes, needles, scalpel blades, and so on) in a puncture-resistant container.
◆ If you need to perform cardiopulmonary resuscitation, use a mask with a one-way valve so you don't breathe the patient's expired air.
◆ If your patient may have active tuberculosis, wear a high-efficiency particulate air respirator, called a HEPA mask.
◆ Keep your vaccinations current, including those for hepatitis B, tetanus, and possibly influenza.
◆ At the end of your work day, remove your clothes as soon as you get home and store them in a safe, contained area until you can wash them.

Primarily in response to fears over acquired immunodeficiency syndrome (AIDS), the Centers for Disease Control and Prevention (CDC) created two sets of guidelines for preventing transmission of infectious diseases: universal precautions and body substance isolation. Both sets of guidelines specified procedures for handling different bodily fluids and using and disposing of medical equipment as well as appropriate types of barrier protection.

In 1996, the CDC established a new set of guidelines called *standard precautions*. These guidelines synthesize the major features of universal precautions and body substance isolation into a set of precautions to be used for all patients, regardless of their infection status. These precautions apply to:

◆ blood
◆ all bodily fluids, secretions, and excretions (except sweat), regardless of whether or not they contain visible blood
◆ broken skin
◆ mucous membranes.

Your agency will provide you with appropriate barriers to protect yourself from these substances. However, you'll be responsible for determining the extent to which barriers are necessary in the home as well as the extent to which family members should use these protective devices.

Gloves are the most common means of barrier protection. If a patient or family member asks you why you're wearing gloves in their home, care-

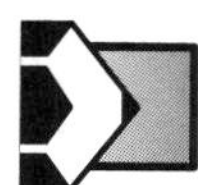

TEACHING POINTS

Infection control checklist

When teaching infection control to patients and their families, especially to someone who has acquired immunodeficiency syndrome (AIDS), be sure to include these instructions:

◆ Keep yourself and your home clean.

◆ Keep your home well ventilated to reduce the risk of airborne disease.

◆ Follow food preparation and handling guidelines scrupulously.

◆ Don't eat unpasteurized milk products.

◆ Wash all dishes in hot, soapy water. You don't need to separate dishes used by a sick person.

◆ If you have a cat or a bird and you have AIDS, are immunocompromised, or are pregnant, ask someone else to clean the litter box or cage. If you must clean it yourself, wear gloves and a mask. Don't clean fish tanks.

◆ Avoid unsafe sex.

◆ Use only your own toothbrush and razor.

◆ Flush all personal wastes down the toilet.

◆ Avoid recreational drugs because they may impair your general health and increase your susceptibility to infection.

◆ Eat a healthy diet.

◆ Get a good balance of sleep, fresh air, exercise, and rest.

◆ If you bathe a sick person or help with personal care, wear gloves.

◆ Clean the bathroom floor, sink, tub, and toilet bowl with bleach solution. Keep mops and rags used in the bathroom separate from those used in the kitchen.

◆ Wear disposable or heavy-duty reusable gloves for cleaning and disinfection procedures.

◆ To clean up spilled blood or bodily fluids, cover the spill with paper towels, pour a 1:10 solution of bleach and water on the towels, and let them sit for 10 minutes. Then wrap the soiled paper towels in newspaper, put them in a plastic bag, and tie it securely. Put this bag in another bag, tie it securely, and put it in the trash.

◆ To clean soiled linens and clothing, wash them by themselves in a 1:10 bleach solution for 30 minutes in the hottest water available. Use your home washing machine, not a public machine.

◆ You can dispose of used needles and syringes in a rigid plastic detergent bottle with a screwtop. When the bottle is full, add enough 1:10 bleach solution to cover the needles. When you've filled the container, cap it, seal the cap in place with tape, and put the bottle in a heavy-duty trash bag for disposal. Do not place the bottle in with other recycled plastics.

fully and politely explain that you must wear gloves with all patients to maintain everyone's safety.

Be careful where and how you discard used gloves. If they're contaminated with blood, treat them as hazardous waste and dispose of them accordingly. If they seem to be clean or they're contaminated with another bodily fluid, you can discard them in a leakproof container (such as a sealed plastic bag) and dispose of them in the household trash. However, if you have any fears that children could remove the gloves from the trash, you'll need to discard them in a safer place. Remember that gloves are not only a mode of disease transmission, but also a choking hazard.

Your agency will also provide you with moisture-proof disposable gowns. If you think you could be splashed by blood or other bodily fluids, wear a gown to keep your clothing from being contaminated. You'll also want to wear one when caring for a heavily draining wound.

In addition to a gown, you'll also want to wear a disposable face mask or safety glasses with side shields if you think you could be splashed by bodily fluids. If you wear glasses already, consider obtaining clip-on side shields. If you wear safety glasses, don't throw them away after use. Instead, wash and dry them for reuse.

If your patient has a disease that can be transmitted by air, such as tuberculosis, wear a high-efficiency particulate air respirator, called a HEPA mask.

◆ DEALING WITH RESTRAINTS

In the past, most health care professionals thought of restraints as a regrettable necessity. Then nurse researchers and others began to discover that restraints commonly failed to meet their stated goal of keeping patients safe. In many cases, all they produced was agitation in the patient and dismay for the family.

Once it became clear that restraints typically weren't helpful, many health care facilities began to reduce or outlaw their use. Legislation enacted in the United States in 1987 formalized and encouraged the trend. Today, restraints are rarely used in professional settings, and then, only the least restrictive devices.

You may find the situation quite different in patients' homes, however. In fact, it's not unusual for families to improvise restraints out of belts, sheets, and clothing. In many cases, health care providers don't even know it's happening. But with careful review and a little imagination, you can probably help reduce the use of restraints in your patients' homes while still keeping your patients safe.

Families use restraints in the home for basically the same reasons nurses once did. They want to prevent falls and wandering and keep patients from sliding out of chairs, pulling at tubes, or harming themselves or others. What they don't know is that they can achieve those goals using more effective and more dignified methods.

Falls

Clearly, falling can cause serious injuries in an elderly or frail patient. However, impress on your patient's family that restraints do little to prevent falls. In fact, because the restrained person works so hard to get out of the restraint, these devices may actually raise the risk of falls or injuries. Some health care professionals believe that injury is even more likely to occur if a restrained person falls, as opposed to an unrestrained person. Plus, routine restraint will lead to deconditioning, in which the patient loses muscular padding over the bones, the ability to keep his balance, and the sense of being able to protect himself from falling.

Rather than restraining an unstable or elderly person, try other tactics. For example, begin gait training. Order supervised walking each day. Instruct caregivers in exercises that can improve the patient's general strength and conditioning. Make sure the patient has an appropriate walking aid. If the patient has osteoporosis or another risk factor for bone fractures, suggest wearing special undergarments into which you can slide protective pads to protect the hips. If the patient does fall, despite these efforts, you or the family will need to respond appropriately. (See *Responding to a fall,* page 100.)

Wandering

If the patient tends to wander, acknowledge to the family that this is a difficult problem, but stress that restraints aren't a good solution. Usually, a patient who wanders is strong and steady on his feet. Restraining him may only increase his frustration and his desire to accomplish a goal he may not be able to explain.

In most cases, a family caregiver won't be able to stay with the patient constantly. Many caregivers try to solve the wandering problem by locking the person in a room or yard. If they're forced to do this, remind them to check on the patient frequently. Also urge them to try to spend as much time with the patient as possible. Tell them to make sure the patient's name and address are on his clothing in case he gets lost.

Another option for some families may be a day care center for the elderly. These facilities perform a great service in providing relief to caregivers as well as socialization, activity, and safety for patients. Also find out if the patient's community has a program to alert police to the patient's medical problem. Alerting police ahead of time enables them to be on the lookout for the person during their patrol. This support can give the family a feeling of greater security.

Sitting posture

If your elderly patient has poor sitting posture, you may arrive at his home to find him restrained by a sheet tied around his waist or shoulders. The problem with this type of restraint is that it restricts respiratory effort. Instead, try having the patient sit on a wedge pillow that's higher in the front than the back. This simple adjustment may solve the problem.

If the patient spends long periods sitting in a wheelchair, explain to him and his family that wheelchair seats were designed for temporary use during transport. For long periods of sitting, he'll need a protective pillow of some kind. Also, if the patient has hemiplegia or a neurologic disorder that causes him to lean to one side, try inserting a small armrest pillow on his weak side. If these simple measures don't solve the problem of sitting posture, consider referring the patient to an occupational therapist for other options.

Self-harm

Patients may wittingly or unwittingly try to harm themselves in many ways. For example, confused patients commonly pull at tubes and drains. Rather than causing the patient increased distress and an increased risk of falling by restraining his hands, try to find another solution. For example, try covering an abdominal tube's exit site with loose clothing or a light, loose abdominal binder. Then be sure to check the skin at the exit site several times each day.

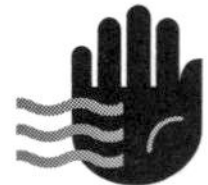

EMERGENCY INTERVENTIONS

Responding to a fall

Imagine that you enter a patient's home for a routine visit and find that the patient has fallen to the floor. What should you do? Here are some guidelines to follow when responding to this potential emergency:

◆ Don't let the patient move, or be moved, unless you must do so to deliver lifesaving treatment or remove him from harm's way.
◆ Call 911 or the local emergency number posted by the patient's phone.
◆ Put on disposable gloves.
◆ Form a quick general impression by looking at the patient's position. Does it suggest injury or pain? Is the patient having trouble breathing? Listen for moaning, snoring, or gurgling sounds. Assess for any unexpected odors in the room, such as chemical or gas fumes, urine, feces, vomitus, or decay.
◆ Check the patient's mental status and level of responsiveness. Use the letters *AVPU* to describe the patient's condition: Alert, responsive to Voice, responsive to Pain, or Unresponsive. Remember that a patient can be disoriented to person, place, or time and still be considered alert.
◆ Assess airway, breathing, and circulation (ABCs) even if the patient isn't in respiratory or cardiac arrest.
◆ You'll know the airway is open if the patient can talk clearly or is crying loudly. It may be obstructed if the patient isn't alert, is supine, or is breathing noisily. If so, open the airway with a jaw-thrust, head-tilt, or chin-lift maneuver. If you find an obstruction, relieve it according to basic life support training.
◆ Look, listen, and feel for breaths. If you detect no breathing, proceed with cardiopulmonary resuscitation (CPR).
◆ Take a carotid pulse for an adult or child, a brachial pulse for an infant. If you find no pulse, proceed with CPR. If you find a pulse, evaluate its rate and the color, temperature, and moisture level of the patient's skin.
◆ If the patient is bleeding, take steps to control it.
◆ Take the patient's blood pressure.
◆ Wait with the patient for the ambulance to arrive.
◆ Reassess the patient's ABCs every few minutes.

If the patient pulls at an I.V. line and seems to risk pulling it out, try rolling gauze lightly over the insertion site and partway up the patient's arm.

Finally, if a confused person is hostile and seems to be in danger of harming himself or others, you should take several actions. First, if this is a change in behavior, know that it may indicate a serious physical problem. Assess the patient for infection, drug toxicity, hypoxia, urine retention, constipation, and other areas of physical decompensation. Notify the patient's doctor and expect further medical evaluation.

If this behavior is chronic, and physical causes have been ruled out, you may want to request a consultation with a geriatrician or a geropsychiatrist. Medication may help the patient to control his behavior.

◆ ARRANGING SAFE TRANSPORT

A homebound patient may need transport to a health care facility for many reasons, ranging from routine doctor and therapy visits to emergency care. Whether that transportation is a car, a taxi, or an ambulance, certain preparations must be made.

Unless you're facing an emergency, allow the patient to choose a service provider. Often, a hospital social worker will give a patient this information before discharge. Just make sure the transportation chosen — paratransit van, taxi, or private car — suits the patient's physical and mental condition. In some communities, ambulance companies will provide a limited number of free nonemergency transports for contributing members. Some insurance carriers reimburse for ambulance transports; have your patient or his caregiver check with the patient's insurance company.

Before the patient leaves the house, make sure he's adequately prepared. (See *What to take during transport*.) The patient and his family should know when the vehicle will arrive at the home; remind them that it may be much earlier than the appointment time. The driver should know exactly where the patient is going and when he needs to be there.

If the patient has had to fast before the appointment, suggest that he take a snack with him to eat after the appointment. It should be convenient and portable, such as peanut butter crackers or a sandwich and something to drink. This type of preparation is essential for a diabetic and for a frail patient because dehydration can lead to orthostatic hypotension, dizziness, and falls.

Suggest that the patient take with him all of his medications, or at least a complete and current list of medications, including nonprescription ones. Also, write the telephone number of the patient's pharmacy on the list, in case the doctor prescribes a new medication.

If indicated, make sure the patient takes a written list of questions he wants to ask the doctor. Also send along a brief summary of the patient's current vital signs and significant findings. You may want to send a doctor's order form with the patient as well, so the doctor can add any new instructions or medications to the patient's record.

Remind the patient's family to consider the weather when preparing the patient for transport. On hot days, they'll naturally dress the patient in cool clothes. However, the doctor's office most likely will be air condi-

What to take during transport

Make sure your patient has these items before transport:

- medication vials or a list of all medications (even nonprescription ones)
- pharmacy phone number
- snack, especially if the patient is diabetic or fasted before the appointment
- list of questions to ask the doctor
- sweater or coat.

tioned, so elderly or frail patients should probably carry a sweater.

For all health care appointments, recommend clothing that's easy to put on and take off. Sleeves should be loose so that blood pressure can be taken and blood can be drawn without disrobing. A two-piece outfit would allow examinations of the upper or lower body without completely disrobing.

If a trip to a health care facility is related to a dramatic change in the patient's condition, prepare the patient and the family for hospitalization. Explore child care and pet care options, if necessary.

◆ ACTIVATING E.M.S.

The emergency medical service (EMS) can be activated by you or by your patients. To help patients activate an emergency response in a timely manner, advise older people to post emergency numbers by the phone. Alternatively, program them into the phone so the patient doesn't have to dial so many numbers. If the patient has a visual impairment, recommend a large-dial telephone.

Make sure that at least one telephone is placed in a low position so the patient can reach it even if he can't stand. If the patient lives alone, suggest that he obtain a telephone alert system. These systems usually require the patient to wear a device around his neck. If he needs help and can't reach a phone, he can push a button on the device. System operators then call the patient to assess his condition. If he doesn't answer the phone, the system activates emergency aid. Urge the patient to ask his insurance company if any part of this service is reimbursable.

If your patient's condition changes dramatically, he has a serious accident, or you come upon an accident in the community, you'll need to activate the emergency response. Usually, that means calling 911. For parts of the United States not yet using 911, you'll need to determine the appropriate local number. (You should also remind the patient to post the number by the phone.)

Whether you call 911 or a local number, follow these important instructions. First, give a short, general description of the situation. Then give the most accurate street address you can or the closest cross streets. Don't use landmarks unless you're sure they can't be confused by the ambulance driver. Be especially careful with the address if you're using a cellular phone to call EMS. That's because the 911 system's caller location service may not work with a cellular phone. No matter what kind of phone you use, don't hang up until the ambulance arrives, in case the dispatcher needs more information.

Whether you're handling a life-threatening emergency or a routine home inspection, it's useful — necessary, perhaps — to remember that you may well be your patients' main source of safety. By taking this role seriously, you can help to keep your patients focused on maximizing the length and quality of their lives.

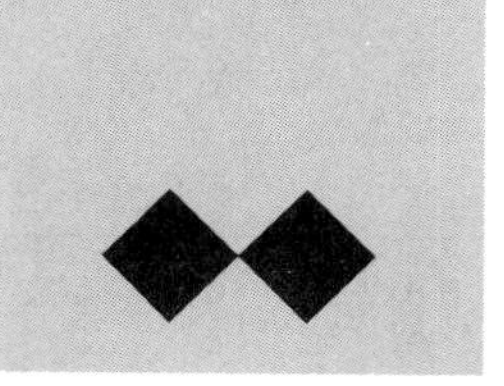

CHAPTER 5

Caring for patients with special needs

In your practice as a home health nurse, you'll meet and care for many patients with widely differing needs and challenges. You'll meet elderly patients struggling to cope with increased dependence and decreased functioning; pregnant patients anxious over the threat of preterm labor; children and parents frightened by the prospect of a chronic childhood illness; and patients battling mental disorders. Indeed, every patient you meet will have a unique combination of problems and needs.

This chapter outlines the basic principles of home care for patients in widely differing populations. By understanding the general needs of these groups, you'll be better able to provide compassionate, high-quality care to each individual.

◆ THE ELDERLY PATIENT

Working with elderly patients requires a special level of compassion and accommodation. As you know, elderly patients tend to tire easily. Their signs and symptoms tend not to mirror those of younger patients with similar problems. They tend to speak and react more slowly than younger patients, and they may tend to think of your visit as a social call as much as a professional health care visit. How you address these and similar issues can make all the difference in how well you succeed with your elderly patients.

Obtaining a history

Before you even begin the process of interviewing and examining an elderly patient, you'll need to quickly take stock of the patient's ability and willingness to cooperate with you. Is the patient short of breath? Hard of hearing? Does the patient seem fatigued or frail? Make sure you can differentiate normal physical changes of aging from abnormal ones that may require intervention even before you start the health history. (See *Recognizing age-related changes*, pages 104 and 105.)

Quickly assess the home environment as well. Is the patient's home in good repair? Do appliances, lamps, and other household devices seem to be functioning properly? Do you see any obvious safety hazards? Do you see accumulating trash, evidence of spoiled food, or other signs of impaired functioning?

Based on your initial intuitive observations, you'll know better how to approach your health history interview. In all cases, remember to prioritize your visit so you obtain the most pertinent and important information first. That way, if necessary, you can leave less important infor-

Recognizing age-related changes

As you examine an elderly patient, expect to see some or all of these age-related changes.

Skin, hair, and nails

◆ Pale, dry skin with wrinkles, decreased elasticity, and spotty pigmentation in sun-exposed areas
◆ More truncal fat, less on extremities
◆ Cool limbs and less perspiration
◆ Nails that grow at a slower rate
◆ Skin lesions, including skin tags; lentigines (liver spots) on face, arms, hands, legs; cherry angiomas; seborrheic keratosis; venous lakes on lips and exposed head areas
◆ Hair on scalp, pubic area, axillae, and limbs becoming grayer, dryer, thinner; possible hair loss in both sexes — in men, typically male-pattern baldness, decreased facial hair; in women, possibly hair growing on upper lip and chin

Eyes and ears

◆ Presbyopia (impairment in near vision with aging), cataracts, and arcus senilis
◆ Possible presbycusis (sensorineural hearing loss starting with high tones and progressing to all tones) and difficulty discriminating consonants during background noise
◆ Elongated earlobes

Nose and mouth

◆ Decreased sense of smell and inability to distinguish between scents
◆ Some erosion of tooth enamel and biting surfaces
◆ Decreased sense of taste, especially sweetness

Respiratory

◆ Slight increase in anterior-posterior thoracic diameter
◆ Initial bibasilar crackles in sedentary older person

Spine

◆ Decrease in height and possible kyphoscoliosis from thinning of intervertebral disks and narrowing of spaces

Cardiovascular

◆ S_4 heart sound
◆ Aortic systolic murmur
◆ Increased tendency to develop systolic hypertension and orthostatic hypotension

Gastrointestinal

◆ Increased abdominal fat and weakened abdominal muscles
◆ Increased risk of constipation, especially with decreased mobility
◆ In men, increased tendency for hernia from inguinal area into scrotum

Musculoskeletal and neurologic

◆ Decreased strength and muscle bulk
◆ Some stiffness and crepitus with joint movement
◆ Some decrease in range of motion, although still within a functional range
◆ Slower movement and longer reaction time

Recognizing age-related changes *(continued)*

Genitourinary
◆ In women (except those on estrogen replacement therapy), decreased size of labia and clitoris, narrowing and shortening of vagina, and pale, thin, dry vaginal mucosa
◆ In men, enlargement of the prostate gland

Immune
◆ Immune system begins losing ability to differentiate between self and nonself, resulting in increased incidence of autoimmune diseases
◆ Immune system loses ability to recognize and destroy mutant cells, accounting for increase in cancer among older people
◆ Decrease in leukocyte count
◆ Slightly reduced size of lymph nodes and spleen

Endocrine
◆ Diminished glucose tolerance and metabolism
◆ Cessation of menstrual activity and start of menopause

mation for your next visit. At each visit, always be sure to obtain any information required by your agency or the reimbursing organization.

Once you've determined that your patient can provide a reasonably accurate history, it's time to start. Keep these important interviewing techniques in mind as you go.

Interviewing techniques

Especially when it comes to interviewing elderly patients, the importance of your ability to use intelligent, appropriate interviewing techniques may be second only to your ability to interpret clinical information.

Try to determine whether the patient has a hearing or vision impairment. If he wears a hearing aid or glasses, make sure it's in use. Whenever possible, sit facing the patient. Eliminate background noise and speak slowly and clearly, in a low-pitched voice. Remember that a comfortable, secure patient will be more likely to relax, pay attention, and cooperate with you.

Frail, older patients usually are most alert and best able to concentrate in the morning rather than later in the day. If possible, visit early. As you begin to converse, watch the patient to ensure that he is following you and understands what you're asking. Then listen to make sure his answers are consistent with information you know to be true.

Does the patient converse logically? Do his explanations make sense? Is he willing to answer your questions fully? Try to determine whether the patient could have a cognitive problem or could be reluctant to disclose certain information. Many older patients are afraid to talk about illnesses and injuries for fear that they'll be forced to leave their homes.

If you feel that your patient has a cognitive impairment or a physical reason for being unable to answer your questions, you may want to consider having a family member join you to provide information that the patient can't. Explain to both of them why you're asking the family member to join the conversation. But be careful not to use this option unless you feel you must. Why? Because the patient may allow another person to answer questions for him, even if he's capable of doing so himself. Or he may become even more afraid to answer your questions truthfully.

Finally, realize that elderly patients have a lot more history to discuss than younger ones. Leave yourself as much time as possible to interview your older patients. Remember that you're forming a relationship in addition to gathering information. As much as possible, listen to your older patients' stories. You'll honor the people telling them and accomplish your home health goals as well.

The medical history

In gathering an older patient's medical history, start by talking about events leading up to the reason for your visit. Remember that the patient's perceptions of the illness and the events surrounding it are as important as the chronological facts of the illness. If the patient digresses, simply ask a focused question to help bring him back on track. In fact, to clarify details, focused or close-ended questions typically provide more specific information than open-ended questions.

Also ask the patient about previous health issues, such as hospitalizations, surgeries, accidents, injuries (including fractures), adult illnesses, and myocardial infarction and other possible precursors of common chronic illnesses (such as diabetes, hypertension, coronary artery disease, valvular heart disease, stroke, arthritis, chronic obstructive pulmonary disease, cancer, and depression).

In most cases, you won't need to spend much time on childhood illnesses and injuries unless they've had some effect on the patient's adult life (such as rheumatic fever or polio).

Current health status

Next, turn to the patient's current condition. Ask him how he'd describe his health. Remember that most older people evaluate their health by their functional abilities. If they can manage day-to-day activities and maintain their independence, they typically describe their health as good. For more specific information, ask close-ended questions pertinent to the patient's diagnosis.

Take time to investigate the patient's medications, both prescription and over-the-counter. In addition to asking the patient what medications he takes, inquire about vitamins, home remedies, laxatives, antacids, sleep aids, and so on. Many patients don't think of these as medications and may not report them unless specifically asked. You can also fill in the details of your patient's medication list by asking how he relieves any symptoms he describes as you go through your interview.

It may be easier for the patient and more helpful for you if the patient actually takes you to the medicine cabinet and the bedside table to look at his medicine containers. In addition to checking storage conditions and possible hoarding or swapping of medicines, you can also make sure the patient's medications are labeled properly and within their freshness dates.

After your medication review, investigate allergies. Ask about possible allergies to medications, foods, animals, or plants. Be sure to describe what you mean by an allergy; many older people think they're allergic to a substance if it gives them a headache or stomachache.

At this point in your interview, it may be helpful to fill in data designed to assess your patient's mental status. Don't try to assess mental status first because you'll only offend a competent older person by asking if he knows what day of the week it is or the city he lives in. Instead, work the mental status information smoothly into your interview a little later. Incorporate such factual information as the patient's address and phone number and the date. Combined with your earlier questions about the medical history, you'll now have a clear picture of the patient's long- and short-term memory, mental status, and reliability.

If at any time you begin to feel that your patient can't provide clear or accurate answers to your questions, consider postponing further questions until someone else can be present. You might also want to do a more extensive mental status assessment at a later time.

If you feel that your interview has been successful and the patient's information has been reliable thus far, continue by turning to the patient's lifestyle and health habits.

Lifestyle and habits

First, find out which adult immunizations the patient has had. Focus particularly on influenza, pneumococcal pneumonia, and tetanus vaccines. Try to determine the dates on which the patient had these vaccines.

Ask about tobacco use, past and present. Don't ask only about cigarettes. Instead, be sure to include the use of a pipe, cigars, chewing tobacco, or snuff. Find out about the frequency and number of years used in each case.

Now turn to alcohol and drug use. Resist the temptation to avoid this topic, because hidden alcoholism is a problem for many elderly people. Various assessment tools have been developed for evaluating alcohol abuse, including the Michigan Alcohol Screen Test (MAST). The MAST-G was developed to evaluate late-onset alcoholism in older adults. (See *Mast-G: Alcoholism screening test for older adults,* pages 108 and 109.)

Based on the answers you get to your screening questions, you may want to ask the patient when he last had a drink. If appropriate, inquire about blackouts, accidents, or injuries he has experienced while drinking and any influence drinking may have had on his work or family life. Also, search for more clues in the patient's home environment. For example, cigarette burns in the upholstery and poor housekeeping, combined with failure to respond to traditional treatments (such as Maalox for GI upset or Elavil for depression), may point to substance abuse.

When asking about drug use, be sure to include sleeping pills, "nerve pills," and pain killers, both prescribed and self-prescribed.

Next, question the patient about exercise, leisure activities, hobbies, and socialization. This topic provides a good lead-in to assessing activities of daily living (ADLs). Using a standard scale or one of your own creation, establish the patient's abilities and independence in walking, eating, grooming and personal hygiene, toileting, using the phone, preparing meals, shopping, banking, doing laundry, and maintaining the home.

Another approach is to ask the patient to describe a typical day from beginning to end and then integrate functional questions into this framework. Look for barriers to the patient's functioning throughout your history interview so you can follow up with possible solutions later.

Whichever method you use to assess your patient's functional abilities, be sure to include inquiries about

MAST-G: Alcoholism screening test for older adults

Use this tool, known as MAST-G, to help assess your older patient for possible alcohol abuse. Score each "yes" answer with one point; give each "no" answer a zero. Five or more "yes" responses indicate that the patient has an alcohol problem.

	YES (1)	**NO (0)**
1. After drinking, have you ever noticed an increase in your heart rate or beating in your chest?	✓	
2. When talking with others, do you ever underestimate how much you actually drink?		✓
3. Does alcohol make you sleepy so that you often fall asleep in your chair?	✓	
4. After a few drinks, have you sometimes not eaten or been able to skip a meal because you didn't feel hungry?		✓
5. Does having a few drinks help decrease your shakiness or tremors?	✓	
6. Does alcohol sometimes make it hard for you to remember parts of the day or night?		✓
7. Do you have rules for yourself that you won't drink before a certain time of the day?		✓
8. Have you lost interest in hobbies or activities you used to enjoy?		✓
9. When you wake up in the morning, do you ever have trouble remembering part of the night before?		✓
10. Does having a drink help you sleep?	✓	
11. Do you hide your alcohol bottles from family members?		✓
12. After a social gathering, have you ever felt embarrassed because you drank too much?		✓
13. Have you ever been concerned that drinking might be harmful to your health?	✓	
14. Do you like to end your evening with a nightcap?		✓
15. Did you find that your drinking increased after someone close to you died?	✓	
16. In general, would you prefer to have a few drinks at home rather than go out to social events?		✓
17. Are you drinking more now than in the past?		✓
18. Do you usually take a drink to relax or calm your nerves?	✓	

MAST-G: Alcoholism screening test for older adults
(continued)

	YES (1)	NO (0)
19. Do you drink to take your mind off your problems?		✓
20. Have you ever increased your drinking after experiencing a loss in your life?	✓	
21. Do you sometimes drive when you've had too much to drink?		✓
22. Has a doctor or a nurse ever said they were worried or concerned about your drinking?		✓
23. Have you ever made rules to manage your drinking?		✓
24. Does having a drink help when you feel lonely?	✓	

Adapted with permission from Beresford, T.P. "Alcoholism in the Elderly," *International Review of Psychiatry* 5:477-83, 1993.

the patient's relationships, including the availability and significance of other people in his life. If the patient needs help in accomplishing certain tasks, find out who provides it.

This line of questioning will help you establish an emergency contact and a person to include when providing demonstrations and patient teaching. It will also give you some idea of the patient's willingness to accept assistance from other people.

Inquiring about contacts with social service agencies or senior centers can also be helpful in assessing available assistance and the patient's willingness to accept it. Remember that even if help is available, the patient may not be willing to accept it.

Also remember to ask whether the patient has any pets, even if you don't see any during your visit. A pet can provide a vital connection for an elderly patient. It also can create practical problems and emotional turmoil if the patient has trouble providing appropriate care or must spend time away from home.

Other areas to explore in the health history include the role of religion in the patient's life and whether the patient has completed advance directives. Also inquire about the level of financial and health-insurance resources available.

Just before turning to the physical examination, perform a complete review of systems. (See *Assessment guide for the elderly patient,* pages 110 and 111.) This part of the interview provides very specific information that you may not have uncovered so far. Keep in mind that elderly patients tend to under-report their symptoms because they think dysfunction is an expected part of getting older.

Physical examination

The physical examination follows the review of systems. In fact, if you have a great deal of experience in interviewing and examining older patients,

Assessment guide for the elderly patient

Use this helpful guide to remember important assessment topics for elderly patients.

General topics
- ◆ Usual weight
- ◆ Gain or loss of 5 to 10 lb (11 to 22 kg) in the past 6 months
- ◆ Clothes that don't fit right
- ◆ Unusual tiredness or weakness
- ◆ Chills, night sweats

Skin
- ◆ Changes in hair or nails
- ◆ Rashes, bruising, color changes
- ◆ Itching, dryness
- ◆ Open sores, lumps

Head
- ◆ Headaches
- ◆ Head injury

Neck
- ◆ Pain or stiffness
- ◆ Swollen glands or lumps
- ◆ Thyroid nodules

Ears
- ◆ Hearing, hearing loss, use of hearing aid
- ◆ Tinnitus, vertigo
- ◆ Impacted earwax

Nose and sinuses
- ◆ Nasal congestion, discharge, itching
- ◆ Nosebleeds, polyps
- ◆ Frequent colds, seasonal or perennial rhinitis
- ◆ Sinus problems

Mouth and throat
- ◆ Presence, absence, and fit of dentures
- ◆ Condition of teeth and gums
- ◆ Bleeding gums, periodontal disease, caries
- ◆ Last dental examination
- ◆ Sore tongue, dry mouth, hoarseness

Chest
- ◆ Cough, wheezing or tightness
- ◆ Sputum, hemoptysis
- ◆ Pneumonia, pleurisy, tuberculosis, bronchitis, asthma, emphysema
- ◆ Last tuberculin test or chest film

Breasts
- ◆ Lumps, pain, discharge from nipples
- ◆ Last mammogram
- ◆ Breast self-examination

Cardiovascular
- ◆ Heart problems, heart murmur, rheumatic fever
- ◆ High blood pressure
- ◆ Chest pain, shortness of breath at rest, during activity, or at night
- ◆ Rapid or irregular heartbeat
- ◆ Swelling of the feet
- ◆ Electrocardiogram or other heart tests

Peripheral vascular
- ◆ Leg cramps at rest, with walking, or at night
- ◆ Swelling of legs or feet
- ◆ Blood clots, varicose veins

Assessment guide for the elderly patient *(continued)*

Gastrointestinal
- Difficulty swallowing
- Nausea, vomiting
- Heartburn, indigestion, reflux, appetite, abdominal pain
- Change in bowel habits
- Hemorrhoids
- Bloody or tarry stools
- Constipation, diarrhea
- Gallbladder or liver problems, such as jaundice, hepatitis

Genitourinary
- Frequency, urgency
- Dysuria, hematuria, polyuria, nocturia
- Incontinence, infections
- Kidney stones

Topics for men
- Hernias
- Penile lesions or discharge, sexually transmitted diseases
- Impotence, current sexual function, sexual preference
- Urinary dribbling, hesitancy

Topics for women
- Age at menopause, post-menopausal bleeding
- Last Papanicolaou test
- Discharge, itching, lumps, sores, sexually transmitted diseases
- Current sexual function, sexual preference

Musculoskeletal
- Joint pain, stiffness
- Arthritis, gout, back problems
- Joint replacement

Neurologic
- Tremors or shaking
- Tingling, numbness, loss of sensation
- Weakness, paralysis, fainting, blackout spells
- Seizures

Hematologic
- Anemia or iron deficiency
- Transfusions
- Bruising or bleeding

Endocrine
- Heat or cold intolerance
- Thyroid problems
- Diabetes

Psychiatric
- Depression
- Nervous problems
- Insomnia, nightmares
- Memory

you may be able to perform the review of systems and the physical examination at the same time. Either way, keep normal age-related changes in mind as you perform your examination.

Most nurses choose a head-to-toe assessment approach within a body-systems framework. If you'd rather use a different approach, do so, as long as you're sure you'll remember to gather all the information you need.

As with the health history, the patient's condition and the reason for your visit will influence both the extent and the approach of your examination. You'll also need to accommodate any specific physical or emotional conditions affecting the patient, such as pain, exhaustion, or limited mobility.

Remember that you already engaged one of the four major assessment techniques when you first entered your patient's home: observation. You've already begun to form impressions based on what you saw, including the patient's height, weight, posture, appearance, and mobility. These are part of the general survey.

If you have access to a scale and the patient can stand on it, obtain his weight. Likewise, try to document at least an estimated height. Even if your patient is bedbound, you can make marks at the head and the foot of the sheet, and then measure between them.

A thorough assessment of your older patient's skin is essential. Look for lesions, pressure sores, edema (presacral in the bedbound patient), and so on. To assess hydration, check skin turgor by gently pinching a fold of skin on the patient's anterior chest, near the clavicle. If it doesn't promptly return to its original flat position, the patient may be dehydrated.

Next, examine the patient's head, eyes, ears, nose, and throat. The patient should hold his head at midline, and his facial features should appear symmetrical. Verify symmetry (and cranial nerve function) by asking the patient to smile, frown, and show his teeth. Assess range of motion (ROM) in the neck and cervical spine by having the patient tilt his head forward and back, then side to side. Finally, have him rotate his head from shoulder to shoulder.

Assess the patient's functional vision by having him read the newspaper. Start with large headlines; then work down to smaller print. If he has corrective lenses, make sure he wears them during your assessment. If the patient holds the paper at arm's length to read it, you'll know that his presbyopia (impairment of near vision with aging) hasn't been adequately corrected.

Also assess the patient's eye health. If the sclera is yellow in a light-skinned person, he could have jaundice (in dark-skinned persons, a yellow tinge is normal). Check the pupillary reaction to light by shining a penlight oblique to the patient's eyes while he looks forward into the distance. Both pupils should constrict equally and at the same time.

If the patient has cataracts, you may be able to see a milky glow in the crystalline lens when you use the oblique light source. You may also observe arcus senilis, which is a light-colored arc around the outer edge of the iris that's normal with aging.

You can evaluate the patient's ability to hear in part by his response when you speak to him in a normal tone of voice. Then hold a watch to his ear and ask if he can hear it ticking. Or whisper a word near the patient's ear and ask what he heard you say. Even if your patient has impaired hearing, you may find that he can hear you quite well in his quiet home, especially if you make an effort to pitch your voice toward the low end of your comfortable range.

If you have an otoscope, assess the patient's ear canals and tympanic membranes. Be sure to check for impacted cerumen, which can affect your patient's ability to hear.

Next, assess the patient's nose and sense of smell. If you find that he has even a slightly impaired sense of smell, make sure that he has a functioning smoke detector in the home.

Assess the patient's mouth, teeth, and gums. If he wears dentures, inspect his mouth with and without them in place. Make sure they fit and that they haven't created lesions in his mouth. Ask the patient to open his mouth and say "Ahhh" so you can check 10th cranial nerve function. Also inspect the mucous membranes for moistness to evaluate hydration. Assess his ability to swallow by asking him to take a sip of water. As he swallows, watch his neck for abnormalities or obvious lumps in the thyroid area.

Next, inspect the chest and back. Assess for symmetry of contour and expansion. Observe the rate and rhythm of respirations. Remember that it's normal for an older person to have a slight increase in anterior-posterior diameter. Palpate for tactile fremitus while the patient says "99." Percuss for resonance on each side. Auscultate, comparing sides, and assess the spine for curvature.

If possible, take blood pressure measurements with the patient standing, sitting, and lying down to assess for orthostatic hypotension. Assess his resting heart rate and apical-radial rate for deficits.

As you would for a younger patient, palpate all pulses, including the brachial, radial, femoral, popliteal, dorsalis pedis, and posterior tibial. Auscultate the carotid arteries and abdominal aorta for bruits. Assess the patient for jugular venous distention, especially if he has a history of heart problems.

Perform an abdominal examination as you would for a younger patient. Keep in mind, however, that an older patient with an acute abdomen may not experience the pain, muscle guarding, and rebound tenderness typically seen in younger people.

Your examination of the musculoskeletal and neurologic systems can be somewhat integrated. In the elderly home care patient, focus on functional strength and motor ability to carry out ADLs. Usually, you'll only need to perform tests that evaluate grasp and resistive strength, ROM, balance, and position sense.

Assessing nutritional status

Another critical area of assessment for elderly patients is nutritional status. With aging comes a decrease in lean body mass and an increase in adipose tissue. Activity levels decline, which means that calorie needs decline as well. However, although the patient needs less food, he needs more quality foods.

Keep in mind that highly convenient foods tend not to be highly nutritious foods. So even if your patient looks overweight, you can't assume that he's adequately nourished. To assess your patient's nutritional status, start by asking what he ate over the previous 24 hours. Ask him if that day accurately represents his usual daily meal pattern and food intake.

You may also want the patient's caregiver to keep a daily journal of the patient's meal patterns and food intake to give you a longer assessment period to review. Comparing this information with the food pyramid as adapted for older persons will give you at least a crude nutritional assessment. (See *An older person's guide to food choices,* page 114.)

Other areas of interest include calcium and fiber intake. Many older people tolerate dairy products poorly and may need a calcium supplement, especially women. Good sources of fiber include dried beans, bran, whole grain products, dried or fresh fruits, and leafy green vegetables. Many elderly people tend to avoid these foods because they fear flatulence or diverticulosis, or they have trouble chewing. Try to determine and address these problems so you can ensure that your patient's dietary fiber intake is adequate.

Because of decreased thirst perception and loss of intracellular fluid with aging, your older patient is especially prone to dehydration. Unless it's medically contraindicated,

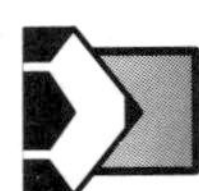

TEACHING POINTS

An older person's guide to food choices

Advise your older patient to use the guide below to help him eat more healthfully. Tell him to have at least the lowest number of suggested servings from each of these food groups every day. (The lower numbers are suggested for older women; the higher numbers are suggested for older men.)

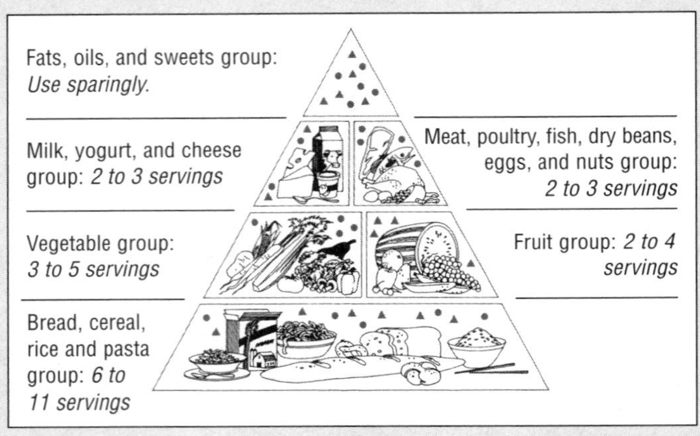

make sure your elderly patient maintains a fluid intake of at least 1⅓ qt (1.3 L) daily.

A more comprehensive nutrition screening tool specific to elderly people is available from the Nutrition Screening Initiative. You can ask the patient or a caregiver to complete the checklist, or you can fill it out yourself by asking the patient the questions shown on the form. (See *Determining nutritional health*.)

If your patient is at risk for nutritional deficiency, you may need to perform additional screening and initiate additional interventions, possibly in association with a community agency that serves elderly citizens, such as the Area Agency on Aging. In a screening of this depth, you'll need to include economic and social factors affecting the patient, as well as his functional abilities and disease states.

Once you've completed your nutritional assessment and identified your patient's risk factors, you can design a plan to address them, or you can consult with nutrition experts in the community for guidance. (See *Responding to your nutritional assessment*, page 116.)

Because elderly patients make up a large percentage of the home health population, it's important for you to understand the unique needs of this growing group. By doing so, you can help improve your patients' quality of life in addition to meeting their immediate health needs.

Determining nutritional health

The warning signs of poor nutritional health are often overlooked. Use this checklist to find out if your patient is at nutritional risk. Remember that warning signs suggest risk but do not represent diagnosis of any condition. Provide the following directions to the patient.

Read the statements below. Circle the number in the yes column for those that apply to you. For each yes answer, give yourself the score shown. Then total your nutritional score.

	YES
I have an illness or condition that made me change the kind or amount of food I eat.	2
I eat fewer than two meals per day.	3
I eat few fruits, vegetables, or milk products.	2
I have three or more drinks of beer, liquor, or wine almost every day.	2
I have tooth or mouth problems that make it hard for me to eat.	2
I don't always have enough money to buy the food I need.	4
I eat alone most of the time.	1
I take three or more different prescribed or over-the-counter drugs a day.	1
Without wanting to, I have lost or gained 10 lb (22.4 kg) in the last 6 months.	2
I am not always physically able to shop, cook, or feed myself.	2
TOTAL	6

IF YOUR NUTRITIONAL SCORE IS:

0 to 2 **Good!** Recheck your nutritional score in 6 months.

3 to 5 **You are at moderate nutritional risk.** See what you can do to improve your eating habits and lifestyle. Your office on aging, senior nutrition program, senior citizens center, or health department can help. Recheck your nutritional score in 3 months.

6 or more **You are at high nutritional risk.** Bring this checklist the next time you see your doctor, dietitian, or other qualified health or social services professional. Talk with them about any problems you may have. Ask for help to improve your nutritional health.

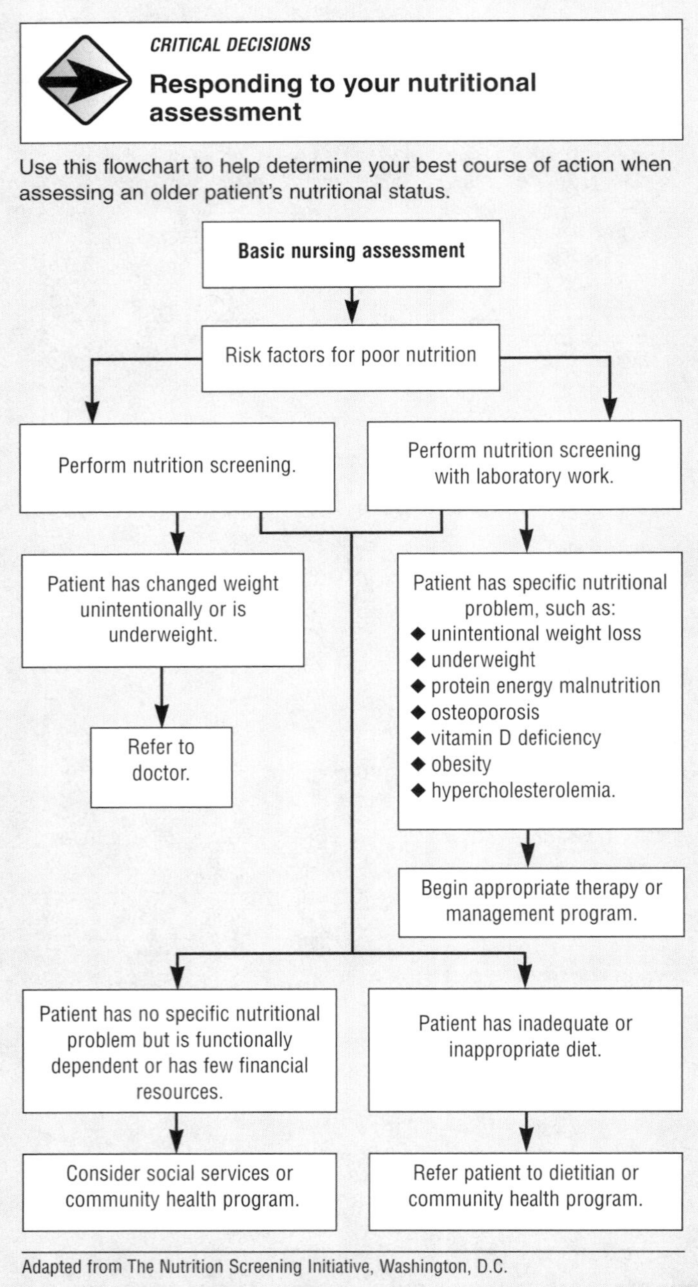

CRITICAL DECISIONS
Responding to your nutritional assessment
Use this flowchart to help determine your best course of action when assessing an older patient's nutritional status.
Basic nursing assessment
Risk factors for poor nutrition
Perform nutrition screening.
Perform nutrition screening with laboratory work.
Patient has changed weight unintentionally or is underweight.
Refer to doctor.
Patient has specific nutritional problem, such as:
◆ unintentional weight loss
◆ underweight
◆ protein energy malnutrition
◆ osteoporosis
◆ vitamin D deficiency
◆ obesity
◆ hypercholesterolemia.
Begin appropriate therapy or management program.
Patient has no specific nutritional problem but is functionally dependent or has few financial resources.
Patient has inadequate or inappropriate diet.
Consider social services or community health program.
Refer patient to dietitian or community health program.

Adapted from The Nutrition Screening Initiative, Washington, D.C.

◆ THE MATERNAL PATIENT

Caring for the maternal patient in her home allows you to accomplish more than you can in an acute care setting. For example, you can establish a more relaxed, casual relationship with your patient, which may encourage her to communicate more freely with you. You can take a more holistic approach in your assessment, one that includes both physical and psychological characteristics. You can respond more specifically to your patient's and her family's needs. Finally, you can incorporate your observations of the patient's home environment into your plan of care for her and her infant.

To care for maternal patients properly, you'll need superior physical assessment skills as well as well-honed skills in teaching patients how to recognize changes in their own bodies and what to do about them. Remember that you'll most likely be caring for low- and high-risk patients, both during and after pregnancy. You can be instrumental in helping your patients know how to recognize and respond to complications before they progress too far.

Prenatal assessment

During your initial prenatal visit and on a regular schedule thereafter, compile an overall health assessment for your patient and her pregnancy. Observe the patient in her environment. Assess the effect of family members and family responsibilities on her mental and physical health. In short, be sure to address the big picture of the pregnant patient's health in addition to performing a standard prenatal assessment.

Naturally, however, the standard prenatal assessment will provide core data for your care. Maternal and fetal assessment in the home setting includes weight, vital signs, uterine growth, urine evaluation, dietary intake, reflexes, physical activity, uterine activity, and fetal status.

Weight gain

In a general sense, the amount of weight gained by your pregnant patient relates to the amount of weight gained by the fetus. So maternal weight gain provides some indicator of fetal well-being in addition to giving you information about the patient's nutritional status.

Ideally, the patient should gain 25 to 30 lb (11 to 14 kg) during her pregnancy. In the second and third trimesters, she should gain about 8 oz to 1 lb (230 to 450 g) per week. Keep in mind that a sudden weight gain, especially during the third trimester, may suggest fluid retention, edema, and pregnancy-induced hypertension. Rapid weight loss may suggest hyperemesis gravidarum, hyperthyroidism, or an eating disorder. Any rapid weight change, especially late in the pregnancy, deserves further investigation.

When assessing your patient's nutritional status, emphasize that she should try to eat foods that contain adequate protein and calories. A good rule of thumb for pregnant patients is to recommend that they increase their daily intake by 300 calories and 10 g of protein.

Review your patient's diet carefully; talk about her food likes and dislikes, the impact of culture or family tradition on her diet, and any unusual dietary needs. Try to find out about her food shopping and preparation habits because they can give you insight into her dietary practices.

Blood pressure and deep tendon reflexes

Check your pregnant patient's blood pressure on a regular basis. Also check her deep tendon reflexes dur-

Measuring fundal height

To monitor fetal growth between weeks 18 and 32, use a flexible (not stretchable) tape measure to determine fundal height. First, with the patient supine, find the point on her abdomen where soft tissue ends and the firm, round fundal edge begins. Now find the notch of the patient's symphysis pubis, and measure between there and the top of the fundus. The length in centimeters approximates gestational age in weeks. After week 32, the measurement doesn't correlate quite as well.

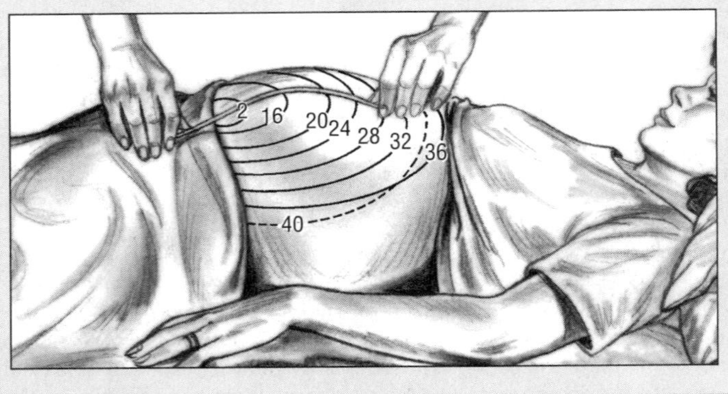

ing every home visit. These procedures are especially important if the patient is at risk for pregnancy-induced hypertension. As with all patients, grade your pregnant patient's reflexes on a scale from 0 (absent or no response) to 4+ (hyperactive or hyperreflexia). Assign a grade of 2+ for normal reflexes and 3+ for reflexes that react more briskly than normal.

Urine profile

Use a chemical reaction strip to evaluate your pregnant patient's urine for protein, glucose, and ketones. You can also use this test as a lead-in to teaching your patient about the complications this test can detect — pregnancy-induced hypertension and gestational diabetes.

Fetal growth and activity

In addition to assessing your patient's weight and diet, you'll also want to assess fetal growth directly through fundal height measurements. Common obstetric practice accepts that after 20 weeks' gestation, fundal height measurement (in centimeters) should coincide with weeks of gestation. (See *Measuring fundal height*.) If you find a discrepancy of more than 2 cm between weeks 20 and 36, arrange for additional investigation to rule out intrauterine growth retardation, macrosomia, or hydramnios.

Late in the pregnancy, from 28 weeks on, instruct your patient to pay attention to how much her fetus moves. Pregnant women are usually very aware of fetal movements. Simply ask your patient to keep track of about how many times the fetus moves each hour. If she reports less than three movements per hour, notify her doctor.

Uterine activity

Whether your patient has a high- or low-risk pregnancy, assess her uterine activity at every home visit. It's especially important to do so if your patient is at risk for preterm labor. Two methods for evaluating uterine activity include palpation and home uterine monitoring.

Mental health

The psychosocial assessment of a pregnant patient and her family is as important as the physical assessment. It should always include the following topics:

- lifestyle patterns, including ADLs, spiritual beliefs, possible substance abuse, and the need for social services, counseling, or financial support
- emotional status, including stress levels and coping patterns, the patient's goals and perceived resources, the family's roles and relationships, patterns of communication, and the adjustment to home care
- environmental conditions, including household safety, sanitation, basic housing needs, and access to a telephone and transportation.

Detecting common prenatal problems

Health problems that arise during pregnancy typically involve one of two categories: concerns that result from a preexisting health problem and concerns induced by the pregnancy. Prenatal patients usually follow treatment started in an acute care facility. Common prenatal health problems include preterm labor, pregnancy-induced hypertension, and diabetes.

Preterm labor

Most women who experience preterm labor receive treatment in an acute care facility. Once stabilized, they can go home for ongoing care. Your interaction with this patient will include health assessment on your part and self-care on the patient's part. You'll need to teach her how to care for herself properly to reduce the risk of preterm delivery.

Start by making sure she knows the signs and symptoms of preterm labor, including menstrual-like or abdominal cramps, a low backache, vaginal pressure, an increase or change in vaginal discharge, leaking of fluid, and uterine contractions.

Bed rest is the most widely used first-level intervention for managing preterm labor. The patient may require 10 to 20 weeks of inactivity to bring the pregnancy as close to term as possible. Begin by instructing your patient to limit her activities and to increase the amount of time she spends resting during the day. Tell her to avoid active sports, heavy housework, and lifting, including lifting children.

If her uterine activity doesn't abate, she'll need to increase the amount of time she spends resting during the day to 2 or 3 hours, possibly more. Also advise her to drink 8 to 10 glasses of nonalcoholic, decaffeinated beverages each day. Tell her to expect to urinate about every 2 hours.

Also tell the patient to avoid sexual arousal and nipple stimulation because this encourages release of oxytocin, which can increase the risk of preterm labor.

If your patient isn't on bed rest, tell her that she can attend childbirth classes if she participates only in the breathing exercises. If the patient is on bed rest, you'll be the one to provide the childbirth information she needs before delivery.

Collaborative preterm assessment

If your home health patient is at risk for preterm labor, you'll need to work together with her to minimize the risk and maintain an ongoing assessment. Here are some of the important steps for you and your patient to take.

- Monitor fetal heart rate.
- Review with the patient the signs and symptoms of preterm labor, including menstrual-like cramps, uterine tightening, an increase or change in vaginal discharge, pelvic pressure, and a low, dull backache.
- Monitor the patient's weight, blood pressure, and pulse as indicated.
- The patient should monitor her uterine contractions two to three times daily for 30 to 60 minutes each time.
- The patient should keep track of fetal movement by the hour.

Many patients at risk for preterm labor are treated with tocolytic medications in addition to bed rest. Once your patient has been stabilized on a parenteral tocolytic drug, she may be weaned to oral terbutaline or ritodrine before being discharged for home care. However, keep in mind that she may receive low-dose parenteral terbutaline at home.

The problem is that long-term maintenance with oral beta-mimetic drugs is associated with breakthrough uterine activity in up to half of the women treated. After prolonged and continuous high-dose therapy, the body's beta receptors become desensitized.

Instead, the doctor may order low-dose, subcutaneous terbutaline delivered continuously in a bimodal system to help prevent desensitivity from developing. This bimodal delivery combines a low-dose, continuous basal rate plus intermittent boluses. The low continuous infusion keeps the uterus relaxed and decreases irritability. The programmed boluses inhibit full uterine contractions and usually are planned to coincide with the woman's peak periods of uterine activity.

Whether your patient is on bed rest alone or bed rest combined with medications, she'll need much support and encouragement. In fact, she'll need to know how to actively cooperate with you in reducing her risk of a preterm birth. (See *Collaborative preterm assessment*.) She may require guidance and direction in planning for outside assistance and support to maintain her home, care for her family, and minimize the effects of boredom and social isolation. To help accomplish these goals, you'll need a sound working knowledge of community resources available to help your patient cope.

Keep in mind that a woman at risk for preterm labor may feel anxious and unprepared for her infant's birth. She'll undoubtedly be frightened about the possibility of a premature baby, and she may even be afraid to finalize her plans for the infant's birth. By helping your patient understand her part in preventing a preterm birth, and by providing appropriate physical and emotional care, you can help increase your patient's chance of making it to full term.

Pregnancy-induced hypertension

A number of factors typically must come into play before a patient with pregnancy-induced hypertension can be cared for at home. For example, the patient and her fetus should be stable, with no evidence of a worsening condition. In addition, she should meet these criteria:

◆ gestational age of more than 20 weeks
◆ blood pressure reading of less than 150/100 mm Hg in the sitting position or less than 140/90 mm Hg in the left lateral position
◆ proteinuria less than 100 mg/L (or less than 1 g/24 hours) evaluated by urine dipstick
◆ no headache, visual disturbances, or epigastric pain that could be related to preeclampsia
◆ no marked edema or clonus
◆ ability to use electronic blood-pressure gauge and urine dipsticks
◆ ability to assess fetal movements accurately.

If you're caring for a patient with pregnancy-induced hypertension, assess her basic knowledge and ability to comply with the treatment regimen. Familiarize her with the basic physiology of blood pressure and hypertension, along with their effects on both mother and fetus. Also teach her how to use blood pressure equipment, how to take her pulse, how to use urine dipsticks, and what warning signs to report to you or her doctor.

These warning signs include visual disturbances, persistent headache, increased swelling, pain in her upper abdomen, symptoms of labor, vaginal bleeding, a sudden gush of vaginal fluid, and severe abdominal pain. In addition to listing these worrisome symptoms, also instruct her how to monitor fetal movement. Tell her to rest in a lateral recumbent position. Finally, urge her to monitor her daily activity level.

Also instruct her to eat a balanced diet each day — one that contains 60 to 70 g of protein; 1,200 mg of calcium; adequate zinc, sodium (2 to 6 g), and magnesium; and at least 6 glasses of water.

In addition to following through on weekly doctor visits and daily to twice-weekly home visits, the patient should also measure and record:

◆ her blood pressure, two to four times daily in both the left lateral and sitting positions
◆ her weight, at about the same time each day
◆ the protein level of her first-voided urine (by dipstick, inserted midstream)
◆ number of fetal movements daily.

Give her clear instructions about what to do if these or other important criteria become abnormal.

Diabetes

The diabetic patient who needs home care is either a gestational diabetic or an existing diabetic whose condition complicates an otherwise normal pregnancy. Before being cared for in a home setting, she must have a stable health status, be able to monitor her blood glucose four to six times a day, and be willing and able to comply with the treatment plan and prescribed medications.

Many patients find it difficult to understand why it's so important to comply with the diabetes treatment plan. Consequently, one of your most important roles will be that of teacher. The goals for all pregnant diabetic patients are to maintain as normal a blood glucose level as possible, to ensure optimal fetal growth, and to avoid maternal or fetal complications.

Start by teaching your patient and her family about diabetes and its potential influence on the pregnancy and its outcome. Show the patient how to use a blood glucose meter, and explain how to interpret the results. Obtain a satisfactory return demonstration. Provide the patient with a schedule showing times when she should test her blood glucose.

If possible, have a nutritionist plan a diet for your patient based on her individual needs and calorie requirements. Then perform follow-up assessments to make sure she's following the diet and that it truly does meet her needs.

For a diabetic patient, prescribed activity levels may range from complete bed rest to complete freedom. Help your patient understand the importance of complying with her plan.

Make sure the patient understands the kinds of complications that can arise from hypoglycemia or hyperglycemia during pregnancy. Above all, emphasize that to help ensure a positive outcome for her pregnancy, she must maintain a balance between her diet, activity level, medications (if any), and blood glucose levels.

Postpartum assessment

Traditionally, the 6-week period following birth is referred to as the puerperium, or postpartum period. During this time, the new mother's body undergoes many physiologic changes that enable her to return to her nonpregnant status. In addition, this period probably will be a time of psychological and social adjustment to the birthing process and the new infant. This time marks the beginning of the child rearing phase of the family life cycle.

Most new mothers spend little time in an acute care setting after delivery. Consequently, most physical and psychosocial changes, and most family adjustment, will take place at home. Home nursing care of the patient and her family will provide you with valuable opportunities for assessment, intervention, and teaching. The concerns and needs of this new mother and her family usually center on the following:

- physiologic recovery and return to prepregnant status
- psychological concerns
- assistance with breast-feeding
- resumption of sexual activity and birth control
- newborn care
- parenting skills.

After an uncomplicated pregnancy and childbirth, the new mother's reproductive system requires a considerable amount of time to recuperate. However, some changes begin within just a few days after birth. If you're providing home care to a postpartum patient, you'll need to follow these changes and assess for potential problems.

The uterus

Just after expelling the placenta, the uterine fundus — now firmly contracted — assumes a position about midway between the umbilicus and the symphysis pubis. Palpating it at this point may feel like palpating a firm orange or grapefruit. (See *Palpating the fundus after delivery*.) By 12 hours after delivery, the fundus rises to the umbilicus or slightly above. Thereafter, it descends 1 to 2 cm (one fingerbreadth) per day. By day 10 after delivery, you should no longer be able to palpate the uterus in the patient's abdomen.

After delivery, the cervix is flabby and thin. It gradually contracts and, by day 7 after delivery, it's thick and nearly closed. Remember that the external os commonly sustains lacerations during delivery. If untreated, they may cause bright red, prolonged bleeding together with a firmly contracted uterus.

Lochia

During the first few days after delivery, the decidua (the spongy layer un-

Palpating the fundus after delivery

By assessing uterine involution after delivery, you can detect complications early and help ensure a normal postpartal recovery. To assess fundal position (with the patient supine), place your right hand at the symphysis pubis to help support the uterus; then palpate the fundus with your left hand (as shown in the illustration).

Document fundal height in centimeters from the umbilicus. For instance, if you palpate the fundus 1 cm below the umbilicus, you'd document it as U-1. While you're palpating, also be sure to assess whether the uterus feels firm or boggy.

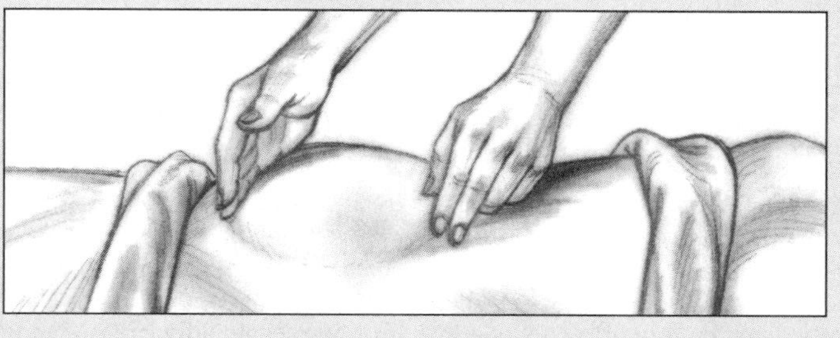

derlying the placenta during pregnancy) sloughs off and is discarded as a discharge called lochia. You'll need to evaluate your patient's lochia for color and content.

For the first 2 or 3 days, lochia contains primarily decidual tissue, epithelial cells, red blood cells, white blood cells, some meconium, vernix caseosa, and lanugo. It's called *lochia rubra* because it's red. Lochia smells similar to normal menstrual flow—it should not have a disagreeable or offensive odor. A foul lochial odor accompanied by fever suggests infection.

By about the 3rd day, the discharge turns into *lochia serosa*, a pale serosanguineous substance that contains decidua, red blood cells, white blood cells, bacteria, and cervical mucus. Lochia serosa may continue until the 10th day following delivery.

At that point, lochia serosa turns to *lochia alba*, a creamy yellow discharge that gradually ceases. It consists primarily of white blood cells, bacteria, some decidual cells, epithelial cells, fat, cervical mucus, and cholesterol. For most patients, lochia alba stops within about 4 weeks after delivery. If your patient's lochia lasts longer than that, consider obtaining further medical evaluation.

Return of ovulation and menstruation

For women who bottle-feed and therefore lactate minimally, ovulation resumes about 10 to 12 weeks after delivery and menstruation resumes about 6 months after delivery. For women who breast-feed and therefore lactate longer, the time may be longer. In general, postpartum amenorrhea in lactating women can range from 6 weeks to more than 2 years, depending on the length of time the woman lactates.

The perineum

Although "perineum" typically refers to the tissue between the vaginal introitus and the anus, your assessment of the perineum after childbirth should include the anus as well. To assess the perineum, place the woman in Sims' position: on her side with her top knee and thigh drawn up and her bottom arm extended along her back. In this position, also called semi-prone, the upper buttock is lifted to make the perineum visible.

Many women experience considerable discomfort from repaired perineal lacerations and episiotomies. They also are at risk for infection and structural alterations. So be sure to assess the perineal area carefully for redness, edema, ecchymosis, discharge, and poor approximation.

The 1st day after delivery, edema and redness are common. However, the edges of the patient's episiotomy or repaired lacerations should be intact. If the delivery caused significant trauma to the patient's perineum, you may see ecchymosis. You should see no discharge. If you do observe vaginal discharge, record its quality (serous, serosanguineous, bloody, or purulent) and quantity.

To promote comfort and reduce swelling, suggest that the patient apply ice to her perineum during the first 24 hours after delivery. Later, warm sitz baths may help promote comfort and increase circulation, which hastens healing. These same measures may also help reduce the discomfort of hemorrhoids, which commonly accompany a vaginal delivery.

Teach the postpartum patient to rinse and wipe her perineum from front to back each time she urinates or defecates to keep from contaminating her vagina and urinary meatus. Show her how to fill a plastic peribottle with warm water and use it as an efficient and soothing way to rinse her perineum clean.

Breasts and infant feeding

Start your evaluation of your patient's breasts by finding out whether the patient will bottle- or breast-feed. You'll also want to assess the mother's knowledge of lactation and ways to suppress lactation. Make sure she knows how to assess the success of her feeding methods.

Physically assess each breast. Note whether your patient is wearing any support. Both breast- and bottle-feeding mothers may be more comfortable wearing a supportive bra.

Breast-feeding. Most new mothers have misconceptions about infant feeding, especially breast-feeding. For example, the new mother may think that all infants are born knowing how to find the nipple and extract milk from it. Consequently, if her infant does not feed readily, she may believe either that the infant isn't hungry or that she's doing something wrong.

Take time to fully assess your patient's knowledge and beliefs about breast-feeding, her ability to nourish her infant adequately, her ability to help her infant grasp the nipple, and her understanding of her infant's hunger and satiety signals.

Remember that just after birth, the mother's breasts produce colostrum. Around the 3rd day postpartum, they begin to produce milk. This milk production will increase with stimulation of the suckling infant. For most women, increases in the vascular and lymphatic systems add to the engorgement around the breasts. They become larger, firmer, and tender or even painful to the touch. By putting

Assessing breast-feeding

When assessing your patient's ability to breast-feed her infant, be sure to include the following areas.

Assess the patient's nipples for:
- ◆ pliability
- ◆ inversion
- ◆ cracks
- ◆ abrasions
- ◆ tenderness
- ◆ pain.

Assess the patient's breasts for:
- ◆ engorgement
- ◆ plugged ducts
- ◆ tenderness
- ◆ pain.

Assess the patient's ability to hold her infant correctly for breast-feeding, including:
- ◆ assuming a comfortable position
- ◆ supporting the infant's head and body
- ◆ bringing the infant close
- ◆ supporting the breast with her other hand.

Assess the infant's ability to suck, including:
- ◆ closing the lips tightly around the areola
- ◆ moving the jaws up and down in a rhythmic pattern
- ◆ keeping the tongue under the nipple.

the infant to the breast frequently (every 2 to 3 hours), the woman will experience milder episodes of engorgement. (These changes also can be suppressed by lactation-suppressant medication administered in the immediate postpartum period.)

You can help your patient prevent or solve many of the problems associated with breast-feeding through planning, patience, and teaching. (See *Assessing breast-feeding*.) Teach your patient that both she and her infant should be positioned comfortably to promote feeding. Show her how to support her breast behind the areola, with all four fingers below and the thumb above. Teach her to direct the nipple into the center of the infant's mouth, with the infant's tongue beneath the nipple. Then the infant's tongue can travel front to back, pressing the nipple against the hard palate, squeezing milk from the breast sinuses.

Tell the new mother that a 2- to 4-hour self-demand schedule is the usual practice for most infants. Tell her to offer both breasts at each feeding, beginning first on the side used last during the previous feeding. Remind her that the infant typically will drain most of the milk in the first 5 to 20 minutes of sucking.

Many nursing mothers worry that the infant isn't interested enough in eating. Reassure the new mother that the infant may not be fully awake. Urge her to unwrap the infant and play with him. Suggest that she rub her fingertips along the infant's back to stimulate him.

To verify adequate nutrition, make sure the infant wets four to six diapers each day, sleeps fairly well, and gains weight at a steady rate. If you're concerned that the infant may not be getting adequate nutrition, advise the mother to put her infant to the breast more often, get more rest herself, and increase the amounts of fluid and protein in her diet.

After feeding, have the patient rinse her nipples with clear water. Tell her about shields that she can wear to protect her outer clothing from milk. Provide plenty of reassurance, encouragement, and patience to help her establish a successful breast-feeding routine.

Bottle-feeding. Mothers who choose to bottle-feed their infants also need reassurance, support, and information about various feeding techniques, formulas, and infant behaviors. As you would with breast-feeding, teach the new mother how to assume a position that supports her and her infant. Show her how to hold the infant close to her body in a semi-reclining position.

Demonstrate to the patient that she should tilt the bottle enough to fill the nipple, and then place the nipple well into the infant's mouth, on top of the tongue. As the infant sucks, tell her to note whether air bubbles rise in the bottle. If the infant seems restless or fussy while feeding, suggest that she remove the nipple from his mouth and burp him by holding him upright on her shoulder or in her lap while stroking or patting his back.

When caring for a family that has chosen bottle-feeding, be sure to assess the home and teach formula preparation techniques carefully. Specifically, make sure the home has an uncontaminated water source and reliable refrigeration. Also ensure that all caregivers will clean their hands and all equipment thoroughly. Remind all caregivers to discard any leftover formula rather than saving it for the next feeding.

Body systems

When caring for the postpartum patient, be sure to provide an ongoing, brief, body-system assessment to make sure the patient is returning, as expected, to her prepregnancy baseline.

Cardiovascular. The increased cardiac output induced by pregnancy begins to resolve shortly after delivery. In fact, the new mother may develop bradycardia for the first 6 to 10 days after delivery. Her pulse rate may go as low as 50 to 70 beats/minute — a normal finding in a postpartum patient. Her blood pressure should remain within the normal adult range.

If your postpartum patient has a very rapid pulse rate, keep in mind that it may suggest postpartum hemorrhage, anxiety, fatigue, infection, fever, or heart disease. If she has hypertension, it may be an extension of pregnancy-induced hypertension. If she has hypotension, it may suggest uterine blood loss.

The patient's total blood volume will return to its nonpregnant level within about 3 weeks postpartum. The clotting factors that increased during pregnancy tend to remain elevated during this period. Be sure to assess your patient's legs for signs of thrombophlebitis (Homans' sign).

Respiratory. The patient's respiratory rate and quality should remain in the normal range following delivery. If the patient had a cesarean section, however, she may experience abdominal pain when trying to breathe deeply or cough. Any postpartum woman who complains of dyspnea, regardless of her delivery method, should be assessed for pulmonary embolism.

Gastrointestinal. The postpartum woman requires adequate nutrition to recover physically and emotionally after childbirth. Make sure your patient's diet contains the appropriate amount of protein and vitamin C, two nutrients that promote healing. Most nonlactating women can obtain adequate vitamins and minerals from their typical diet.

In contrast, lactating women usually require about 500 to 1,000 additional calories each day to be able to supply the necessary milk and nutrients. Lactating women also need increased fluids: 2½ to 3 qt (2.5 to 3 L) each day to produce ample breast milk.

Whether your patient delivers vaginally or by cesarean section, she may experience sluggish bowels for several days following delivery as a result of the anesthesia, diminished muscle tone, poor fluid intake, or the fear of pain from an episiotomy or surgical excision. Urge your patient to eat plenty of fresh fruits and vegetables, plus four or five dried prunes each day, to help avoid constipation and resume a normal bowel pattern.

Urinary. If your patient gave birth in an acute care facility, she wasn't discharged until she could void unassisted. That's because many women have trouble resuming a normal urinary pattern because of perineal lacerations, hematomas, generalized swelling, bruising of the perineum, and a reduced sensation of bladder fullness. Expect the patient to void as much as 3,000 ml of urine per day for the first 3 to 5 days after delivery.

Mental health

In addition to caring for your postpartum patient's body, you'll need to attend to her mental status and that of her family. To assess mental status, observe family interactions, watch individuals carrying out their roles and responsibilities, and perform specific assessments as needed. (See *Postpartum psychosocial assessment*, page 128.)

When assessing a postpartum patient's mental status, keep in mind that she may be reluctant to talk about it. In fact, she may react as though she thinks your questions are intrusive and inappropriate. Tell her that many women have difficulty adjusting to the reality of an infant. Explain that many women experience mood swings and emotional lability, usually from the combination of sleep deprivation and dramatic hormonal changes. By doing so, you may help her become comfortable enough to tell you how she feels.

Usually, the "postpartum blues" last 2 or 3 weeks, and then they resolve on their own. They may include some tearfulness, feeling down, feeling guilty or inadequate, and feeling unable to cope with infant care. You can help your patient get through these feelings. If you observe more severe and long-lasting difficulties, however, notify the patient's doctor.

◆ THE NEONATAL PATIENT

Now more than ever, neonates — even high-risk neonates — may receive the bulk of their health care at home from a visiting nurse. But remember: Caring for a neonate at home involves much more than simply performing a physical assessment. It also requires counseling, support, and sometimes extensive teaching for the new mother, possibly the whole family.

Assessing the normal neonate

When you set out to care for a new infant at home, start by reviewing the infant's discharge plan. Acquaint yourself with the hospital course, discharge medications, and care instructions. See if you can estimate the parents' (or parent's) caregiving skills, confidence level, and need for teaching and support, even before you arrive for your visit.

Once you arrive at the home, of course, you'll have a much clearer picture of the needs of both infant

Postpartum psychosocial assessment

To assess the postpartum patient's psychosocial status and adaptation to the maternal role, explore her feelings by asking questions like the ones shown here. Remember to keep all questions open-ended. If a patient hesitates to answer any question, clarify and reword it; if she still seems resistant, go to the next question.

Daily activities

◆ How well are you managing your daily activities?
◆ How do you feel about your appetite and the amount of sleep you're getting?
◆ How would you rate your effectiveness in managing your responsibilities?

Impact of childbirth events

◆ What thoughts and feelings do you have when you look back at your childbirth experience?
◆ How do you think you handled the experience?
◆ What aspects of the experience stand out in your mind and why?

Mother-infant interaction

◆ How do you feel about yourself as a mother?
◆ How do you think your infant feels about you as a mother?
◆ What thoughts and feelings do you have when you are with your infant?
◆ What concerns do you have about your infant's health and safety? How do you handle these concerns?

Social activities and support

◆ What stage have you reached in resuming your social activities and responsibilities with other adults?
◆ How is your relationship with your infant's father?
◆ Since delivery, which social activities have you engaged in that were pleasurable? Which were not pleasurable?

Self-esteem

◆ How would you rate yourself right now in terms of goodness?
◆ How well do you feel you are adjusting?
◆ What thoughts and feelings have you had about your physical attractiveness since the delivery?
◆ What is your predominant mood these days?
◆ How do you view your future?

Adapted with permission from Affonso, D.D. "Assessment of Maternal Postpartum Adaption," *Public Health Nursing* 4(1):12, 1987.

and parents. At each home visit, be sure to assess the "big picture" of the infant's home and caregivers in addition to characteristics and needs specific to the infant.

For example, you'll want to assess the parents' ability to provide routine care (such as bathing, feeding, diapering, stimulation, and cord and circumcision care). You'll want to solicit information about the infant's

Assessment findings for the normal neonate

Axillary temperature
- 97.7° to 98.6° F (36.5° to 37° C)

Pulse
- 120 to 160 beats/minute
- Strong and regular

Respirations
- 30 to 50 breaths/minute
- Normal breath sounds
- No retractions or grunting
- Irregular rhythm

Skin
- Warm
- No jaundice or rashes
- Good turgor

Activity
- Extremities move normally
- Alert demeanor

Head
- Shape normalizing
- Symmetrical, with flat fontanels

Abdomen
- Bowel sounds present
- Soft, undistended

Umbilical cord
- Dry base
- Becoming atrophied
- No odor or redness

Circumcision
- No oozing
- Normal urine stream
- Healing as expected

Feeding
- Effective sucking and burping
- Appropriate volume consumed

Elimination
- 6 to 10 wet diapers daily
- Stools reflect feeding method in color, consistency, and number

feeding patterns, urinary and bowel elimination patterns, and sleep-wake patterns. You'll also want to examine the infant directly to assess nutritional status, healing of the umbilicus and circumcision site, and so on.

Obtain information for insurance and other financial matters, and have the parents sign any necessary forms. At the first visit and all subsequent visits, ask the parents what their main concerns are and then address those concerns.

Make every effort to build rapport with the parents, so they'll feel comfortable telling you about their fears and concerns. Don't use medical jargon when you speak to them. Be attentive and nonjudgmental. Remember that the home, unlike the health care facility, is the family's territory; an intrusive, domineering approach will make them resent you.

Physical status

At your first visit, obtain a health history and baseline information about the neonate's vital signs, physical status, growth, and development. (See *Assessment findings for the normal neonate.*) Also perform a physical assessment. During later visits, take vital signs and assess for changes in the neonate's condition.

If the neonate needs medications, review the dosages and schedules with the parents. If the schedules are inconvenient and tiring, with nighttime doses and many separate dosage times, consider asking the doctor to modify them.

For the neonate receiving phototherapy, assess for signs of treatment efficacy, such as improvement in the color of skin and mucous membranes. Also check for dehydration, an adverse effect of phototherapy, which may manifest as lethargy, poor feeding, and excessive, watery stools.

Parenting skills

One of the benefits of neonatal home care is that you have the opportunity to watch the mother and other family members interact with the newborn. This interaction is crucial to normal growth and development. Note the degree of eye contact between parent and neonate. Watch how often the mother fondles, kisses, and vocalizes with the neonate.

Keep in mind that problems in parent-infant bonding sometimes manifest in behavior problems, such as sleep disturbances, feeding disorders, failure to gain weight, and refusal to feed. Especially if you detect potential problems, you may want to implement a specific assessment tool to assess the mother-neonate relationship.

Also assess the mother's and family's ability to perform routine neonatal health care. Provide information about infant growth and development. Offer anticipatory guidance about feeding problems, the crying baby, umbilicus and circumcision care, and what problems should prompt a call to you or the doctor.

If the neonate needs specialized care, such as phototherapy, evaluate the mother's and family's understanding of why it's necessary, what it should accomplish, and the steps needed to perform it. Make sure they know how to properly operate and store needed equipment and medical supplies. Also, make sure they know how to examine the neonate for problems related to the use of such equipment.

As the parents become more familiar and comfortable with neonatal care, expect their caregiving skills to improve. If they don't, or you see new problems developing, provide additional teaching sessions.

Support systems

Although the discharge planner at the neonate's acute care facility will make a preliminary assessment of support available to the family after discharge, you'll be able to assess that support system in action.

Determine how much physical support the parents need and how much they're receiving. Try to mobilize whatever family support may be available. Reinforce the discharge teaching given to the patient and her partner in the acute care facility.

Whenever possible, prompt parents to contact a parent support group. Besides offering first-hand knowledge and advice from experienced parents, these groups often provide much-needed reassurance and encouragement.

The birth of a child causes dramatic changes in family dynamics and relationships. Acknowledge this fact and reassure the family that those changes are normal. Help family members adapt by asking them what they enjoy most in their new roles. Ask them to describe how the newborn has changed their relationships. To help minimize conflicts and misunderstandings, encourage a nonjudgmental discussion of the perceived roles and responsibilities of all involved family members.

The home environment

Assess whether the home is safe and suitable for a newborn. Is it adequately heated and ventilated? Are there sources of safe water and refrigeration? Is the newborn safe from potentially toxic substances such as lead-based paint? If you feel that parents need to make improvements in the home environment to keep their infant safe and healthy, think carefully about how to frame your comments tactfully before giving advice.

Also determine whether the family has a plan for handling emergencies. If not, help them construct one. Especially if they don't have a telephone, you'll need to help them devise rapid, suitable methods to obtain emergency help. Make sure that parents and all other caregivers know how to administer cardiopulmonary resuscitation (CPR) to an infant and under what circumstances to seek immediate medical attention.

Assessing the high-risk neonate

Families of high-risk neonates need stalwart psychosocial support in addition to expert nursing care, especially if their newborn was sick enough to need intensive care before discharge. Usually, although parents are relieved that their infant is well enough to come home, they have doubts about their abilities to provide the kind of care their child needs. You'll need to offer them frequent encouragement and positive reinforcement. As always, make every effort to establish rapport with the parents so they'll feel free to discuss their concerns openly with you.

Physical status

Obtain baseline information about the neonate and the family. Then augment the routine assessment by investigating the neonate's specific problem. The typical high-risk neonate is preterm or of low birth weight and has one or more of the following disorders: respiratory distress, bronchopulmonary dysplasia, apnea of prematurity, patent ductus arteriosus, hearing or visual impairment, hydrocephalus, intraventricular hemorrhage, seizures, or necrotizing enterocolitis. Congenital anomalies and the effects of maternal substance abuse also may place the neonate at high risk for serious health problems.

Clearly, you'll have to take extra care to focus your physical assessments on the infant's specific problems in addition to providing typical neonatal assessments. (See *Focused assessment for the high-risk neonate,* pages 132 and 133.) As with any neonate, ongoing visits should focus on detecting changes in the neonate's physical status and the parents' ability to provide needed care.

Support systems

In addition to assessing the neonate, you'll need to assess parents and other family members to make sure they're coping physically, emotionally, and possibly financially with the addition of a high-risk neonate to the family. In this stressful situation, the availability of support and respite can make all the difference between coping and not coping.

Begin by determining whether the parents have a secondary source of care for their infant. Many have trouble finding reliable, knowledgeable helpers (extended-family members may be too frightened to offer) and can't afford to pay for professional nursing care beyond that included in your home visits. Help the family determine whether any local perinatal centers provide respite care. Also help them find out whether respite care is available through community programs. Keep in mind, however, that

Focused assessment for the high-risk neonate

Problem	Focused assessment areas	Parent teaching
Respiratory disorder	◆ Vital signs and changes from baseline ◆ Breath sounds ◆ Skin color ◆ Respiratory pattern ◆ Signs of respiratory distress ◆ Respiratory secretions ◆ Medications and their effectiveness ◆ Dietary intake and growth	◆ Disorder and related anatomy and physiology ◆ Signs and symptoms of respiratory distress ◆ Purpose of interventions ◆ Assessment of respiratory status ◆ Signs of possible respiratory infection and distress ◆ Medication administration ◆ Treatments, such as chest physiotherapy, oxygen therapy, suctioning, and mechanical ventilation ◆ When to notify health care provider
Hydrocephalus	◆ Head circumference ◆ Mental status ◆ Neck range of motion ◆ Eye movements ◆ Fontanels ◆ Shunt functioning	◆ Disorder and related anatomy and physiology ◆ Purpose of shunt ◆ How to monitor level of consciousness ◆ Measurement of head circumference ◆ Checking fontanels ◆ When to notify health care provider
Seizures	◆ Vital signs ◆ Level of consciousness ◆ Motor and ocular responses to stimulation ◆ Signs and symptoms of seizures ◆ Anticonvulsant therapy ◆ Drug level monitoring	◆ Disorder and related anatomy and physiology ◆ Signs and symptoms of seizures ◆ Maintaining seizure log ◆ Assessment of neurologic status ◆ Emergency interventions ◆ Seizure and safety precautions ◆ Anticonvulsant therapy regimen ◆ When to notify health care provider

Focused assessment for the high-risk neonate *(continued)*

Problem	Focused assessment areas	Parent teaching
Visual impairment	◆ Vision screening ◆ Examination of lids, pupils, sclera, and conjunctiva ◆ Pupillary response ◆ Presence of nystagmus, strabismus ◆ Focusing ability	◆ Disorder and related anatomy and physiology ◆ Home stimulation program ◆ Safety measures ◆ When to notify health care provider
Acquired immunodeficiency syndrome	◆ Overall physical examination ◆ Facial features ◆ Achievement of growth and development milestones ◆ Signs and symptoms of infection ◆ Signs and symptoms of neurologic abnormalities	◆ Disorder and related anatomy and physiology ◆ Care required ◆ Infection control measures ◆ Sensory stimulation ◆ When to notify health care provider
Maternal substance abuse	◆ Reflex responses ◆ Crying pattern ◆ Activity level ◆ Feeding patterns ◆ Muscle tone	◆ Effects of substance abuse ◆ Care required ◆ Signs and symptoms of associated problems and complications ◆ When to notify health care provider

these programs rarely provide helpers trained specifically to care for high-risk neonates.

Find out whether there are any local support groups for parents of high-risk neonates, especially neonates with the same problem. Not only will members of such a group be able to provide parents with caregiving advice, but they also may know of other sources of respite care and assistance.

As you provide ongoing care for a high-risk neonate, continue to assess the parents and other family members to make sure they have realistic expectations of themselves and each other. Many parents feel that they should be able to provide round-the-clock care for their high-risk neonate while also keeping house, attending to other children, and meeting their own personal needs. Eventually, these unrealistic expectations may boil over into arguments, health problems, and possible splintering of the family.

Specialized equipment

Besides routine and basic care, the high-risk neonate typically requires sophisticated, complex care at home. Examples of that care include apnea monitoring, suctioning, chest physiotherapy, oxygen therapy, tracheostomy care, mechanical ventilation, enteral or parenteral nutrition, medication administration, and developmental stimulation programs.

It's up to you to make sure that parents understand the purpose, care, and operation of all equipment needed to provide care for the neonate, as well as how to make sure it's producing the desired results. Carefully assess the parents' understanding of needed equipment, and instruct them as appropriate. In addition, assess the neonate to determine the effectiveness of therapy. (See *Assessment guidelines for the neonate who needs special equipment.*)

Remember that new parents may feel overwhelmed by the responsibility of providing specialized care to a newborn, even care that you consider to be fairly simple. Help new parents learn what to do by demonstrating it to them and then asking them to try it. Repeat this process as many times as you need to. Even if their efforts fall short at first, encourage them. Convey a sense of trust and confidence that they'll be able to provide the care their child needs.

The home environment

As with all neonates, be sure to assess whether the home has adequate facilities and space for caregiving. Check for sufficient electrical outlets and adequate shelving or other storage areas for supplies. (Warn parents not to store anything directly over the neonate's bed.)

Consider whether the family might benefit from installing ramps to move the infant and equipment more easily into and out of the house. Also observe for evidence that home health care may be disrupting family functioning; if so, assess whether the parents should consider converting a downstairs room into the child's bedroom to give them privacy from home health personnel.

Make sure the family has an adequate emergency plan. If the family has telephone service, suggest that they post important emergency numbers near every phone. If the home lacks a phone, find out if the parents have made other arrangements for obtaining help in an emergency. To help ensure prompt emergency intervention, make sure they've notified the local police and fire departments, in writing, about their infant's condition, medications, and treatments, as well as the names of the doctor and acute care facility to which emergency personnel should transport the child in an emergency.

Likewise, they should ask the telephone and electric companies to place them on a priority service list, give them advance warning of interrupted service, and provide them with priority reinstatement of service after unexpected interruptions.

Also make sure parents and all other caregivers know how to administer infant CPR correctly and when to seek immediate medical attention for a problem. If necessary, consider posting infant CPR instructions by the neonate's bed.

Nursing considerations

For all neonates — sick and well — your goals for home care include managing or correcting any problems detected during assessment and ensuring that parents and caregivers are providing safe, appropriate care.

Assessment guidelines for the neonate who needs special equipment

The table below shows key assessment guidelines for neonates who require special medical equipment. At each home visit, verify that all equipment is functioning properly. Conduct a rapid review of functional patterns and body systems; then focus on the neonate's specific problem.

Equipment and indications	Health history and physical assessment data	Equipment-related data
Apnea monitor Apnea of prematurity, respiratory compromise, tracheostomy use, acute drug withdrawal, family history of apnea or sudden infant death	◆ Vital signs ◆ Respiratory status ◆ Frequency and duration of predischarge apneic episodes ◆ Need for resuscitation ◆ Any associated signs or precipitating factors ◆ History of pallor, cyanosis, or hypotonia ◆ History of apnea or bradycardia, its frequency and duration, and type of stimulation required to arouse the neonate	◆ All needed supplies are in the home, including leadwires, patches, and instruction manual. ◆ Grounded outlet is available for the monitor. ◆ Monitor settings are appropriate and accurate. ◆ Monitor is placed on a hard surface at the bedside and has sufficient ventilation. ◆ Electrodes are placed correctly on sides of chest wall.
Oxygen therapy Respiratory or cardiac disorder	◆ Vital signs ◆ Respiratory status ◆ Skin color changes, such as peripheral cyanosis, and signs of respiratory distress	◆ Concentration and liter flow are accurate. ◆ Recommended equipment is in use. ◆ Correct number of hours of daily oxygen therapy are given. ◆ Equipment is functioning properly. ◆ Oxygen source has adequate supply level. ◆ Humidity source (if prescribed) is in use. ◆ Humidifier is functioning properly with correct settings. ◆ Prescribed delivery method is in use.

(continued)

Assessment guidelines for the neonate who needs special equipment *(continued)*

Equipment and indications	Health history and physical assessment data	Equipment-related data
Tracheostomy Upper airway obstruction, respiratory failure from mechanical or neurologic problems, chronic aspiration, long-term mechanical ventilation	◆ Vital signs ◆ Respiratory status ◆ Quality, color, viscosity, and odor of tracheal secretions ◆ Condition of skin at tracheostomy site	◆ Humidification source (compressor with nebulizer or cascade, room humidifier, or tracheostomy humidifying filter) is in proper use. ◆ Tracheostomy tubes and suction catheter are correct size.
Mechanical ventilator Respiratory disorder	◆ Vital signs (compare observed respiratory rate against ventilator rate) ◆ Skin color, respiratory pattern, and rise and fall of chest with each breath	◆ Ventilator settings are correct. ◆ Bellows are functioning correctly. ◆ Alarm lights are on. ◆ Connections are secure. ◆ Tubing isn't kinked. ◆ Humidifier is filled. ◆ Backup power supply is available.
Enteral or parenteral nutrition therapy Inability to ingest adequate calories by mouth	◆ Nutritional status (such as growth parameters and daily tube or I.V. intake) ◆ Skin condition around tube or I.V. insertion site	◆ Feeding pump is functioning correctly. ◆ Administration method, feeding technique, and frequency and duration of feeding are appropriate. ◆ Formula (enteral or I.V.) is appropriate. ◆ Placement, size, and type of tube are correct. ◆ Neonate is positioned correctly. ◆ Refrigeration is available for solution storage. ◆ Home sanitation is adequate to allow sterile procedures.

Make sure that the neonate has a source of primary pediatric care, that all care is coordinated, and that the family's resources are adequate to provide appropriate, ongoing care. If necessary, help the family obtain a pediatrician. Also facilitate communication and coordination among care providers.

Be prepared to help the family through financial crises triggered by the neonate's care requirements, especially if the neonate is sick. For example, mechanical ventilation may substantially increase the family's electric bill. Or perhaps the home lacks adequate plumbing, running water, hot water, or electricity. In all such cases, make sure a social service agency has been contacted. Financial and other assistance for such problems may be available through charities, religious organizations, and city, county, state, and federal social services departments.

Family risk factors

The birth of a child can disturb roles and relationships in even the most stable families, at least temporarily. You'll need to evaluate family members for signs of stress, depression and, possibly, resentment. Expect parents to show signs of exhaustion and possibly marital strain. Assess siblings for overt or covert signs of jealousy and resentment of the neonate. Also explore family dynamics, strengths, and weaknesses.

Especially for the family of a high-risk neonate, discharge from the acute care facility may herald a new crisis. Keep in mind that parents of a neonate with a chronic or disabling condition must pass through the stages of grief to deal with the loss of what they hoped would be a "perfect" child before they can accept the real one. These stages typically include denial, anger, bargaining, depression, and acceptance. If possible, determine which stage of grief each parent is in and how the parent attempts to cope with the feelings it produces.

Studies show that parents of special-needs children don't necessarily experience reduced marital satisfaction or a higher likelihood of separation. Indeed, many parents of such children report a strengthening of the marital relationship over time. Nonetheless, a high-risk neonate's condition undoubtedly will cause tremendous stress in the relationship, especially at first.

Assess for overt signs of marital stress, such as arguments, and more subtle indications, such as sarcasm, terse conversations, and a reluctance to acknowledge the partner's presence. If stress is apparent or you suspect it, consider tactfully suggesting that the couple seek counseling.

Parental disappointment or grief over a sick neonate's medical condition or physical appearance may raise family risk factors as well, including poor parent-infant bonding. If the interactions you observe seem to suggest poor bonding, reinforce your teaching about neonatal behavioral states, communication cues, growth and developmental patterns, and sleep-wake patterns. Also encourage parents to express their feelings freely, without fear of being judged as bad people or bad parents.

Remember that some cases of poor parent-infant interaction may reflect child neglect or abuse. If you suspect this problem, you'll need to contact the local child protective services agency.

Helping siblings adjust

The addition of a new family member may cause siblings to feel neglected and unloved, especially if the neonate's care is demanding and time-consuming. If your family assessment reveals changes in a sibling's behavior or attitudes, you'll need to take action.

Start by making sure siblings understand that they didn't cause a sick infant's illness, even if they had bad thoughts about the infant before it was born. Also take time to explain, as clearly and simply as you can, what's wrong with the newborn. Uninformed siblings tend to be less sure of what parents expect of them and less confident about how to behave around the infant. They may even feel that their own identity is threatened.

Encourage parents to let siblings participate in the infant's care at a level appropriate to each sibling's developmental stage. Doing so can help each sibling feel more involved in the family and more important as a family member. (Watch to make sure that parents don't load siblings with too much responsibility.) Finally, urge parents to regularly spend time alone with each sibling to convey the feeling that each child has a special place in the family.

◆THE PEDIATRIC PATIENT

Before home care is deemed appropriate for a child, the doctor usually determines whether the child's condition warrants home care and whether the family is capable of understanding and providing what the child needs. The child must have a primary doctor. And family members must have the resources, both physical and emotional, to maintain the family's function and coping strategies.

You may be called upon to provide pediatric home care for many reasons, including postsurgical care, terminal illness, and such chronic illnesses as asthma, cystic fibrosis, and cancer.

Assessing the child

Assessing a child at home is much the same as assessing a child in an acute care setting. You'll need to tailor it to the child's specific age and illness. (See *Age-appropriate assessment*.) However, working in the child's home may confer some benefits over those you receive in the typical acute care setting.

For example, caring for a child at home typically gives you easier access to information about his family and how it functions. It also provides you with increased opportunities to teach the child's parents about health promotion, signs of health and illness, and expected milestones of growth and development. Providing this anticipatory guidance can exert a lasting effect on the child's and the family's health.

At your first home visit, you'll want to obtain a complete history and physical examination. Remember to provide the child and family with the same level of privacy you'd ensure in an acute care facility.

At subsequent meetings, focus on detecting any changes in the child's physical and emotional condition. Evaluate his ongoing response to his illness and treatments. Also monitor the child's growth and development. Be sure to document specific milestones reached or not reached.

In addition to assessing the child, you'll also need to assess his caregivers to make sure that they're continuing to provide appropriate care. Watch how caregivers interact with the child. Watch his reactions to them. Remember that changes in the child's condition can change the family's ability to provide care. If the child's condition worsens, for example, he may need more frequent nursing vis-

Age-appropriate assessment

Children at different ages have different needs. In addition to the routine physical assessment you perform for any child, make sure you include information that's age-specific in your assessments.

Age	Focused assessment areas
Toddler and preschooler	◆ Safe play area away from steps ◆ Screens and locks on windows and doors ◆ Lead-free paint on all painted surfaces ◆ Appropriate items and activities for stimulation and learning ◆ Safety locks on kitchen cabinets and medicine cabinets ◆ Safety covers on unused electrical outlets ◆ Medicines and toxic materials stored safely
School age and adolescent	◆ Provisions for schooling ◆ Socialization and interaction with peers ◆ Medication reminder system ◆ Lead-free paint on all painted surfaces

its. If he needs additional specialized equipment, the family may feel incapable of coping with the increased needs.

As in all health care settings, your assessment of the pediatric home care patient will have ramifications for other aspects of his care, including the preparation of his environment.

Preparing the home environment

When cared for at home, a child may need many of the same environmental aids he would receive in an acute care facility. For example, he may need a hospital bed. If his parents can't afford to buy or rent one, you may be able to adapt an existing bed. Try placing wooden or concrete blocks under the bed to elevate it. Slide a piece of plywood under the mattress if it needs to be more firm. Insert pillows under the end of the mattress to raise the child's head. And improvise by making a bed tray out of a cardboard box.

If the child's bedroom is removed from the home's center of activity, remember that the child may become lonely. If appropriate, encourage him to join the family for activities by resting on the couch or a lounge chair or by sitting in the kitchen. Also encourage family members to include the child in as many activities as possible, even if it means moving his bed to a more public place. Perhaps the family could bring a television into the child's room and have everyone gather there to watch it; a temporary table could be set up in the room so that everyone can eat meals with the child.

Urge family members to let the child perform as much of his own personal care as possible to maintain his sense of control, wellness, and self-esteem. If possible, locate the child's bed near a bathroom. Make adaptations as needed, such as using a basin for bathing, a detachable fixture in the shower, or a chair to sit on while bathing.

Finally, make sure your patient's home environment is safe. In addition to the usual home safety procedures, see if the local fire department has a sticker to place on the window of a disabled child's room, thus calling attention to the room if a fire breaks out. The child also should be able to reach the phone, for socialization in addition to emergency access. Make sure the child knows how to activate the emergency medical system in the area.

Ensuring mobility and independence

Encourage as much mobility and independence as the child's condition permits. Help parents determine what adaptations they can make to maintain the child's mobility. For example, if the child is confined to a wheelchair, they may need to install ramps in the home. Handrails along staircases can help as well.

In the kitchen and bathroom, parents can keep all of the child's things on lower shelves. If necessary, they can also keep a pair of long tongs or a "third hand" nearby so the child can reach items on higher shelves. Safety rails by the toilet and in the bathtub can help the child with transfers. Placing a microwave oven on a low table can allow the child to warm up meals and prepare snacks independently. Placing a board across the wheelchair's arms can provide the child with a workspace or table surface on which to do things.

Giving medications and treatments

Most children who receive home care need medications. Usually, they're given orally; however, sometimes they're given parenterally, by injection (subcutaneous or intramuscular), or intravenously through a peripheral or central venous access device. You'll need to ensure that family members understand how and when to administer the child's medications, especially when they're given parenterally. (See *Teaching parents to administer medications*.)

The treatments needed by pediatric home care patients are as varied as the patients themselves. Commonly, however, they include efforts to promote respiratory function. These treatments can range from incentive spirometry and oxygen therapy to tracheostomy care and mechanical ventilation. In each of these situations, parents need education about all aspects of the child's care.

One of your biggest challenges will be teaching the parents of a ventilator-dependent child. You'll need to provide plenty of teaching until the parents are completely comfortable with the ventilator. Remember that this machine is frightening to a layperson and requires continuous monitoring. In fact, parents commonly grow fatigued from lack of sleep and the daily stress of the responsibility. It severely limits their ability to leave the house, even for such necessary trips as grocery shopping. Be sure to assess the parents' level of functioning in addition to the child's.

Maintaining nutrition and elimination

Children receiving home care need as much or more dietary supervision as those in acute care facilities. Why? Because home care patients rarely

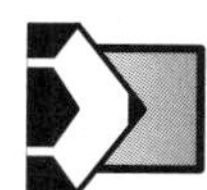

TEACHING POINTS

Teaching parents to administer medications

When teaching parents about safe medication administration, be sure to include these tips:

◆ Store all medications in their original labeled containers.
◆ Discard any unused, outdated, or previously prescribed medications by flushing them down the toilet.
◆ Keep all medications out of the reach of children.
◆ Prepare medications under good light to minimize the chance of error.
◆ Use a calendar or chart to track doses and to avoid double doses.
◆ Don't give over-the-counter medications without checking with the child's doctor.

If the parent must administer I.V. drugs, be sure to include these tips:

◆ Check the I.V. site for signs of infection or infiltration.
◆ Dilute the medication properly and double-check the correct dosage.
◆ Use sterile technique and maintain the sterility of all equipment.
◆ Administer the medication continuously or intermittently, as ordered.
◆ Dispose of used needles and syringes properly.

have access to a dietitian, as they would in an acute care setting. Also, the child may resort to unhealthy food habits out of boredom or a need for attention. Be sure to evaluate the quantity and quality of the child's diet to make sure he's receiving adequate nutrition and fiber.

If the child needs enteral or parenteral nutrition, carefully teach family members about the purpose of the treatment, needed equipment, administration procedures, signs and symptoms of problems or complications, and care needed before, during, and after the treatment.

If the child can ambulate to the bathroom for elimination, encourage him to do so. Installing handrails in the hallway leading to the bathroom may be helpful if the child needs assistance. If the child can't ambulate to the bathroom, advise the parents to buy or rent a bedpan or portable commode from a medical equipment company or local pharmacy. An overbed trapeze can allow the child to raise and lower himself in bed and help with self-care.

If necessary, you may need to catheterize the child to alleviate urine retention. If he'll need this procedure frequently, you can teach parents or the child himself how to perform intermittent clean catheterization to eliminate the need for continuous catheterization. Children with inadequate renal function can be managed at home with continuous ambulatory peritoneal dialysis.

Providing wound care

If your patient needs wound care, teach parents how to provide it using aseptic technique. If the dressing will be changed frequently, consider using Montgomery straps or a stockinette to secure the dressing and reduce skin irritation. Stress that parents should wash their hands thoroughly before and after a dressing change to reduce the risk of infection.

Promoting growth and development

Children receiving home care need stimulation and education just like other children. If their medical condition allows, arrange home tutoring or a special program with the local school.

During other times, encourage the child to work on age-appropriate projects, such as needlecraft, planning family menus, reading magazines, listening to tapes, or watching videotapes on science or nature. If possible, try to find projects that stimulate learning in addition to simply passing the time.

Also encourage children to perform self-care activities and to contribute to the household routine as much as possible. Doing so will help lift some of the burden from caregivers in addition to helping the child see himself as a functioning member of the family.

Assessing family function

When an ill child is in the home, you'll notice that the child's needs can disrupt normal family routines and shift the focus of attention away from other family members and onto the child. Over time, this shift can create physical and emotional problems for the entire family — even the sick child.

If you observe such problems, encourage communication among all members of the family. Urge them to identify and share their feelings about the situation. Help them work together to solve problems and redefine roles and responsibilities. By doing so, you'll help the child as well as the family.

◆THE MENTALLY ILL PATIENT

As in other areas of health care, home health nurses are seeing more mentally ill patients than ever before, and their illnesses are more profound than ever. In fact, you may be charged with assessing a mentally ill patient's response to a new medication in addition to stabilizing symptoms that, not long ago, would have been stabilized in an acute care facility. You also may provide the primary link between the patient, the family, and other members of the health care team.

When providing mental health care in the patient's home, you'll discover that boundary issues can arise more easily than they do in a more formal setting. You'll need to be especially careful to establish a well-defined role for yourself and a relationship that's truly therapeutic for the patient. In simple terms, you'll want to create a relationship where the patient knows you're helping him reach a goal; don't let the patient become overly dependent on you.

In addition to working with the patient, include family members as appropriate. They commonly play a vital role in stabilizing the patient and verifying your assessment.

Also be sure to investigate possible organic problems or medical treatments that could underlie what seems to be a mental illness. Observe for key signs and symptoms, and examine the patient using inspection, palpation, percussion, and auscultation. Remember that a patient caught up in a medical problem may have signs of depression or anxiety and fail to recognize or validate them. Whether he recognizes it or not, a patient with

Tips for success in the psychiatric interview

To make the most of your psychiatric interview, follow these guidelines.

◆ Keep your goals clearly in mind. Remember that an interview isn't a random discussion. You must pursue your goal of obtaining information from the patient, screening for abnormalities, or investigating a suspected psychiatric condition, such as depression or suicidal thoughts.

◆ Never allow personal values or attitudes to obstruct your professional judgment.

◆ Pay attention to unspoken signals. Throughout the interview, listen carefully for indications that the patient is anxious or distressed. You may find important clues in the patient's method of self-expression and in the subjects he avoids.

◆ Always consider the patient's cultural beliefs and values. A person who blames misfortune on "bad juju" might be considered delusional in the United States but would seem quite normal in Nigeria. When dealing with patients from an unfamiliar culture, consult with an outside resource before drawing any conclusions.

◆ Don't make assumptions about how past events affected the patient's emotional status. Try to discover what each event meant to the patient and how he perceived it.

◆ Monitor your reactions to make sure the patient doesn't provoke an emotional response strong enough to interfere with your professional judgment. Remember that it's natural for you to be influenced by your patient's affect. A depressed patient may make you feel depressed, and an anxious patient may make you anxious. A violent, psychotic patient may make you fearful.

◆ Remember that identifying too closely with a patient may threaten your therapeutic relationship, disrupt your objectivity, or cause you to avoid or reject the patient. If you recognize in yourself strong prejudices toward a patient, seek assistance from another health care professional.

mental illness needs a complete evaluation and appropriate treatment.

The psychiatric interview

A systematic psychiatric interview helps you acquire broad information about the patient. The interview should include a description of the patient's behavioral disturbances, a thorough emotional and social history, and mental status tests.

Using this information, you'll be able to assess the patient's psychological functioning, understand his coping methods and their effect on his psychosocial growth, build a therapeutic alliance that encourages the patient to talk openly, and develop an accurate care plan.

A supportive atmosphere

The success of your interview hinges on your ability to listen objectively and to respond with empathy. (See *Tips for success in the psychiatric interview*.) The patient must feel comfortable enough to discuss his problems with you. Remember that you may need to use a variety of intuitive methods to help the patient arrive at this comfort level.

That's because patients may be angry and argumentative. They may be too withdrawn to explain why they need help. They may refuse to accept that they need help. They may come from cultural backgrounds that frown on discussing intimate details with a stranger, even a nurse. Adolescents may refuse to discuss many topics in front of their parents. In all of these scenarios, you'll need to listen carefully to the patient and respond with sensitivity to draw him out.

If the patient can't provide answers to important questions or appears unreliable, ask for permission to interview family members or friends.

The chief complaint

When you feel that the patient is willing to talk openly with you, ask what he thinks is wrong and what he expects to accomplish through treatment. A person with low self-esteem may seek a better self-image. A schizophrenic may want to stop his hallucinations. Some patients may not know what to expect and may not think anything is wrong. At the very least, help such patients see the benefits of dealing with their problems openly.

However the patient describes his problem and his goals for treatment, document them in his own words as the chief complaint. When possible, fully discuss the patient's complaint, its severity and persistence, and whether it occurred abruptly or insidiously. If discussing a recurrent problem, ask the patient what prompted him to seek help at this time.

A psychosocial history

Also discuss past mental health disorders, such as episodes of delusions, violence, or attempted suicide. Ask if the patient has ever undergone psychiatric treatment and what happened as a result. Even though the patient may be reluctant to respond, such questions may elicit early warnings of depression, dementia, suicide risk, psychosis, or adverse medication effects.

Also be sure to discuss psychosocial issues, including the patient's beliefs, relationships, lifestyle, coping skills, diet, sleep patterns, and use of alcohol, drugs, or tobacco. Discuss the patient's ability to function socially. Have the patient describe school, work, religious practices, community life, hobbies, and sexual activity.

As much as possible, take an in-depth look at the patient's personality. Look for indications of stumbling blocks during the maturation process. Also assess how the patient copes with stress. Can he control impulses and demonstrate good judgment? How strong is his sense of identity? Look for areas of strength through evidence of the patient's adaptability, talents, accomplishments, and ability to find emotional support.

Next, discuss important life changes. Explore how the patient coped with such changes as a recent marriage, divorce, illness, job loss, or death of a loved one. How did the patient feel when these changes occurred?

Family history

Now move on to questions about family customs, child-rearing practices, and emotional support the patient received during childhood. This line of questioning may reveal important insights about environmental influences on the patient's development.

Watch carefully how the patient reacts while disclosing his family history. For example, when a patient tells you about his parents' divorce, can you detect feelings of jealousy, hostility, or unresolved grief? Likewise, watch how the patient describes the emotional health of his relatives. Is there a family history of substance abuse, alcoholism, suicide, psychiatric hospitalization, child abuse, or violence?

Ask about physical disorders as well. A family history of diabetes mellitus or thyroid disorders, for instance, can point out the need to investigate a possible organic basis for the patient's emotional signs and symptoms.

Mental status

Often included as part of the psychiatric interview, the mental status examination (MSE) is a tool for assessing psychological dysfunction and for identifying the causes of psychopathology. You may need to administer part or all of this examination, so you'll need to be familiar with its components and its implications. The MSE can provide you with a wide-ranging impression of the patient's mental health.

Level of consciousness. Begin by assessing the patient's level of consciousness, a basic brain function. Identify the intensity of stimulation needed to arouse the patient. Does the patient respond to a normal conversational tone of voice? A loud voice? Or does it take a light touch, vigorous shaking, or painful stimulation to rouse the patient?

Describe the patient's response to stimulation, including the degree and quality of movement, content and coherence of speech, and level of eye opening and eye contact. Finally, describe the patient's actions once the stimulus is removed.

An impaired level of consciousness may indicate a tumor, abscess, hematoma, hydrocephalus, electrolyte or acid-base imbalance, or toxicity from liver or kidney failure, alcohol, or drugs.

General appearance. The patient's appearance also provides information about mental status. Describe his weight, coloring, skin condition, odor, body build, and obvious physical impairments. Note discrepancies between the patient's feelings about his health and your observations. Answer the following questions:

- Is the patient's appearance appropriate to his age, sex, and situation?
- Are his skin, hair, nails, and teeth clean?
- Is his manner of dress appropriate?
- If the patient wears cosmetics, are they appropriately applied?

A disheveled appearance may indicate self-neglect or a preoccupation with other activities. A pale, emaciated, sad appearance may indicate depression. Posture and gait may reveal physical and emotional disorders. For example, a slumped posture may indicate depression, fatigue, or suspicious feelings. An uneven or unsteady gait suggests physical abnormalities or the influence of drugs or alcohol.

Behavior. Describe the patient's demeanor and way of relating to others. When entering the room, does the patient appear sad, somber, joyful, manic? Does he use appropriate gestures? Does he acknowledge your initial greeting and introduction? Does he keep an appropriate distance between himself and others? Does he have distinctive mannerisms, such as tics or tremors? Does he gaze directly at you, at the floor, or around the

Signs of mood disorders

◆ Lability of affect; rapid, dramatic fluctuation in the range of emotion
◆ Flat affect; unresponsive range of emotion, possibly an indication of schizophrenia or Parkinson's disease
◆ Inappropriate affect; inconsistency between expression (affect) and mood (for example, a patient who smiles when discussing an anger-provoking situation)

room? Does he maintain eye contact with you?

When responding to your questions, is the patient cooperative, mistrustful, embarrassed, hostile, overly revealing? Describe the patient's level of activity. Is he tense, rigid, restless, calm? An inability to sit still may indicate anxiety.

Note any extraordinary behavior. Disconnected gestures may indicate that the patient is hallucinating. A patient who hears voices may appear to speak to someone who isn't there, or you may see him tilt his head as though listening. Pressured, rapid speech and a heightened level of activity may suggest bipolar disorder.

Speech. Consider the content and quality of the patient's speech, taking special notice of:
◆ illogical choice of topics
◆ irrelevant or illogical answers to your questions
◆ speech defects, such as stuttering
◆ excessively fast or slow speech
◆ sudden interruptions
◆ inappropriate speech volume
◆ altered voice tone and modulation
◆ slurred speech
◆ an excessive number of words (overproductive speech)
◆ minimal, monosyllabic responses (underproductive speech).

Also note how much time elapses before the patient responds to your questions. If he communicates only with gestures, determine whether this is an isolated behavior or part of a pattern of diminished responsiveness.

Mood and affect. *Mood* refers to a person's pervading feeling or state of mind. *Affect* refers to a person's expression of his mood. Variations in affect are referred to as range of emotion. To assess mood and affect, begin by asking the patient about his current feelings. Also look for indications of mood in facial expression and posture. Pay attention to how often and how rapidly the patient's mood changes. (See *Signs of mood disorders*.)

Remember that mood swings may result from a physiologic disorder. Medications, recreational drug or alcohol use, stress, dehydration, electrolyte imbalance, or disease may all induce mood changes. After childbirth and during menopause, women may be more likely to experience depression.

Intellectual performance. Emotionally distressed patients may be unable to reason abstractly, make judgments, or solve problems. To develop a picture of the patient's intellectual abilities, use the following series of simple tests. Note that these tests screen for organic brain syndromes as well. If you suspect an organic syndrome, make sure the patient receives appropriate follow-up testing.

Orientation. Ask the patient the time, date, place, and his name.

Immediate and delayed recall. Assess the patient's ability to recall something that just occurred and to remember events after a reasonable amount of time passes. For example, to test immediate recall, say, "I want you to remember three words: apple, house, and umbrella. What are the three words I want you to remember?" To test delayed recall, ask the patient to repeat the same words after 5 or 10 minutes have gone by.

Recent and remote memory. Ask the patient about an event he experienced in the past few hours or days. Make sure you know the correct response or can validate it with a family member. Remember that the patient may fabricate plausible answers to mask a memory deficit.

Assess the patient's ability to remember events in the more distant past, such as where he was born or attended high school. Recent memory loss with intact remote memory may indicate an organic disorder.

Attention span. Assess the patient's ability to concentrate on a task for an appropriate length of time. If the patient has a poor attention span, remember to provide him with simple, written instructions for health care.

Comprehension. Assess the patient's ability to understand material, retain it, and repeat the content. To test comprehension, ask him to read part of a news article and explain what he read.

Abstract thinking. To test the patient's ability to think abstractly, ask the meaning of a common proverb, such as, "People in glass houses shouldn't throw stones." The patient should say something like, "Don't criticize others for what you do yourself." If the patient gives a concrete answer, such as, "Houses shouldn't be made out of glass," he may have mental retardation, severe anxiety, organic brain syndrome, or schizophrenia. (Schizophrenics may also give elaborate or bizarre answers.) If he can't give an answer, he may have a low intellectual ability or brain damage. Remember that people don't gain the ability to think abstractly until about age 12.

You can use other well-known proverbs as well, such as, "A stitch in time saves nine." Keep in mind, however, that some familiar American sayings may confuse people from other cultures.

General knowledge. To determine the patient's store of common knowledge, ask questions appropriate to his age and level of learning, for example, "Who is the President of the United States?"

Judgment. Assess the patient's ability to evaluate choices and to draw appropriate conclusions. Ask, "What would you do if you found a stamped, addressed, sealed airmail letter lying on the sidewalk?" The answer "Track down the recipient" would indicate impaired judgment. Questions that emerge naturally during conversation (for example, "What would you do if you ran out of medication?") may also help you evaluate the patient's judgment. Details of the patient's history might as well. Pay attention to how the patient handles interpersonal relationships and work and financial responsibilities.

Insight. For this phase of the MSE, consider whether the patient sees himself realistically. Is he aware of his illness and its circumstances? Ask such questions as, "What do you think has caused your anxiety?" or "Have you noticed a recent change in yourself?"

Keep in mind that patients will have varying degrees of insight depending on the topic of conversation. For example, an alcoholic patient may admit to a drinking problem but blame it on his work. Severe lack of insight may indicate psychosis.

Perception. Perception refers to interpretation of reality as well as use of the senses. Recently, proponents of the cognitive theory of depression have suggested that depression arises from distorted perception. Depressed patients perceive themselves as worthless, the world as barren, and the future as bleak.

In sensory perceptive disorders, the patient may experience *hallucinations*, in which he perceives nonexistent external stimuli, or *illusions*, in which he misinterprets external stimuli. Tactile, olfactory, and gustatory hallucinations usually indicate organic disorders.

Not all visual and auditory hallucinations are psychological disorders. For example, heat mirages, visions of a recently deceased loved one, and illusions evoked by environmental effects or experienced just before falling asleep don't indicate abnormalities. Constant visual and auditory hallucinations may, however, give rise to bizarre behavior. Disorders associated with hallucinations include schizophrenia and acute organic brain syndrome after withdrawal from alcohol or barbiturate addiction.

Thought content. Assess the patient's thought patterns as expressed throughout the examination. Are his thoughts well connected to reality? Are his ideas clear? Do they progress in a logical sequence? Observe him for indications of morbid thoughts, preoccupations, or abnormal beliefs.

Delusions. Usually associated with schizophrenia, delusions are grandiose or, more commonly, persecutory false beliefs. Occasionally, delusions are seen in patients with psychotic depression or dementia. Delusions may be obvious ("The FBI is after me"), or they may have a slight basis in reality.

Obsessions and compulsions. Some patients suffer intense preoccupations, called *obsessions*, that interfere with daily living. They may think constantly about hygiene, for example. They also may have *compulsions*, which are behaviors in response to obsessions. For example, the patient may constantly wash his hands. Patients often cannot control compulsive behavior without great effort.

Observe also for suicidal, self-destructive, violent, or superstitious thoughts; recurring dreams; distorted perceptions of reality; and feelings of worthlessness.

Sexual desire

Changes in the patient's sex drive can provide valuable information in a psychological assessment. However, you'll need to sharpen your interview skills to prepare yourself for patients who are uncomfortable discussing their sexuality. Avoid language that implies a heterosexual orientation. Introduce the subject tactfully but directly.

Competence

Finally, when conducting a psychiatric interview, remember to look at the big picture as much as possible. Think about the patient's overall competence. Can he understand reality and the consequences of his actions? Does he understand the implications of his illness, its treatment, and the consequences of avoiding treatment?

Always use extreme caution when assessing changes in competence. Unless the patient's behavior strongly indicates otherwise, always assume that a patient is competent. Remember that, legally, only a judge has the power or right to declare a person incompetent to make decisions about his personal health, safety, and finances.

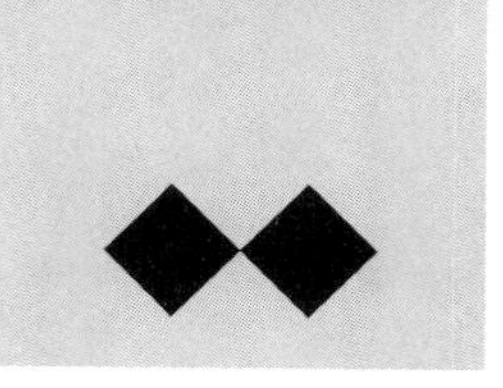

CHAPTER 6

Ensuring accurate diagnostic tests

As you've seen so far, the home differs from other health care settings in many important ways. When it comes to diagnostic tests, however, one guiding principle holds true for all settings: Your results are only as reliable as your methods.

In a patient's home, it's up to you to ensure accurate results for diagnostic tests by understanding the ordered test and its purpose, determining the best time to collect the specimen, using the most appropriate collection method, and finding the safest way to transport the specimen to the laboratory.

This chapter outlines steps for collecting urine and blood specimens, managing other diagnostic tests, and making sure samples make it to the laboratory safely. It also provides descriptions and reference information for various common tests.

By following the guidelines presented here and referring regularly to the chapter's reference section, you can ensure that all your patients' diagnostic tests are done properly and that the results are as accurate as possible.

◆ OBTAINING A URINE SPECIMEN

You may need to collect a urine specimen in one of several ways, depending on the test's purpose and whether or not your patient has an indwelling urinary catheter. Types of urine collection methods include the random specimen, clean-catch specimen, straight-catheter specimen, indwelling catheter specimen, and timed specimen. These specimens provide a wide range of diagnostic data, including white blood cell (WBC) counts, the presence of red blood cells (RBCs) or bacteria, specific gravity, and measurements of hormones, proteins, and electrolytes.

Random specimen

Commonly used for routine urinary function tests, the random specimen isn't invasive and requires the least precision and preparation on the part of the patient and the nurse. To collect it, simply have the patient urinate into a specimen container or into a clean bedpan or urinal. Be sure to provide privacy.

If the patient uses a bedpan or urinal, put gloves on and pour at least 120 ml of urine into a specimen container. Tighten the container's lid and label it with the patient's name, doctor's name, and date and time of collection. Place the specimen in a leakproof bag and clean all reusable equipment items.

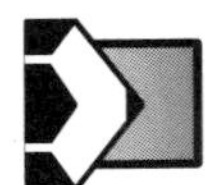

TEACHING POINTS

Obtaining a clean-catch urine specimen

If you need to collect a clean-catch urine specimen, be sure to tell your patient that the doctor ordered a special kind of test that requires what's called a clean-catch specimen. Emphasize that the patient will need to follow certain procedures when collecting the specimen. Otherwise, the results may not be accurate. Then provide the patient with cleaning pads and a specimen cup, and offer these instructions.

◆ Start by washing your penis or vulva with soap and water. Rinse and dry yourself.

◆ Next, wipe your penis or vulva with the special cleaning pads. (Tell a male patient to clean the tip of the penis first, then to wipe in a circular pattern around the glans. Tell a female patient to clean from the front of the vaginal area to the back. She should use one pad to clean one side, then use a fresh pad to clean the other side.)

◆ Now you can collect the specimen. To do so properly, start urinating before you start collecting. Once you've started the urine stream, insert the specimen cup into the stream to catch your sample.

◆ Try to collect as much urine as possible once the first part of the urine stream has passed into the toilet.

◆ When you're finished, place the specimen container on a stable surface nearby. Clean yourself and wash your hands. Then, if you're able, place the lid on the container and tighten it.

If you don't think your patient will be able to safely tighten the lid on the specimen cup, suggest leaving the open container in the bathroom. You can cover the specimen when the patient leaves the bathroom.

Clean-catch specimen

If the doctor thinks the patient could have a urinary tract infection (UTI), you'll need to supervise collection of a clean-catch, midstream specimen. This collection method helps ensure that the sample isn't contaminated with flora from the patient's genitalia or anus.

There are two secrets to obtaining an uncontaminated (clean-catch) urine specimen: First, clean the genitals thoroughly and, second, wait until the urine stream has started before collecting the specimen. If you think your patient can handle these steps accurately, you'll simply need to explain the procedure and provide the appropriate tools. (See *Obtaining a clean-catch urine specimen*.)

If you don't think your patient will be able to obtain the specimen accurately, you'll have to help. Clean the patient's perineum, position the patient to avoid contamination, then clean and dry the perineum again after you collect the specimen.

Remember to use a sterile specimen container for a clean-catch specimen. If you don't have one, you can improvise by boiling a small jar and its lid for 5 minutes and letting them cool. Once the specimen is in the container and the patient is cleaned up, tighten the lid on the specimen container. Then apply a label that documents the patient's name, doctor's name, and date and time of collection. Make sure you also indicate that the container contains a clean-catch specimen. Then place the specimen container in a leakproof bag for transport.

Straight-catheter specimen

If you need to catheterize the patient to collect a urine specimen, remember to follow strict sterile technique. Catheterize the patient according to accepted sterile practice, and collect a sufficient amount of urine into a sterile specimen container. Close the container tightly, remove the catheter, and make sure the patient is comfortable.

Then apply a label to the specimen container that includes the patient's name, doctor's name, date and time of collection, and method of collection. Place the container in a leakproof bag, and deliver it to the laboratory.

Aspirating a urine specimen

To obtain a urine specimen from your patient's indwelling urinary catheter, use a 21 G or 22 G needle about 1" long on a 10-ml (2.5 cm) syringe. After wiping the aspiration port with an alcohol swab, uncap the needle on the syringe and insert it into the aspiration port at a 90-degree angle. Aspirate the urine specimen and inject it into a specimen cup. Then unclamp the drainage tubing.

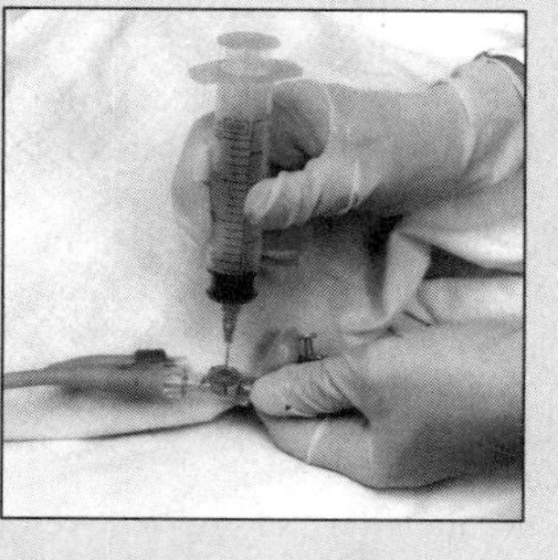

Indwelling catheter specimen

If you need a urine specimen from a patient who has an indwelling urinary catheter, you'll need to take the specimen from the catheter itself. Here's how.

Start by telling the patient that you need to take a specimen of urine from the catheter. Then clamp the catheter's drainage tubing. If the catheter has an aspiration port, you'll be taking the specimen from there. About 30 minutes after clamping the tubing, put gloves on, wipe the aspiration port with an alcohol swab, and aspirate the specimen. (See *Aspirating a urine specimen.*) Inject it into a sterile container.

If the catheter doesn't have an aspiration port and is made of self-sealing rubber, you can take the sample directly from the catheter, just above the point where it connects with the drainage tubing. Wipe the area with an alcohol pad, and insert the needle at a 45-degree angle. Never insert the needle into the catheter shaft because you could puncture the lumen that leads to the catheter balloon. Inject the aspirated urine into a sterile specimen container.

Don't insert a needle into a catheter that isn't made of rubber, because you'll make it leak. In this case, you'll have to wipe the junction of the catheter and drainage tubing with an alcohol pad, then disconnect the tubing and let the catheter drain into a sterile container. Don't let the catheter touch the inside of the container. When you have your specimen, wipe both the catheter and the drainage tubing with alcohol and reconnect them.

Make sure you close the lid of the specimen container tightly. Then apply a label that includes the patient's name, doctor's name, date and time of collection, and method of collection (indwelling catheter aspiration or drainage). If the specimen will be cultured, be sure to list any antibiotics the patient is taking on your laboratory request form. Place the labeled container in a leakproof bag before transporting it to the laboratory.

To help ensure accurate results for this test, try to obtain the specimen shortly after the patient receives a new catheter. That way, you'll avoid obtaining a specimen from contaminated catheter tubing.

No matter which method you use to obtain the specimen, don't forget to unclamp the drainage tubing when you're finished.

Timed sample

Because the body excretes hormones, proteins, and electrolytes in small, variable amounts throughout the day and night, tests to measure these substances usually require the patient to collect urine over a specified period of time. Although the time frame may vary with the test being done, you're most likely to need a 24-hour specimen. Obtaining one will require you to teach the patient verbally and in writing how to collect and store the specimen correctly.

Start by telling the patient that he'll need to save all his urine over a 24-hour period. Unless the doctor directs otherwise, tell the patient not to exercise, drink coffee or tea, or take any drugs just before or during the collection period.

Tell the patient that he'll need to start the collection with an empty bladder. In other words, have him void, and then immediately start the collection period. End it 24 hours later with one final voiding. (Make sure the 24-hour collection ends at a time when the laboratory will be open.)

In the meantime, have the patient store the urine container in a brown bag in the refrigerator, away from food items. Check with the laboratory to see if you need to add a preservative to the container. Emphasize to the patient that missing even one urination will invalidate his test results. And warn him not to contaminate the sample with stool or toilet tissue.

At the end of the 24-hour period, pack the container in ice, label it appropriately, and send it to the laboratory.

Other specimens

On occasion, you may need to collect a second-voided urine specimen, a first-morning specimen, or a fasting specimen. For a second-voided specimen, have the patient void and discard the urine. Then give him at least one glass of water to stimulate urine production. After 30 minutes, collect a urine specimen using the random specimen method.

For first-morning and fasting specimens, have the patient void when he retires for the night. Then collect his first voiding in the morning. If he needs to urinate at night, have him write down the time. Then label his morning specimen container with something like "Urine specimen, 2:15 a.m. to 8:00 a.m." For a fasting sample, tell the patient not to eat or drink anything after midnight.

◆ OBTAINING A BLOOD SAMPLE

Many diagnostic tests rely on a sample of the patient's blood. In the home environment, the sample will almost always involve venous blood, which you'll draw by performing a venipuncture. Occasionally, you may need to draw a sample of arterial blood, usually for arterial blood gas (ABG) analysis.

Venous sample

Venipuncture involves piercing a vein with a needle and allowing blood to flow into a syringe or evacuated tube. Prepare for your venipuncture by making sure you have a tourniquet, gloves, a syringe or needle holder, evacuated color-top tubes, alcohol pads, povidone-iodine pads, needles of the appropriate gauge (usually 20G, 21G, and 25G), labels, laboratory request forms, 2″ × 2″ gauze pads, and adhesive tape or bandages. Select the appropriate tubes and label them with the patient's name, medical record number, date and time of the sample, and test needed. (See *Guide to color-top collection tubes,* pages 154 to 156.)

Now wash your hands and put on a pair of gloves. Remember that you must follow standard precautions. As necessary, briefly tell the patient about the process of drawing blood. Look at the patient's arms to find possible venipuncture sites. The antecubital fossa is the most common location for venipuncture, but you can use other locations on the hand, wrist, or arm if you need to.

Try to avoid using leg veins for venipuncture because puncturing them raises the risk of thrombophlebitis. Also avoid using any extremity that:

- has an active, infected wound
- is edematous
- has an arteriovenous shunt
- is on the same side as a mastectomy
- had a previous hematoma
- has a vascular injury.

Once you've selected a likely site, open the needle and attach it to the holder. Then apply the tourniquet about 2″ (5 cm) above the site. (To reduce the risk of hematoma, don't use a tourniquet if the patient has full, bounding veins.) Make it tight enough to impede venous flow but not tight enough to impede arterial flow. If the veins don't become engorged, ask the patient to open and close his fist a few times to help the veins distend. Then have him make a fist and hold it.

If the veins still don't fill and you can't find a good venipuncture site, you can try placing a warm cloth over the patient's arm for about 5 minutes. The heat will help the veins distend and become more prominent.

When you've settled on a particular vein, open a packet containing an alcohol or povidone-iodine pad and begin cleaning the area. If you're using povidone-iodine, start at the center and clean outward in a circular pattern. Don't wipe off the povidone-iodine with alcohol. If you're using alcohol, apply it to the skin with friction for at least 30 seconds. Then allow the skin to air-dry before performing the venipuncture.

When the skin has dried, immobilize the area by pressing down just beneath the puncture area. Grasp the needle holder so the needle is bevel up, with the shaft parallel to the skin. Then glide the needle into the vein. Hold the needle steady with one hand while you smoothly push a tube into

(Text continues on page 157.)

Guide to color-top collection tubes

The colors of collection tubes can vary from laboratory to laboratory. This guide lists the most commonly used collection tubes. Consult your laboratory for its specific collection tube requirements.

RED

Red-top *tubes contain no additives. Draw volume may be 2 to 20 ml. These tubes are used for tests performed on serum samples.*

ABO blood typing
Acetaminophen
Acetylcholine receptor antibodies
Alpha-fetoprotein
Androstenedione
Angiotensin-converting enzyme
Antibody screening
Anticonvulsants
Antidepressants, plasma
Antidiuretic hormone
Antideoxyribonucleic acid antibodies
Antiglobulin, direct
Antimicrobials
Antimitochondrial antibodies
Anti–smooth-muscle antibodies
Antistreptolysin-O
Antithyroid antibodies
Arginine
Barbiturates
Bronchodilators
Ceruloplasmin
Cold agglutinins
Creatinine clearance
C-reactive protein
Crossmatching
D-xylose absorption
Estrogens
Ethanol, blood
Extractable nuclear antigen antibodies
Febrile agglutination tests
Ferritin
Fluorescent treponemal antibody absorption
Fungal serology
Haptoglobin
Heterophil agglutination
Hexosaminidase A and B
Human chorionic gonadotropin
Human placental lactogen
Hypnotics
HIV antibody, serum enzyme
Immunoglobulins A,G, and M
Immune complex assays
Insulin
Iron and total iron-binding capacity
Isocitrate dehydrogenase
Isopropanol
Leucine aminopeptidase
Leukoagglutinins
Long-acting thyroid stimulator
Lupus erythematosus cell preparation
Luteinizing hormone, plasma
Lyme disease test
Methanol
Myoglobin
5'-Nucleotidase
Ornithine carbamoyltransferase
Parathyroid hormone (parathormone)
Phenothiazines
Prothrombin consumption time
Radioallergosorbent test
Rh typing
Rheumatoid factor
Rubella antibodies
Salicylates
Thyroid-stimulating hormone, neonatal
Thyroxine
Thyroxine-binding globulin
Tranquilizers

Guide to color-top collection tubes *(continued)*

RED *(continued)*
Transferrin
Triiodothyronine (T_3)
Venereal Disease Research Laboratory test
Vitamin A and carotene
Vitamin B_2
Vitamin D_3

MARBLE

Marble-top *tubes contain a silicone gel to separate serum from cells.*

Acid phosphatase
Alanine aminotransferase
Alkaline phosphatase
Amylase
Aspartate aminotransferase
Bilirubin
Blood urea nitrogen
Calcium
Carcinoembryonic antigen
Chloride
Cholesterol, total
Cholinesterase
Creatine
Creatine kinase
Creatinine
Cryoglobulins
Digitalis glycosides
Folic acid
Follicle-stimulating hormone
Free thyroxine and free triiodothyronine
Gamma-glutamyltransferase
Gastrin
Growth hormone/somatropic hormone
Growth hormone suppression (glucose loading)
Hepatitis B surface antigen
Hydroxybutyric dehydrogenase
Lactate dehydrogenase
Lipase
Lipoprotein-cholesterol fractionation
Magnesium
Phosphates
Phospholipids
Potassium
Prolactin
Protein electrophoresis
Sodium
T_3 resin uptake
Testosterone
Thyroid-stimulating hormone
Triglycerides
Tubular reabsorption of phosphate
Urea clearance
Uric acid
Vitamin B_{12}

LAVENDER

Lavender-top *tubes contain EDTA. Draw volume may be 2 to 10 ml. These tubes are used for tests performed on whole blood samples.*

ABO blood typing
Adrenocorticotropic hormone (corticotropin)
Antidiuretic hormone
Complete blood count
Coombs' direct test
Erythrocyte sedimentation rate
Glucagon
Glucose-6-phosphate dehydrogenase
Heinz bodies
Hematocrit
Hemoglobin,glycosylated
Hemoglobin, total
Hemoglobin, unstable
Hemoglobin electrophoresis
Lead
Lipoprotein phenotyping

(continued)

Guide to color-top collection tubes *(continued)*

LAVENDER *(continued)*

Plasma renin activity
Platelet count
Platelet survival
Pyruvate kinase
Red blood cell count
Red cell indices
Reticulocyte count
Rh typing
Sickle cell test (hemoglobin S)
White blood cell count
White blood cell differential

GREEN

***Green-top** tubes contain heparin. Draw volume may be 2 to 15 ml. These tubes are used for tests performed on plasma samples.*

Amino acid scan
Ammonia
Androstenedione
Angiotensin-converting enzyme
Calcitonin (thyrocalcitonin)
Catecholamines
Chromosomal analysis
Erythropoietic porphyrins
Galactose-1-phosphate uridyltransferase
Insulin intolerance
Insulin clearance
Lymphocyte transformation
Osmotic fragility
Para-aminohippuric acid excretion
Rapid adrenocorticotropic hormone
Red blood cell survival time
Terminal deoxynucleotidyl transferase
Uroporphyrinogen I synthase

BLUE

***Blue-top** tubes contain sodium citrate and citric acid. Draw volume may be 2.7 or 4.5 ml. These tubes are used for coagulation studies requiring plasma samples.*

Activated partial thromboplastin time
Euglobulin lysis time
Fibrinogen
Hemoglobin derivatives
One-stage assay: Extrinsic coagulation system
One-stage assay: Intrinsic coagulation system
Plasminogen
Platelet aggregation
Protein C
Protein S
Prothrombin time
Thrombin time
Tissue thromboplastin inhibitor study (lupus anticoagulation)

BLACK

***Black-top** tubes contain sodium oxalate. Draw volume may be 2.7 or 4.5 ml. These tubes are used for coagulation studies performed on plasma samples.*

Plasma vitamin C
Fibrin split products

GRAY

***Gray-top** tubes contain a glycolytic inhibitor (such as sodium fluoride, powdered oxalate, or glycolytic/microbial inhibitor). Draw volume may be 3 to 10 ml. These tubes are used most often for glucose determinations in serum or plasma samples.*

Glucose serum (all types)
Insulin tolerance
Lactic acid and pyruvic acid
Tolbutamide tolerance

place. Ask the patient to release his fist if he's been holding it. Because of the vacuum in the tube, blood should flow freely into it.

Collect as many tubes of blood as you need for your test. When you've filled the final tube, remove it from the needle holder. Position a gauze pad over the puncture site and, while holding it in place, gently remove the needle from the patient's arm. Have the patient place two fingers over the gauze pad, then bend his arm at the elbow to create pressure on the puncture site. Ask him to hold the pressure for at least 2 minutes or until the bleeding stops. If he takes an anticoagulant or has a clotting disorder, tell him to maintain firm pressure for at least 5 minutes to help prevent hematoma formation. Then apply a small bandage over the site. Discard all used items according to standard precautions.

If you're using a syringe instead of evacuated tubes, remember to begin drawing blood slowly. If you pull the plunger back too rapidly, you'll collapse the vein, reducing your chance of obtaining an adequate sample. Once you've drawn blood into the syringe, you can transfer it to the appropriate testing containers.

Before you leave the patient's home, reassess the puncture site to make sure a hematoma hasn't formed. If it has, apply warm soaks to the site.

Arterial sample

If the patient needs ABG analysis, you'll have to perform an arterial puncture to obtain a sample of arterial blood. Usually, you'll use the radial, brachial, or femoral artery.

If you intend to use the radial artery, first perform Allen's test to make sure the patient has a patent ulnar artery. (See *Performing Allen's test,* page 158.) Then explain to the patient a little about an arterial puncture. Urge him to breathe normally during the puncture. Tell him that it's normal to feel a brief cramping or throbbing pain at the puncture site. Reassure him that you'll be removing only a small amount of blood.

If your patient is on oxygen, don't draw an arterial sample within 15 minutes of starting, stopping, or changing his therapy. If you're supposed to run the test on room air, stop the oxygen flow and wait 15 or 20 minutes before performing the puncture. Don't suction the patient just before performing an arterial puncture.

To perform the puncture, wash your hands and put gloves on. If you'll be using the radial artery, place the patient's wrist on a small rolled towel, palm up. Find the artery and palpate it. You should feel a strong pulse. Clean the puncture site with povidone-iodine or alcohol in the same manner described for performing a venipuncture.

Palpate the artery with the index and middle fingers of your nondominant hand while you hold the syringe with your dominant hand, bevel up, at a 30- to 45-degree angle over the puncture site (as shown below). When puncturing the brachial artery, hold the needle at a 60-degree angle. Puncture the artery with a smooth motion, following the vessel's path.

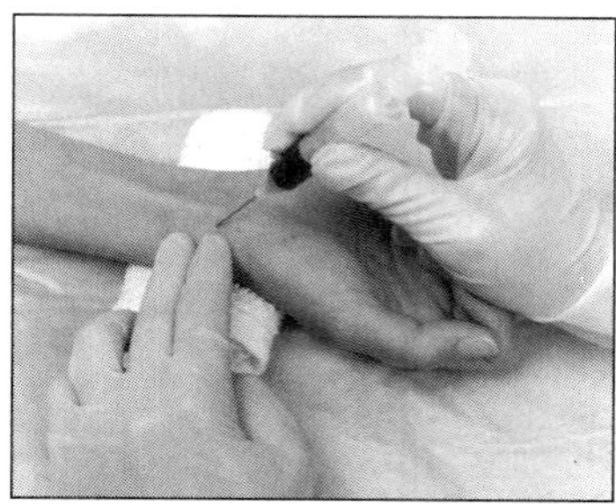

Blood should begin flowing on its own into the heparinized syringe. You shouldn't have to pull back on the

Performing Allen's test

Before performing an arterial puncture of your patient's radial artery, you'll need to perform Allen's test to be sure his ulnar artery can bring plenty of oxygenated blood to his hand after the puncture. Here's what to do.

Rest the patient's arm on the mattress or a table. Make sure it's below heart level. Now ask the patient to make a fist while you occlude both his radial and ulnar arteries (as shown below). Hold this position for a few seconds.

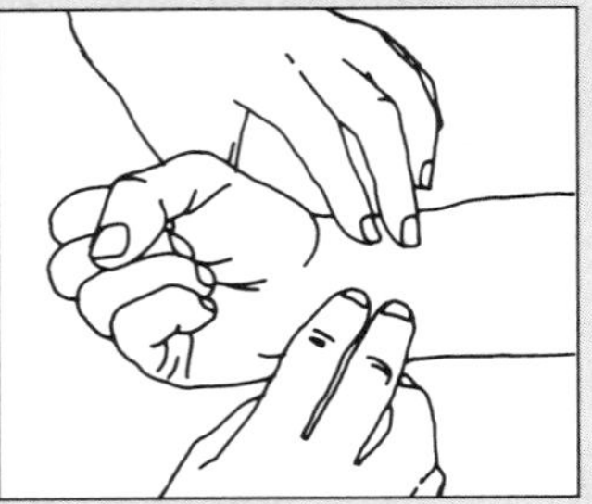

Without removing your fingers from the patient's arteries, ask him to unclench his fist and hold his hand in a relaxed position (as shown above right). Look at the color of his palm. It should be blanched because pressure from your fingers has blocked arterial blood from passing to his palm through the radial and ulnar arteries.

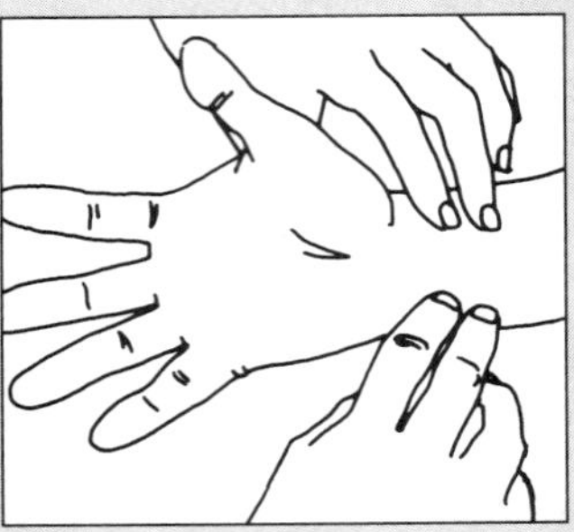

Finally, release pressure on the ulnar artery while maintaining pressure on the radial artery (as shown below). If the ulnar artery is patent, you'll see his palm flush. If that happens, you can proceed with the arterial puncture.

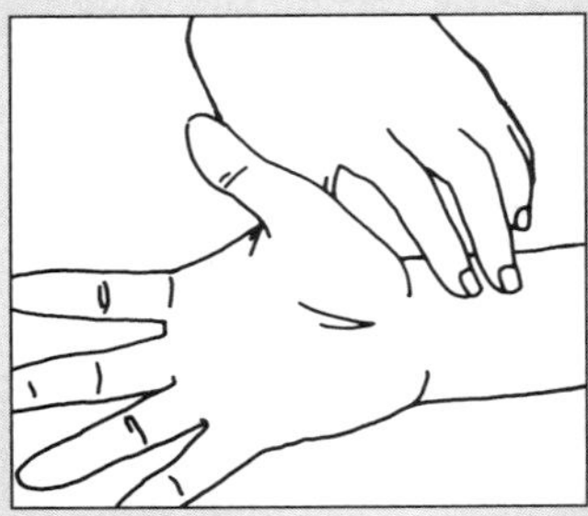

If the patient's palm doesn't flush when you release the ulnar artery, you'll have to perform Allen's procedure on the other wrist to see if you can use that arm for the arterial puncture.

plunger when you're drawing arterial blood. Once you've collected a 5-ml sample, withdraw the needle and press a gauze pad firmly on the site for at least 5 minutes. If the patient takes an anticoagulant or has a blood dyscrasia, bleeding probably won't stop for 10 or 15 minutes. Then tape a gauze pad firmly over the site.

Try to avoid having the patient apply pressure to an arterial puncture site. If he doesn't apply enough pressure, or doesn't apply it long enough, he may develop a large, painful hematoma that could thwart future arterial punctures at that site. For that reason, you're better off applying the pressure yourself or asking a team member to do it, if someone's at the home with you.

If you see air bubbles inside the syringe, you'll need to remove them because they can alter the results of the test for partial pressure of arterial oxygen (PaO_2). Hold the syringe upright and slowly eject some of the blood onto a gauze pad.

After inserting the needle into a rubber stopper to keep blood from leaking out, label the sample, pack it in ice, attach a laboratory request form, and deliver it to the laboratory right away.

◆ MANAGING OTHER TESTS

You may be called upon to perform a variety of other tests in the patient's home, such as sputum tests, stool tests, and cultures of wound exudate, among others. Many are described in detail later in the chapter. Naturally, each has its own requirements.

Many diagnostic tests require the patient to fast beforehand or to abstain from specific foods and beverages. In such cases, you can ensure accurate results only by giving the patient ample verbal and written instructions. Make your instructions as specific as possible. For example, be sure to address the following issues:

◆ Rather than simply telling the patient to fast overnight, tell him how many hours to go without eating before the test.

◆ Tell the patient whether or not he should take his regular medications during the fasting time before his test. If the test requires that the patient take no medications, give him that information in enough time for him to comply.

◆ If the patient must alter his diet before the test, explain exactly how he should alter it and for how long. If he must consume or avoid certain foods or beverages, provide him with a written list so he can remember.

◆ If the patient must drink a specific solution for the test, arrange a way for him to obtain the needed solution in plenty of time to prepare for the test. If possible, arrange to have a backup supply as well, in case the solution is damaged, lost, or destroyed by accident.

◆ ENSURING SAFE SPECIMEN TRANSPORT

The final step in ensuring accurate diagnostic tests for your home care patients is making the trip from the patient's home to the laboratory or the laboratory's deposit site. In general, the best way to achieve success in the transport phase is to be prepared ahead of time.

For example, contact the laboratory before you draw the specimen. Ask about any specific precautions you should take to make sure the specimen stays viable. Find out if it should be transported in a particular kind of container. If the sample needs to be kept cool, obtain a cooling container from the laboratory ahead of time. Also, make sure the laboratory knows when the sample will arrive.

When transporting any specimen, make sure it's in a secure location in your car. Keep a spill kit in your home care bag in case of a mishap. Keep the specimen at the proper temperature, and be sure to drop it off within the laboratory's specified time frame. If you'll be unavoidably delayed, contact the laboratory and find out if you can do anything to keep the specimen viable for a longer time.

If you know that a specimen has been contaminated, don't take it to the laboratory for analysis. You'll have to arrange with the patient to collect another specimen to replace the contaminated one.

◆ INTERPRETING COMMON TEST FINDINGS

A large part of your ability to ensure accurate diagnostic testing for your patients lies in collecting and transporting viable blood and urine specimens. To better understand your patients' conditions and manage care appropriately, you'll also need to understand normal test values and the implications of abnormal values. The rest of this chapter provides descriptions of some of the most common and important diagnostic tests you'll perform in your patients' homes.

Activated partial thromboplastin time

Activated partial thromboplastin time (APTT) measures clotting factors (except platelets) in the intrinsic pathway. Specifically, it measures the time needed for the patient's blood to clot after calcium and phospholipid emulsions are added to the sample. A clotting factor such as kaolin may be added as well to shorten the clotting time.

Purpose

The APTT test is used to:

◆ screen for bleeding tendencies
◆ screen for clotting factor deficiencies in the intrinsic pathway
◆ monitor heparin therapy.

Procedure-related nursing care

Tell the patient that you'll need to draw a blood sample from one of his veins, probably in his arm or hand. Review the steps of the venipuncture process with him. Reassure the patient that you'll remove only a small amount of blood. If the patient takes heparin, tell him that his doctor may want to repeat this test regularly to monitor his blood's clotting status.

Perform the venipuncture and fill a 7-ml blue-top tube. Then gently invert the tube several times to disperse the additive. Place the tube in a cooler and transport it to the laboratory. An insufficient blood sample, inadequate mixing with the additive, and improper transportation of the sample to the laboratory all contribute to incorrect test results.

If the patient takes an anticoagulant, exert firm pressure on the puncture site until the bleeding stops — usually for 5 to 10 minutes. If a hematoma develops at the site, apply warm, wet compresses.

Reference values

Once the clotting agents are added to the sample at the laboratory, a fibrin clot will form, usually within 25 to 36 seconds. If the patient is on anticoagulant therapy, the clot will take longer to form. The attending doctor should be contacted to specify the values for the type of therapy being administered.

Implications of results

A prolonged APTT might indicate:

◆ a deficiency of certain plasma clotting factors
◆ long-term warfarin (Coumadin) therapy
◆ the presence of heparin
◆ the presence of fibrin split products, fibrinolysins, or circulating anticoagulants, which are antibodies to specific clotting factors.

Alanine aminotransferase

Alanine aminotransferase (ALT) is one of two specialized enzymes that catalyze a reversible amino group transfer reaction in the Krebs cycle. Thus, ALT is necessary for tissue energy production.

ALT accumulates in the bloodstream when liver cells are damaged. It appears in hepatocellular cytoplasm and, in small amounts, in the kidneys, heart, and skeletal muscles. Depending on the laboratory, this test may be referred to as alanine transaminase or serum glutamic-pyruvic transaminase (SGPT).

Purpose

ALT levels are used to:

◆ detect and evaluate treatment of acute hepatic disease, especially hepatitis and cirrhosis not accompanied by jaundice

◆ help distinguish hepatic tissue damage from myocardial tissue damage when used in conjunction with the aspartate aminotransferase (AST) test

◆ assess the hepatotoxicity of certain medications.

Procedure-related nursing care

Explain to the patient that this test measures how well his liver is functioning. Tell him that you'll need to draw a blood sample from one of his veins, probably in his arm or hand. Review the steps of the venipuncture process with him. Reassure the patient that you'll remove only a small amount of blood.

Perform the venipuncture and fill a 7-ml red-marble-top tube. To prevent hemolysis, place the specimen in a sturdy container. ALT levels are stable in serum for up to 3 days if stored at room temperature. Make a note on the laboratory slip if the patient takes a hepatotoxic or cholestatic medication, such as methotrexate, chlorpromazine, salicylates, or narcotics. Ideally, these medications should be withheld before drawing the blood sample.

If a hematoma develops at the venipuncture site, apply warm, wet compresses. Have the patient resume his hepatotoxic medication if it was withheld before the test.

Reference values

Normally, serum ALT levels range from 10 to 35 U/L.

Implications of results

Occasionally, marginal elevations occur in acute myocardial infarction as a result of secondary hepatic congestion or release of some ALT from myocardial tissue. Slight to moderate elevations might appear in conditions that produce acute hepatocellular injury, such as active cirrhosis and drug-induced or alcoholic hepatitis.

Moderate to high ALT levels might indicate infectious mononucleosis, chronic hepatitis, intrahepatic cholestasis or cholecystitis, early or improving acute viral hepatitis, or severe hepatic congestion caused by heart failure.

Extremely high ALT levels (up to or over 50 times the normal range) indicate viral or severe drug-induced hepatitis or other hepatic disease with liver tissue necrosis. Ingestion of or exposure to lead or carbon tetrachloride causes direct injury to hepatic cells, leading to sharp elevations of ALT.

Many medications produce hepatic injury by interfering with cellular metabolism. Falsely elevated ALT levels can be seen in patients who use barbiturates, chlorpromazine, griseofulvin, isoniazid, methyldopa, nitrofurantoin, para-aminosalicylic acid, phenothiazines, phenytoin, salicylates, and tetracycline. Narcotic analgesics, such as morphine, codeine, and meperidine, might also cause false ALT elevations by increasing intrabiliary pressure. Rough handling of the blood sample also may interfere with accurate ALT levels.

Alkaline phosphatase

Alkaline phosphatase (ALP) is an enzyme that influences bone calcification and the transport of lipid metabolites. Most active at a pH of 9.0, it reflects the combined activity of several ALP isoenzymes found in the liver, bones, kidneys, intestinal lining, and placenta. ALP is particularly sensitive to mild biliary obstruction. This test measures ALP levels.

Purpose

ALP levels are used to:

◆ assess the effectiveness of vitamin D therapy used for deficiency-induced rickets

◆ detect focal hepatic lesions, such as tumors or abscesses, which cause biliary obstruction

◆ detect skeletal diseases characterized by marked osteoblastic activity

◆ supplement information from other liver function studies and GI enzyme tests.

Procedure-related nursing care

Explain to the patient that this test is used to assess liver or bone function. Tell him to abstain from food and fluids for at least 8 hours before the test. Tell him that you'll need to draw a blood sample from one of his veins, probably in his arm or hand. Review the steps of the venipuncture process with him. Reassure the patient that you'll remove only a small amount of blood.

Perform the venipuncture and fill a 7-ml red-marble-top tube. Handle the specimen gently to prevent hemolysis, which can alter the test results. Deliver the blood specimen to the laboratory immediately after you draw it. It should be analyzed within 4 hours. ALP activity increases at room temperature because its pH rises.

If a hematoma develops at the venipuncture site, apply warm, wet compresses.

Reference values

Normal ALP levels may vary, depending on the laboratory method used. Typically, total serum ALP levels measured by chemical inhibition range as follows:

◆ *Men: 98 to 251 U/L*

◆ *Women: 81 to 312 U/L (depending on age)*

Implications of results

Significantly elevated ALP levels probably indicate skeletal disease or an extrahepatic or intrahepatic biliary obstruction causing cholestasis. Other acute hepatic diseases also cause ALP levels to increase before serum bilirubin levels change.

Moderately increased ALP levels may reflect acute biliary obstruction from hepatocellular inflammation caused by active cirrhosis, mononucleosis, or viral hepatitis. It also could result from osteomalacia or deficiency-induced rickets.

Sharply increased ALP levels might indicate complete biliary obstruction caused by malignant or infectious infiltrations or fibrosis. These high levels are common in Paget's disease and occasionally occur in extensive bone metastasis or hyperparathyroidism. Metastatic bone tumors caused by pancreatic cancer will raise ALP levels without a corresponding increase in serum alanine aminotransferase levels.

Keep in mind that many factors can raise ALP levels. For example, ALP can rise after recent ingestion of vitamin D. Levels may rise greatly if the patient had a recent infusion of albumin that was made from placental venous blood. ALP also rises during the third trimester of pregnancy. Patients with healing long-bone fractures have increased levels, as do infants, children, adolescents, and women over age 45.

Rough handling of the blood specimen can interfere with accurate ALP determination.

Medications that influence liver function or result in cholestasis, such as barbiturates, chlorpropamide, isoniazid, methyldopa, oral contraceptives, phenothiazines, phenytoin, and rifampin, can cause mild ALP elevations. Patients sensitive to halothane might experience drastic increases in ALP.

Although rarely seen, low ALP levels signify hypophosphatasia and protein or magnesium deficiency. Clofibrate decreases levels as well.

Amylase, serum

Amylase is an enzyme synthesized primarily in the pancreas and salivary glands. It's secreted into the GI tract and helps digest starch and glycogen in the mouth, stomach, and intestines. Alterations in serum amylase levels can indicate acute pancreatic disease.

Purpose

Serum amylase levels are used to:

- ◆ assess pancreatic injury caused by abdominal surgery or trauma
- ◆ diagnose acute pancreatitis
- ◆ distinguish acute pancreatitis from other causes of abdominal pain that might require immediate surgery.

Procedure-related nursing care

Explain to the patient that this test is used to measure pancreatic function. Instruct the patient to abstain from alcohol for at least 24 hours before the test. Tell him that you'll need to draw a blood sample from one of his veins, probably in his arm or hand. Review the steps of the venipuncture process with him. Reassure the patient that you'll remove only a small amount of blood.

Perform the venipuncture and fill a 7-ml red-marble-top tube. Handle the specimen gently to prevent hemolysis, which can alter the test results. If a hematoma develops at the venipuncture site, apply warm, wet compresses.

Document on the laboratory slip any drugs the patient might have ingested recently that could affect the amylase level, including aspirin, asparaginase, azathioprine, corticosteroids, ciproheptadine, narcotic analgesics, oral contraceptives, rifampin, sulfasalazine, and thiazide or loop diuretics.

This test should be done before other diagnostic or therapeutic procedures, especially if the patient complains of acute right upper quadrant abdominal pain.

Reference values

More than 20 methods are available to measure serum amylase levels, all with different normal ranges. That means serum amylase values vary widely depending on the method used. Typically, levels for adults 18 years or older range from 25 to 115 U/L

Implications of results

High serum amylase levels occur 4 to 12 hours after the onset of acute pancreatitis. Over the next 48 to 72 hours, the levels return to normal. If the doctor suspects pancreatitis but the patient has normal serum amylase levels, an analysis of urine amylase levels should be performed.

Moderately elevated serum amylase levels may result from obstructions of the common bile duct, pancreatic duct, or Vater's ampulla. They also may result from pancreatic injury from a perforated peptic ulcer, pancreatic cancer, acute salivary gland disease, ectopic pregnancy, peritonitis, ovarian or lung cancer, and impaired renal function.

Slightly elevated levels have been seen in patients who are asymptomatic or are responding in an unusual manner to treatment. Additional tests, such as amylase fractionation, will help determine the source of the amylase.

Falsely elevated serum amylase levels have been associated with ingestion of large amounts of alcohol, use of certain medications, recent peripancreatic surgery, a perforated or abscessed ulcer or intestine, a spasm at the sphincter of Oddi, or macroamylasemia.

Decreased serum amylase levels may result from chronic pancreatitis, cirrhosis, hepatitis, pancreatic cancer, and toxemia of pregnancy.

Arterial blood gas analysis

Arterial blood gas (ABG) analysis is used to evaluate gas exchange in the lungs by measuring the partial pressure of arterial oxygen (PaO_2) and the partial pressure of arterial carbon dioxide ($PaCO_2$). PaO_2 shows how much oxygen the lungs are delivering to the blood. $PaCO_2$ shows how efficiently the lungs are eliminating carbon dioxide from the body.

ABG analysis also allows you to check for acidosis or alkalosis by measuring blood pH, hydrogen ion concentration, oxygen content, oxygen saturation (SaO_2), and bicarbonate (HCO_3^-) levels. Acidosis is indicated by decreased blood pH, increased hydrogen ions, and decreased bicarbonate. Alkalosis is indicated by increased pH, decreased hydrogen ions, and increased bicarbonate.

Purpose

ABG analysis is used to:

- ◆ assess the efficiency of mechanical ventilation
- ◆ determine acid-base balance in the blood
- ◆ evaluate the efficiency of pulmonary gas exchange
- ◆ monitor respiratory therapy.

Procedure-related nursing care

Explain to the patient that this test is used to measure his respiratory function. Tell the patient that you'll need to draw a blood sample from one of his arteries, probably in his wrist. Review the steps of the arterial puncture with him. Reassure the patient that you'll remove only a small amount of blood.

If Allen's test is normal, perform the arterial puncture and fill a heparinized syringe. Pack the sample in a bag of ice before transporting it to the laboratory.

If you used the radial artery, apply pressure to the puncture site for at least 5 minutes. If you used the femoral artery or if the patient is on anticoagulant therapy, hold the puncture site for at least 10 minutes. After applying pressure, tape a gauze pad firmly over the puncture. Don't wrap the tape around the limb.

On the laboratory request, note whether the patient was breathing room air or supplemental oxygen when you drew the sample. If he was receiving oxygen, include the flow rate. If he was on mechanical ventilation, write the fraction of inspired air and tidal volume. For all ABG samples, document the patient's rectal temperature and respiratory rate at the time you collected the sample.

After the puncture, stay with the patient so you can monitor his vital signs. Assess the limb for signs and symptoms of circulatory impairment, including discoloration, numbness, pain, swelling, and tingling. Check the puncture site for continued bleeding.

Reference values

Normally, ABG values should be within the following ranges:

- *pH: 7.35 to 7.45*
- *PaO_2: 75 to 100 mm Hg*
- *$PaCO_2$: 35 to 45 mm Hg*
- *O_2 content: 15% to 23%*
- *SaO_2: 94% to 100%*
- *HCO_3^-: 22 to 26 mEq/L*

Implications of results

A blood pH over 7.42 indicates alkalosis; under 7.35, it indicates acidosis. A PaO_2 below 50 mm Hg indicates hypoxia. Even a PaO_2 between 50 and 75 mm Hg might signal hypoxia, depending on the patient's age and concentration of inspired oxygen. Patients over age 60 may normally have a PaO_2 below 75 mm Hg.

A $PaCO_2$ over 45 mm Hg indicates hypoventilation or hypercapnia. Levels below 35 mm Hg indicate hyperventilation or hypocapnia. An elevated $PaCO_2$ can be caused by use of bicarbonate, ethacrynic acid, hydrocortisone, metolazone, prednisone, and thiazides. A low $PaCO_2$ might be caused by use of acetazolamide, methicillin, nitrofurantoin, and tetracycline.

Patients with a PaO_2 between 60 and 100 mm Hg should have an SaO_2 above 85%. If the SaO_2 drops, the PaO_2 has probably dropped below 50 mm Hg.

An HCO_3^- value above 26 mEq/L can indicate either respiratory acidosis or metabolic alkalosis. Respiratory acidosis can be caused by central nervous system depression from drugs, injury, disease, or hypoventilation from respiratory, cardiac, musculoskeletal, or neuromuscular illness. Metabolic acidosis is seen in patients who have lost hydrochloric acid from prolonged vomiting or gastric suctioning, loss of potassium from increased renal excretion (or diuretic therapy), steroid overdose, or excessive alkali ingestion.

An HCO_3^- value below 22 mEq/L can indicate either respiratory alkalosis or metabolic acidosis. Respiratory alkalosis can be caused by hyperventilatory states or respiratory stimulation from drugs, disease, hypoxia, fever, or gram-negative bacteremia. Metabolic acidosis can be caused by bicarbonate depletion that stems from excessive diarrhea, renal disease, or small-bowel fistulas. Or it can stem from excessive acid production, as in hepatic disease and endocrine disorders, or inadequate acid secretion from renal disease.

Low PaO_2, O_2 content, and SaO_2 with a high $PaCO_2$ can result from conditions that impair respiratory function, such as respiratory muscle weakness or paralysis, respiratory center inhibition, and airway obstruction. Other low readings might result from bronchiole obstruction secondary to asthma or emphysema, an abnormal ventilation-perfusion ratio from partially blocked alveoli or pulmonary capillaries, or damaged or fluid-filled alveoli, as seen in hemorrhage or near drowning.

If inspired air contains a low oxygen content, the PaO_2, O_2 content, and SaO_2 decrease while the $PaCO_2$ remains normal. This finding is common in pneumothorax, impaired diffusion between alveoli and blood, and in an arteriovenous shunt, in which blood bypasses the lungs.

A low O_2 content with a normal PaO_2, SaO_2, and $PaCO_2$ may be seen in severe anemia, decreased blood volume, and reduced hemoglobin (Hb) oxygen-carrying capacity.

Exposing the sample to room air will alter the PaO_2 and $PaCO_2$ levels. Results will also be adversely affected if the syringe isn't heparinized, the sample isn't placed in a bag of ice, or the sample isn't taken to the laboratory immediately. An extremely elevated $PaCO_2$ with a severely low PaO_2 may indicate that venous blood has been mixed into the arterial sample.

Aspartate aminotransferase

Aspartate aminotransferase (AST) is one of two hepatic enzymes that catalyze conversion of the nitrogenous portion of an amino acid to an amino acid residue. This reaction is necessary for energy production via the Krebs cycle.

AST is found in the cytoplasm and mitochondria of many cells, primarily in the heart, kidneys, liver, pancreas, skeletal muscles and, in minimal amounts, the red blood cells.

When cellular damage occurs, AST is released into the plasma. Consequently, it can serve as an indication of hepatic and cardiac disease.

Depending on the laboratory, this test may also be known as aspartate transaminase or serum glutamic-oxaloacetic transaminase (SGOT).

Purpose

AST levels are used to:

- aid in identifying and diagnosing acute hepatic disease
- detect a recent myocardial infarction (MI), in conjunction with creatine kinase and lactate dehydrogenase levels
- monitor the progress of patients receiving treatment for cardiac or hepatic disease.

Procedure-related nursing care

Explain to the patient that this test is used to measure heart and liver function. Tell him that you'll need to draw a blood sample from one of his veins, probably in his arm or hand, over 3 consecutive days. Review the steps of the venipuncture process with him. Reassure the patient that you'll remove only a small amount of blood.

Perform the venipuncture and fill a 7-ml red-marble-top tube. Handle the sample gently to prevent hemolysis, which can alter the test results. If a hematoma develops at the venipuncture site, apply warm, wet compresses.

Transport the sample to the laboratory immediately. If you think the patient may have ingested a medication that could affect the test results, document it on the laboratory request. Include such medications as antitubercular drugs (isoniazid, para-aminosalicylates, and pyrazinamide), chlorpropamide, codeine, methyldopa, morphine, and phenazopyridine.

Make sure you note the time at which you drew the first sample. Then make arrangements with the patient to draw another sample at the same time on each of the next 2 days.

Reference values

Normal AST levels range from 8 to 20 U/L in males and from 5 to 40 U/L in females. Children's values are typically higher.

Implications of results

AST levels fluctuate with cellular necrosis. Levels may rise slightly early in the course of a disease and peak during the most acute phase. Increasing AST levels indicate worsening disease and subsequent tissue damage. Decreasing levels indicate disease resolution and tissue repair. Thus, you can track cellular damage and repair by carefully monitoring AST levels.

Slight elevations in the AST level may appear after the first few days of a biliary duct obstruction. Low to moderate elevations (2 to 5 times the normal level) may suggest hemolytic anemia, metastatic hepatic tumors, acute pancreatitis, pulmonary emboli, alcohol withdrawal syndrome, or fatty liver.

Moderate to high AST levels (5 to 10 times the normal level) may indicate Duchenne's muscular dystrophy, dermatomyositis, or chronic hepatitis. They also may be seen in the prodromal or resolution stages of diseases that typically cause high AST elevations.

High AST elevations (10 to 20 times the normal level) may arise after severe MI, severe infectious mononucleosis, and alcoholic cirrhosis. High levels also are seen during the prodromal or resolution stages of illnesses that cause extremely high levels.

Extremely high elevations (more than 20 times the normal level) may indicate acute viral hepatitis, severe skeletal trauma, extensive surgery, drug-induced hepatic injury, or severe passive hepatic congestion.

Medications known to affect the liver can elevate AST levels. They include chlorpropamide, opiates, methyldopa, erythromycin, sulfonamides, pyridoxine, dicumarol, antitubercular agents, large doses of acetaminophen, salicylates, and vitamin A. Strenuous exercise and muscle trauma after I.M. injections can raise AST levels as well.

Inappropriate handling of the blood sample can lead to hemolysis and affect test results. Failure to draw subsequent AST values at the same time of day can also interfere with test results.

Bilirubin, serum

Bilirubin, the primary pigment in bile, is the major byproduct of hemoglobin catabolism. It's formed in the reticuloendothelial system. Once formed, it then binds with albumin and is transported to the liver as unconjugated bilirubin. While in the liver, it joins with glucuronic acid to form bilirubin glucuronide and bilirubin diglucuronide for excretion into bile as conjugated bilirubin.

A properly functioning hepatobiliary system and a normal turnover rate of red blood cells (RBCs) is essential for the effective conjugation and excretion of bilirubin.

Levels of serum bilirubin are especially significant in neonates because unexcreted unconjugated bilirubin can accumulate in the brain, leading to irreparable brain damage.

Purpose

Serum bilirubin levels are used to:

- aid in the differential diagnosis of jaundice and monitor the progress of treatment
- aid in diagnosing biliary obstruction and hemolytic anemia
- evaluate hepatobiliary and erythropoietic functions
- determine whether a neonate requires treatment.

Procedure-related nursing care

Explain to the patient or the parents of a newborn that this test is used to evaluate liver function and the condition of RBCs. Instruct the patient or parents to withhold food and fluids for at least 4 hours before the test. Explain that you'll need to draw a blood sample from a vein, probably in the arm or hand. If the patient is a newborn, tell the parents that you'll draw from the infant's heel. Review the steps of the venipuncture process. Reassure the patient or parents that you'll remove only a small amount of blood.

Perform the venipuncture and fill a 7-ml red-top or red-marble-top tube. If the patient is an infant, perform a heelstick and fill a microcapillary tube with blood to the designated level. Handle the sample gently to prevent hemolysis, which can affect test results. Also protect the sample from sunlight.

Document on the laboratory request any drugs the patient might have ingested recently that could interfere with serum bilirubin levels. Then transport the sample to the laboratory immediately.

If a hematoma develops at the venipuncture site, apply warm, wet compresses.

Reference values

In an adult, the normal indirect serum bilirubin level is 1.1 mg/dl or less; the normal direct serum bilirubin level is less than 0.5 mg/dl. In a neonate, the normal total serum bilirubin level is 1 to 12 mg/dl.

Implications of results

Elevated indirect serum bilirubin levels can indicate liver damage, severe hemolytic or pernicious anemia, hemolysis, a transfusion reaction, hemorrhage, or hepatocellular dysfunction related to viral hepatitis or congenital enzyme deficiencies, such as Gilbert's or Crigler-Najjar syndromes.

Elevated direct serum bilirubin levels typically indicate biliary obstruction. The obstruction blocks direct bilirubin from its normal path through the liver to the biliary tree, causing it to overflow into the bloodstream. The biliary obstruction may be inside the liver (from viral hepatitis, cirrhosis, or a chlorpromazine reaction) or outside the liver (from gallstones or cancer of the gallbladder or pancreas). Bile duct disease also can increase direct serum bilirubin levels.

If a biliary obstruction goes untreated, indirect bilirubin levels may also increase because of hepatic damage. In severe, chronic hepatic damage, direct bilirubin levels eventually return to normal or near-normal while indirect bilirubin levels remain elevated.

Blood urea nitrogen

This test measures the nitrogen fraction of urea, the major endproduct of protein metabolism. Formed in the liver from ammonia and excreted by the kidneys, urea accounts for 40% to 50% of the blood's nonprotein nitrogen. The blood urea nitrogen (BUN) level reflects protein intake and renal excretory capacity. However, the serum creatinine test is a more reliable indicator of uremia.

Purpose

BUN levels are used to:

- ◆ aid in diagnosing renal disease
- ◆ evaluate renal function
- ◆ assess hydration status.

Procedure-related nursing care

Explain to the patient that this test is used to evaluate kidney function. Instruct the patient to avoid a diet high in meat for 2 to 3 days before the test. Tell him that you'll need to draw a blood sample from one of his veins, probably in his arm or hand. Review the steps of the venipuncture process with him. Reassure the patient that you'll remove only a small amount of blood.

Perform the venipuncture and fill either a 7-ml or a 10- to 15-ml red-top or red-marble-top tube (depending on laboratory preference). Handle the sample gently to prevent hemolysis, which can alter test results.

Be sure to document on the laboratory request form any drugs the patient recently ingested that could interfere with BUN levels. They include chloramphenicol, tetracycline, growth hormone, and nephrotoxic drugs (aminoglycosides, amphotericin B, and methicillin). Then transport the sample to the laboratory immediately.

If a hematoma develops at the venipuncture site, apply warm, wet compresses.

Reference values

BUN levels normally range from 8 to 20 mg/dl. Elderly patients may have slightly higher levels.

Implications of results

Low BUN levels reflect malnutrition, overhydration, or severe hepatic damage. Chloramphenicol and growth hormone can falsely lower BUN levels.

Elevated BUN levels reflect renal disease, reduced renal blood flow (caused by dehydration), urinary tract obstruction, and conditions that increase protein catabolism such as burns. Nephrotoxic drugs (aminoglycosides, amphotericin B, corticosteroids, and methicillin) and tetracycline can elevate BUN levels.

Calcium, serum

Calcium is a cation that helps regulate and promote neuromuscular and enzyme activity, bone development, and blood coagulation. In the presence of vitamin D, the body absorbs calcium from the GI tract and excretes it in urine and feces. Over 98% of the body's calcium is located in the bones and teeth. However, calcium can shift in and out of these structures if the blood doesn't contain enough calcium to help regulate other body mechanisms. This test measures the amount of calcium in the blood.

Purpose

Serum calcium levels are used to help diagnose arrhythmias, blood-clotting deficiencies, acid-base imbalance, and neuromuscular, skeletal, and endocrine disorders.

Procedure-related nursing care

Explain to the patient that this test is used to measure calcium levels in the blood. Tell him that you'll need to draw a blood sample from one of his veins, probably in his arm or hand. Review the steps of the venipuncture process with him. Reassure the patient that you'll remove only a small amount of blood.

Perform the venipuncture without a tourniquet, if possible, and fill a 7-, 10-, or 15-ml red-top or marble-top tube.

Document any signs or symptoms that could indicate hypercalcemia, such as deep bone pain, flank pain, muscle hypotonicity, nausea, dehydration, or vomiting. Also document any signs or symptoms that could indicate hypocalcemia, such as circumoral peripheral tingling, muscle twitching, facial muscle spasm, tetany, muscle cramping, seizure, or arrhythmias.

If a hematoma develops at the venipuncture site, apply warm, wet compresses.

Reference values

Normal serum calcium levels in adults range from 8.9 to 10.1 mg/dl or from 4.5 to 5.5 mEq/L.

Implications of results

Slightly decreased serum calcium levels can occur in Cushing's syndrome, renal failure, acute pancreatitis, peritonitis, and excessive laxative use. Low levels (hypocalcemia) indicate hypoparathyroidism, total parathyroidectomy, or malabsorption syndrome.

Abnormally high serum calcium levels (hypercalcemia) may indicate hyperparathyroidism, parathyroid tumor, Paget's disease of the bone, multiple myeloma, metastatic cancer, multiple fractures, or prolonged immobilization. High levels may also result from:

- inadequate calcium excretion, as in adrenal insufficiency and renal disease
- excessive calcium ingestion, as in overuse of calcium carbonate antacids
- thiazide diuretics
- excessive intake of vitamin D, androgens, calciferol-activated calcium salts, progestins, estrogens, or thiazides.

Chloride, serum

The serum chloride test measures serum levels of chloride, the major anion in extracellular fluid. Chloride helps regulate blood volume and arterial pressure by interacting with sodium (the major extracellular cation) to control osmotic pressure. Chloride also affects acid-base balance. Excessive loss of chloride through gastric juices or other secretions can cause hypochloremic metabolic alkalosis. Excessive intake or retention of chloride can lead to hyperchloremic metabolic acidosis.

Purpose

Serum chloride is used to:

- detect acid-base imbalance
- help evaluate fluid status and extracellular cation-anion balance.

Procedure-related nursing care

Explain to the patient that this test is used to measure the chloride content of blood. Tell him that you'll need to draw a blood sample from one of his veins, probably in his arm or hand. Review the steps of the venipuncture process with him. Reassure the patient that you'll remove only a small amount of blood.

Perform the venipuncture and fill a 7-, 10-, or 15-ml red-top or red-marble-top tube. Handle the sample gently to prevent hemolysis, which can alter the test results.

Document any signs or symptoms that could indicate either a low or high serum chloride level. In hypochloremia, look for muscle hypertonicity, tetany, and a reduced respiratory rate. In hyperchloremia, look for pending stupor, weakness, and rapid, deep respirations.

If a hematoma develops at the venipuncture site, apply warm, wet compresses.

Reference values

Normal serum chloride levels range from 100 to 108 mEq/L.

Implications of results

Low serum chloride levels (hypochloremia) have been associated with low sodium and potassium levels. Underlying causes of hypochloremia include prolonged vomiting, gastric suctioning, intestinal fistula, chronic renal failure, and Addison's disease. Conditions that lead to excess extracellular fluid, such as heart failure and edema, can cause dilutional hypochloremia.

Increased serum chloride levels (hyperchloremia) may result from severe dehydration, complete renal shutdown, head injury leading to neurogenic hyperventilation, and primary aldosteronism.

Serum chloride levels are decreased by thiazides, furosemide, ethacrynic acid, bicarbonates, or prolonged I.V.

infusions of dextrose and water. Increased levels may be caused by ammonium chloride, cholestyramine, boric acid, oxyphenbutazone, phenylbutazone, or excessive I.V. infusions of sodium chloride.

Cholesterol, total

The total cholesterol test measures the circulating levels of the body's two forms of cholesterol: free cholesterol and cholesterol esters. Cholesterol is absorbed from the diet and synthesized in the liver and other body tissues. It's needed to form adrenocorticoid steroids, bile salts, androgens, and estrogens. A diet high in saturated fat increases cholesterol levels by stimulating the absorption of lipids from the intestine. High serum cholesterol levels may be associated with an increased risk of coronary artery disease. A diet low in saturated fat decreases the cholesterol level.

Purpose

Total cholesterol levels are used to:

- ◆ assess the risk of coronary artery disease
- ◆ evaluate fat metabolism
- ◆ help diagnose nephrotic syndrome, pancreatitis, hepatic disease, hypothyroidism, and hyperthyroidism.

Procedure-related nursing care

Explain to the patient that this test is used to assess the body's ability to metabolize fat. Instruct the patient to abstain from food and fluids for at least 12 hours and to not ingest alcohol for at least 24 hours before the test. Tell him that you'll need to draw a blood sample from one of his veins, probably in his arm or hand. Review the steps of the venipuncture process with him. Reassure the patient that you'll remove only a small amount of blood.

Perform the venipuncture and fill a 7-ml red-top or red-marble-top tube. Arrange for the sample to be transported to the laboratory immediately. If a hematoma develops at the venipuncture site, apply warm, wet compresses. Instruct the patient to resume his regular eating pattern.

Reference values

Total cholesterol levels vary with age. The normal adult range is between 150 and 200 mg/dl. Levels of 280 mg/dl or greater are elevated.

Implications of results

Low total cholesterol levels (hypocholesterolemia) are commonly associated with malnutrition, malabsorption, cellular necrosis of the liver, and hyperthyroidism. Further testing is indicated to pinpoint the definitive cause of low total cholesterol levels.

Elevated total cholesterol levels (hypercholesterolemia) may indicate an increased risk of coronary artery disease in addition to incipient hepatitis, lipid disorders, bile duct blockage, nephrotic syndrome, obstructive jaundice, pancreatitis, and hypothyroidism.

Certain drugs can raise cholesterol levels, including epinephrine, chlorpromazine, trifluoperazine, oral contraceptives, and trimethadione. Total cholesterol levels are lowered by cholestyramine, clofibrate, colestipol, dextrothyroxine, haloperidol, neomycin, niacin, and chlortetracycline. Androgens can either increase or decrease total cholesterol.

Complete blood count

The complete blood count (CBC) measures all blood elements: hemoglobin concentration, hematocrit (HCT), red blood cells (RBCs), white blood cells (WBCs), WBC differential, and stained RBC and platelet examination. A CBC is used to evaluate conditions in which the HCT doesn't parallel the RBC count. For more information on each of the CBC components, refer to each specific test.

Purpose

The CBC is used to:

◆ compare the status of specific blood elements

◆ detect anemia and determine its severity

◆ indicate whether further diagnostic studies are needed.

Procedure-related nursing care

Explain to the patient that this test is used to assess the different components of blood. Tell him that you'll need to draw a blood sample from one of his veins, probably in his arm or hand. Review the steps of the venipuncture process with him. Reassure the patient that you'll remove only a small amount of blood.

Perform the venipuncture and fill a 5-ml lavender-top tube. Invert the tube several times to thoroughly mix the additive within it. Arrange for the sample to be transported to the laboratory immediately. If a hematoma develops at the venipuncture site, apply warm, wet compresses.

Reference values

Except for the white blood cell count, values vary depending on age, sex, sample, and geographic location. Normally, blood element levels should be within the following ranges:

Hemoglobin

◆ *Men: 14 to 18 g/dl*

◆ *Women: 12 to 16 g/dl*

Hematocrit

◆ *Men: 42% to 54%*

◆ *Women: 38% to 46%*

Red blood cells

◆ *Men: 4.6 to 6.2 million/µl*

◆ *Women: 4.2 to 5.4 million/µl*

White blood cells

◆ *Men: 4,000 to 10,000/µl*

◆ *Women: 4,000 to 10,000/µl*

Implications of results

See the "Implications of results" section in the appropriate test entry.

Creatine kinase

Creatine kinase (CK) is an enzyme found primarily in muscle cells and brain tissue. It catalyzes the transfer of a phosphate group from adenosine triphosphate to creatine, creating energy in the process. Because of this process, CK reflects tissue catabolism. Elevated CK levels indicate cellular trauma.

The total CK value represents three separate isoenzymes: CK-BB, found in brain tissue; CK-MB, found in cardiac muscle; and CK-MM, found in skeletal muscle. Consequently, the CK value can be broken down to isolate the specific muscle type undergoing cellular degeneration.

Purpose

CK levels are used to:

◆ detect musculoskeletal disorders that don't have a neurogenic origin (Duchenne's muscular dystrophy or early dermatomyositis)

◆ diagnose acute myocardial infarction (MI) and reinfarction

◆ evaluate possible causes of chest pain

◆ monitor the severity of myocardial ischemia after cardiac surgery, catheterization, or cardioversion.

Procedure-related nursing care

Explain to the patient that this test is used to assess either heart or muscle function. Tell him that you'll need to draw a blood sample from one of his veins, probably in his arm or hand. Review the steps of the venipuncture process with him. Reassure the patient that you'll remove only a small amount of blood.

If the sample is being drawn to evaluate a musculoskeletal disorder, tell the patient to avoid exercising for at least 24 hours before the test. If the patient is scheduled to receive an I.M. injection, draw the sample beforehand or at least 1 hour afterward. If possible, withhold aminocaproic acid, lithium, and alcohol before the test. If that's not possible, be sure to note their use on the laboratory request.

Perform the venipuncture and fill a 7-ml red-top or red-marble-top tube. Arrange for the sample to be transported to the laboratory at once.

If a hematoma develops at the venipuncture site, apply warm, wet compresses. Instruct the patient to resume taking his medications.

Reference values

Normal total CK values range from 52 to 336 U/L for men and from 38 to 176 U/L for women. Elevations are possible in very muscular people. Normal isoenzyme values are:

- *CK-BB: Undetectable*
- *CK-MB: Undetectable to 7 U/L*
- *CK-MM: 5 to 70 U/L*

Implications of results

Total CK levels may increase in acute cerebrovascular disease, alcoholic cardiomyopathy, cerebral ischemia, carbon monoxide poisoning, malignant hyperthermia, muscular dystrophy, polymyositis, severe hypokalemia, and viral myositis. They also can increase in response to aminocaproic acid, large doses of alcohol, halothane, lithium, succinylcholine, cardioversion, I.M. injections, invasive procedures, recent vigorous exercise or massage, severe coughing, and trauma.

Detectable CK-BB values may indicate brain tissue injury, renal failure, severe shock, or widespread malignant tumors. A CK-MB value greater that 5% of the total CK value indicates an acute MI. This level will begin to rise 2 to 4 hours after the initial infarct, peak in 12 to 24 hours, and then return to normal over the next 24 to 48 hours. If the level remains high, suspect an ongoing infarction.

Elevated CK-MM levels result from skeletal muscle damage secondary to trauma or from such diseases as muscular dystrophy and hypothyroidism.

The test results will be altered if the sample isn't refrigerated or sent to the laboratory immediately. Don't refrigerate the sample for more than 2 hours; after that time, the results won't be accurate.

Creatinine clearance

This test determines how efficiently the kidneys remove creatinine from the blood. The end product of creatine, creatinine appears in amounts proportionate to total muscle mass and is usually unaffected by urine volume, regular physical activity, or diet. The rate of clearance is measured according to the number of milliliters of blood cleared by the kidneys in 1 minute. Both blood and urine specimens are needed for this test.

Purpose

Creatinine clearance rate is used to:

- assess renal glomerular filtration
- monitor the progression of renal insufficiency.

Procedure-related nursing care

Explain to the patient that this test is used to assess kidney function. Instruct the patient to avoid excessive amounts of meat, tea, and coffee for 2 to 3 days before the test. Also have him avoid strenuous physical activity during the test period.

Tell the patient that you'll need a timed urine specimen and at least one sample of venous blood. Teach the patient how to obtain a urine specimen over the ordered time frame, usually 2, 6, 12, or 24 hours. Tell him that you'll also need to draw a blood sample from one of his veins, probably in his arm or hand. Review the steps of the venipuncture process with him. Reassure the patient that you'll remove only a small amount of blood.

Perform the venipuncture any time during the urine collection period, and fill a 7-ml red-top tube. Deliver it to the laboratory right away. Instruct the patient to refrigerate his collected urine or keep it on ice during the collection period. At the end of the collection period, send the urine to the laboratory immediately.

If a hematoma develops at the venipuncture site, apply warm, wet compresses.

Reference values

Normal creatinine clearance values at age 20 have the following ranges:
- *Men: 85 to 146 ml/minute*
- *Women: 81 to 134 ml/minute*

Creatinine clearance normally decreases by 6 ml/minute for each decade after age 20.

Implications of results

Decreased creatinine clearance rates may result from reduced renal blood flow caused by shock or renal artery obstruction, acute tubular necrosis, acute or chronic glomerulonephritis, advanced bilateral renal lesions (as seen in polycystic kidney disease), renal tuberculosis, cancer, or nephrosclerosis. Decreased rates also may indicate heart failure or severe dehydration.

Increased creatinine clearance has no specific diagnostic significance.

Medications known to interfere with the results of this test include amphotericin B, thiazide diuretics, furosemide, and aminoglycosides.

Creatinine, serum

The serum creatinine test is a more accurate measure of renal function than blood urea nitrogen level because renal impairment is virtually the only cause of elevated serum creatinine. Creatinine is a nonprotein product of creatine metabolism. It appears in amounts proportionate to the amount of muscle mass. Because the kidneys easily excrete creatinine, serum levels are directly related to the renal glomerular filtration rate (GFR).

Purpose

Serum creatinine levels are used to:
- assess renal GFR
- screen for renal damage.

Procedure-related nursing care

Explain to the patient that this test is used to assess kidney function. Tell him that you'll need to draw a blood sample from one of his veins, probably in his arm or hand. Review the steps of the venipuncture process with him. Reassure the patient that you'll remove only a small amount of blood.

Perform the venipuncture and fill either a 7-ml or 10- to 15-ml red-top or red-marble-top tube. Arrange for the sample to be transported to the laboratory immediately. Note on the laboratory request if the patient has ingested ascorbic acid, barbiturates, or diuretics over the past 24 hours.

If a hematoma develops at the venipuncture site, apply warm, wet compresses.

Reference values

Normal serum creatinine levels range from 0.8 to 1.2 mg/dl in men and from 0.6 to 0.9 mg/dl in women.

Implications of results

Decreased serum creatinine levels may indicate advanced muscular dystrophy. Increased levels indicate renal disease in which at least half the nephrons are damaged. Increased levels also have been associated with gigantism, hyperthyroidism, and acromegaly. Ascorbic acid, barbiturates, diuretics, and known nephrotoxic drugs also can increase creatinine levels.

Culture, blood

Blood cultures are used to identify and treat bacteremia and septicemia. The procedure requires inoculation of a culture medium with a blood sample and an adequate incubation period.

Purpose

Blood culture is used to:
- ◆ confirm a diagnosis of bacteremia
- ◆ identify the causative pathogen in bacteremia and septicemia.

Procedure-related nursing care

Explain to the patient that this test is used to determine if he has an infection in his bloodstream. Tell him that you'll need to draw a blood sample (or several) from one of his veins, probably in his arm or hand. Review the steps of the venipuncture process with him. Reassure the patient that you'll remove only a small amount of blood.

Before you perform the venipuncture, be sure to obtain two culture bottles (one vented for aerobic and one unvented for anaerobic) in addition to your usual venipuncture equipment. Clean the expected venipuncture site carefully, starting with an alcohol pad and then a povidone-iodine swab. Let the skin dry for at least 1 minute. Meanwhile, clean the tops of the culture bottles with alcohol or povidone-iodine.

When you perform the venipuncture, draw 10 to 20 ml of blood into a syringe. Then change the needle on the syringe and inject about half of the drawn blood into the first culture bottle. Withdraw the syringe, change the needle, and inject the remaining blood into the second bottle. Complete the necessary steps to prepare the culture bottles according to the laboratory's instructions. Arrange for the sample to be transported to the laboratory immediately.

If a hematoma develops at the venipuncture site, apply warm, wet compresses.

Normal findings

Blood normally is sterile.

Implications of results

It can take up to 72 hours to isolate most organisms, so the laboratory will usually hold negative cultures for up to a week before pronouncing them truly negative. Keep in mind that even positive cultures don't always confirm septicemia. Common blood pathogens include *Neisseria meningitidis, Streptococcus pneumoniae, Haemophilus influenzae, Staphylococcus aureus, Pseudomonas aeruginosa*, and Enterobacteriaceae. Previous or ongoing antimicrobial therapy might cause a false-negative result.

An incorrect collection technique can invalidate the results of a blood culture. In fact, because 2% to 3% of blood cultures are contaminated, you'll want to take special care to perform this test properly.

Culture, sputum

A sputum culture reveals the presence of bacteria in the lungs.

Purpose

A sputum culture is used to:

◆ identify the cause of a pulmonary infection

◆ guide the diagnosis and management of lung disease.

Procedure-related nursing care

Explain to the patient that this test will help determine whether he has a lung infection. Tell him whether the specimen will be collected by a deep cough and expectoration, by tracheal suctioning, or by bronchoscopy.

If you'll be asking the patient to produce a sputum specimen, instruct him to increase his fluid intake the night before the test (earlier if possible). Ahead of time, show the patient how to generate a deep cough by taking three deep breaths and forcefully expelling air in a cough on the final breath. Remind the patient that he needs to try to produce the specimen first thing in the morning, before he brushes his teeth or uses mouthwash.

Make sure you have gloves, a sterile container, and a leakproof bag. Put on the gloves, instruct the patient to perform a deep cough, collect the specimen, and close the container. Label it with the type of specimen, date, time, and any antimicrobial drugs the patient takes. Place the specimen in the leakproof bag and have it delivered to the laboratory immediately.

Normal findings

Sputum typically contains oropharyngeal organisms. However, the type and amount of the organisms detected can indicate infection. Further diagnostic studies may be needed.

Implications of results

Pathogens known to be found in sputum include *Streptococcus pneumoniae, Mycobacterium tuberculosis,* Enterobacteriaceae, *H. influenzae, S. aureus*, and *P. aeruginosa*.

Culture, stool

Although even normal stool contains several potentially pathogenic organisms, a stool culture is valuable for identifying organisms that can cause overt GI disease. In addition, stool cultures can be used to detect viruses that cause aseptic meningitis.

Purpose

Stool culture is used to:

◆ identify pathogens

◆ identify carrier states

◆ aid in the treatment of diseases

◆ assist in diagnosing severe infectious disease

◆ prevent possibly fatal complications.

Procedure-related nursing care

Explain to the patient that this test is used to determine whether he has a GI infection. Tell the patient that the test may require you to collect a stool specimen from him on 3 consecutive days.

To perform the test, make sure you have gloves, a waterproof container with a tight-fitting lid (or a rectal swab and sterile collection and transport system), a leakproof bag, a tongue blade and, if necessary, a bedpan. Before collecting the specimen, put on gloves. Collect the specimen directly into the container, if possible, and close the lid tightly. If the patient is not ambulatory, collect the specimen in the bedpan and use the tongue blade to transfer a sample into the container.

If you need to collect the specimen with a rectal swab, insert the swab past the patient's rectal sphincter, gently rotate it, and withdraw it. Place the swab into the container. Whichever method you use, be sure to include in the culture container any mucus or blood you see. Place the stool sample container in the leakproof bag.

If the patient can collect the specimen before your visit, instruct him to collect it in a clean container with a tight-fitting lid. Tell him to then wrap the container in a plastic bag and brown paper bag and keep it in the refrigerator (separate from food items) until you arrive. Label the specimen with the patient's name, the date, and the time it was collected.

Normal findings

Normally, stool contains such anaerobic bacteria as non-spore-forming bacilli, clostridia, and anaerobic streptococci. It also typically contains a much smaller percentage of aerobic bacteria, including gram-negative bacilli, gram-positive cocci, and yeasts.

Implications of results

The most common disease-causing organisms in the GI tract include *Shigella, Salmonella, and Campylobacter jejuni*. Less common organisms include *Vibrio cholerae, Clostridium botulinum, C. difficile*, and *C. perfringens*. *C. botulinum* indicates food poisoning. Patients undergoing long-term antimicrobial therapy may have large numbers of *S. aureus* or yeast, indicating an infection. The presence of enteroviruses may indicate aseptic meningitis.

The presence of urine in the specimen could injure or destroy some enteric pathogens, so take care to avoid contaminating the sample with urine.

Culture, urine

Urine cultures are used primarily to diagnose urinary tract infections (UTIs), especially those originating in the bladder.

Purpose

Urine culture is used to:

◆ diagnose a UTI

◆ monitor microorganism colonization in the bladder after insertion of an indwelling urinary catheter.

Procedure-related nursing care

Explain to the patient that this test will determine whether he has a UTI. Tell him that you'll need a clean-catch urine specimen and tell him how to collect it. Emphasize the need to thoroughly clean the external genitalia beforehand.

If the patient can't collect the specimen, you may need to catheterize him to obtain an uncontaminated specimen. If so, be sure to use the correct catheterization package for the procedure. If an indwelling catheter is present, follow appropriate procedures for obtaining a specimen from the catheter.

Obtain the urine specimen (at least 3 ml), and seal the specimen container tightly with a sterile lid. Place the specimen in a leakproof bag for transport. If delivery of the culture must be delayed for over 30 minutes, store the specimen at 39.2° F (4° C) unless you're using a urine transport tube that contains a preservative.

Normal findings

Normally, urine is sterile. The laboratory will report this result as "no growth." Keep in mind, however, that a specimen might contain a variety of organisms captured as urine traversed the urethra or contacted the external genitalia.

Implications of results

Counts of 100,000 or more of a single bacterial species per milliliter of urine indicate a probable UTI. Counts under 100,000 may be significant as well, depending on the patient's age, sex, history, and other health conditions. Counts under 10,000 usually suggest a contaminated specimen. Other factors can reduce the count as well, including fluid- or medication-induced diuresis and antimicrobial therapy.

The presence of two or more organisms, especially those of vaginal or skin origin, suggests a contaminated specimen. Multiple organisms have also been seen in patients with prolonged indwelling urinary catheterization or those with a urinary diversion. If you receive doubtful results, you'll probably need to repeat the test.

Culture, wound

A wound culture microscopically analyzes a specimen of wound exudate to detect aerobic organisms (in a superficial wound) or anaerobic organisms (in a wound with little or no perfusion). You'll probably perform a wound culture if your patient has a fever, inflammation, and damaged, draining tissue.

Purpose

Wound culture is used to identify infectious organisms in a wound.

Procedure-related nursing care

Explain to the patient that this test can help determine whether his wound is infected. Tell him that you'll collect a specimen of drainage from the wound, either with a cotton swab or a syringe.

Before the test, make sure you have sterile cotton swabs and tubes that allow aerobic or anaerobic analysis, sterile gloves, saline solution or sterile water, and a leakproof bag. To obtain reliable results from a wound culture, clean the wound first with saline solution or sterile water. Then collect the specimen in one of several ways.

If you're using a cotton swab, insert it deeply into the wound, rotate it gently, and place it immediately into the culture tube. Alternatively, express exudate from the wound and pick up as much as possible by using a "Z" stroke to cover the entire wound.

If you're using a syringe, aspirate 1 to 5 ml of exudate from the wound and either inject it into the appropriate culture tube or insert the needle into a rubber stopper and leave the exudate in the syringe.

Place the culture tube or syringe into the leakproof bag, and have the specimen transported to the laboratory immediately. Document on the laboratory request the date, time, and wound site. If necessary, take specimens from several different areas of the wound.

Normal findings

A result of "no organisms" indicates a clean wound.

Implications of results

The most common aerobic organisms found in wounds include *Staphylococcus aureus*, group A beta-hemolytic streptococci, *Proteus*, *Es-*

cherichia coli, other Enterobacteriaceae, and some *Pseudomonas* species. The most common anaerobic organisms include *Clostridium* and *Bacteroides* species.

Erythrocyte sedimentation rate

The erythrocyte sedimentation rate (ESR) measures the time it takes for red blood cells (RBCs) in a whole blood sample to settle to the bottom of a vertical tube. This test provides the earliest indication of a disease process when other signs may still be normal.

The ESR rises significantly in inflammatory disorders caused by infection or autoimmune mechanisms. It also may be prolonged in localized inflammation and cancer.

Purpose

ESR is used to:

◆ aid in diagnosing occult diseases, such as connective tissue disease, tissue necrosis, and tuberculosis

◆ monitor inflammatory and malignant diseases.

Procedure-related nursing care

Explain to the patient that this test is used to help check for certain disorders that could affect his RBCs. Tell him that you'll need to draw a blood sample from one of his veins, probably in his arm or hand. Review the steps of the venipuncture process with him. Reassure the patient that you'll remove only a small amount of blood.

Perform the venipuncture and fill either a 7-ml lavender-top, a 4.5-ml black-top, or a 4.5-ml blue-top tube. Check with the laboratory to see which tube you should use. Once you've collected the sample, gently invert the tube to thoroughly mix the sample with the additive. Arrange for the sample to be transported to the laboratory immediately because it must be tested within 2 hours of collection.

If a hematoma develops at the venipuncture site, apply warm, wet compresses.

Reference values

Normally, the ESR ranges between 0 and 10 mm/hour in men and 0 to 20 mm/hour for women. Rates gradually increase with age.

Implications of results

A low ESR is seen in polycythemia, sickle cell anemia, hyperviscosity, and low plasma fibrinogen or globulin levels. An elevated ESR is seen in pregnancy, anemia, acute or chronic inflammation, tuberculosis, paraproteinemias (such as multiple myeloma), rheumatic fever, rheumatoid arthritis, and certain cancers.

Glucose, fasting plasma

This test, also known as a fasting blood glucose, measures the level of glucose in the plasma after the patient has abstained from food and fluids for 12 to 14 hours. During a fast, plasma glucose levels normally decrease. This decrease stimulates release of the hormone glucagon. Glucagon increases plasma glucose levels by stimulating gluconeogenesis and inhibiting glycogen synthesis. The secretion of insulin normally stops the rise in glucose levels. However, in patients with diabetes, absent or deficient insulin permits glucose levels to remain elevated.

Purpose

Fasting plasma glucose is used to:

◆ screen for diabetes mellitus

◆ help evaluate patients with known or suspected hypoglycemia

◆ help determine the insulin requirements for patients with diabetes

and those who need parenteral or enteral nutrition
◆ monitor medication or diet therapy in patients with diabetes mellitus.

Procedure-related nursing care

Explain to the patient that this test is used to measure the amount of glucose in his blood. Tell the patient to abstain from food and fluids for 12 to 14 hours before the test. To avoid falsely elevated results, tell him not to take any of the following medications during that time: acetaminophen, chlorthalidone, thiazide diuretics, furosemide, triamterene, oral contraceptives, benzodiazepines, phenytoin, phenothiazines, lithium, epinephrine, arginine, dextrothyroxine, diazoxide, nicotinic acid, corticosteroids, beta blockers, ethanol, clofibrate, insulin, oral antidiabetic agents, MAO inhibitors, and ethacrynic acid.

Explain that you'll need to draw a blood sample from one of his veins, probably in his arm or hand. Review the steps of the venipuncture process with him. Reassure the patient that you'll remove only a small amount of blood.

Perform the venipuncture and fill a 5-ml gray-top tube. Arrange for the sample to be transported to the laboratory immediately. If you'll be delayed, be sure to refrigerate the sample. If a hematoma develops at the venipuncture site, apply warm, wet compresses. Instruct the patient to resume taking any medications withheld before the test.

Reference values

Normal fasting plasma glucose levels after a 12- to 14-hour fast range from 70 to 100 mg/dl when measured by the glucose oxidase and hexokinase methods.

Implications of results

Abnormally low values can result from hyperinsulinism, insulinoma, von Gierke's disease, functional or reactive hypoglycemia, myxedema, adrenal insufficiency, congenital adrenal hyperplasia, hypopituitarism, and malabsorption syndrome. Glycolysis from failure to adequately refrigerate the sample can cause a falsely low result.

Elevated levels may indicate diabetes mellitus, pancreatitis, recent acute illness, Cushing's syndrome, acromegaly or pheochromocytoma. They're also seen in hyperlipoproteinemia, chronic hepatic disease, nephrotic syndrome, brain tumor, sepsis, or gastrectomy with dumping syndrome.

To confirm diabetes mellitus, you'll need to obtain two or more fasting plasma glucose levels of at least 126 mg/dl, according to the American Diabetes Association's 1997 guidelines.

Glucose, 2-hour postprandial plasma

This test is used to monitor the body's metabolic response to a carbohydrate challenge. It involves measuring blood glucose levels 2 hours after ingesting a high-carbohydrate meal.

Purpose

The 2-hour postprandial plasma test is used to:
◆ confirm diabetes mellitus in patients with signs and symptoms of the disorder
◆ identify disorders associated with abnormal glucose metabolism
◆ monitor the effectiveness of medication or diet therapy in patients with diabetes mellitus.

Procedure-related nursing care

Explain to the patient that this test can either confirm a diagnosis of diabetes or determine how well he's reacting to treatment. Instruct the patient to eat a high-carbohydrate breakfast and then fast for 2 hours. Remind him to avoid smoking and engaging in any strenuous activity after eating.

Tell the patient that you'll need to draw a blood sample from one of his veins, probably in his arm or hand, 2 hours after his high-carbohydrate meal. Review the steps of the venipuncture process with him. Reassure him that you'll remove only a small amount of blood.

Perform the venipuncture and fill a 5-ml gray-top tube. Arrange for the sample to be transported immediately to the laboratory, or refrigerate the sample until the test can be run. If a hematoma develops at the venipuncture site, apply warm, wet compresses.

Reference values

For people without diabetes, the results are usually less than 145 mg/dl by the glucose oxidase or hexokinase method. Levels are slightly elevated in people over age 50.

Implications of results

Reduced glucose levels are seen in patients with hyperinsulinism, insulinoma, von Gierke's disease, functional or reactive hypoglycemia, myxedema, adrenal insufficiency, congenital adrenal hyperplasia, hypopituitarism, malabsorption syndrome, and some cases of hepatic insufficiency.

Levels of 200 mg/dl or more indicate diabetes mellitus. High values are also seen in pancreatitis, Cushing's syndrome, acromegaly, and pheochromocytoma. Other disorders in which this test is elevated include hyperlipoproteinemia, chronic hepatic disease, nephrotic syndrome, brain tumor, sepsis, gastrectomy with subsequent dumping syndrome, eclampsia, anoxia, and seizure disorders. Certain medications can cause falsely elevated results as well. (See "Glucose, fasting plasma.")

Glucose tolerance test, oral

This test measures the carbohydrate metabolism after ingesting a dose of glucose. It's considered the most sensitive test for evaluating borderline diabetes mellitus.

Purpose

The oral glucose tolerance test is used to:

◆ aid in diagnosing hypoglycemia and malabsorption syndrome

◆ confirm a diagnosis of diabetes mellitus.

Procedure-related nursing care

Explain to the patient that this test is used to measure how his body reacts to the foods he eats. Tell him to maintain a high-carbohydrate diet and to avoid smoking, caffeine, and alcohol for 3 days before the test. Also tell him to abstain from food and fluids for 10 to 16 hours before the test begins.

Tell him that you'll need to draw several blood samples from veins in his arms or hands. Review the steps of the venipuncture process with him. Reassure the patient that you'll remove only a small amount of blood each time.

Begin the test by drawing a fasting plasma glucose sample in a 7-ml gray-top tube. Collect a urine specimen at the same time. Then have the patient drink an oral glucose solution. Urge him to drink all the solution within 5 minutes. Record the time that the patient drank the solution.

Be prepared to draw subsequent blood samples in 7-ml gray-top tubes at 30 minutes, 1 hour, 1½ hours, 2 hours, and 3 hours after he drank the solution. (Some doctors continue the test for 5 hours.) Collect urine specimens at the same time intervals.

Instruct the patient to lie down if he begins to feel faint at any time during the test. If he develops severe symptoms of hypoglycemia, draw a blood sample, discontinue the test, and provide the patient with a glass of orange juice.

Refrigerate the samples until the test is complete. Document the time that you drew each blood sample on the appropriate laboratory slips. Then take the clearly labeled samples to the laboratory immediately. If hematomas develop at the venipuncture sites, apply warm, wet compresses.

Reference values

Normal plasma glucose levels peak at 160 to 180 mg/dl within 1 hour after ingesting the glucose solution and return to fasting level or lower within 3 hours. After 2 hours, the normal level is less than 126 mg/dl.

Implications of results

Decreased glucose tolerance levels are seen in hyperinsulinism, malabsorption syndrome, Addison's disease, hypothyroidism, and hypopituitarism.

Glucose levels that equal or exceed 200 mg/dl at 2 hours confirm diabetes mellitus in a nonpregnant adult. Gestational diabetes is confirmed if two plasma glucose levels equal or exceed a fasting value of 105 mg/dl, a 1-hour value of 190 mg/dl, a 2-hour value of 165 mg/dl, or a 3-hour value of 145 mg/dl.

Increased values are also associated with Cushing's syndrome, pheochromocytoma, central nervous system lesions, liver cirrhosis, myocardial or cerebral infarction, hyperthyroidism, and high anxiety states.

Hematocrit

One of the components of the complete blood count, hematocrit (HCT) measures the percentage of packed red blood cells (RBCs) in a whole blood sample. The HCT level depends on the number of RBCs but also is influenced by the size of RBCs.

Purpose

HCT levels are used to:

- ◆ help calculate RBC indices
- ◆ aid in diagnosing polycythemia, anemia, and hydrational states
- ◆ monitor blood loss and evaluate blood replacement
- ◆ monitor fluid imbalance.

Procedure-related nursing care

Explain to the patient that this test is used to evaluate his circulating blood, especially his RBCs. Tell him that you'll need to draw a blood sample from one of his veins, probably in his arm or hand. Review the steps of the venipuncture or fingerstick process with him. Reassure the patient that you'll remove only a small amount of blood.

Perform the venipuncture and fill a 5-ml lavender-top tube. Gently invert the tube to make sure the blood and anticoagulant mix adequately in the tube. If you perform a fingerstick instead, fill a capillary tube that has a red band on the anticoagulant end until it's about two-thirds full. Then plug the top of the capillary tube with clay.

Arrange for the sample to be transported to the laboratory immediately. If a hematoma develops at the venipuncture site, apply warm, wet compresses. Put pressure over the fingerstick site until the bleeding stops.

Reference values

For men, the HCT level normally ranges from 42% to 54%. For women, it ranges from 38% to 46%. Values may vary, depending on the patient's age or sex, the type of sample, and the laboratory's testing procedure.

Implications of results

Low HCT levels indicate anemia, hemodilution, or a recent massive blood loss. Elevated counts indicate polycythemia or hemoconcentration from blood loss or dehydration. Conditions that cause the RBCs to swell, such as elevated blood glucose or sodium values, may increase the HCT level as well. Remember that failing to adequately mix the anticoagulant with the sample can adversely affect your results.

Hemoglobin, glycosylated

This test involves the measurement of three minor types of hemoglobin (Hb): HbA_{1a}, HbA_{1b}, and HbA_{1c}. These are variants of HbA, a hemoglobin formed by glycosylation (a molecular process in which glucose becomes incorporated into HbA).

Because glycosylation occurs constantly during the RBC's 120-day lifespan, this test reflects the patient's average blood glucose level during the previous 2 to 3 months. This makes glycosylated Hb a good test for measuring the effectiveness of a patient's diabetes treatment.

Purpose

Glycosylated Hb is used to monitor the effectiveness of diabetes therapy.

Procedure-related nursing care

Explain to the patient that this test is used to assess the effectiveness of diabetes treatment. Tell him that you'll need to draw a blood sample from one of his veins, probably in his arm or hand. Review the steps of the venipuncture process with him. Reassure the patient that you'll remove only a small amount of blood.

Perform the venipuncture and fill a 5-ml lavender-top tube. Gently invert the tube several times to mix the blood sample with the anticoagulant in the tube. Arrange for the sample to be transported to the laboratory immediately. If a hematoma develops at the venipuncture site, apply warm, wet compresses.

Reference values

Test values are reported as percentages of total Hb:

- *glycosylated Hb: 5.5% to 9%*
- *HbA_{1a}: About 1.6%*
- *HbA_{1b}: About 0.8%*
- *HbA_{1c}: 5.5% to 9%*

You may see HbA_{1a} and HbA_{1b} reported together, as one value.

Implications of results

In diabetes, total glycosylated Hb levels range from 10.9% to 15.5%. HbA_{1c} ranges between 8% and 11.9%. HbA_{1a} and HbA_{1b} make up about 2.5% to 3.9%. As therapy continues and control becomes more consistent, the levels will approach normal Hb ranges.

Hemoglobin, total

Included in the complete blood count, the total hemoglobin (Hb) test measures grams of Hb in a deciliter of whole blood. The Hb values correlate closely with the red blood cell count.

Purpose

The total Hb test is used to:

- assess the severity of anemia or polycythemia

◆ monitor response to anemia therapy.

Procedure-related nursing care

Explain to the patient that this test is used to assess his response to anemia therapy. Tell him that you'll need to draw a blood sample from one of his veins, probably in his arm or hand. Review the steps of the venipuncture process with him. Reassure the patient that you'll remove only a small amount of blood.

Perform the venipuncture and fill a 7-ml lavender-top tube. Gently invert the tube several times after filling to thoroughly mix the blood with the additive. Arrange for the sample to be transported to the laboratory immediately. If a hematoma develops at the venipuncture site, apply warm, wet compresses.

Reference values

Normal values range from 14 to 18 g/dl in men and from 12 to 16 g/dl in women. Levels usually are higher in neonates and infants.

Implications of results

Low hemoglobin may indicate anemia, a recent hemorrhage, or hemodilution caused by fluid retention. Elevated total Hb levels suggest hemoconcentration from dehydration or polycythemia.

HIV Type 1 and Type 2 antibody serum enzyme immunoassays

This test detects antibodies to the two known types of human immunodeficiency virus (HIV) in serum. This test does not differentiate between HIV-1 and HIV-2 reactivity. Positive findings are confirmed by the Western blot assay or other tests. Because this test is highly sensitive, it is used to screen for HIV infection and to test all donated blood.

Purpose

The serum enzyme immunoassay HIV antibody test is used to:

◆ screen donated blood for HIV
◆ aid in diagnosing HIV infection.

Procedure-related nursing care

Explain to the patient that this test is used to determine whether he's infected with HIV. Provide adequate pretest counseling to explain the reasons that the patient needs the test. Tell him that you'll need to draw a blood sample from one of his veins, probably in his arm or hand. Review the steps of the venipuncture process with him. Reassure the patient that you'll remove only a small amount of blood.

Perform the venipuncture and fill a 10-ml red-top tube. Arrange for the sample to be transported immediately to the laboratory. If a hematoma develops at the venipuncture site, apply warm, wet compresses.

Reference values

Persons not infected by HIV will test negative for HIV antibodies. Those who test negative but practice high-risk behaviors or know they've been exposed to the virus should be retested in 6 months and 1 year.

Implications of results

A positive result means that the person's body has been infected with HIV and has mounted an antibody reaction against it. Emphasize to the patient that an HIV infection doesn't mean he has AIDS. Historically, however, AIDS has developed within about 10 years in most infected people. Make sure the patient gets appropriate counseling and treatment to keep HIV levels low.

Keep in mind that false-positive results may occur in people with autoimmune disorders, such as systemic lupus erythematosus, or in people with antibodies to human leukocyte antigens.

Lactate dehydrogenase

The enzyme lactate dehydrogenase (LD) catalyzes conversion of muscle pyruvic acid into lactic acid. Because LD appears in almost all body tissues, cellular damage elevates total serum LD levels. However, five tissue-specific isoenzymes can also be identified and measured:

- ◆ LD_1 and LD_2 — appear in the heart, RBCs, and kidneys
- ◆ LD_3 — appears in the lungs
- ◆ LD_4 and LD_5 — appear in the liver and in skeletal muscle.

LD commonly is used to detect myocardial infarction (MI). That's because LD_1 and LD_2 levels rise 12 to 48 hours after an MI begins, peak in 2 to 5 days, and return to normal in 7 to 14 days.

Purpose

LD levels are used to:

- ◆ aid in diagnosing MI, pulmonary infarction, anemia, and hepatic disease
- ◆ monitor the patient's response to some chemotherapies
- ◆ support creatine kinase (CK) test results when diagnosing MI or when CK-MB samples are drawn too late (more than 24 hours after the onset of acute MI).

Procedure-related nursing care

Explain to the patient that this test helps assess his heart muscle. Tell him that you'll need to draw a blood sample from one of his veins, probably in his arm or hand. If an MI is suspected, tell the patient that you'll be drawing samples on 3 consecutive mornings. Review the steps of the venipuncture process with him. Reassure the patient that you'll remove only a small amount of blood.

Perform the venipuncture and fill a 7-ml red-top or red-marble-top tube. Draw each sample on schedule to avoid missing a peak isoenzyme level. Arrange for the samples to be transported to the laboratory immediately. Keep the sample at room temperature if transport to the laboratory is delayed. If a hematoma develops at the venipuncture site, apply warm, wet compresses.

Reference values

Total LD levels normally range from 46 to 90 U/L. Each isoenzyme has normal values as well.

- ◆ *LD_1: 14% to 26% of total*
- ◆ *LD_2: 29% to 39% of total*
- ◆ *LD_3: 20% to 26% of total*
- ◆ *LD_4: 8% to 16% of total*
- ◆ *LD_5: 6% to 16% of total*

Implications of results

Recent surgery or pregnancy as well as a number of other diseases can cause elevated total LD levels. In addition, total LD may remain normal even though certain isoenzymes are abnormal. Consequently, isoenzyme electrophoresis usually is necessary to pinpoint a diagnosis.

For example, in acute MI, LD_1 levels may rise above LD_2 levels within 12 to 48 hours after the onset of symptoms, a condition called a flipped LD ratio. LD_2, LD_3, and LD_4 levels may be elevated in granulocytic leukemia, lymphomas, and platelet disorders.

Magnesium, serum

An electrolyte essential to neuromuscular function, magnesium is found primarily in bone and intracellular fluid and, in smaller quantities, extracellular fluid. It helps transport sodium and potassium across cell membranes and, because of its additional effect on parathyroid hormone secretion, influences intracellular calcium levels. Absorbed by the small intestine, magnesium is excreted through the feces and urine. This test measures the amount of magnesium in serum.

Purpose

Serum magnesium levels are used to:

◆ assess neuromuscular or renal function

◆ evaluate electrolyte status.

Procedure-related nursing care

Explain to the patient that this test measures the amount of magnesium in the blood. Instruct him to avoid milk of magnesia or Epsom salts for at least 3 days before the test. Tell him that you'll need to draw a blood sample from one of his veins, probably in his arm or hand. Review the steps of the venipuncture process with him. Reassure the patient that you'll remove only a small amount of blood.

Perform the venipuncture, without a tourniquet if possible, and fill a 7-ml red-top or red-marble-top tube. Handle the sample gently to prevent hemolysis, which can alter the test results. Arrange for the sample to be transported to the laboratory immediately. If a hematoma develops at the venipuncture site, apply warm, wet compresses.

Reference values

Normal serum magnesium levels range from 1.7 to 2.1 mg/dl (atomic absorption) or from 1.5 to 2.5 mEq/L.

Implications of results

Decreased magnesium levels (hypomagnesemia) are common in chronic alcoholism, diarrhea, malabsorption syndrome, faulty absorption after bowel resection, prolonged bowel or gastric aspiration, acute pancreatitis, primary aldosteronism, severe burns, hypercalcemic conditions, and excessive use of diuretics. Patients with hypomagnesemia may experience leg and foot cramps, hyperactive deep tendon reflexes (DTRs), cardiac arrhythmias, muscle weakness, seizures, twitching, tetany, and tremors.

Increased magnesium levels (hypermagnesemia) commonly occur in renal failure and adrenal insufficiency. Patients with high levels might experience lethargy, flushing, diaphoresis, decreased blood pressure, a slow or weak pulse, diminished DTRs, muscle weakness, and slow, shallow respirations.

Occult blood, fecal

Usually, fecal occult blood can be detected only by microscopic analysis or through the use of chemical additives, as in the guaiac or orthotolidin tests. Small amounts of blood (2 to 2.5 ml/day) in the feces are considered normal; the chemical tests are designed to detect greater-than-normal amounts.

Purpose

The fecal occult blood test is used to:

◆ aid in the early diagnosis of colorectal cancer

◆ detect GI bleeding.

Procedure-related nursing care

Explain to the patient that this test is used to see if there's any blood in his stool. Instruct him to eat a high-fiber diet, and to avoid red meat, poultry, fish, turnips, horseradish, iron preparations, bromides, iodides, nonsteroidal anti-inflammatory drugs, colchicine, salicylates, steroids, and ascorbic acid for at least 2 days before the test.

You'll need to obtain three stool specimens. Tell the patient how to collect them, and remind him not to contaminate the specimens with toilet paper or urine. If the test will be conducted in the laboratory, transport each specimen promptly. Don't refrigerate the specimens.

If you'll be performing the test in the patient's home, use a commercial occult-blood test. Select a small amount of feces from at least two separate areas of the specimen. Then apply 2 drops of developer to the paper over the specimen. Wait 1 minute and note the color of the paper. After you complete the test, tell the patient that he can resume his normal diet.

Normal findings

Less than 2.5 ml of blood should be present. If this is the case, the test paper will turn green.

Implications of results

If there's blood in the patient's stool, the paper will turn blue within about 60 seconds. Possible causes of a positive test include GI bleeding from varices, peptic ulcer disease, cancer, ulcerative colitis, dysentery, or hemorrhagic disease. If the blue color appears more than 60 seconds after the test begins, consider it a weak positive result that may or may not indicate a significant disease process. In this case, consider further testing.

Keep in mind that a high intake of vitamin C can cause false-negative results even in the presence of significant GI bleeding.

Phosphates, serum

The primary anion in intracellular fluid, phosphate helps store and use body energy, regulate calcium levels, facilitate carbohydrate and lipid metabolism, and maintain acid-base balance. This electrolyte is essential to bone formation. It's absorbed in the small intestine and excreted in urine.

Because of the reciprocal relationship between phosphate and calcium, excretion of phosphate increases or decreases in inverse proportion to serum calcium levels. Abnormal levels are more likely to be caused by faulty excretion than malabsorption.

Purpose

Serum phosphate levels are used to:
- ◆ aid in diagnosing renal disorders and acid-base imbalance
- ◆ detect endocrine, skeletal, and calcium disorders.

Procedure-related nursing care

Explain to the patient that this test measures the amount of phosphate in his blood. Tell him that you'll need to draw a blood sample from one of his veins, probably in his arm or hand. Review the steps of the venipuncture process with him. Reassure the patient that you'll remove only a small amount of blood.

Perform the venipuncture and fill a 7-ml red-top or red-marble-top tube. Handle the specimen gently to prevent hemolysis, which can alter the test results. Arrange for the sample to be transported to the laboratory immediately. If a hematoma develops at the venipuncture site, apply warm, wet compresses.

Reference values

Normally, serum phosphate levels in adults range from 2.5 to 4.5 mg/dl (atomic absorption) or from 1.8 to 2.6 mEq/L.

Implications of results

Decreased phosphate levels (hypophosphatemia) may result from malnutrition, malabsorption, hyperparathyroidism, osteomalacia, acute alcoholism, hypokalemia, or renal tubular disease or as an adverse effect of treatment for diabetic acidosis. In addition, prolonged vomiting, diarrhea, vitamin D deficiency, extensive I.V. infusions of dextrose 5% in water, and phosphate-binding antacids, insulin, and epinephrine also can cause falsely low values.

Elevated phosphate levels (hyperphosphatemia) may accompany skeletal diseases, myelogenous leukemia, sarcoidosis, bone tumors, healing fractures, hypoparathyroidism, acromegaly, diabetic acidosis, high intestinal obstruction, or renal failure. Excessive intake of vitamin D, the use of anabolic steroids and androgens, and a hemolyzed sample all can cause falsely elevated results.

Platelet count

Platelets, the smallest formed elements in blood, are vital in promoting coagulation. By supplying phospholipids to the intrinsic thromboplastin pathway, platelets contribute to the formation of a hemostatic plug.

Purpose

The platelet count is used to:

◆ evaluate platelet production

◆ assess the effects of chemotherapy or radiation therapy on platelet production

◆ aid in diagnosing thrombocytopenia or thrombocytosis

◆ confirm a visual estimate of platelets and morphology from a stained blood film.

Procedure-related nursing care

Explain to the patient that this test is used to measure how well his blood will clot. Tell him that you'll need to draw a blood sample from one of his veins, probably in his arm or hand. Review the steps of the venipuncture process with him. Reassure the patient that you'll remove only a small amount of blood.

Perform the venipuncture and fill a 7-ml lavender-top tube. Gently invert it several times to mix the blood with the anticoagulant. Arrange for the sample to be transported to the laboratory immediately. If a hematoma develops at the venipuncture site, apply warm, wet compresses.

Reference values

Normal platelet counts range from 140,000 to 400,000/µl in adults and from 150,000 to 450,000/µl in children.

Implications of results

Decreased platelet counts (thrombocytopenia) can be caused by aplastic or hypoplastic bone marrow, infiltrative bone marrow disease (such as cancer or leukemia), megakaryocytic hypoplasia, ineffective thrombopoiesis from folic acid or vitamin B_{12} deficiency, pooling of platelets in an enlarged spleen, increased platelet destruction from drugs or immune disorders, disseminated intravascular coagulation, or mechanical injury to the platelets.

Medications known to decrease the platelet count include acetazolamide, acetohexamide, antineoplastics, brompheniramine maleate, carbamazepine, chloramphenicol, ethacrynic acid, furosemide, gold salts, hydroxychloroquine, indomethacin, isoniazid, mephenytoin, methimazole, methyldopa, oral diazoxide, oxyphenbutazone, penicillamine, phenytoin, phenylbutazone, pyrimethamine, quinidine sulfate, quinine, salicylates, streptomycin, sulfonamides, thiazide, and thiazide-like diuretics. Heparin causes transient reversible thrombocytopenia.

Elevated platelet counts can be caused by hemorrhage, infectious disorders, cancer, iron deficiency anemia, recent surgery, pregnancy, splenectomy, and inflammatory disorders. Sustained elevated counts may accompany primary thrombocythemia, myelofibrosis with myeloid metaplasia, polycythemia vera, and chronic myelogenous leukemia. Platelet counts also can be elevated because of cold temperatures, strenuous exercise, excitement, and impending menstruation.

Potassium, serum

The major intracellular cation, potassium helps to maintain cellular osmotic equilibrium and to regulate muscle activity (by maintaining electrical conduction in cardiac and skeletal muscles), enzyme activity, and acid-base balance. This electrolyte is affected by secretion of adrenal steroid hormones and by fluctuations in pH, serum glucose levels, and serum sodium levels.

Potassium has a reciprocal relationship with sodium; when one increases, the other decreases. Potassium can't be stored by the body; it's readily excreted by the kidneys, making potassium deficiency quite common.

Purpose

The serum potassium test is used to:

◆ check for hyperkalemia or hypokalemia
◆ monitor renal function, acid-base balance, and glucose metabolism
◆ evaluate neuromuscular and endocrine disorders
◆ detect the origin of cardiac arrhythmias.

Procedure-related nursing care

Explain to the patient that this test is used to measure the amount of potassium in his blood. Tell him that you'll need to draw a blood sample from one of his veins, probably in his arm or hand. Review the steps of the venipuncture process with him. Reassure the patient that you'll remove only a small amount of blood.

Perform the venipuncture, telling the patient not to make a fist after you apply the tourniquet. Fill either a 7-ml red-top or red-marble-top tube or a 10- to 15-ml red-top tube. Handle the specimen gently to avoid hemolysis, which can alter the test results. Arrange for the sample to be transported to the laboratory immediately. If a hematoma develops at the venipuncture site, apply warm, wet compresses.

Reference values

Normally, serum potassium levels range from 3.8 to 5 mEq/L.

Implications of results

Low potassium levels (hypokalemia) often are associated with aldosteronism or Cushing's syndrome, long-term diuretic therapy, or excessive licorice ingestion. Other factors that deplete potassium include I.V. infusions that don't contain supplemental potassium, and administration of insulin and glucose.

Elevated potassium levels (hyperkalemia) are common in patients with burns, crushing injuries, diabetic ketoacidosis, renal failure, Addison's disease, or myocardial infarction. Other factors that can elevate potassium levels include rapid potassium infusions, penicillin G therapy, or renal toxicity secondary to the use of amphotericin B, methicillin, or tetracycline.

Protein, urine

Normally, the renal glomerular capillary membrane permits only proteins of low molecular weight to enter the filtrate. Renal tubules then reabsorb most of these proteins, eventually excreting in urine an amount of protein undetectable by screening tests. When glomerular capillary membranes sustain damage, however, they allow proteins to be excreted in urine. That's why this test is valuable in helping to diagnose renal disease.

Purpose

Urine protein levels are used to:

◆ aid in diagnosing renal disease

◆ aid in diagnosing preeclampsia in pregnant women.

Procedure-related nursing care

Explain to the patient that this test detects whether he has protein in his urine. Tell him that he'll need to collect all his urine over a 24-hour period, and carefully explain how he should do so. Provide an appropriate container for the specimen, and instruct the patient to keep it refrigerated throughout the collection period. After 24 hours, arrange for the specimen to be transported to the laboratory immediately.

Reference values

A normal 24-hour urine sample contains 150 mg or less of protein.

Implications of results

Small amounts or urine protein are common in renal diseases in which glomerular involvement isn't a factor, as in chronic pyelonephritis. Moderate levels of urine protein (0.5 to 4 g in 24 hours) suggest other types of renal disease, such as acute or chronic glomerulonephritis, amyloidosis, toxic nephropathies, diabetes, or heart failure. Large amounts of urine protein (more than 4 g in 24 hours) are seen in patients with nephrotic syndrome.

If the patient ingests sodium bicarbonate, penicillin, sulfonamides, iodine contrast media, or cephalosporins, he may have falsely elevated levels of urine protein. Highly dilute urine may decrease protein levels, resulting in falsely negative results.

Prothrombin time

Prothrombin time (PT) measures the time required for a fibrin clot to form in a plasma sample after the introduction of calcium ions and tissue thromboplastin (factor III). This time is then compared to the time of a control sample. PT measures prothrombin activity and evaluates the extrinsic coagulation system, including factors V and VII, as well as prothrombin and fibrinogen levels.

Purpose

The PT test is used to:

◆ aid in diagnosing conditions associated with abnormal bleeding

◆ detect deficiencies of specific clotting factors

◆ evaluate the extrinsic coagulation system

◆ monitor a patient's response to oral anticoagulant therapy

◆ monitor the effects of diseases that cause abnormal clotting.

Procedure-related nursing care

Explain to the patient that this test is used to assess how fast his blood clots. Tell him that you'll need to draw a blood sample from one of his veins, probably in his arm or hand. Review the steps of the venipuncture process with him. Reassure the patient that you'll remove only a small amount of blood.

Perform the venipuncture and fill a 7-ml blue-top tube. Avoid excessive probing while collecting the sample. Gently invert the tube several times after filling to mix the additive throughout the blood sample. Place the sample in a cooler, and arrange for immediate transport to the laboratory. If a hematoma develops at the venipuncture site, apply warm, wet compresses.

Reference values

Normal PT is reported in relation to an international normalized ratio (INR) and should be between 2.0 and 3.0.

Implications of results

Prolonged PT may suggest hepatic disease or clotting deficiencies. It also may indicate vitamin K deficiency in patients not receiving anticoagulant therapy. If the patient is on anticoagulant therapy, PT is usually maintained at between one and one and one-half times the normal value.

In addition, prolonged PT has been seen in patients receiving corticotropin, anabolic steroids, cholestyramine resin, I.V. heparin, indomethacin, mefenamic acid, methimazole, oxyphenbutazone, para-aminosalicylate, phenylbutazone, phenytoin, propylthiouracil, quinidine, quinine, thyroid hormones, vitamin A, or excessive alcohol.

Either reduced or elevated times may occur with the use of antibiotics, barbiturates, hydroxyzine, sulfonamides, salicylates, mineral oil, or clofibrate. Reduced PT can result from the use of antihistamines, chloral hydrate, digitalis glycosides, diuretics, griseofulvin, vitamin K, and xanthines, such as caffeine and theophylline.

Red blood cell count

This test, a part of the complete blood count, measures the number of red blood cells (RBCs) in a cubic millimeter of whole blood. Also called an erythrocyte count, it can be used to calculate two RBC indices: mean corpuscular volume and mean corpuscular hemoglobin (Hb). These indices reveal RBC size and the concentration and weight of Hb.

Purpose

RBC count is used to:

◆ aid in diagnosing anemia and polycythemia

◆ help compute RBC indices.

Procedure-related nursing care

Explain to the patient that this test is used to assess the number of RBCs in his body. Tell him that you'll need to draw a blood sample from one of his veins, probably in his arm or hand. Review the steps of the venipuncture process with him. Reassure the patient that you'll remove only a small amount of blood.

Perform the venipuncture and fill a 7-ml lavender-top tube. Gently invert the tube several times after filling to adequately mix the blood with the anticoagulant. Arrange for the sample to be transported to the laboratory immediately. If a hematoma develops at the venipuncture site, apply warm, wet compresses.

Reference values

Normal RBC counts vary with the patient's age and sex. For men, values normally range from 4.5 to 6.2 million/µl. For women, they range from 4.2 to 5.4 million/µl. People living at higher altitudes usually have higher RBC concentrations.

Implications of results

Low RBC counts usually suggest anemia, fluid overload, or recent hemorrhage. Elevated counts may indicate primary or secondary polycythemia or dehydration. Further studies, such as stained RBC examination, hematocrit, total Hb levels, RBC indices, and white blood cell counts, are needed to confirm a suspected diagnosis.

Red blood cell indices

Red blood cell (RBC) indices provide additional information about the size, hemoglobin (Hb) concentration, and weight of an average RBC. The mean corpuscular volume (MCV) is the ratio of hematocrit (HCT) to RBCs and gives the average RBC size. The mean corpuscular Hb (MCH) is the ratio of Hb to RBCs and gives the weight of Hb in an average RBC. Mean corpuscular Hb concentration (MCHC) is the ratio of Hb weight to HCT and gives the concentration of Hb in 100 ml of packed RBCs.

Purpose

RBC indices are used to help diagnose and classify anemias.

Procedure-related nursing care

Explain to the patient that this test is used to assess components of his RBCs. Tell him that you'll need to draw a blood sample from one of his veins, probably in his arm or hand. Review the steps of the venipuncture process with him. Reassure the patient that you'll remove only a small amount of blood.

Perform the venipuncture and fill a 7-ml lavender-top tube. Gently invert the tube after filling to mix the anticoagulant with the blood. Arrange for the sample to be transported to the laboratory immediately. If a hematoma develops at the venipuncture site, apply warm, wet compresses.

Reference values

Normal RBC indices are as follows:

- *MCV: 84 to 99 fl/RBC*
- *MCH: 26 to 32 pg/RBC*
- *MCHC: 30 to 36 g/dl*

Implications of results

Low MCV and MCHC indicate microcytic hypochromic anemias caused by iron deficiency anemia, sideroblastic anemia, or thalassemia. Elevated MCV is seen in macrocytic anemias caused by megaloblastic anemia that results from folic acid or vitamin B_{12} deficiency, inherited disorders of DNA synthesis, or reticulocytosis.

Sodium, serum

Sodium maintains the osmotic pressure of extracellular fluid, affects water distribution in the body, and helps promote neuromuscular function. In addition, sodium is needed for acid-base balance and influences chloride and potassium levels. Sodium is absorbed by the intestines and excreted in urine. It's regulated by aldosterone, which inhibits sodium excretion and promotes reabsorption by the renal tubules. Decreased sodium levels promote water excretion; increased levels lead to water retention. This test measures the amount of sodium in blood.

Purpose

Serum sodium levels are used to:

- evaluate fluid-electrolyte and acid-base balances
- evaluate neuromuscular, renal, and adrenal function

◆ evaluate the effects of diuretic therapy on serum sodium levels.

Procedure-related nursing care

Explain to the patient that this test is used to measure the amount of sodium in his blood. Tell him that you'll need to draw a blood sample from one of his veins, probably in his arm or hand. Review the steps of the venipuncture process with him. Reassure the patient that you'll remove only a small amount of blood.

Perform the venipuncture and fill either a 7-ml or a 10- to 15-ml red-top or red-marble-top tube. Handle the sample gently to prevent hemolysis, which can alter the test results. Make note of any medications or substances that could alter the test results by encouraging excretion or retention of sodium. Then arrange for the sample to be transported to the laboratory immediately. If a hematoma develops at the venipuncture site, apply warm, wet compresses.

Reference values

Normal serum sodium levels range from 135 to 145 mEq/L.

Implications of results

Low sodium levels (hyponatremia) can result from inadequate sodium intake or excessive sodium loss caused by diaphoresis, GI suctioning, diuretic therapy, diarrhea, vomiting, adrenal insufficiency, burns, or chronic renal insufficiency with acidosis.

High sodium levels (hypernatremia) can result from inadequate water intake, water loss that exceeds sodium loss (as in diabetes insipidus), impaired renal function, prolonged hyperventilation, or sodium retention.

Triglycerides, serum

The serum triglyceride test measures the amount of triglycerides — the main form in which lipids are stored — in the blood. Triglycerides are made up of one molecule of glycerol bonded to three molecules of fatty acids. The breakdown of triglycerides leads to the production of fatty acids. In combination with carbohydrates, triglycerides provide energy for metabolism.

Purpose

Serum triglyceride levels are used to:
◆ determine the risk of coronary artery disease
◆ identify disorders associated with altered triglyceride levels
◆ screen for hyperlipidemia.

Procedure-related nursing care

Explain to the patient that this test is used to measure the amount of fat-producing elements in his blood. Tell him that you'll need to draw a blood sample from one of his veins, probably in his arm or hand. Review the steps of the venipuncture process with him. Reassure the patient that you'll remove only a small amount of blood.

Instruct the patient to abstain from food and fluids for 12 to 14 hours and alcohol for 24 hours before the test. In addition, tell the patient to avoid taking corticosteroids, estrogen, and certain diuretics before the test.

Perform the venipuncture and fill a 7-ml red-marble-top tube. Arrange for the sample to be transported to the laboratory immediately. If a hematoma develops at the venipuncture site, apply warm, wet compresses. Instruct the patient to resume his normal diet and medication schedule after the test.

Reference values

Normal serum triglyceride levels usually range from 40 to 160 mg/dl in men and from 35 to 135 mg/dl in women.

Implications of results

Mild to moderate triglyceride elevations indicate biliary obstruction, diabetes mellitus, nephrotic syndrome, endocrinopathies, or excessive consumption of alcohol. Marked increases suggest congenital hyperlipoproteinemia and require further testing. Elevated levels have been associated with coronary artery disease or long-term use of corticosteroids, oral contraceptives, estrogen, ethyl alcohol, furosemide, or miconazole.

Decreased serum triglyceride levels are rare but can occur in malnutrition or abetalipoproteinemia.

Uric acid, serum

This test is used to measure uric acid, the byproduct of purine. Purine is present in nucleic acids and is derived from dietary and endogenous sources. It's excreted from the body by renal glomerular filtration and tubular secretion.

Purpose

Serum uric acid levels are used to:

◆ confirm a diagnosis of gout
◆ help detect renal dysfunction.

Procedure-related nursing care

Explain to the patient that this test is used to measure the level of uric acid in his blood. Tell him that you'll need to draw a blood sample from one of his veins, probably in his arm or hand. Review the steps of the venipuncture process with him. Reassure the patient that you'll remove only a small amount of blood. Instruct the patient to abstain from food and fluids for at least 8 hours before the test.

Perform the venipuncture and fill a 7-ml red-top or red-marble-top tube. Handle the specimen gently to prevent hemolysis, which can alter the test results. Arrange for the sample to be transported to the laboratory immediately. If a hematoma develops at the venipuncture site, apply warm, wet compresses.

Reference values

Normal uric acid levels range from 4.3 to 8 mg/dl in men and from 2.3 to 6.6 mg/dl in women.

Implications of results

Increased uric acid levels have been associated with impaired renal function and gout. Elevations also may accompany heart failure, acute infectious diseases, hemolytic or sickle cell anemia, hemoglobinopathies, polycythemia, leukemia, lymphoma, metastatic cancer, and psoriasis. Other factors that can increase uric acid include starvation, a high-purine diet, stress, alcohol abuse, and the use of loop diuretics, beta-adrenergic blockers, corticosteroids, thiazides, furosemide, salicylates, vincristine, or aspirin (in low doses).

Decreased uric acid levels may suggest defective renal tubular reabsorption or acute hepatic injury.

Urinalysis, routine

Urinalysis is used to screen for urinary and systemic disorders. The test evaluates the physical characteristics of urine specific gravity, pH, protein, glucose, ketone bodies, bilirubin, urobilinogen, hemoglobin, blood nitrites, and white blood cells. Abnormal findings suggest a disease process and indicate the need for further testing.

Purpose

Routine urinalysis is used to:

◆ help detect metabolic or systemic disease

◆ screen for renal or urinary tract disorders.

Procedure-related nursing care

Explain to the patient that this test uses a sample of his urine to evaluate aspects of his health. Tell him to avoid strenuous exercise before the test. Also tell him to avoid excessive ingestion of carrots, rhubarb, and beets because they can change the color of his urine. And warn him to avoid excessive amounts of meat and cranberry juice because they can lower his urine pH.

Tell the patient how to collect a random or clean-catch specimen of at least 10 ml. Ideally, have him collect the first-voided morning urine. If you can't send the specimen to the laboratory right away, refrigerate it until you can get it there.

Normal findings

Normal routine urinalysis includes the following:

◆ *Color: Straw-colored and clear*

◆ *Odor: Aromatic but not indicative of disease*

◆ *Specific gravity: 1.005 to 1.035*

◆ *pH: 4.5 to 8.0*

◆ *Protein, glucose, ketones, or other glucose elements: None*

◆ *RBCs: 0 to 2*

◆ *WBCs: 1 to 5*

◆ *Epithelial cells, crystals: Few*

◆ *Yeast, parasites, casts, bacteria: None.*

Implications of results

Each constituent of the urinalysis can reveal possible alterations in the patient's health.

Color. A change in urine color may result from drugs or diet. It also may result from metabolic, inflammatory, or infectious diseases.

Odor. In diabetes mellitus, starvation, and dehydration, urine odor is slightly fruity. In urinary tract infections (UTIs), the odor is fetid. Other conditions that cause distinctive urine odors include maple syrup urine disease and phenylketonuria.

Turbidity. Turbid urine could be caused by red blood cells, white blood cells, bacteria, fat, or chyle. It may reflect renal infection.

Specific gravity. Specific gravity under 1.005 is seen in diabetes insipidus, nephrogenic diabetes insipidus, acute tubular necrosis, and pyelonephritis. Specific gravity that remains at 1.010 regardless of fluid intake occurs in chronic glomerulonephritis with severe renal damage. Specific gravity over 1.020 is seen in nephrotic syndrome, dehydration, acute glomerulonephritis, heart failure, liver failure, and shock.

pH. Acid urine is associated with renal tuberculosis, pyrexia, phenylketonuria, alkaptonuria, and all forms of acidosis. Alkaline urine may result from Fanconi's syndrome, UTI, or metabolic or respiratory alkalosis.

Protein. Protein in the urine suggests renal disease, renal failure, or multiple myeloma.

Glucose. Glycosuria usually indicates diabetes mellitus, but it also may be caused by pheochromocytoma, Cushing's syndrome, or increased intracranial pressure.

Ketones. Ketonuria occurs in diabetes mellitus when cellular energy exceeds the availability of glucose. In the absence of glucose, the body metabolizes fatty acids instead of carbohydrates. Ketone bodies accumulate in plasma and are excreted in the urine. Ketones can also appear in urine during starvation, diarrhea, or vomiting.

Cells. Red blood cells in the urine indicate bleeding in the GU tract as a result of infection, obstruction, inflammation, trauma, tumors, glomerulonephritis, renal hypertension, lupus nephritis, renal tuberculosis, renal vein thrombosis, hydronephrosis, pyelonephritis, scurvy, malaria, parasitic infection of the bladder, subacute bacterial endocarditis, polyarteritis nodosa, or hemorrhagic disorders. White blood cells in the urine suggest urinary tract inflammation, such as cystitis or pyelonephritis. Excessive numbers of epithelial cells have been associated with renal tubular degeneration.

Casts. Excessive amounts of casts indicate renal disease.

Crystals. Although urine normally contains some crystals, numerous calcium oxalate crystals suggest hypercalcemia.

Other components. Yeast and parasites in the urine suggest a GU tract infection. The most common parasite in urine sediment is *Trichomonas vaginalis*, a protozoan that commonly causes vaginitis, urethritis, and prostatovesiculitis.

White blood cell count

Included in the complete blood count, the white blood cell (WBC) count reports the number of WBCs in a cubic millimeter of whole blood. The count can vary by as much as 2,000/µl as a result of strenuous exercise, stress, or digestion.

Purpose

WBC count is used to:

- ◆ detect the presence of infection or inflammation
- ◆ determine the need for further tests
- ◆ monitor a patient's response to chemotherapy or radiation therapy.

Procedure-related nursing care

Explain to the patient that this test is used to measure his body's ability to fight infection. Tell him that you'll need to draw a blood sample from one of his veins, probably in his arm or hand. Review the steps of the venipuncture process with him. Reassure the patient that you'll remove only a small amount of blood. Instruct him to avoid strenuous exercise or heavy meals for 24 hours before the test.

Perform the venipuncture and fill a 7-ml lavender-top tube. Handle the sample gently to prevent hemolysis, which can alter the test results. Arrange for the sample to be transported to the laboratory immediately. If a hematoma develops at the venipuncture site, apply warm, wet compresses.

Reference values

Normal WBC counts range from 4,000 to 10,000/µl.

Implications of results

Low WBC counts (leukopenia) may indicate bone marrow depression from a variety of causes, such as viral infection, toxic reaction, treatment with antineoplastics, ingestion of mercury or other heavy metals, and exposure to benzene or arsenic. They also typically accompany the flu, typhoid fever, measles, infectious hepatitis, mononucleosis, and rubella.

High WBC counts (leukocytosis) are seen in infections, such as abscesses, meningitis, appendicitis, or tonsillitis. They also may result from leukemia or tissue necrosis due to burns, myocardial infarction, or gangrene.

White blood cell differential

The white blood cell (WBC) differential provides more specific information about a patient's immune function because it differentiates the distribution and morphology of the WBCs. The count represents the relative number of each type of WBC in the blood.

Purpose

The WBC differential is used to:

- ◆ assess the severity of allergic reactions (eosinophil count)
- ◆ detect allergic reactions
- ◆ detect and identify various types of leukemia
- ◆ detect parasitic infections
- ◆ determine the stage and severity of an infection
- ◆ evaluate the body's ability to resist and overcome infections.

Procedure-related nursing care

Explain to the patient that this test assesses how well his body can fight infections. Tell him that you'll need to draw a blood sample from one of his veins, probably in his arm or hand. Review the steps of the venipuncture process with him. Reassure the patient that you'll remove only a small amount of blood. Instruct him to avoid strenuous exercise for 24 hours before the test.

Perform the venipuncture and fill a 7-ml lavender-top tube. Gently invert the tube after filling to adequately mix the sample. Avoid shaking the tube to prevent hemolysis, which can alter the test results. Arrange for the sample to be transported to the laboratory immediately. If a hematoma develops at the venipuncture site, apply warm, wet compresses.

Reference values

Normally, WBC types have the following ranges:

- ◆ *Neutrophils: 1,950 to 8,400/µl (47.6 % to 76.8%)*
- ◆ *Eosinophils: 12 to 760/µl (0.3% to 7%)*
- ◆ *Basophils: 12 to 200/µl (0.3% to 2%)*
- ◆ *Lymphocytes: 660 to 4,600/µl (16.2% to 43%)*
- ◆ *Monocytes: 12 to 760/µl (0.6% to 9.6%)*

Implications of results

Altered results of the WBC differential are seen in a wide variety of illnesses. For example, increased neutrophils may result from burns, cancer, chickenpox, childbirth, diabetic acidosis, eclampsia, endocarditis, excessive exercise, gonorrhea, acute gout, acute hemorrhage, herpes, myocardial infarction, myositis, osteomyelitis, otitis media, pregnancy in the third trimester, rheumatic fever, rheumatoid arthritis, Rocky Mountain spotted fever, salpingitis, septicemia, smallpox, surgery, thyrotoxicosis, uremia, and vasculitis.

Decreased neutrophils may result from bone marrow depression, brucellosis, cytotoxic drugs, folic acid deficiency, hepatic disease, hepatitis, influenza, measles, infectious mononucleosis, mumps, radiation therapy, rheumatoid arthritis, rubella, systemic lupus erythematosus, typhoid fever, tularemia, and vitamin B_{12} deficiency.

Increased eosinophils can result from adrenocortical hypofunction, amebiasis, pernicious anemia, angioneurotic edema, asthma, collagen vascular disease, dermatitis, eczema, excessive exercise, hay fever, herpes, Hodgkin's disease, hookworm, chronic myelocytic leukemia, metastasis or necrosis of a solid tumor, pemphigus, polyarteritis nodosa, psoriasis, roundworm, scarlet fever, sensitivity to a food or drug, serum sickness, splenectomy, trichinosis, and ulcerative colitis.

Decreased eosinophils can result from burns, Cushing's syndrome, mental distress, shock, a stress response from trauma, and surgery.

Increased basophils can result from chronic hemolytic anemias, Hodgkin's disease, chronic hypersensitivity states, chronic myelocytic leukemia, systemic mastocytosis, myxedema, nephrosis, polycythemia vera, and ulcerative colitis.

Decreased basophils can result from hyperthyroidism, ovulation, pregnancy, and stress.

Increased lymphocytes can result from brucellosis, cytomegalovirus, German measles, hepatitis, hypoadrenalism, immune diseases, lymphocytic leukemia, infectious mononucleosis, mumps, pertussis, syphilis, thyrotoxicosis, tuberculosis, and ulcerative colitis.

Decreased lymphocytes can result from adrenal corticosteroid excess, heart failure, immunosuppressant therapy, lymphatic circulation defect, renal failure, and advanced tuberculosis.

Increased monocytes can result from certain cancers, subacute bacterial endocarditis, hepatitis, monocytic leukemia, lymphomas, malaria, polyarteritis nodosa, rheumatoid arthritis, Rocky Mountain spotted fever, systemic lupus erythematosus, and tuberculosis.

Decreased monocytes can result from hairy-cell leukemia or prednisone treatment.

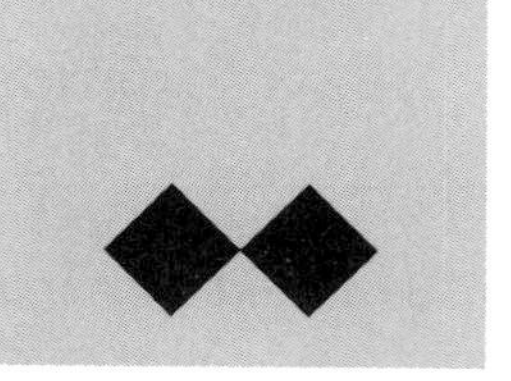

CHAPTER 7

Managing common conditions

As a home health nurse, you'll be called upon to handle a wide variety of clinical situations, many of which were once managed in acute care settings. However, even though you need to be ready to respond with skill to many patient needs, you may find yourself spending most of your time with patients who have a limited number of relatively common disorders.

As the nurse coordinating the patient's care, you are responsible for assessing the patient, formulating the plan of care, evaluating the patient's compliance, teaching the patient and his caregivers, and adjusting the plan of care as appropriate. This chapter presents important information to help you manage some of the disorders most common in home health nursing.

◆ ACQUIRED IMMUNODEFICIENCY SYNDROME

A number of years after being infected with the human immunodeficiency virus (HIV), the body's $CD4^+$ T lymphocytes (T cells) begin to disappear. The resulting immunodeficiency predisposes the HIV-infected person to opportunistic infections, unusual cancers, and other abnormalities (such as severe diarrhea and wasting), which we've come to recognize as acquired immunodeficiency syndrome (AIDS).

Although many of these opportunistic infections respond to medications, they tend to recur eventually, or the patient becomes intolerant of the therapy. Researchers continue to make progress in developing drugs designed to keep HIV in check, but AIDS is still considered an incurable and ultimately fatal disease.

Assessment findings

Just after being infected with HIV, the person either may have no signs and symptoms or may experience a mononucleosis-like syndrome for 3 to 6 weeks. Afterward, he'll likely remain asymptomatic for years.

Initial symptoms usually include fever, rigors, arthralgia, myalgia, a maculopapular rash, urticaria, abdominal cramps, and diarrhea. Symptoms of aseptic meningitis may occur as well, such as a severe headache and stiff neck. Assessment may disclose palpable lymph nodes in two or more extrainguinal sites.

As AIDS progresses, the patient will develop opportunistic infections — such as Kaposi's sarcoma or *Pneumocystis carinii* pneumonia — and neurologic symptoms from HIV encephalopathy. Behavioral, cognitive, and motor changes develop from progressive dementia in about one-third

Recognizing AIDS-related dementia

A common condition in patients with acquired immunodeficiency syndrome (AIDS), dementia can result from tumors of the central nervous system (CNS) and from opportunistic infections, such as toxoplasmosis, cytomegalovirus, cryptococcosis, tuberculosis, and syphilis.

Although dementia is characterized by certain signs and symptoms (see "Dementia" later in the chapter), it can be tough to discern in patients who have AIDS. Why? Because it starts out with subtle signs and symptoms that can be easily confused with depression and other psychological problems.

Relatively early in the course of AIDS-related dementia, findings may include nothing more than mild forgetfulness and a decline in appearance and grooming. Over time, they expand to include apathy, dysphoria, generalized weakness, fatigue, a blunted or flat affect, social withdrawal, somatic preoccupation, anxiety, loss of interest in usual activities, subtle personality changes, anorexia, hypersomnia, distractibility, and psychomotor slowing.

As the disorder progresses, signs and symptoms become more recognizable as dementia. They may include memory impairment, amnesia, or language disturbance. Cognitive, behavioral, and affective changes develop. Fine motor skills (such as handwriting) and concentration deteriorate. The patient may complain of numbness, tingling, and pain in his hands and feet. His gait may become unsteady.

Medications

Most AIDS patients take medications to offset the symptoms of dementia, including:

◆ psychotropic medications for symptoms of CNS involvement, such as anxiety, psychosis, or depression

◆ antidepressants for treating depression

◆ benzodiazepines for anxiety and insomnia

◆ antipsychotics, such as trifluoperazine (Stelazine) and haloperidol (Haldol), for agitation (The dose will be lower than normal because of patient's brain damage.)

◆ lithium for patients with manic symptoms. (Levels must be monitored carefully if infection has impaired the patient's renal function.)

Nursing care

When caring for a patient with AIDS-related dementia, you'll want to promote his safety and independence with interventions such as those that follow:

◆ Establish trust with the patient. Orient him to reality by recounting the date, time, place, and recent activities, as needed. Place a clock, a calendar, and pictures of significant others within his view.

◆ Encourage the patient to verbalize his fears, concerns, and needs.

Recognizing AIDS-related dementia *(continued)*

◆ Speak in short, clear sentences. Ask questions that have yes-or-no answers.
◆ Remove hazards from the environment to help prevent injuries.
◆ Set limits gently but immediately on inappropriate behavior.
◆ Assess the patient's level of confusion and disorientation at every visit to help determine the progress of his illness.

of AIDS patients. (See *Recognizing AIDS-related dementia*.)

Implementation

When caring for a patient who has AIDS or is HIV-positive, you'll want to prevent infection, promote an optimal nutritional status, and prevent transmission of the infection to others. Specific interventions include the following:

◆ Administer prescribed treatment as symptoms occur and the disease progresses.
◆ Provide meticulous skin and mouth care, especially for the debilitated patient. Give saline or bicarbonate mouthwashes for rinsing the mouth. Avoid glycerine swabs because they dry mucous membranes.
◆ Monitor for signs and symptoms of new opportunistic infections or other signs of disease progression. Institute treatments as ordered.
◆ Promote optimal nutrition, increasing intake as needed to meet greater metabolic needs during periods of stress, recovery, and adjuvant treatment.
◆ Encourage oral intake of food and fluids. Adjust fluid intake during periods of diarrhea. Monitor intake, output, and weight for changes.
◆ Provide nutritional supplements as necessary and as tolerated. Remember that total parenteral nutrition is controversial for AIDS patients because of the increased risk of infection associated with high glucose levels in the feeding solution.
◆ Follow standard precautions at all times, and tell caregivers to do the same.
◆ Educate the patient and family members, sexual partners, and friends about AIDS and its transmission. Tell the patient not to donate blood, blood products, organs, tissues, or sperm.
◆ Urge the patient to inform potential sexual partners and health care workers of his HIV status. Explain safe sexual practices.
◆ Encourage the use of prescribed analgesics to promote comfort.
◆ Plan rest periods to conserve the patient's energy.
◆ Review and reinforce the patient's treatment regimen and its adverse effects, as needed.
◆ Assess patient compliance with and response to all treatments.
◆ Encourage the patient and his family to discuss their feelings, concerns, and fears. Help the patient develop effective coping strategies to deal with an altered body image, the emotional burden of a serious illness, and the threat of death.
◆ As the patient approaches the terminal stage of his illness, encourage him to choose hospice care; then involve him in it as soon as possible so he can establish a trusting relationship with the hospice staff.

◆ ALZHEIMER'S DISEASE

A primary, progressive, degenerative disorder, Alzheimer's disease affects the cerebral cortex, especially the frontal lobe. It accounts for more than half of all cases of dementia. Over time, it causes massive impairment of intellectual, perceptual, motor, sensory, and affective functioning. In most cases, the affected person dies from debilitating brain involvement after an average of 8 years.

Only after death is it possible to confirm Alzheimer's disease. Consequently, diagnosis can be made only by ruling out other disorders. Symptoms produced by Alzheimer's are easily confused with such other illnesses as depression, cerebral arteriosclerosis, and chronic poisoning.

Treatment for Alzheimer's disease is palliative and supportive. It commonly involves psychostimulators (such as methylphenidate) to enhance mood, antidepressants, and low doses of neuroleptics or anxiolytics to treat severe agitation, paranoid behavior, or aggression. Patients also may benefit from hyperbaric oxygen therapy to increase oxygen to the brain, aroma therapy to ease labile emotions and mood swings, and massage to aid relaxation. Dietary modifications can help prevent further damage to the nervous system; they include avoiding free amino acids and other excitotoxins and maintaining steady blood glucose levels.

Assessment findings

Initially, the typical Alzheimer's patient shows very minor changes, including subtle memory loss and forgetfulness. Social skills and behavior are unaffected. Then, over time, the person will begin to lose short-term memory. He'll have trouble learning and retaining new information as well as difficulty concentrating. He may show a decline in personal grooming and dressing.

The patient also will develop progressive difficulty in communicating, making judgments, and thinking abstractly. He'll develop a severe deterioration in memory, motor function, and language. Eventually, he'll be unable to speak or write.

He may be restless, hostile, paranoid, depressed, possibly agitated and violent. He'll exhibit repetitive behaviors. His sleep may be disturbed. He'll be disoriented to person, place, and time. Family members may report that he has mood swings or that he laughs or cries suddenly.

A neurologic examination may reveal that the patient has an impaired sense of smell — a common early symptom. It may also reveal tremors and impaired stereognosis (inability to recognize and understand the form and nature of objects by handling them). The patient may pucker or grimace.

Implementation

When caring for a patient with Alzheimer's disease, you'll want to promote his safety, nutrition, and independence. You'll also need to help him and his family with coping skills. (See *Living with Alzheimer's disease.*) Specific interventions include the following:

◆ Provide a safe environment in which the patient can maintain as much independence as possible. Remove hazardous objects and obstacles to decrease the risk of injury and falls.

◆ Assess the home for safety problems, such as dark halls and walkways and safety rails in bathrooms. Explain steps the caregiver should take to ensure home safety.

◆ Establish an effective communication system with the patient and his

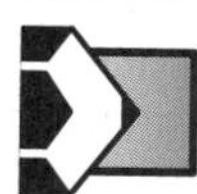

TEACHING POINTS

Living with Alzheimer's disease

If you care for a patient with Alzheimer's disease, you'll need to provide considerable teaching for his family in addition to fostering an appropriate environment for the patient. Be sure to include these topics:

◆ Teach the patient's family about Alzheimer's disease. Tell them that its cause is unknown. Review the signs and symptoms of the disease. Explain that, over time, the patient will lose his memory and physical abilities.

◆ Educate the family about diagnostic tests, medications, and treatments the patient may need. Teach the family about the patient's medications, including purpose, actions, dosages, and adverse effects.

◆ Teach the family about the importance of exercise in preventing constipation, decreasing restlessness and boredom, and promoting sleep. Suggest simple activities the patient might enjoy.

◆ Explain the importance of proper nutrition. Urge the family to provide small meals of foods the patient enjoys to encourage him to eat without feeling overwhelmed. If the patient's motor skills are impaired, tell them to cut his food to make it easier to handle. Inform them that plates with rim guards, built-up utensils, and cups with lids and spouts can be very helpful.

◆ Emphasize the importance of allowing the patient as much independence as possible. Creating a routine for the patient encourages his security and familiarity.

◆ Teach the family how to bathe, feed, and dress the patient.

◆ Encourage them to toilet the patient every 4 hours to prevent nighttime waking.

◆ Show them how to help the patient when he's walking.

◆ Teach the family about seizure precautions. If the patient is at risk for seizures, keep padded tongue blades at his bedside, and teach the family how to use them.

◆ Show the family how to reorient the patient, and mention how important it is to listen to his repetitive storytelling. Tell them that retelling life stories will help the patient feel that his life is in order.

◆ Teach the family about caregiver exhaustion and burnout. Encourage caregivers to acknowledge their needs and to get support wherever they can. Decreasing stress and fatigue, and having strong family support, facilitate problem solving and healthy coping mechanisms.

◆ Provide information about Alzheimer's support groups and respite care.

◆ Provide emotional support to the patient and his family. Encourage them to talk about their concerns. Listen carefully to them, and answer their questions honestly and completely.

◆ Make sure the family knows when to contact the doctor and whom to call in an emergency.

family to help them adjust to the patient's altered cognitive abilities.

◆ Use a soft tone and a slow, calm manner when you speak to the patient, and explain to the caregivers the need for speaking in this manner. Remember that the patient's thought processes have been slowed, impairing his ability to communicate verbally.

◆ Help the patient find a way to communicate. Explain it to the caregivers and encourage them to support him in this process. If the patient is aphasic, he may be able to communicate in alternate modes, such as nodding when he hears the correct word, pointing to a written word, or picking out a picture.

◆ Help the patient learn to perform activities of daily living at a pace slow enough to decrease his anxiety and frustration. Explain to caregivers the importance of providing simple, safe tasks that promote self-esteem. Remind them that music and exercise programs can be both enjoyable and physically stimulating.

◆ Provide the patient with activities that stimulate as many senses as possible, including sight, touch, smell, and memory. Explain the need for these activities to caregivers.

◆ Help the patient maintain a consistent routine to reinforce good habits and decrease anxiety.

◆ Ensure that medications are administered as ordered. Note their effects. Teach caregivers about the medications and the need to monitor these effects.

◆ If the patient has trouble swallowing, ask the pharmacist if crushing his medications or mixing the contents of capsules with soft food would interfere with the medications' effectiveness. Tell the caregiver to consult the pharmacist about medication administration problems.

◆ Encourage proper nutrition. Assess the patient's food preferences, and try to include them in his daily meal plan. Teach caregivers to offer finger foods or sandwiches that the patient can eat while walking around. Instruct them to help the patient if he needs it but to allow him to eat as independently as possible. Also instruct them to assist with oral hygiene.

◆ Urge caregivers to weigh the patient every week and note any change in weight.

◆ Encourage the patient to exercise and remain active during the day, then to relax as bedtime approaches. Have caregivers steer him away from stimulants, such as tea, coffee, cola, and chocolate.

◆ Provide environmental cues to improve the patient's orientation and reduce confusion. For example, place calendars and clocks around the house. Post signs with arrows pointing to the bathroom. Label all rooms, drawers, and frequently used items. If the patient needs sensory or mobility aids, make sure he uses them.

◆ Reorient the patient to person, place, and time whenever you interact with him. Reminders about meal times and bedtime provide structure and orientation. Display family pictures, including pictures of the patient, throughout the house. Inform the patient about current events slowly; repeat yourself as necessary.

◆ Make sure the patient wears an identification bracelet that displays his name and address.

◆ As appropriate, consult local respite care services to prevent caregiver exhaustion.

◆ Inform family members about support groups for families dealing with Alzheimer's disease.

◆ ASTHMA

A chronic reactive airway disorder, asthma involves episodic, reversible airway obstruction that includes bronchospasm, increased mucus secretion, and mucosal edema. Signs and symptoms range from mild wheezing, coughing, and dyspnea to life-threatening respiratory failure. Evidence of airway obstruction may or may not persist between acute episodes.

Asthma may result from sensitivity to specific external allergens (called extrinsic asthma) or from internal, nonallergenic factors (called intrinsic asthma). Many asthmatics, especially children, have characteristics of both types.

The best treatment for asthma is to identify and avoid trigger factors. Drug therapy usually involves bronchodilators and is most effective when administered shortly after the onset of signs and symptoms. Drugs used include rapid-acting epinephrine, terbutaline, aminophylline, theophylline and theophylline-containing oral preparations, oral sympathomimetics, corticosteroids, aerosolized sympathomimetics (such as albuterol), and anti-inflammatory drugs (such as cromolyn sodium and triamcinolone).

Assessment findings

Physical findings vary with the severity of the attack. (See *Determining asthma's severity*, page 206.) Usually, children begin an attack with wheezing, throat-clearing, or coughing that progresses to a deeper cough, then red-faced coughing spasms. As mucus is produced, the cough becomes more moist.

The most important aspect of auscultating the chest is determining whether the patient has equal and effective air exchange. Also keep in mind that, in severe bronchospasm, the wheezing actually may stop as the airways close down. It may seem that the attack is easing, yet the child will be in severe distress.

Percussion may produce hyperresonance. Palpation may reveal vocal fremitus. Auscultation may disclose tachycardia, tachypnea, mild systolic hypertension, harsh respirations with expiratory and inspiratory wheezing, a prolonged expiratory phase, and diminished breath sounds. A peak flow meter (at home) or spirometry (in the office) identifies the severity of the attack. Pulse oximetry determines the degree of hypoxia.

Cyanosis, lethargy, and confusion indicate the onset of life-threatening status asthmaticus and respiratory failure.

Implementation

When caring for a patient with asthma, you'll want to promote airway exchange and tissue perfusion, prevent infection, maintain hydration, safeguard nutrition, and assist with coping. Specific interventions include the following:

- Assess all body systems, especially respiratory. On each home visit, evaluate nutrition, hydration, weight, and skin turgor and condition.
- Review and reinforce the patient's drug regimen.
- If the patient uses a theophylline bronchodilator, monitor his plasma drug levels, as ordered, because oral absorption of theophylline may vary. Some medications, such as erythromycin, also affect drug levels.
- Encourage the patient to maintain adequate hydration and nutrition.
- If the patient is a child, help parents learn to respond early to oncoming attacks, to assess the child's condition accurately, and to seek appropiate health care. (See *Living with asthma,* page 207.)

Determining asthma's severity

Use the characteristics listed below to help determine the severity of your patient's asthma.

Mild asthma

- Brief wheezing, coughing, dyspnea with activity
- Infrequent nocturnal coughing or wheezing
- Adequate air exchange
- Intermittent, brief (<1 hour) wheezing, coughing, or dyspnea once or twice a week
- Asymptomatic between attacks

Diagnostic test results

- FEV_1 or peak flow 80% of normal values
- pH normal or increased
- PaO_2 normal or decreased
- $PaCO_2$ normal or decreased
- Chest X-ray normal

Other assessment findings

- Positive response to bronchodilator therapy within 24 hours
- No sleep interruption
- No hyperventilation
- Minimal evidence of airway obstruction
- Minimal or no increase in lung volume

Moderate asthma

- Respiratory distress at rest
- Hyperpnea
- Marked coughing, wheezing
- Air exchange normal or below normal
- Exacerbations that may last several days

Diagnostic test results

- FEV_1 or peak flow 60% to 80% of normal values; may vary 20% to 30% with symptoms
- pH typically decreased
- PaO_2 increased
- $PaCO_2$ typically decreased
- Chest X-ray showing hyperinflation

Other assessment findings

- Symptoms occurring more than twice weekly
- Coughing and wheezing between episodes
- Diminished exercise tolerance
- Possible sleep interruption
- Increased lung volume

Severe asthma

- Marked respiratory distress
- Marked wheezing or absent breath sounds
- Pulsus paradoxus >10 mm Hg
- Chest wall contractions
- Continuous symptoms
- Frequent exacerbations

Diagnostic test results

- FEV_1 or peak flow less than 60% of normal values; may normally vary 20% to 30% with routine medications and up to 50% with exacerbations
- pH normal or reduced
- PaO_2 decreased
- $PaCO_2$ normal or increased
- Chest X-ray that may show hyperinflation
- Other assessment findings
- Frequent severe attacks
- Daily wheezing
- Poor exercise tolerance
- Frequent sleep interruption
- Bronchodilator therapy doesn't completely reverse airway obstruction
- Markedly increased lung volume

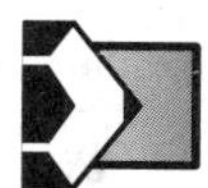

TEACHING POINTS

Living with asthma

If you care for a child with asthma, you'll need to provide support and teaching for the child and especially for his parents. Use these ideas as a start.

◆ Teach the child and his parents about trigger factors that can cause an asthma attack.

◆ Help parents evaluate their home for triggers that could cause their child to have an attack.

◆ Provide suggestions for ways to minimize trigger factors in the home or reduce their effect. Stress that most acute asthma attacks can be thwarted by minimizing the child's exposure to his triggers.

◆ Teach the child and his parents how to use a metered-dose inhaler. If necessary, recommend a spacer device and show them how to use it.

◆ Discuss signs and symptoms of an impending asthma attack. Then give the child and his parents some ideas to help minimize it.

◆ Teach parents how and when to activate the emergency medical system.

◆ Review the child's medications and when and how to use them. Instruct the parents to call the doctor if symptoms persist after initial interventions.

◆ Advise the parents to inform the child's teacher and the school nurse of his asthma.

◆ Encourage parents to allow their child to perform whatever activities he feels comfortable performing. Help them see the drawbacks of being overly protective.

◆ Offer support and encouragement to the patient and family. Listen to their fears and concerns. Help the patient plan a lifestyle incorporating diet, exercise, rest, and elimination of exacerbating factors.

◆ Assess the patient's compliance with therapy, and suggest ways to improve it.

◆ CANCER

The cancers you're most likely to encounter as a home health nurse include lung, breast, prostate, and colon. Naturally, each has its own care requirements. Keep in mind, however, that you'll be providing similar types of basic care and support no matter what kind of cancer the patient has.

Lung cancer

The leading cause of cancer deaths in the United States, lung cancer typically forms on the wall or epithelium of the bronchial tree. Risk factors include tobacco smoking, exposure to carcinogenic and industrial air pollutants (such as asbestos, arsenic, chromium, coal dust, iron oxides, nickel, radioactive dust, and uranium), and genetic predisposition.

Because there are no effective screening tests for lung cancer and signs and symptoms are often absent in the early stages, most patients have extensive disease at the time of diagnosis. Only about 13% of patients with lung cancer survive 5 years beyond diagnosis. Most treatments — combinations of surgery, radiation, and chemotherapy — are palliative.

Breast cancer

About one in eight American women develop breast cancer, usually after age 50. Occasionally, it affects men as well. Risk factors include close-family history, increasing age, long menstrual cycle with early menarche or late menopause, first pregnancy after age 35, high-fat diet, history of endometrial or ovarian cancer, radiation therapy, estrogen therapy, antihypertensive therapy, alcohol and tobacco use, and fibrocystic disease.

About half of breast cancers develop in the upper outer quadrant. The disease spreads through the axillary lymphatic system, the bloodstream, or by direct extension. Common sites of metastasis include the liver, brain, bone, lung, and chest wall. Therapy may include a combination of surgery, radiation, chemotherapy, and hormonal therapy.

Survival depends largely on the stage at which the cancer is detected. It ranges from 94% for localized disease (stage I) to 18% for disease with distant metastasis at diagnosis (stage IV). The overall survival rate currently is 76% in the United States.

Prostate cancer

The most common cancer in American men, prostate cancer is also the second leading cause of male cancer death. Risk factors for prostate cancer include age (it seldom develops before age 40) and infection. Androgens may play a role as well, by speeding tumor growth.

Treatment may include radiation therapy, surgery, and hormone therapy, although many health professionals find treatment controversial because of the advanced age of many men at the time of diagnosis and the cancer's slow progression. The 5-year survival rate for localized prostate cancer is 70%; after metastasis (usually to bone), it's less than 35%.

Colorectal cancer

The second most common visceral cancer in the United Sates and Europe, colorectal cancer is equally distributed between men and women. It occurs more frequently in those over age 40. About half the tumors are sessile lesions of the rectosigmoid area; the rest are polypoid lesions.

Risk factors for colorectal cancer include excess animal fat (particularly beef) and low fiber in the diet. Other factors include digestive diseases, a history of ulcerative colitis, and familial polyposis. If treated before metastasis, the 5-year survival rate is about 80% for rectal cancer and more than 85% for colon cancer. Treatment typically involves surgery to remove the tumor, adjacent tissues, and involved lymph nodes. The patient may also receive chemotherapy, radiation therapy, or both.

Assessment findings

As you know, assessment findings relate specifically to the type of cancer involved.

Lung cancer

The patient's chief complaint may include coughing (including coughing up blood), dyspnea, and sometimes hoarseness. You may notice that the patient becomes short of breath with minimal or no exertion. You also may notice signs and symptoms of superior vena cava syndrome: finger clubbing, edema of the upper body, weight

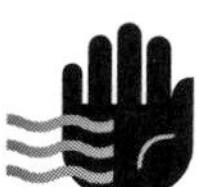

EMERGENCY INTERVENTIONS

Treating superior vena cava syndrome

Superior vena cava syndrome arises when blood can't flow normally through the superior vena cava. This large, thin-walled vein is easily compressed by enlarging lymph nodes or tumors of the mediastinum and right lung. When the syndrome is untreated or progresses rapidly, it may lead to respiratory arrest.

If you detect superior vena cava syndrome, perform the following interventions right away.

- ◆ Elevate the head of the bed to Fowler's or high Fowler's position, or prop the patient up with pillows.
- ◆ Administer oxygen therapy, as ordered, to help reduce cardiac output and decrease venous pressure.
- ◆ Notify the doctor and, if the patient's condition is severe (for example, if he's in acute respiratory distress), activate the emergency medical system.
- ◆ Administer diuretics cautiously, as ordered, to control edema of the face and upper extremities.
- ◆ Monitor the patient's fluid and electrolyte balance.
- ◆ Monitor for signs and symptoms of a worsening condition, which include progressive respiratory distress, cyanosis, increased edema of the head and upper extremities, and mental status changes.

loss, fatigue, and dilated chest and abdominal veins. (See *Treating superior vena cava syndrome*.)

Palpation may reveal enlarged lymph nodes and an enlarged liver. Percussion may reveal dullness over the lung fields in a patient with pleural effusion, which is common in lung cancer. Auscultation may disclose decreased breath sounds, wheezing, and a pleural friction rub (with pleural effusion).

Breast cancer

Commonly, the patient reports that she detected a painless lump or mass in her breast or that she noticed a thickening of breast tissue. Otherwise, the disease most commonly appears on a mammogram before a lesion becomes palpable. The patient's history may reveal several risk factors for breast cancer.

Diagnostic tests commonly performed during the initial staging work-up for breast cancer include biopsy, ultrasound, chest X-ray to pinpoint metastasis in the chest, liver function tests to detect metastasis, hormone receptor assay to determine whether the tumor is estrogen- or progesterone-dependent, and scans of bone, brain, and liver.

If the patient will have chemotherapy with doxorubicin, a cardiotoxic drug, she may need a baseline multiple-gated acquisition scan as well.

Prostate cancer

Early prostate cancer produces few signs and symptoms. With more advanced disease, the patient's history

Responding to radiation therapy

Although it works to cure patients in the long run, in the short run radiation therapy can cause considerable discomfort, usually from skin reactions. The skin reacts — usually 2 to 3 weeks into therapy — because radiation damages or destroys epidermal basal cells in the treatment field.

To help your patient weather the discomfort, you'll need to provide sound nursing care and compassionate teaching, starting with these measures.

- Review your patient's treatment regimen. Explain expected adverse effects and the procedures used to minimize discomfort.
- Describe the effects of radiation, including its potential effect on skin.
- As applicable, mention that radiation is most likely to produce a skin reaction or worsen a reaction in areas where two skin surfaces rub together, such as under the arm; where skin is broken, including at surgical incisions; and in areas of inflammation.
- Encourage the patient to use prescribed analgesics to promote comfort.
- If necessary, explain the need for skin care at the affected site.
- Gently clean the affected skin with mild soap, tepid water, and a soft cloth.
- Urge the patient to avoid wearing tight clothing over the treatment area.
- Suggest that the patient or family launder the patient's clothing in a gentle detergent.
- Instruct the patient to avoid putting very hot or very cold water on the treatment area.
- Tell the patient to avoid exposing the treatment area to the sun.
- Warn the patient to avoid using creams, ointments, perfumes, lotions, or deodorants in the treatment field.
- Urge the patient to avoid shaving with a blade in the treatment field; instead, encourage use of an electric razor.
- Tell the patient to inspect the skin at least daily at the entrance and exit site of the radiation beam and to report changes to the nurse and radiologist.
- Report skin reactions to the patient's doctor.

may reveal urinary problems, such as dysuria, frequency, retention, and hematuria. He may complain of back, hip, or other bone pain — a possible indicator of metastasis.

Inspection may reveal edema of the scrotum or leg in advanced disease. Digital rectal examination may reveal a nonraised, firm, nodular mass with a sharp edge (in early disease) or a hard lump (in advanced disease).

The initial diagnosis and staging work-up probably will include a digital rectal examination, a blood test for prostate-specific antigen, transrectal prostatic ultrasonography, and a bone scan.

Colorectal cancer

Signs and symptoms depend on the tumor's location and the extent of disease. All colon and rectal tumors tend to cause changes in bowel habits ranging from diarrhea to obstipation, blood in stools (ranging from bright red to black and tarry). These signs may be accompanied by weakness, a dull achiness in the abdomen or rectum, and weight loss. As the tumor grows and encroaches on abdominal organs, the patient may develop abdominal distention and intestinal obstruction. Anemia may develop from continued bleeding.

Implementation

When caring for a patient with cancer, try to minimize fear and stress, promote coping, maintain skin and tissue integrity, minimize pain, help the patient adapt to body changes, promote self-care and independence, prevent treatment-associated complications, and manage adverse effects. Specific interventions include the following:

◆ Encourage the patient and family to express their feelings and concerns. In response, provide information and support.

◆ Help the patient identify coping strategies used successfully in the past.

◆ Promote optimal nutrition. Urge the patient to increase intake as needed to meet the increased metabolic demand during postoperative recovery and treatment.

◆ If the patient has lung cancer, assess respiratory status. Monitor arterial blood gases and pulse oximetry. Place the patient in semi-Fowler's position to ease respirations when appropriate. Administer oxygen and antimicrobial therapy, as ordered. Teach the patient to cough and deep-breathe every hour. Increase fluid intake to at least 2 qt (2 L) per day. Explain to the patient and family the need to follow this treatment regimen.

◆ If the patient has prostate cancer, address issues of impotence and urinary incontinence. Watch for common adverse affects of radiation to the prostate, including proctitis, diarrhea, bladder spasms, nocturia, urinary frequency, rectal irritation, and tenesmus. Make sure that the patient and his caregivers know the common adverse effects and understand how to manage them. Remember that internal radiation of the prostate almost always causes cystitis for the first 2 to 3 weeks of therapy.

◆ If the patient has breast cancer and has had surgery, instruct her in range-of-motion exercises to promote mobility and stimulate vascular and neurologic functioning on the affected side. Urge her to perform a monthly breast self-examination on the remaining breast. Offer information and referral to a local breast cancer support group.

◆ If the patient has colorectal cancer, collaborate with an enterostomal therapist for effective teaching and coping strategies.

◆ If the patient had radiation therapy, instruct him in how to care for the radiation site. (See *Responding to radiation therapy*.)

◆ If the patient had chemotherapy, assess for adverse reactions as appropriate. They commonly include a decreased white blood cell count, decreased platelet count, decreased red blood cell count, diarrhea, nausea, and vomiting. Make sure the patient understands the adverse reactions and how to alleviate them.

◆ Certain agents used to treat cancer may cause partial or total hair loss. As appropriate, encourage your patient to consider wearing a turban or scarf. The patient may also want to purchase a wig before hair loss occurs.

◆ Help the patient adjust to body changes associated with surgery or treatment. Offer support and encouragement.

◆ Encourage participation in all postoperative care and activities of daily living.
◆ Encourage the use of prescribed analgesics to promote comfort.
◆ Review the patient's treatment regimen and adverse effects as needed.

◆ CEREBROVASCULAR ACCIDENT

Also known as a stroke, cerebrovascular accident (CVA) results from a sudden interruption of blood flow in one or more vessels supplying the brain. The longer blood doesn't flow, the more profound is the resulting brain damage. About 500,000 people have CVAs each year in the United States; half of them die as a result. That makes CVA the third leading cause of death in the United States and the most common cause of neurologic disability.

Major causes of CVA include cerebral thrombosis, embolism, and hemorrhage. Risk factors include a history of transient ischemic attack, atherosclerosis, hypertension, arrhythmias, rheumatic heart disease, diabetes mellitus, gout, postural hypotension, cardiac enlargement, high serum triglyceride levels, lack of exercise, use of oral contraceptives, smoking, and a family history of CVA.

Treatment for CVA commonly includes physical rehabilitation, diet changes and medications to help decrease risk factors, possibly surgery, and care measures designed to help the patient adapt to neurologic deficits, such as speech impairment and paralysis.

Assessment findings

Clinical features of CVA vary with the artery affected, the severity of the damage, and the extent of collateral circulation that develops to help the brain compensate for a decreased blood supply. The patient's history may reveal one or more risk factors for CVA, a gradual or sudden onset of hemiparesis or hemiplegia, loss of consciousness, aphasia, or other communication problems.

Physical examination will identify deficits caused by the CVA, possibly including an altered level of consciousness, hemiparesis or hemiplegia, flaccid paralysis with decreased deep tendon reflexes (in the early phase), hemianopia on the affected side, altered visual-spatial relationships (in patients with left-sided hemiplegia), urinary incontinence, sensory losses, and expressive or receptive aphasia.

Remember that the effects of a CVA appear on the side opposite the damage. In other words, CVAs that damage the right side of the brain will produce signs and symptoms on the left side of the body, and vice versa. However, a CVA that causes cranial nerve damage produces signs of cranial nerve dysfunction on the same side as the hemorrhage.

Many diagnostic tests are used to determine the location and extent of CVA damage. They include cerebral angiography, digital subtraction angiography, computed tomography scan, positron emission tomography, magnetic resonance imaging, transcranial Doppler ultrasonography, cerebral blood flow studies, ophthalmoscopy, and EEG.

Implementation

When caring for a patient with a CVA, you'll want to maintain a patent airway and oxygenation, prevent the complications of decreased mobility, ensure the patient's safety, foster as much independence as possible, promote nutrition, and facilitate coping. (See *Living with a CVA*.) Specific interventions include the following:

◆ Perform a complete assessment, paying special attention to the neurologic examination. Assess level of consciousness (LOC) and orientation as well as neurologic function on the affected side.

◆ Monitor the patient's blood pressure, LOC, pupillary changes, motor function (voluntary and involuntary), sensory function, speech, skin color, temperature, signs of increased intracranial pressure, and nuchal rigidity or flaccidity.

◆ Evaluate the patient's response to the plan of care; medications; physical, occupational, or speech therapy; and home health aide intervention.

◆ Depending on the patient's LOC, position him to prevent aspiration. Suction secretions as needed, and maintain a patent airway. Teach caregivers how to position the patient, how to determine when suctioning is necessary, and how to perform the procedure.

◆ Position the patient in correct alignment. Encourage the use of high-topped sneakers to prevent footdrop and a convoluted foam, flotation, or pulsating mattress to prevent pressure ulcers.

◆ To decrease the possibility of pneumonia, advise caregivers to turn the patient at least every 2 hours and to encourage coughing and deep breathing to the extent possible. Urge caregivers to offer the urinal or bedpan every 2 hours to prevent skin breakdown secondary to incontinence.

◆ Promote a safe environment to prevent injury. Explain the importance of having bed rails and keeping them up at all times; apply padding if necessary. Don't encourage caregivers to use restraints.

◆ Help the patient perform bilateral range-of-motion exercises, and teach

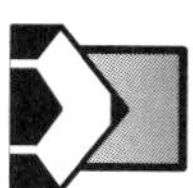

TEACHING POINTS

Living with a CVA

If your patient has a cerebrovascular accident (CVA), the health care team will need to provide wide-ranging teaching and assistance to help him and his family cope with lingering deficits. Here are some general teaching ideas:

◆ Reinforce the methods and goals of rehabilitation.

◆ Remind family members to encourage the patient to be as independent as possible.

◆ Teach the patient and his caregivers about all his medications, including their names, dosages, times of administration, and possible adverse effects and interactions. Instruct caregivers to call the patient's doctor if he experiences adverse reactions.

◆ Teach caregivers to recognize the signs of continuing or impending CVA.

◆ Help caregivers keep the patient's environment as safe as possible.

◆ Review emergency measures with the patient and caregivers.

◆ Talk with caregivers about the need for respite. Suggest options for obtaining support and help.

◆ Refer the patient and family to local groups and national organizations for support and information.

◆ Emphasize the need to keep all follow-up appointments.

caregivers to help with these exercises.

◆ Establish and maintain communication with the patient and caregivers; encourage them to express their fears and concerns. Respond with support and information.

◆ Evaluate the patient's ability to swallow. Explain the need for a soft diet and help with feeding, as necessary.

◆ Assess the patient's self-care ability and determine the availability of capable support people. Direct the patient to support groups as needed.

◆ Obtain appropriate assistive devices. Collaborate with the physical therapist, occupational therapist, and speech therapist as indicated. Reinforce the therapists' instructions about exercise, activities of daily living, and how to use assistive devices.

◆ To reduce the risk of another CVA, teach the patient and family about risk factors. For example, explain measures to reduce atherosclerosis. If needed, refer the patient to a smoking cessation or weight loss program. Teach all patients the importance of following a low-cholesterol, low-salt diet and increasing activity levels.

◆ CESAREAN DELIVERY

A patient may undergo cesarean (surgical) delivery for a number of reasons, including a difficult or dangerous fetal presentation, failure of labor to progress, genital herpes, cephalopelvic disproportion, placenta previa, abruptio placenta, or fetal distress. The procedure may be scheduled ahead of time or may be performed on an emergency basis.

When caring for a patient after cesarean delivery, remember that your patient is both postoperative and postpartum, with all the needs of each condition. In addition, the patient may have strong emotional responses to a cesarean delivery, including fear, guilt, and grief for loss of a "normal" pregnancy and birth experience. The patient may have difficulty bonding with her new infant because of the anesthesia, pain, or separation.

Assessment findings

During your home visit, carefully assess the following:

◆ Ensure that the breasts are well-supported by a brassiere that fits well. The breasts should be nontender and show no signs of inflammation. Nipples should be intact, without cracks, and not unduly sore.

◆ If the patient is breast-feeding, have her demonstrate or describe the technique that she uses to place the baby on the breast and to remove the baby from the breast. It's common for new mothers to have trouble with breast-feeding after a cesarean delivery because the infant's weight may rest on her incision.

◆ If the patient is not breast-feeding, check the breasts to ensure that they aren't engorged. Make sure that the patient is taking lactation suppressants properly if they were prescribed.

◆ The uterine fundus should be firm and descending below the umbilicus at a rate of about 1 cm daily.

◆ The incision should be dry, well-approximated, and only slightly red; if present, sutures or steristrips should be in place.

◆ Examination of the lochia should show normally progressive involution. Ask the patient if the lochia color is progressing from rubra to serosa to alba and if it is occurring in decreasing amounts. It should have a fleshy odor and no clots.

◆ Normal bowel elimination patterns should be reestablished. Hemorrhoids, if present, should not cause undue discomfort and should be decreasing in size.

◆ Urinary elimination should be normal and occur without burning. The patient should have no difficulty initiating the stream.
◆ The patient's legs should be nontender, and Homans' sign should be negative bilaterally.
◆ The patient should be able to maintain good body alignment when ambulating.

Implementation

When caring for a patient after cesarean delivery, you'll want to promote tissue integrity, ensure the patient's safety, maintain hydration, facilitate effective breast-feeding, and encourage mother-infant bonding. Specific interventions include the following:
◆ Assess the patient thoroughly, including vital signs, bowel elimination, lochia, fundal position, incision and dressing, pain, breast condition, and emotional response.
◆ Make sure the patient is performing incentive spirometry, deep breathing, and coughing exercises, as needed. Also encourage her to perform leg exercises and wear antiembolism stockings, as ordered.
◆ Provide emotional support as appropriate.
◆ Perform incision care and change the dressing as ordered. Teach the patient about wound care, and show her how to care for her incision, including dressing changes, as needed.
◆ Offer support and assistance for breast-feeding, bottle-feeding, and self-care.
◆ Assess the infant's respiratory rate, vital signs, and signs of distress.
◆ Monitor the infant for signs of hypoglycemia. Perform a heelstick to determine blood glucose levels, as ordered.
◆ Promote family bonding.
◆ Help the patient maintain adequate hydration and nutrition.
◆ Teach the patient about the importance of adequate rest.
◆ Teach the patient how to assess her fundus and lochia.
◆ Teach the patient routine infant care, and answer any questions she may have.
◆ Teach the patient about prescribed medications, adverse reactions, and when to contact the doctor.

◆ CHRONIC OBSTRUCTIVE PULMONARY DISEASE

In chronic obstructive pulmonary disease (COPD), or chronic airflow limitation, the patient has irreversible airway obstruction associated with varying degrees of chronic bronchitis, emphysema, or asthma. Cigarette smoking is the most common cause of COPD. It affects men more than women, presumably because men once smoked more heavily than women.

The most effective treatment for COPD includes smoking cessation and avoidance of other air pollutants. Antibiotics can be used for recurring infections. Bronchodilators may relieve bronchospasm and facilitate mucus clearance. Ultrasonic or mechanical nebulizer treatments may help loosen and mobilize secretions, as will increased fluids. Some patients respond to corticosteroids. Diuretics may be used to treat edema. Supplemental oxygen may be necessary. Pulmonary rehabilitation may restore some function.

Assessment findings

The patient's history typically reveals a long-time smoker with frequent upper respiratory tract infections. The patient also typically reports progressively worsening shortness of breath.

Inspection usually reveals a cough, often with gray, white, or yellow spu-

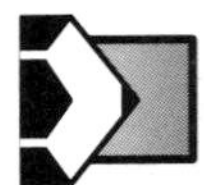

TEACHING POINTS

Living with COPD

If you care for a patient with chronic obstructive pulmonary disease (COPD), you'll need to help him maintain as much respiratory function as possible while also helping to head off complications. Start with the following ideas:

◆ Promote as much self-care and independence as possible for the patient, including teaching him and his family how to perform procedures and use and care for equipment.

◆ Show the patient and family how to perform postural drainage and chest percussion and vibration. Instruct the patient to maintain each position for 10 minutes, if possible, before a caregiver performs chest percussion and the patient coughs.

◆ Teach the patient coughing and deep-breathing techniques to enhance ventilation and remove secretions.

◆ Review all of the patient's medications, including names, purposes, dosages, administration times, and possible adverse effects. Teach the patient how to use an inhaler. Advise him to immediately report adverse reactions to the doctor.

◆ Encourage the patient to maintain good nutrition by eating high-calorie, protein-rich meals and drinking plenty of fluids to prevent dehydration and help loosen secretions.

◆ If the patient smokes, encourage him to stop. Teach him about the hazards of smoking, and provide him with smoking cessation resources, including community-based smoking cessation programs, the names of over-the-counter cessation aids, and sources of counseling.

◆ Explain measures the patient can use to decrease his risk of repeated upper respiratory tract infections. For example, tell him to avoid using antibiotics indiscriminately for minor infections; such use could allow antibiotic-resistant bacteria to colonize his upper airway. Also encourage the patient to obtain a pneumococcal pneumonia vaccination (one lasts a lifetime) and an annual influenza vaccination.

tum. The patient may appear cyanotic and may use accessory muscles for breathing. Vital signs usually indicate tachypnea and tachycardia. Palpation may reveal close pedal edema and neck vein distention. Auscultation findings include abnormal breath sounds, such as crackles, a prolonged expiratory time, and wheezing.

Diagnostic tests include chest X-rays, pulmonary function tests, arterial blood gas measurements, sputum culture, pulse oximetry, and electrocardiogram.

Implementation

When caring for a patient with COPD, you'll want to improve gas exchange, promote effective breathing patterns, maintain nutrition, increase fluid volume, minimize fatigue, decrease anxiety, and promote comfort. (See *Living with COPD.*) Specific interventions include the following:

◆ Assess for changes in baseline respiratory function. Evaluate sputum quality and quantity, restlessness, increased tachypnea, and altered breath sounds.

◆ Administer oxygen, bronchodilators, and nebulizer treatments as ordered. Teach the patient how to self-administer oxygen and perform nebulizer treatments.

◆ Urge the patient to avoid irritants that stimulate secretions, such as cigarette smoke and dust.

◆ Encourage a diet of soft foods high in calories and protein. Provide nutritional supplements as necessary. Urge the patient to drink at least 2 qt (2 L) of fluids each day. Collaborate with the dietitian as indicated, and monitor the patient's weight at least weekly.

◆ Stress the importance of daily activity, and encourage the caregiver to provide diversional activities as appropriate. Alternate activities with periods of rest to prevent fatigue.

◆ Monitor the patient's response to pulmonary rehabilitation, as appropriate.

◆ Encourage the patient and his family to express their fears and concerns. Respond with support and information.

◆ Evaluate the patient's response to the plan of care and medications.

◆ Teach the patient to recognize signs and symptoms of complications or exacerbation.

◆ Explain how and when to activate the emergency medical system.

◆ Reinforce teaching about the disease process and its treatment, including diet, postural drainage, and breathing exercises.

◆ CYSTIC FIBROSIS

A chronic, progressive disease, cystic fibrosis is transmitted as an autosomal recessive trait. A defect in the chloride ion channel disturbs ion and water transport across the cell membrane, resulting in abnormally thick mucus. It plugs the respiratory tract, increasing the risk of infection, lung damage, and eventual respiratory failure. It also clogs the pancreatic ducts, resulting in pancreatic insufficiency. It can cause bronchiectasis, pneumonia, atelectasis, hemoptysis, dehydration, distal intestinal obstructive syndrome, malnutrition, gastroesophageal reflux, rectal prolapse, nasal polyps, and cor pulmonale.

Treatment aims to help the patient lead as normal a life as possible. Specific treatments depend on the organ system involved. Pancreatic enzymes taken with meals and snacks can help offset pancreatic enzyme deficiencies. Chest physiotherapy and nebulizer treatments can help loosen pulmonary secretions. Dornase alfa, a pulmonary enzyme given by aerosol nebulizer, helps to thin airway mucus, improving lung function and reducing the risk of infection.

Assessment findings

Diagnosis usually results from an infant's failure to grow properly despite a voracious appetite. Parents usually report noticing that the infant has light colored, frothy, foul-smelling steatorrhea. If undiagnosed before his first upper respiratory infection, the child may present with a persistent cough and possible wheezing. Hyponatremic dehydration may be the presenting symptom in hot weather or in a child with a fever.

The sweat test continues to be the initial diagnostic test because the disorder causes excessive secretion of sodium and chloride in the sweat. Ge-

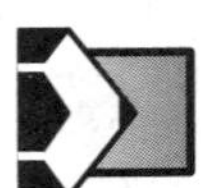

TEACHING POINTS

Living with cystic fibrosis

If you care for a patient with cystic fibrosis, you'll need to provide extensive teaching for the family in addition to expert care for the patient. Start with the following ideas.

◆ Teach the parents how to assess the child's condition, including counting the sleeping respiratory rate and observing for retractions, color change, mucus characteristics (color, consistency, amount), and the frequency and type of cough (dry, moist, productive, bronchial, throat-clearing).

◆ Stress to parents that children with cystic fibrosis are at risk for hyponatremic dehydration during hot weather, strenuous exercise, and fevers. Have them increase the child's salt and fluid intake during these times to help prevent this problem.

◆ Urge parents to maintain a smoke-free environment for their child, particularly in their own home.

◆ Teach or review chest physiotherapy and postural drainage positions, and have parents demonstrate the procedure for you.

◆ Help the parents find alternatives to cupped hands for chest physiotherapy, such as using a small, light-weight plastic cup or bowl. Mechanical percussors are also available.

◆ Teach the patient and family about prescribed medications, including nebulizer therapy. Discuss adverse reactions and what to do about them.

◆ Review breathing exercises with the child and family.

◆ Teach the patient and family to recognize signs of infection and sudden changes in the patient's condition — and when to report them to the doctor.

◆ Warn parents that hemoptysis and pneumothorax can occur spontaneously in patients with advanced pulmonary disease. Outline the signs and symptoms of these complications, and tell parents what to do if they arise.

netic testing also may be done. Pulmonary function tests and chest X-rays are helpful in staging the disease but are not specific to cystic fibrosis.

Depending on the stage of the disease, you may notice muscle wasting, a bronchial cough, wheezing, and possibly vomiting during coughing. The child may have clear breath sounds or crackles and wheezes. He may display dyspnea on exertion or decreased activity tolerance, along with an increased breathing effort that includes retractions. He may show decreased pulmonary function, thick sputum (yellow, green, or blood-tinged), clubbed fingers, an excessive appetite (at or before diagnosis), decreased appetite with pulmonary infections, an enlarged liver, and tarry stools.

Implementation

When caring for the patient with cystic fibrosis, you'll want to promote effective breathing, ensure adequate nutrition and hydration, facilitate effective coping, and safeguard the patient from injury and infection. (See *Living with cystic fibrosis*.) Specific interventions include the following:

◆ Monitor I.V. antibiotic therapy. If the patient is administering the medications, verify compliance.

◆ If the patient has an I.V. access device, assess the integrity of the catheter. Perform dressing changes, as necessary. Flush the device according to agency policy.

◆ Ensure that the patient is taking all prescribed medications and supplements properly, including pancreatic enzyme supplements and multiple vitamins.

◆ Teach the patient and caregivers to adjust pancreatic enzyme capsule dosage according to fat intake and the character and volume of bowel movements. Explain that the goal is to produce one or two stools of normal color and consistency each day.

◆ Monitor the patient's nutritional and fluid intake. Stress the importance of supplemental enzyme therapy and a well-balanced diet high in calories, protein, and salt.

◆ Assess pulmonary status, air exchange, and effort of breathing.

◆ Help parents and child obtain necessary equipment and supplies. If needed, also help them obtain assistance in administering the three or four chest physiotherapy treatments needed each day.

◆ Evaluate the patient's and parents' ability to perform chest physiotherapy.

◆ Encourage the parents to obtain an air conditioner for their child's room.

◆ Note the patient's weight and assess weight gain. Adjust the diet as needed.

◆ Teach the patient and caregivers to replace salt and water during hot weather and during a fever.

◆ DEGENERATIVE JOINT DISEASE

Degenerative joint disease (DJD), commonly known as osteoarthritis, causes deterioration of the joint cartilage and formation of reactive new bone at marginal and subchondral joint areas. This chronic degeneration results from a breakdown of chondrocytes, most often in the hips and knees.

DJD occurs equally in both sexes. More than half of people over age 30 have some features of primary osteoarthritis, and nearly all people over age 60 have radiographic evidence of the disorder. Fewer than half experience symptoms.

Depending on the site and severity of joint involvement, disability can range from minor limitation of the fingers to near immobility in persons with hip or knee disease. Progression rates vary; joints may remain stable for years in early stages of degeneration.

To relieve pain, improve mobility, and minimize disability, treatment includes medications (usually aspirin or nonsteroidal anti-inflammatory drugs), rest, physical therapy, assistive mobility devices, corticosteroid injections, and possible surgery.

Physical therapy includes massage, moist heat, paraffin dips for the hands, supervised exercise to decrease muscle spasms and atrophy, and protective techniques for reducing joint stress.

Assessment findings

The patient usually complains of gradually increasing signs and symptoms. Many have a predisposing event such as traumatic injury. Most com-

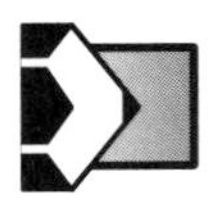

TEACHING POINTS

Living with DJD

If you care for a patient with degenerative joint disease (DJD), you'll need to find ways to help him minimize pain and maximize mobility. Here are some ideas:

◆ Review prescribed range-of-motion (ROM) exercises with the patient and his family. Determine how much help the patient needs to perform the exercises. Then show family members how to provide that help appropriately.

◆ Urge the patient to comply with the prescribed frequency of ROM exercises. Although they may be uncomfortable, the exercises will help maintain mobility. Many patients with DJD perform ROM exercises twice daily.

◆ Help the patient and family perform progressive resistance exercises to increase the patient's muscle strength.

◆ Encourage the patient to plan for adequate rest throughout the day. Suggest planning periods of rest between activities, and discuss energy conservation methods, such as simplifying work procedures and protecting joints. Advise against overexertion.

◆ Help the patient figure out how to relieve specific discomforts. For example, using a firm mattress or bed board may lessen morning pain from lumbosacral spinal joints.

monly, the patient has deep, aching joint pain, particularly after exercise or weight bearing on the affected joint. Rest may relieve the pain.

Additional complaints include stiffness in the morning and after exercise, aching during weather changes, a "grating" feeling when the joint moves, contractures, and limited movement. These symptoms tend to be worse in patients with poor posture, obesity, or occupational stress.

Inspection may reveal joint swelling, muscle atrophy, deformity of the involved area, and gait abnormalities (when the disease affects the hips or knees). Palpation may reveal joint tenderness and warmth without redness, grating with movement, joint instability, and limited movement.

Diagnostic tests may include X-rays of the affected joints, synovial fluid analysis, radionucleotide bone scan, arthroscopy, magnetic resonance imaging, and neuromuscular tests.

Implementation

When caring for a patient with degenerative joint disease, you'll want to encourage self-care, minimize impairment and decreased mobility, control pain, and promote effective individual coping. (See *Living with DJD*.) Specific interventions include the following:

◆ Assess pain at regular intervals. Note its location and intensity, precipitating factors, alleviating factors, and any identifiable patterns. Encourage the use of pain medications as ordered.

◆ Encourage the patient to perform as much self-care as possible. Give pain medications before the patient undertakes activities, and allow sufficient time and space for the patient to complete them. Encourage use of assistive devices, as needed. Collaborate with the physical and occupational therapist as needed, and reinforce the plan of care.

◆ Evaluate the patient's response to pain medication. Review the adverse effects, as needed, and urge the patient to report them promptly.

◆ Assess the patient's home for safety, and report any problems to the patient and caregiver for repair or replacement.

◆ Coordinate care with the physical therapist, occupational therapist, home health aide, social worker, dietitian, chaplain, and other referred professionals.

◆ Recommend elastic supports or braces if needed. As indicated, check all assistive devices, such as crutches, canes, braces and walkers. Reinforce their proper use and positioning to prevent injury.

◆ Provide emotional support and reassurance to help the patient cope with reduced mobility. Allow him to voice his feelings. In response, offer information and support. If necessary, refer the patient for individual counseling.

◆ Evaluate the patient's response to treatment.

◆ DEMENTIA

Dementia may result from many causes and may be primary or secondary. Primary dementia is progressive and irreversible. It results from such conditions as Alzheimer's disease, multi-infarct dementia, and Pick's disease. Secondary dementia results from another process, such as infection, trauma, toxic or metabolic disturbance, tumor, neurologic disease, normal-pressure hydrocephalus, and acquired immunodeficiency syndrome. Symptoms of some secondary dementias abate when the underlying cause is corrected.

Assessment findings

Whether primary or secondary, dementia is characterized by progressive deterioration in intellectual functioning, memory, and the ability to learn new skills and solve problems. Personality traits change. Judgment, insight, and morals decline as the disease progresses.

The multiple cognitive deficits include memory impairment and at least one of the following: aphasia, apraxia, agnosia, or a disturbance in executive functioning. Cognitive impairments may associate with mood and sleep disturbances and with anxiety. The patient may have hallucinations (especially visual) and delusions (usually persecutory).

Diagnostic tests include the mental status examination and neuropsychological testing. (See chapter 5 for more information.) Standardized rating scales can measure the severity of impairment in personal care, intellectual functioning, and the ability to use the telephone, dishwasher, and other tools and implements. Visual-spatial function can be assessed by asking the patient to copy such drawings as a circle, overlapping pentagons, and a cube. Computed tomography or magnetic resonance imaging may show cerebral atrophy, focal brain lesions (such as cortical stroke), tumor, subdural hematoma, ischemic brain injury, and hydrocephalus.

Although coexisting medical conditions require specific treatment measures, treatment for dementia typically is supportive. In general, barbiturates and benzodiazepines should be avoided because they can worsen cognition. Low doses of antipsychotics can be used for agitation. Short-acting benzodiazepines can be used for insomnia, but they may cause further memory deficits the follow-

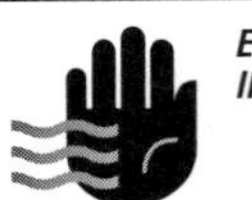

EMERGENCY INTERVENTIONS

Responding to a fall

If the patient falls, respond quickly and accurately, as follows:

◆ Maintain a patent airway using a chin-lift or jaw-thrust maneuver.
◆ Assess breathing and circulation.
◆ Obtain vital signs.
◆ Apply direct pressure to areas of bleeding.
◆ Call 911 for transport to the hospital for evaluation.
◆ Do not move the patient.
◆ Keep the patient's neck immobilized.
◆ Reassure the patient and stay with him until help arrives.
◆ Once he's stable and safe, notify his doctor.

ing day. Support groups can help families cope.

Implementation

When caring for a patient with dementia, you'll want to promote his safety and independence. Specific interventions include the following:

◆ Ask family members to identify the patient's daily habits and recreational preferences for inclusion in the patient's care.
◆ Introduce yourself every time you visit the patient, and repeat your name throughout your visit. Communicate in clear, simple, concrete sentences.
◆ Always give careful explanations to the patient before you provide care. This helps to remind the patient and prevents undue anxiety.
◆ Help the patient maintain a daily routine that's similar to his old one. Doing so will help decrease anxiety and minimize memory deficits. Stress the importance of these activities to the patient and caregivers.
◆ Explain the need to maintain the patient's nutrition, exercise, and stimulation during the day to help him sleep and avoid wandering during the night. Provide safe opportunities for wandering during the day.
◆ Stress the importance of providing frequent cues for orientation to day, date, place, and time. Tell the patient and caregiver to place memory clues (including clocks, calendars, pictures, notes, and arrows to the most used rooms) in common locations. Explain the need to provide instructions in short, simple, repetitive sentences.
◆ Approach the patient with understanding, and validate his fears and concerns; instruct caregivers to do the same.
◆ Ask family members to describe the extent to which memory disturbances influence the patient's functioning, including shopping, working, cooking, paying bills, and returning home without getting lost. Also inquire about the patient's ability to plan activities, make a budget, and perform other tasks of daily life.
◆ Tell family members to assess the patient's behavior. If he suddenly becomes restless and seems to be searching for something, he may be looking for the bathroom.
◆ If the patient wanders, make sure caregivers understand the importance of ensuring that the patient always wears identification that includes his name, address, and telephone number. If the identification is on a bracelet, make sure the patient can't remove it.

◆ Encourage the family or caregivers to notify local police and neighbors that the patient has a history of wandering. Provide police with recent photos of the patient.
◆ Urge the family to install complex, difficult-to-reach locks on all doors and child-proof doorknob covers on all doors that lead outside. Also urge them to install motion detectors outside to warn them if the patient leaves the house. (See *Responding to a fall*.)

◆ DIABETES MELLITUS

A chronic disease of absolute or relative insulin deficiency or resistance, diabetes mellitus is characterized by disturbances in carbohydrate, protein, and fat metabolism. The disorder occurs in two primary forms: type 1 (insulin-dependent) and the more prevalent type 2 (non-insulin-dependent). A number of secondary forms exist. They result from such conditions as pancreatic disease, pregnancy, hormonal or genetic syndromes, or ingestion of certain drugs or chemicals. (See *Responding to gestational diabetes*, page 224.)

Treatment aims to optimize blood glucose levels and decrease complications. For type 1 diabetes, treatment focuses on insulin replacement, diet, and exercise. For the obese patient with type 2 diabetes, weight reduction is an important goal. Treatment for both types requires strict adherence to a diet that's carefully planned to meet the patient's nutritional needs while controlling blood glucose levels.

Assessment findings

The patient with type 1 diabetes typically reports that symptoms developed quickly. The patient with type 2 typically reports vague symptoms that have developed gradually. The patient probably has a family history of diabetes, gestational diabetes, delivery of a baby weighing more than 9 lb (4 kg), a severe viral infection, endocrine disease, recent stress or trauma, or use of drugs that increase serum glucose levels.

Patients with either type of diabetes may report symptoms associated with hyperglycemia, such as polyuria, polydipsia, polyphagia, weight loss, and fatigue. Or they may complain of weakness; vision changes; frequent skin infections; dry, itchy skin; sexual problems; and vaginal discomfort — all signs of hyperglycemia.

Inspection may show retinopathy or cataract formation. Skin changes, especially on the legs and feet, may represent impaired peripheral circulation. Muscle wasting and loss of subcutaneous fat may be evident if the patient has type 1 diabetes. The patient with type 2 diabetes typically presents with obesity, particularly in the abdominal area.

Palpation may detect poor skin turgor and dry mucous membranes related to dehydration. Decreased peripheral pulses, cool skin temperature, and decreased reflexes may also be palpable. Auscultation may reveal orthostatic hypotension. Patients with diabetic ketoacidosis may have a characteristic fruity breath odor due to increased acetone production.

Fasting and random serum glucose levels are the primary tool for diagnosing and monitoring diabetes mellitus. Oral glucose tolerance tests are also used.

Chronic complications of diabetes mellitus include cardiovascular disease, peripheral vascular diseases, retinopathy, neuropathy, diabetic dermopathy, and peripheral and autonomic neuropathy. Hyperglycemia impairs the patient's resistance to infection because the glucose content

Responding to gestational diabetes

Gestational diabetes is a condition that develops in 2% to 3% of pregnant women, usually at midterm. It's probably caused by the placental hormone lactogen and high levels of other hormones. Risk factors for gestational diabetes include obesity, age over 30, history of having babies over 10 lb (4.5 kg), unexplained fetal loss, previous congenital anomalies, and a family history of diabetes.

The gestational diabetic will need insulin (by intermittent injection or continuous subcutaneous infusion pump) when and if dietary control isn't sufficient to regulate blood glucose levels. Insulin dosages are adjusted to keep fasting blood sugar levels between 100 and 115 mg/dl and postprandial levels between 120 and 138 mg/dl. Oral antidiabetic agents typically aren't used because they cross the placenta and may be teratogenic.

Gestational diabetes usually resolves after delivery, but it may raise a woman's risk of developing diabetes later in life. If you care for a woman with gestational diabetes, you'll need to provide her with ample education in addition to promoting safety, tissue integrity, and proper nutrition. Use the following topics as a start:

◆ Monitor the patient's vital signs and measure fundal height.

◆ Assess fetal heart tones and uterine activity. Teach the patient how to assess fetal well-being by counting fetal movements.

◆ As needed, teach the patient and family about her condition, glucose monitoring procedures, and treatment regimen. Explain the signs and symptoms of hypoglycemia. If they develop, tell her to eat a snack made of complex carbohydrates and low sugars, such as milk and crackers. This tactic helps prevent rebound hyperglycemia and more severe hypoglycemia.

◆ Urge the patient to monitor her blood glucose levels at prescribed times, usually after fasting, after eating, and at bedtime. Occasionally she may need to check her blood glucose level at 2 a.m. because hypoglycemia is especially likely to occur at this time.

◆ Monitor the patient's blood glucose level, and encourage her to maintain adequate nutrition while adhering to her prescribed diet. Most patients consume 1,800 to 2,200 calories divided between three meals and three snacks to help keep glucose levels constant. The diet should be low in saturated fats and cholesterol and high in fiber.

◆ Advise the patient to increase her fiber intake to help decrease the possibility of postprandial hyperglycemia.

of the epidermis and urine encourages bacterial growth. Thus, the patient is susceptible to skin and urinary tract infections and vaginitis.

Implementation

When caring for a patient with diabetes mellitus, you'll want to promote self-care and independent manage-

ment of the disease, encourage adequate nutrition and activity, prevent complications of the disease, and nurture effective individual coping. Specific interventions include the following:
◆ Stress the importance of carefully adhering to the prescribed program. As necessary, discuss and review diet (including food exchange lists), medications, exercise, monitoring techniques, hygiene (especially foot care), and sick day rules.
◆ Assess the patient's record of blood glucose levels performed before meals and at bedtime or as prescribed. Perform a blood glucose measurement during your visit.
◆ Draw blood for glycosylated hemoglobin level and serum electrolyte levels, as ordered.
◆ Collaborate with a dietitian to plan a diet that includes recommended levels of calories, protein, carbohydrates, and fats, based on the patient's individual requirements.
◆ Explain the interaction between diabetes control and food intake, medication therapy, exercise, and stress (both psychological and physiologic).
◆ Encourage the patient and family to verbalize their feelings about diabetes and its effects on lifestyle and life expectancy.
◆ Offer emotional support and a realistic assessment of the patient's condition. Stress that, with proper treatment, diabetics can have a near-normal lifestyle and life expectancy. Help the patient develop or enhance coping strategies.
◆ Monitor for acute complications, especially hypoglycemia. Review signs and symptoms of hypoglycemia and hyperglycemia. Instruct the patient and family on how to recognize and prevent hypoglycemia. Review appropriate actions to take if the patient develops hypoglycemia or hyperglycemia. (See *Treating hypoglycemia*.)
◆ Monitor for chronic complications, including effects on the peripheral and autonomic nervous system and on the cardiovascular system (such as cerebrovascular, coronary artery,

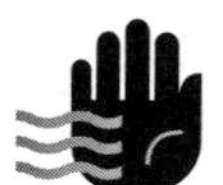

EMERGENCY INTERVENTIONS

Treating hypoglycemia

If your patient develops hypoglycemia, you'll need to respond right away with the following interventions:
◆ Administer an oral form of simple sugar, such as 4 oz (120 ml) of orange juice, 6 Lifesavers or jelly beans, a lump of sugar, or 2 tablespoons of raisins.
◆ If severe hypoglycemia persists, repeat in 10 to 15 minutes.
◆ After the symptoms have subsided, give a protein source, such as half of a cheese sandwich, a glass of milk, or peanut butter crackers.
◆ If the patient is unconscious, activate the emergency medical system and give the patient nothing by mouth to prevent aspiration. (Some practitioners place a thin layer of cake icing in the buccal area of the mouth and along the lower lip to increase blood glucose levels.)
◆ Teach the patient and family members how to respond to hypoglycemia.

and peripheral vascular impairment). Monitor for signs of diabetic neuropathy. Also watch for signs and symptoms of urinary tract and vaginal infections.

◆ Evaluate the patient's response to the plan of care and medications; confer with the doctor if adjustment are needed.

◆ Refer the patient and family to counseling, as appropriate. Encourage participation in a support group.

◆ HIP FRACTURE

Hip fracture is a general term used to describe fractures of the head, neck (intracapsular fracture), or trochanteric area (extracapsular fracture) of the femur. The condition is most common among elderly women, mainly as a result of osteoporosis. Hip fractures are usually associated with a fall.

Assessment findings

The patient will report pain in the affected hip, usually caused by a fall, and may not be able to bear weight on that leg. In addition, the patient may report changes in sensation on the affected side, including numbness and tingling. On inspection, the affected leg appears shorter, and there may be external rotation of the affected limb.

The diagnosis of fractured hip is confirmed by X-ray. Treatment may include temporary traction to relieve pain until surgery can take place (or if surgery is contraindicated). Closed reduction with a hip spica cast may be used to treat fractures of the intratrochanteric area. Other hip fractures may be treated with open reduction and internal fixation using various prosthetic devices.

Implementation

When caring for a patient with a hip fracture, you'll want to control pain, promote early mobility, and prevent complications. Specific interventions include the following:

◆ Assess the patient's condition. Note vital signs, mobility, and states of surgical inversion. Check the affected leg for color, edema, warmth, and pulses. Assess the joint for range of motion and pain with movement.

◆ Initiate interdisciplinary referrals (physical therapist, occupational therapist, vocational therapist).

◆ Assess pain at regular intervals. Note its location and intensity, precipitating factors, alleviating factors, and any identifiable patterns. Teach the patient and caregivers pain evaluation techniques.

◆ As ordered, encourage mobility. Teach the patient to administer pain medications ahead of time, so they can start working before you ambulate the patient. Encourage quadriceps setting exercises. Collaborate with the physical therapist as necessary. Review, reinforce, and encourage compliance with the prescribed exercise regimen.

◆ Urge the patient to perform coughing and deep-breathing exercises to prevent upper respiratory congestion. Reinforce the importance of using incentive spirometry.

◆ Encourage the patient to use prescribed pain medications, and evaluate their effect. Explain possible adverse effects, and encourage the patient to report them promptly.

◆ Many falls and hip fractures result from the patient's inability to see stairs and obstacles. Thus, you'll want to urge family members to maintain a safe environment, for example, to clear obstacles from walking areas and highlight the edges of stairs. Also urge the patient to have regular eye examinations and to wear appropriate prescriptive lenses.

◆ Remind the patient that the prosthetics used in hip replacement will be picked up by metal detectors used for security purposes (such as at airports and courthouses). If the manufacturer provides one, urge the patient to carry an identification card describing the implant.

◆ Teach incisional care and asepsis, signs of infection to report, and transfer and pivoting techniques. Explain how to make the home safe.

◆ HYPERBILIRUBINEMIA, NEONATAL

An elevation of serum bilirubin, hyperbilirubinemia leads to jaundice. The disorder can be physiologic or pathologic. Physiologic jaundice is the most common and disappears in a few days, usually without treatment. It typically occurs on the second to fourth day after birth and is caused by the breakdown of red blood cells and immature liver function.

If the bilirubin level rises above 10 mg/dl, the doctor will consider treatment. Brain damage may occur at levels above 20 mg/dl. Complications — chiefly kernicterus — are rare but may be deadly.

Assessment findings

Jaundice usually isn't apparent until bilirubin reaches 7 mg/dl. Once it does, you can see jaundice easily by pressing the skin on the cheek, tip of nose, or abdomen and then releasing the pressure and observing the color. The infant also may have cephalhematoma, bruising, or petechiae.

Early feedings and adequate intestinal elimination prevent bilirubin buildup and may obviate treatment. The decision of when and how to treat it is generally determined by the serum bilirubin level, the neonate's age, and the underlying cause. Phototherapy is the usual treatment of choice. Exchange transfusions, albumin infusion, and drug therapy also may be considered.

Implementation

When caring for a patient with hyperbilirubinemia, you'll want to promote hydration, protect tissue integrity, ensure adequate nutrition, and provide safety. (See *Responding to hyperbilirubinemia*, page 228.) Specific interventions include the following:

◆ Perform a complete physical assessment, noting particularly the degree and extent of jaundice. Inspect the sclerae carefully. Check the mucosa and skin after blanching with finger pressure.

◆ Perform heelsticks to obtain blood samples for serum bilirubin as ordered.

◆ Monitor the intake and output record kept by the parents.

◆ Assess for adequate feedings (to prevent dehydration). Determine 24-hour elimination patterns, and identify urine and stool characteristics. Record the number and color of voidings and stools per day.

◆ Assess for neurosensory findings that could indicate worsening, such as lethargy, loss of Moro reflex, a shrill cry, bulging fontanels, or opisthotonos.

◆ Assess the degree, extent, and timing of jaundice, as well as periodic serum bilirubin levels.

◆ Have the infant's mother take his temperature every 2 to 4 hours.

◆ Encourage the new mother to feed her newborn every 2 to 3 hours and to provide water supplements.

◆ If the infant is receiving phototherapy, teach the parents to record the time of treatment and length of exposure, to use shields to protect the infant's eyes (removing them every 2

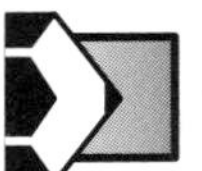

Responding to hyperbilirubinemia

If you care for an infant with hyperbilirubinemia, you'll need to provide teaching to the infant's parents. Use these ideas as a start:
◆ Explain to parents what hyperbilirubinemia is, what causes it, how it was detected in the acute care facility, and what treatments are available for it.
◆ Explain the treatment being used specifically for their infant. Describe the phototherapy unit (bililight or biliblanket) and its management.
◆ Tell parents not to worry if the treatment causes their infant to produce green stool; explain that it simply indicates elimination of the excess bilirubin.
◆ Encourage parents to feed the infant every 2 to 4 hours, and to offer water or dextrose 5% in water between feedings to help avoid dehydration.
◆ Stress the importance of maintaining the infant's oral intake. Tell the infant's mother not to skip any feedings because fasting will stimulate production of more bilirubin.

to 4 hours to inspect the infant's eyes and allow him visual stimulation), and to shield the penis and scrotum of a male infant.

◆ Instruct the mother to turn the infant every 2 hours to provide overall skin exposure.
◆ Explain the need to maintain the infant's body temperature and protect him from drafts.
◆ Teach the new mother how to maintain her milk supply if the phototherapy interrupts breast-feeding,
◆ Provide emotional support to the parents and family.
◆ Emphasize the importance of repeated serum bilirubin testing and follow-up doctor visits.

◆ HYPERTENSION

This disorder is marked by a sustained elevation of systolic pressure at or above 140 mm Hg, or a sustained elevation of diastolic pressure at or above 90 mm Hg. The two major types of hypertension are essential (also called primary or idiopathic) and secondary, which results from renal disease or another identifiable cause. Malignant hypertension is a severe, fulminant form that may be fatal.

Although essential hypertension has no cure, drugs and modifications in diet and lifestyle help control it. Generally, nondrug treatment, such as lifestyle modification, is tried first, especially in early, mild cases. If this is ineffective, treatment progresses in a stepwise manner to include various types of antihypertensive medications. (See *Managing antihypertensive therapy*.)

Assessment findings

In many cases, the hypertensive patient has no symptoms; instead, the disorder is revealed incidentally during evaluation for another disorder or during routine blood pressure screening.

When symptoms do occur, they reflect the effect of hypertension on or-

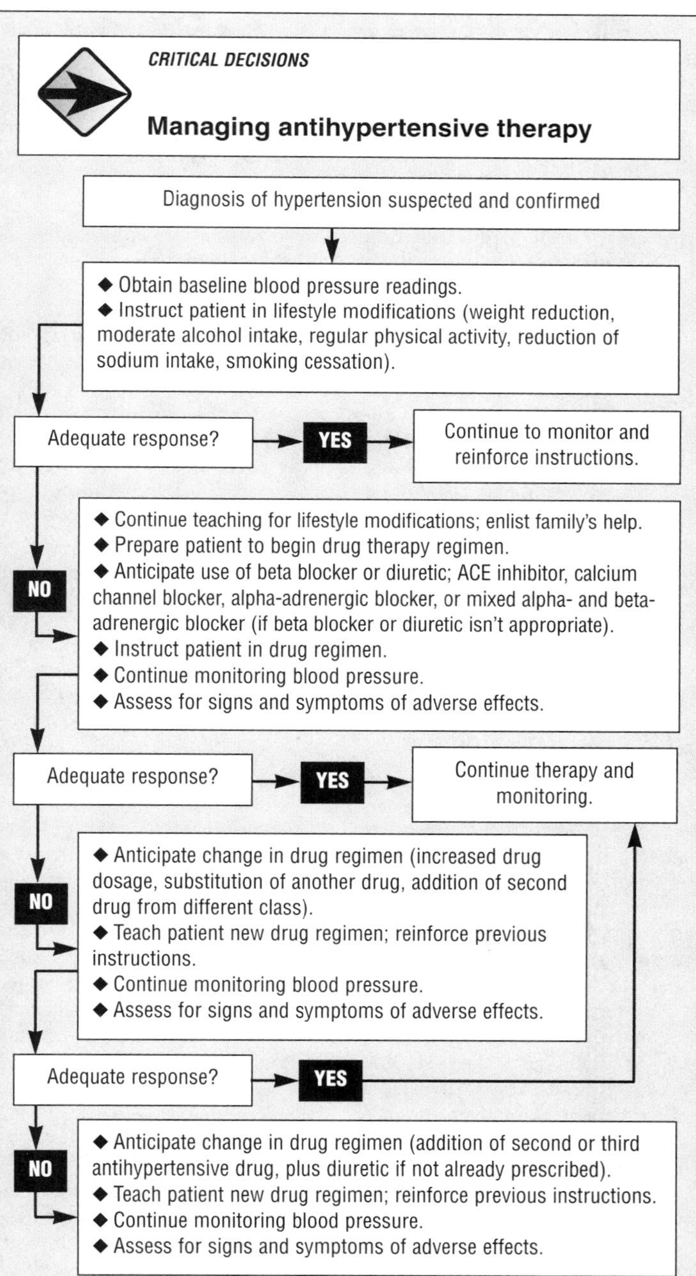
CRITICAL DECISIONS
Managing antihypertensive therapy
Diagnosis of hypertension suspected and confirmed
◆ Obtain baseline blood pressure readings.
◆ Instruct patient in lifestyle modifications (weight reduction, moderate alcohol intake, regular physical activity, reduction of sodium intake, smoking cessation).
Adequate response?
YES
Continue to monitor and reinforce instructions.
NO
◆ Continue teaching for lifestyle modifications; enlist family's help.
◆ Prepare patient to begin drug therapy regimen.
◆ Anticipate use of beta blocker or diuretic; ACE inhibitor, calcium channel blocker, alpha-adrenergic blocker, or mixed alpha- and beta-adrenergic blocker (if beta blocker or diuretic isn't appropriate).
◆ Instruct patient in drug regimen.
◆ Continue monitoring blood pressure.
◆ Assess for signs and symptoms of adverse effects.
Adequate response?
YES
Continue therapy and monitoring.
NO
◆ Anticipate change in drug regimen (increased drug dosage, substitution of another drug, addition of second drug from different class).
◆ Teach patient new drug regimen; reinforce previous instructions.
◆ Continue monitoring blood pressure.
◆ Assess for signs and symptoms of adverse effects.
Adequate response?
YES
NO
◆ Anticipate change in drug regimen (addition of second or third antihypertensive drug, plus diuretic if not already prescribed).
◆ Teach patient new drug regimen; reinforce previous instructions.
◆ Continue monitoring blood pressure.
◆ Assess for signs and symptoms of adverse effects.

gan systems. For example, vascular involvement may cause nosebleeds, bloody urine, weakness, and blurred vision. Cardiac involvement may cause chest pain, dyspnea, and peripheral edema. Ophthalmoscopic evaluation may reveal hemorrhages, exudates, papilledema, and possible hypertensive retinopathy. Palpation of the carotid artery may disclose stenosis or occlusion. Palpation of the abdomen may reveal a pulsating mass, suggesting an abdominal aneurysm.

Diagnostic tests used to evaluate hypertension include urinalysis; excretory urography; serum potassium, blood urea nitrogen, and creatinine levels; electrocardiogram, and chest X-ray.

Implementation

When caring for a patient with hypertension, you'll want to encourage needed lifestyle changes, monitor the patient's response to antihypertensive therapy, and promote coping skills. Specific interventions include the following:

- Assess the patient. Measure vital signs and weigh the patient. Assess level of responsiveness and complaints of headache, dizziness, nausea, vomiting, vision changes, and epistaxis. Auscultate for heart sounds and breath sounds. Palpate pulses (carotid, femoral, radial, and pedal).
- Help the patient examine and modify his lifestyle. Suggest that he try stress-reduction measures and an exercise program, particularly aerobic walking, to improve cardiac status and reduce obesity and serum cholesterol levels.
- Encourage the patient to change his diet. Tell him to avoid high-sodium foods, table salt, and foods high in cholesterol and saturated fats. Help the obese patient plan a weight-loss diet. Provide written teaching materials if possible.
- Assess for compliance with lifestyle changes and medication therapy. Warn the patient that uncontrolled hypertension may cause a stroke or heart attack.
- To encourage compliance with antihypertensive therapy, suggest establishing a daily routine for taking medications.
- Monitor blood pressure with the patient lying down, sitting up, and standing up. Record and report any differences.
- Monitor for signs and symptoms of adverse reactions to medication therapy, especially orthostatic hypotension. Explain orthostatic hypotension to the patient and caregivers. If it occurs, tell them to institute safety measures, such as having the patient change positions slowly and sit up in bed before standing up.
- Teach the patient to use a blood pressure cuff and to record the readings at least twice weekly so the doctor can review them at every follow-up visit. Tell the patient to take his blood pressure at the same time each day, with similar activities preceding each measurement.
- Teach the patient about the disorder and its care and treatment as appropriate. Stress the need for follow-up care.
- Advise the patient to avoid high-sodium antacids and over-the-counter cold and sinus medications because they may contain harmful vasoconstrictors.

◆ HYPERTENSION, PREGNANCY-INDUCED

A potentially life-threatening disorder, pregnancy-induced hypertension usually develops after the 20th week of pregnancy. It most often occurs in nulliparous women and may be nonconvulsive or convulsive.

The nonconvulsive form of the disorder is called *preeclampsia*. It's marked by the onset of hypertension after 20 weeks of gestation. It develops in about 7% of pregnancies and may be mild to severe. The incidence is significantly higher in low socioeconomic groups.

The convulsive form is called *eclampsia*. It develops between 24 weeks of gestation and the end of the first postpartal week. The incidence is higher among women who are pregnant for the first time, have multiple fetuses, and have a history of vascular disease.

Complications include generalized arteriolar vasoconstriction, which may decrease blood flow through the placenta and maternal organs, possibly causing intrauterine growth retardation, placental infarcts, and abruptio placentae. Severe eclampsia is marked by hemolysis, elevated liver enzyme levels, and a low platelet count (HELLP syndrome). A unique form of coagulopathy is also associated with this disorder.

Other possible complications include stillbirth of the neonate, seizures, coma, premature labor, renal failure, and hepatic damage in the mother.

Assessment findings

A patient with mild preeclampsia typically reports a sudden weight gain of more than 3 lb (1.36 kg) per week in the second trimester or more than 1 lb (0.45 kg) per week in the third trimester.

The patient's history reveals hypertension, as evidenced by blood pressure readings of 140/90 mm Hg or above. Alternatively, the patient may have an increase of 30 mm Hg or more above her normal systolic pressure or 15 mm Hg or more above her normal diastolic pressure, measured on two occasions at least 6 hours apart.

Inspection detects generalized edema, especially of the face. Palpation may reveal pitting edema of the legs and feet. Deep tendon reflexes may indicate either hyporeflexia or hyperreflexia.

As preeclampsia worsens, the patient may develop oliguria (urine output of 400 ml/day or less), blurred vision caused by retinal arteriolar spasm, epigastric pain or heartburn, irritability, and emotional tension. She may complain of a severe frontal headache.

In severe preeclampsia, blood pressure readings rise to 160/110 mm Hg or higher on two occasions, 6 hours apart, while the patient is on bed rest. Ophthalmoscopic examination may reveal vascular spasm, papilledema, retinal edema or detachment, and arteriovenous nicking or hemorrhage.

Preeclampsia can suddenly progress to eclampsia with the onset of seizures. The patient with eclampsia may appear to cease breathing, then suddenly take a deep, stertorous breath and resume breathing. The patient may then lapse into a coma, lasting a few minutes to several hours. Awakening from the coma, the patient may have no memory of the seizure.

Laboratory test findings reveal proteinuria (more than 300 mg/24 hours [1+] with preeclampsia, and 5 g/24 hours [5+] or more with severe eclampsia). Test results may suggest the HELLP syndrome. Ultrasonography, stress and nonstress tests, and biophysical profiles evaluate fetal well-being.

Therapy for preeclampsia is designed to halt the disorder's progress. Some doctors advocate the prompt induction of labor, especially if the patient is near term. Others follow a

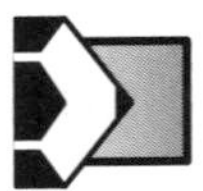

Responding to pregnancy-induced hypertension

If you care for a patient with pregnancy-induced hypertension, you'll need to assess her carefully, reassure her repeatedly, and teach her how to respond to her condition. Start with ideas like these:

◆ Instruct the patient to maintain bed rest, as ordered. Advise her to lie in a left lateral position to increase venous return, cardiac output, and renal blood flow.

◆ Stress the importance of adequate nutrition in the prenatal period. Advise the patient to avoid foods high in sodium.

◆ Teach the patient and family to identify and report signs of preeclampsia and eclampsia, such as headache, weight gain, edema, and oliguria.

◆ If the patient must undergo premature delivery, point out that infants whose mothers had pregnancy-induced hypertension usually are small for gestational age, but may be healthier than other premature babies of the same weight, possibly because they've developed adaptive stress responses in utero.

◆ Emphasize the importance of keeping all prenatal appointments with the doctor.

more conservative approach that includes complete bed rest in the left lateral lying position to enhance venous return, plus antihypertensive drugs (such as methyldopa and hydralazine).

If the patient's blood pressure does not respond to bed rest and antihypertensive therapy and persistently rises above 160/100 mm Hg, or if central nervous system irritability increases, the doctor may order magnesium sulfate to promote diuresis, reduce blood pressure, and prevent seizures.

Adequate nutrition, good prenatal care, and control of preexisting hypertension during pregnancy can decrease the incidence and severity of preeclampsia. Early recognition and prompt treatment of preeclampsia can prevent its progression to eclampsia.

Implementation

When caring for a patient with pregnancy-induced hypertension, you'll want to promote tissue integrity, maintain the patient's fluid balance, and ensure safety. (See *Responding to pregnancy-induced hypertension.*) Specific interventions include the following:

◆ During each home visit, assess the patient and immediately report changes in blood pressure, pulse rate, respiratory rate, fetal heart rate, vision, level of consciousness, deep tendon reflexes, and urine output (dipstick for protein). Note shortness of breath and the degree and location of any edema. Also watch for headache unrelieved by medication.

◆ Ask the patient about early warning signs of pelvic inflammatory disease, such as epigastric pain, headache, and vision disturbances.

◆ Ask the patient about signs of abruptio placentae, such as vaginal bleeding, sustained abdominal pain, uterine tenderness and firmness, and increasing fundal height.

◆ Explain the purposes of the treatment regimen and the importance of complying with it.

◆ Teach the patient how to assess her blood pressure, body weight, urine output, edema, and fetal movement. Also show the patient how to assess her urine for protein daily.

◆ Explain the need for a diet that is high in protein and relatively low in salt.

◆ Teach the patient to recognize and report danger signs immediately.

◆ Ensure that the patient understands the actions, dosage, and possible adverse effects of prescribed medications, such as magnesium sulfate.

◆ PNEUMONIA

An acute inflammation of lung parenchyma, pneumonia can result from infection by viruses, bacteria, fungi, protozoans, mycobacteria, mycoplasmas, or rickettsia. It may be classified as primary, secondary, or aspiration pneumonia. Its location may be classified as bronchopneumonia, lobular pneumonia, or lobar pneumonia.

Patients who have normal lungs and adequate immune systems usually recover fully from pneumonia. In debilitated patients, however, bacterial pneumonia ranks as the leading cause of death. Pneumonia also is the leading cause of death from infectious disease in the United States.

Risk factors for bacterial and viral pneumonia include chronic illness and debilitation, cancer (particularly lung cancer), abdominal and thoracic surgery, atelectasis, viral respiratory infections, chronic respiratory disease, influenza, smoking, malnutrition, alcoholism, sickle cell disease, tracheostomy, exposure to noxious gases, aspiration, and immunosuppressive therapy.

Risk factors for aspiration pneumonia include advanced age, nasogastric tube feedings, an impaired gag reflex, poor oral hygiene, and a decreased level of consciousness.

Assessment

In bacterial pneumonia, the patient may report pleuritic chest pain, a cough, excessive sputum production, and chills. Assessment may reveal fever with shaking chills, plus a productive cough.

Sputum characteristics can help pinpoint the cause of pneumonia. For example, creamy yellow sputum suggests staphylococcal pneumonia; green sputum denotes pneumonia caused by *Pseudomonas* organisms; and sputum that looks like currant jelly indicates pneumonia caused by *Klebsiella*. (Clear sputum means that the patient does not have an infective process.)

Diagnostic tests include chest X-rays, which disclose infiltrates, thus confirming the diagnosis; Gram stain and culture and sensitivity tests for sputum; blood cultures; white blood cell count; arterial blood gas (ABG) analysis; and pulse oximetry. In certain cases, bronchoscopy, transtracheal aspiration, or pleural fluid cultures may be performed.

Antimicrobial therapy should begin as soon as possible. Supportive measures include humidified oxygen therapy for hypoxia, bronchodilator therapy, antitussives, a high-calorie diet and adequate fluid intake, limited activity, and analgesics to relieve pleuritic chest pain. If respiratory failure occurs, mechanical ventilation may be necessary.

Implementation

When caring for a patient with pneumonia, you'll want to maximize gas exchange, improve airway clearance, maintain nutrition, ensure fluid volume, decrease anxiety, and promote comfort. Specific interventions include the following:

◆ During each visit, perform a complete physical assessment of the patient, focusing on the respiratory system.

◆ Look for signs and symptoms of distress. Monitor his ABG values and pulse oximetry levels, as appropriate.

◆ Administer oxygen, bronchodilators, and antimicrobial therapy as ordered.

◆ Instruct the patient and caregivers in ordered treatments, such as oxygen therapy, chest physiotherapy, medications or procedures. Monitor the patient's response to treatments. Reinstruct him as necessary.

◆ Encourage the patient to sit upright to promote lung expansion. When he's in bed, encourage semi-Fowler's position.

◆ Perform chest physiotherapy — including postural drainage, percussion, and vibration — every 4 hours as tolerated. Urge the patient to cough and deep-breathe every hour while awake.

◆ Advise the patient to consume 2 to 3 qt (2 to 3 L) of fluids daily to help liquefy secretions. Administer I.V. fluids as ordered, if necessary, to prevent dehydration.

◆ Assess for signs and symptoms of dehydration (low urine output, dry skin, sunken eyes).

◆ Encourage a high-calorie, high-protein diet of soft foods. Provide nutritional supplements as necessary. Collaborate with the dietitian as indicated.

◆ Assess the patient's pain, and encourage him to use prescribed analgesics to promote comfort.

◆ Urge the patient to avoid irritants that stimulate secretions, such as cigarette smoke and dust.

◆ Discuss ways to avoid spreading the infection to others. Explain careful hygiene measures, especially disposal of all materials that contain respiratory secretions. Also demonstrate and encourage thorough, repeated hand washing.

◆ Encourage the patient and his family to express their fears and concerns. Respond with support and information.

◆ When the patient recovers, encourage him to receive the pneumococcal pneumonia vaccination (once for life) and an annual influenza vaccination.

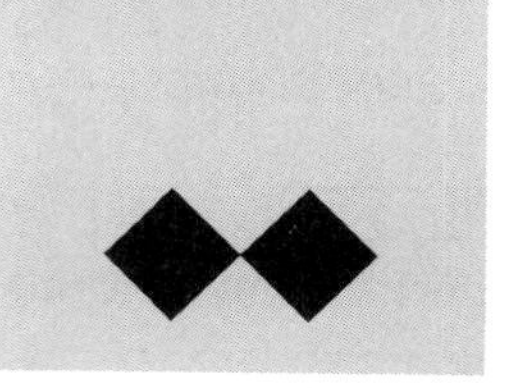

CHAPTER 8

Performing procedures

In every health care setting, procedures performed in a timely and accurate manner form the foundation of successful nursing practice. In the home, it's critical that you be able to perform procedures with expertise and virtually no supervision in a highly variable environment.

This chapter outlines a collection of important procedures you'll need to know for home practice. It includes special adaptations to increase your effectiveness in the home and describes crucial steps to reduce the risk of disease transmission in the home.

◆ BLOOD TRANSFUSION

If your home health agency accepts orders for home-based blood transfusions (some agencies don't), you may be called upon to perform this complex but relatively uncommon procedure from time to time.

Equipment and preparation

Before performing a home-based blood transfusion, you'll most likely need special training or certification in infusion techniques. You'll also need clear documentation that the patient qualifies for the transfusion. Your documentation should include:

- evidence that the patient has had previous successful transfusions
- evidence that the patient can't be transported safely to an acute care facility or outpatient surgical center
- evidence that the patient's hemoglobin and hematocrit levels justify a transfusion rather than a more conservative therapy, such as iron supplements
- evidence that the patient's blood has been typed and cross-matched.

Contact the blood bank to find out when the blood will be ready for transport to the patient's home, and check your agency's policy to find out who's responsible for transporting it. Most blood banks use refrigerated transportation equipment to make sure the blood stays at the proper temperature. Finally, coordinate with the blood bank and the patient so you can perform the transfusion at the optimal time.

When you arrive at the patient's home, gather all the equipment you'll need to perform the procedure. (See *Equipment for performing a home transfusion*, page 236.) When the blood arrives, double-check the doctor's order to see how long the blood should infuse. And make sure the patient has signed a consent form.

Implementation

Before you begin, explain to the patient what you'll be doing. Help him into a position that will be comfortable for the length of the transfusion. Wash your hands and arrange all your equipment within easy reach.

After putting on clean gloves, a gown, and goggles, measure the pa-

Equipment for performing a home transfusion

Before you start a home-based blood transfusion, make sure you have the following equipment on hand:
- ◆ blood transfusion sets (filter, tubing, drip chamber)
- ◆ venipuncture equipment, including an 18G or 19G angiocatheter
- ◆ I.V. infusion pole
- ◆ Y-connector I.V. tubing
- ◆ sterile normal saline for infusion (at least a 250-ml bag)
- ◆ gloves, gown, and face shield
- ◆ povidone-iodine and alcohol swabs
- ◆ sharps container
- ◆ plastic trash bag
- ◆ blood transportation container to return the empty infusion bag and tubing to the blood bank.

You'll also want the following emergency equipment on hand so you can respond appropriately if your patient has a transfusion reaction:
- ◆ epinephrine, either 1:1,000 1-ml ampules or 1:10,000 10-ml prefilled syringes
- ◆ diphenhydramine hydrochloride, either 25-mg or 50-mg ampules
- ◆ 1-ml and 3-ml syringes (two or three of them) with 25G ⅝″ needles
- ◆ adult oral airway
- ◆ urine specimen cup.

tient's vital signs and record your results as "preinfusion." Check the expiration date on the blood container and record it. Also make note of the blood's appearance; check it for bubbles, cloudiness, darkening, or sediment. Make sure the patient's documented blood type and Rh factor are clearly marked on the blood container.

Prepare the blood for transfusion by opening the Y-connector I.V. transfusion set. Close the clamp and spike the 250-ml bag of sterile normal saline solution. Next, open the port on the blood bag, and spike it with the other set of tubing. Hang both the bag of normal saline solution and the blood bag on the I.V. pole.

Now open the line on the saline bag, and squeeze the drip chamber until it's half full. Open the clamp on the transfusion tubing, and prime it with normal saline solution. Clamp the normal saline bag and hang the tubing on the pole, protecting the transfusion end from contamination.

Explain to the patient how you'll be inserting the angiocatheter. Use at least a 19G catheter to allow free passage of red blood cells. Once the angiocatheter is in place, flush it with saline solution and attach the transfusion end of the tubing directly to the angiocatheter. Then clamp the normal saline bag, and open the blood transfusion clamp.

Stay with the patient for at least 15 minutes to make sure the transfusion is proceeding smoothly. Then adjust the flow rate to administer the blood within the ordered period of time. The maximum time for infusing a unit of blood is 4 hours.

Place blood-contaminated items and used sharps in the sharps container. Place other used items in the plastic trash bag. Then remove your gown, gloves, and goggles, and wash your hands. Don't discard your goggles unless they're disposable.

Continue to assess the patient and measure his vital signs at least hourly. When the transfusion is completed, wash your hands and put on fresh gloves, gown, and goggles. Clamp the transfusion tubing and turn on the normal saline solution infusion to flush the line and the angiocatheter. Once they're flushed, clamp the normal saline line.

Depending on the patient and the order, you may need to remove the entire angiocatheter from the vein with tubing intact, or you may disconnect the transfusion tubing and place a cap over the venous access site. For the latter, flush the angiocatheter with saline and then heparin, according to your agency's policy.

Place the empty blood bag, normal saline solution, Y-connector tubing, and possibly the angiocatheter in the blood transportation container to be returned to the blood bank. Finally, measure your patient's vital signs and record them as "posttransfusion." Document the patient's response to the transfusion, the appearance of the angiocatheter site, and whether you removed the angiocatheter or left it in place.

Special considerations

Despite the highly sophisticated cross-matching procedures in use today, your patient still could have a transfusion reaction. It might result from an antigen-antibody reaction, a hemolytic reaction to incompatible blood, or blood contaminated with *Pseudomonas*, *Staphylococcus*, or other bacteria that can survive cold temperatures.

A reaction that takes place during or up to 96 hours after a transfusion probably stems from an antigen-antibody or a hemolytic reaction. Reactions caused by contaminated blood can go undetected for days, weeks, or months. (See *Recognizing a transfusion reaction*.) Make sure the patient and his caregivers know what signs and symptoms to watch for and how to respond appropriately. (See *Handling a transfusion reaction,* page 238.)

Recognizing a transfusion reaction

Signs and symptoms of an antigen-antibody transfusion reaction include:

- chills
- facial swelling
- laryngeal edema
- pruritus
- urticaria
- wheezing
- fever
- nausea
- vomiting
- lower back pain.

Signs and symptoms of a reaction to bacteria-contaminated blood include:

- chills
- fever
- vomiting
- abdominal cramping
- diarrhea
- shock
- signs of renal failure.

Signs and symptoms of a hemolytic reaction to incompatible blood include:

- chest pain
- dyspnea
- facial flushing
- fever
- shaking chills
- hypotension
- flank pain
- burning sensation along the transfusion vein
- possible shock and renal failure.

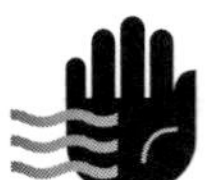

EMERGENCY INTERVENTIONS

Handling a transfusion reaction

A transfusion reaction is a medical emergency. If you think your patient is having a reaction, stop the transfusion and assess his cardiopulmonary status and vital signs. If possible, have someone contact the emergency medical service immediately; if not, do so yourself. Then do the following:

◆ Get ready to begin cardiopulmonary resuscitation if necessary.

◆ Prepare epinephrine for subcutaneous (S.C.) or I.V. administration. If you're using the 1:1,000 formula for S.C. administration, prepare a dose of 0.1 to 0.5 ml. Repeat the S.C. dose every 10 to 15 minutes if the patient hasn't experienced cardiovascular collapse. If you're using the 1:10,000 formula for I.V. administration, prepare for a dose of 0.5 to 1 mg. If the patient is facing cardiovascular collapse, begin rapid infusion of normal saline solution to maintain his blood pressure and administer the epinephrine I.V.

◆ Prepare and administer diphenhydramine hydrochloride, 10 to 50 mg, by the I.V. or I.M. route.

◆ Stay with the patient until the emergency team arrives.

◆ If possible, obtain a urine specimen for analysis.

◆ Contact the patient's doctor for additional orders.

◆ Once the emergency team stabilizes the patient and prepares him for transport to an acute care facility, make sure the patient's family knows what's happening and where the patient is going.

◆ Return the blood bag, tubing, and all laboratory tags to the blood bank for analysis.

◆ Discard used S.C., I.V., and I.M. equipment in the sharps container. Discard other equipment and personal protective gear in a plastic bag, and wash your hands.

◆ Document the date and time of the reaction and the signs and symptoms the patient experienced. Also note all medications administered, including the dosage, the route, and the patient's response. Document the time you called the emergency medical service and the time of their arrival.

◆ Complete an incident report according to agency policy.

◆ CHEST PHYSIOTHERAPY

Chest physiotherapy (PT) involves four techniques: postural drainage, chest percussion, chest vibration, and exercises (deep breathing, coughing, or both). Used in combination, these activities help to mobilize and eliminate secretions, reexpand lung tissue, and promote the efficient use of respiratory muscles. Chest PT is especially effective for patients with bronchiectasis, cystic fibrosis, and other disorders that produce copious amounts of mucus.

Postural drainage uses gravity to help drain peripheral pulmonary secretions into the large bronchi or trachea, where they're easier for the patient to expel. In this procedure, the patient is placed in a series of positions, each of which drains a particular area of lung tissue. Typically, the lower and middle lobes drain best when the patient assumes a head-down position, and the upper lobes drain best when the patient stays head-up.

Chest percussion and vibration can help increase the effectiveness of postural drainage. Percussion involves rhythmically clapping your cupped hands over specific lung segments (as shown below). This technique helps to dislodge trapped mucus from alveoli and bronchioles.

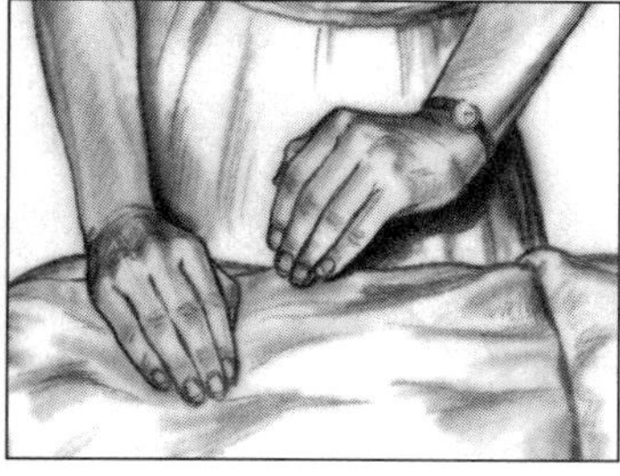

Chest vibration, commonly used together with percussion, can help loosen additional trapped mucus from minor airways. This technique involves placing your hands over specific long segments and rapidly moving them to and fro (as shown below).

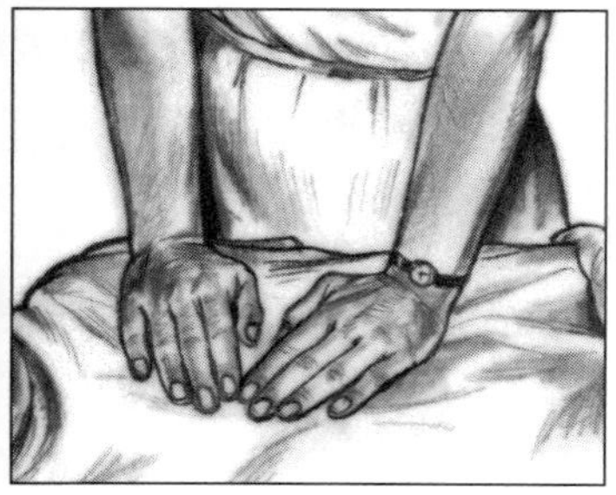

It can be used instead of percussion for patients who can't withstand the discomfort sometimes associated with percussion, such as those recovering from major surgery and those who have acute pain.

Deep-breathing and coughing exercises help the patient expectorate loosened secretions. When performed just after postural drainage or chest percussion and vibration, these exercises can help the patient attain a more effective cough while expending less energy.

Equipment and preparation

Ideally, you'll want to use a tilt table, a postural drainage table, or an adjustable hospital bed when performing chest PT. If you don't have access to one of these implements, however, you can make do with pillows, foam wedges, or both. Also make sure you have the following: ◆ stethoscope ◆ emesis basin and facial tissues ◆ suction equipment, if necessary ◆ oral hygiene equipment.

Make sure your suction equipment is working, and arrange your supplies conveniently nearby.

Implementation

Before you begin, explain what you'll be doing, including the hand motions and sensations involved in percussion and vibration. Tell the patient that you'll be asking him to take deep breaths and cough at certain times throughout the procedure. Make sure he hasn't ingested food or fluids for at least 60 minutes, preferably 90, before you begin.

Wash your hands and measure the patient's blood pressure, pulse, and respiratory rate. Auscultate his lungs to identify any specific areas of reduced or adventitious breath sounds. Then help him loosen any tight clothing from around his chest, neck, or abdomen.

If you have a tilt table, find a convenient location in which to set it up. If you don't have one, find a place next to a sofa or bed where you can

Positions for chest physiotherapy

The following illustrations depict postural drainage positions and the lung areas they drain.

Lower lobes: Posterior basal segments
Elevate the foot of the bed 30 degrees. Have the patient lie prone with his head lowered. Position pillows under his chest and abdomen. Percuss his lower ribs on both sides of his spine.

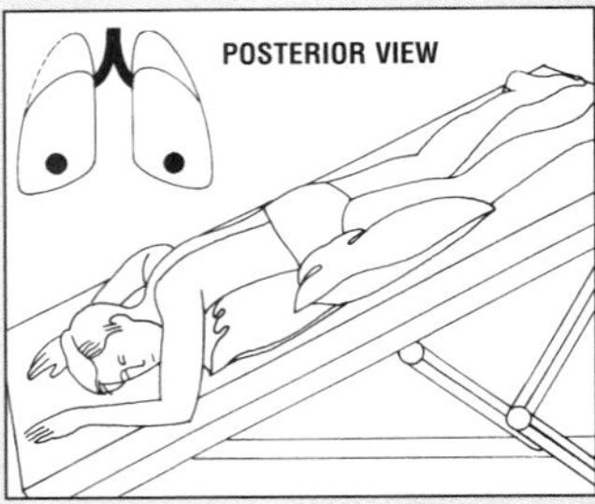

Lower lobes: Lateral basal segments
Elevate the foot of the bed 30 degrees. Instruct the patient to lie on his abdomen, with his head lowered and his upper leg flexed over a pillow for support. Then have him rotate a quarter turn upward. Percuss his lower ribs on the uppermost portion of his lateral chest wall.

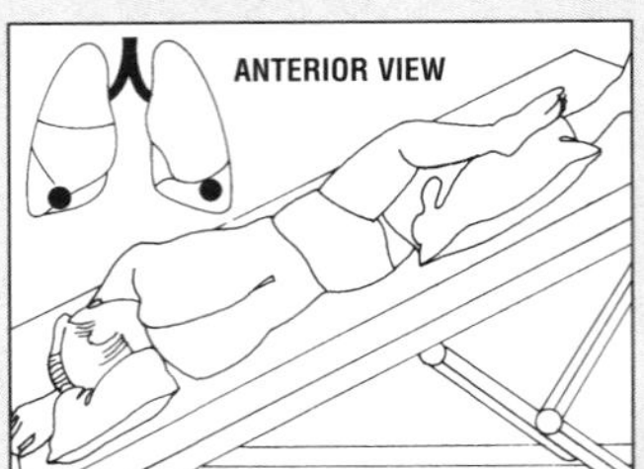

Lower lobes: Anterior basal segments
Elevate the foot of the bed 30 degrees. Instruct the patient to lie on his side, with his head lowered. Then place pillows as shown. Percuss with a slightly cupped hand over his lower ribs, just beneath the axilla. If an acutely ill patient has trouble breathing in this position, adjust the bed to an angle he can tolerate. Then begin percussion.

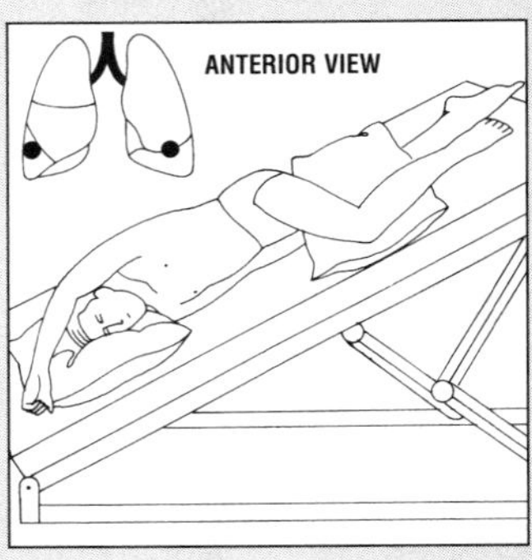

Lower lobes: Superior segments
With the bed flat, have the patient lie on his abdomen. Place two pillows under his hips. Percuss on both sides of his spine at the lower tips of his scapulae.

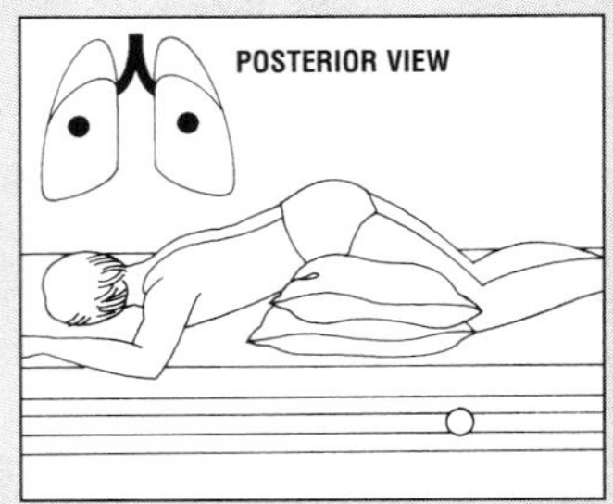

Positions for chest physiotherapy *(continued)*

Right middle lobe: Medial and lateral segments
Elevate the foot of the bed 15 degrees. Have the patient lie on his left side, with his head down and knees flexed. Then have him rotate a quarter turn backward. Place a pillow beneath him. Percuss with your hand moderately cupped over the right nipple. For a woman, cup your hand so that its heel is under her armpit and your fingers extend forward beneath her breast.

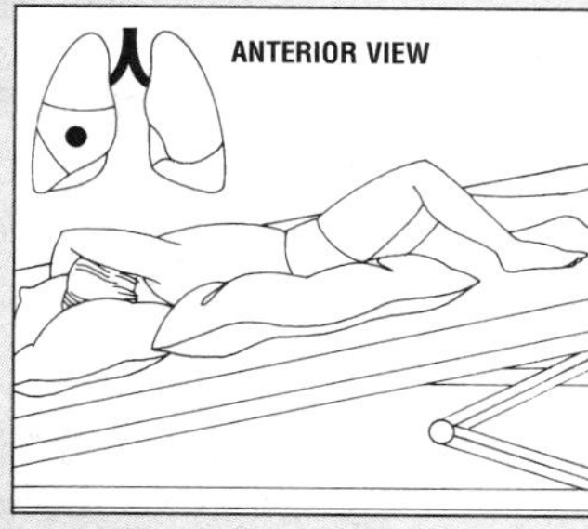

Left upper lobe: Superior and inferior segments, lingular portion
Elevate the foot of the bed 15 degrees. Have the patient lie on his right side, with his head down and knees flexed. Then have him rotate a quarter turn backward. Place a pillow behind him, from shoulders to hips. Percuss with your hand moderately cupped over his left nipple. For a woman, cup your hand so that its heel is beneath her armpit and your fingers extend forward beneath her breast.

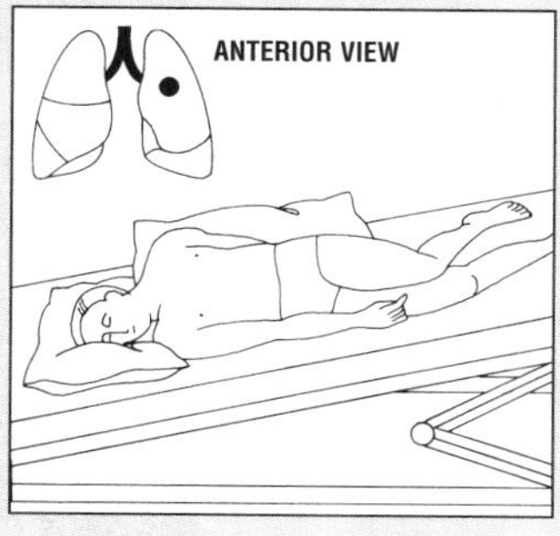

Upper lobes: Anterior segments
Make sure the bed is flat. Have the patient lie on his back with a pillow folded under his knees. Then have him rotate slightly away from the side being drained. Percuss between his clavicle and nipple.

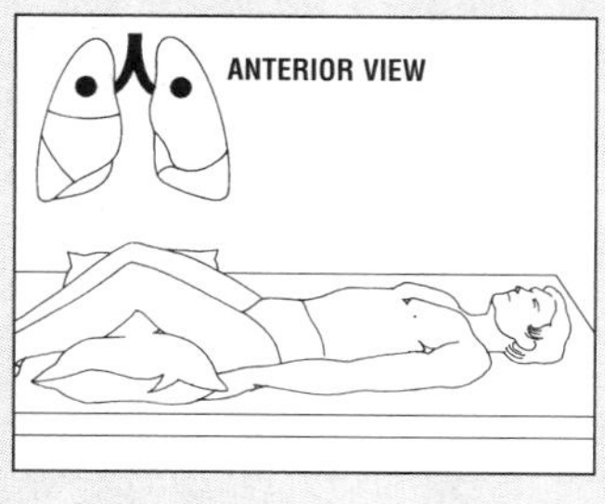

(continued)

use foam wedges or pillows to create a gradual slope to the floor. Place the facial tissues, emesis basin, and suction equipment on the floor near where the patient's head will be.

Ideally, you'll want to drain the lower lung lobes first, then the right middle lobe, and finally the upper lobes. Help the patient into each position in turn. (See *Positions for chest physiotherapy*.)

Positions for chest physiotherapy *(continued)*

Upper lobes: Apical segments
Keep the bed flat. Have the patient lean back at a 30-degree angle against you and a pillow. Percuss with a cupped hand between his clavicles and the top of each scapula.

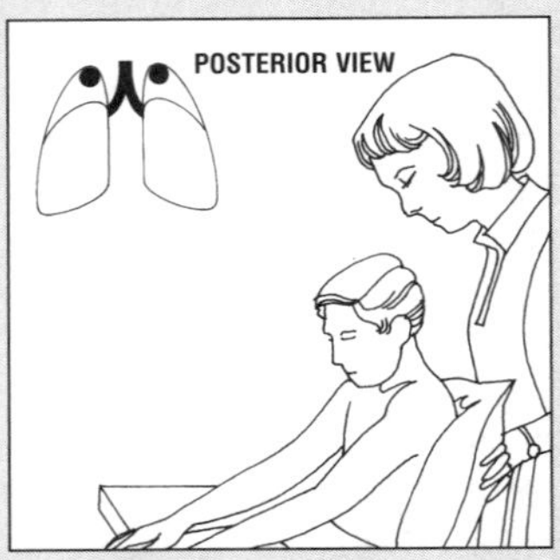

Upper lobes: Posterior segments
Keep the bed flat. Have the patient lean over a pillow at a 30-degree angle. Percuss and clap his upper back on each side.

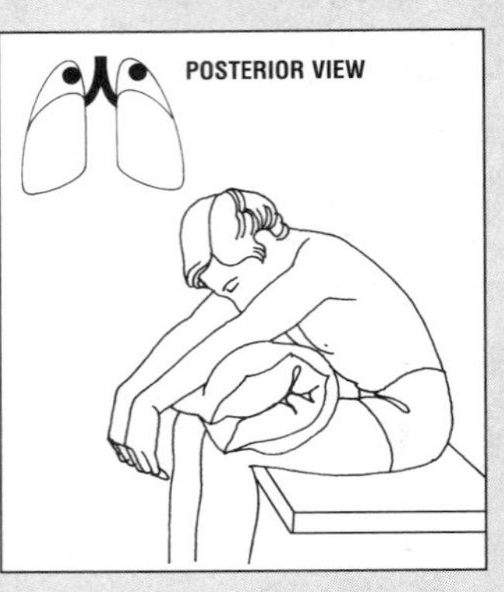

Remember that you'll achieve maximum success with drainage if the patient can stay in each position for 10 to 15 minutes. During that time, you'll perform percussion and vibration. Percuss for 1 to 2 minutes, and then vibrate while the patient exhales for four or five breaths.

Many patients find it difficult or impossible to maintain postural drainage positions for the optimal length of time. Be sure to assess your patient's tolerance frequently; be especially alert for dyspnea, cyanosis, or pain. Over time, as the patient's tolerance increases, he may be able to spend more time in each position.

When you've completed postural drainage, help the patient to a sitting position slowly to prevent light-headedness and possible fainting. Make him comfortable. Then coach him in deep-breathing and coughing exercises to help him expectorate the loosened secretions. Follow these steps:

◆ Tell the patient to inhale deeply through his nose, and then exhale in three short huffs.

◆ Have him repeat the deep inhalations, and then cough at least three times through a slightly opened mouth. Be sure to provide tissues or an emesis basin as needed.

◆ Tell the patient to continue the deep breathing and coughing for a full minute, and then rest for about 2 minutes and repeat the exercise.

◆ If the patient is too weak to expel the mucus, you'll have to suction him. (See "Tracheal suctioning" later in the chapter.)

When you've completed the deep-breathing and coughing exercises, offer the patient oral hygiene. Remove items used during chest PT, disinfect those that are reusable, and wash your hands. Auscultate the patient's lungs to evaluate the effectiveness of the procedure.

In your home care record, document the positions you used for postural drainage, the length of time the patient tolerated each position, the amount and character of mucus expelled, and the patient's breath sounds before and after the procedure.

Special considerations

If your patient has trouble tolerating postural drainage positions, you may need to modify them. Stop any position that causes cyanosis, dyspnea, or significant changes in the patient's mental status. If the patient tires quickly, reduce the time spent in each position because fatigue leads to shallow respirations, reduced cough strength, and hypoxia.

Encourage the patient to increase his fluid intake after chest PT and for up to 90 minutes before the next session. Tell him that extra fluids will help to moisten and loosen mucus. If your patient is on intermittent inhaler or nebulizer therapy, tell him to take his medication before undergoing chest PT because the procedure can induce bronchospasm.

Always use caution when percussing near the spine, liver, kidneys, or spleen because you could injure these organs. Make sure the patient is wearing light clothing, or use a towel over the areas being percussed. Avoid percussing over buttons, zippers, or snaps because they could irritate the skin. Also remind the patient to remove any jewelry because it could cause scratches or bruises during percussion.

Chest PT is contraindicated for patients with active pulmonary bleeding, hemoptysis, fractured ribs, lung contusions, pulmonary tuberculosis, untreated pneumothorax, acute asthma or bronchospasm, lung abscess or tumor, bone metastasis, head injury, or recent myocardial infarction or epidural spinal infusions.

Parts of a gastrostomy feeding button

A gastrostomy feeding button extends through the patient's abdominal wall, leaving only a flat plug visible on the skin's surface. Inside the abdominal cavity, there's a mushroom dome and an antireflux valve, as shown in the illustration below.

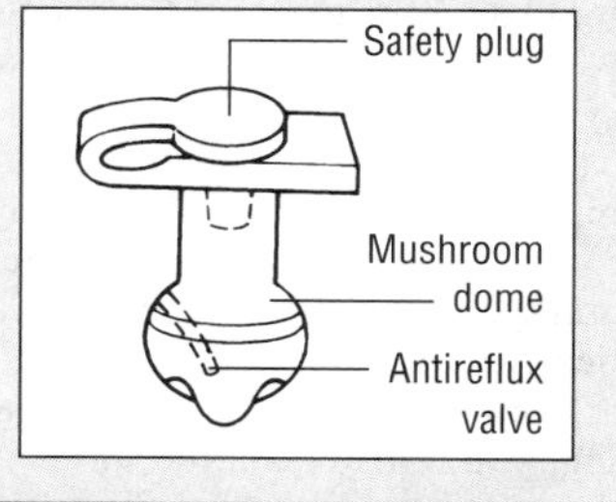

◆ ENTERAL FEEDINGS

Patients unable to sustain adequate nutrition by mouth may need enteral feedings instead. In these feedings, liquid sustenance is infused into the stomach or small intestine. Conditions that typically create a need for enteral feedings include GI disorders, coma, extensive burns, or simply a need for nutritional supplements. Enteral feedings can be delivered either through a nasogastric (NG) tube or across the abdominal wall through a gastrostomy tube or feeding button. (See *Parts of a gastrostomy feeding button*.)

Usually, you'll use an NG tube only if the patient needs short-term nutritional support. He may come home from an acute care facility with the tube in place, or you or his doctor may need to insert the tube.

Patients who need long-term enteral nutrition usually receive it through a gastrostomy tube. Because the insertion procedure typically takes place under anesthesia, your patient will probably have the gastrostomy tube or feeding button in place when discharged from the acute care facility. Gastrostomy feeding buttons are ideal for patients who will be returning to independent living but still require long-term enteral nutrition.

Equipment and preparation

To prepare for an NG feeding, gather the following equipment: ◆ prescribed formula at room temperature ◆ administration device (soft-bulb syringe, irrigation syringe, feeding bag) ◆ administration pump (for feedings over several hours) ◆ water at room temperature ◆ stethoscope ◆ oral hygiene supplies ◆ gloves ◆ plastic trash bag.

To prepare for a gastrostomy feeding, you'll also need the following dressing supplies: ◆ clean 4″ × 4″ gauze pads ◆ cotton-tipped applicators ◆ topical antiseptic ◆ adhesive tape ◆ basin.

To prepare for a patient who has a gastrostomy feeding button, you'll also need to take along a spare button (a precaution) and supplies to clean the button: ◆ cotton-tipped applicators ◆ pipe cleaner ◆ mild soap.

Implementation

Begin by explaining the procedure to the patient. Arrange all your equipment in a convenient work area, and provide the patient with mouth care.

NG tube

To deliver an NG tube feeding, help the patient to a sitting or near-sitting position (at least a 45-degree angle) and wash your hands. Then auscultate for bowel sounds. If you don't hear any, don't give the feeding. Instead, contact the patient's doctor.

Next, assess NG tube placement in one of two ways. Either attach a syringe to the end of the tube and aspirate tube contents, or place your stethoscope over the patient's gastric region and listen for a "whooshing" sound while you inject about 20 cc of air into the tube. If the patient has more than 100 ml of residual gastric contents, withhold the feeding for 30 to 60 minutes and then reassess. Notify the patient's doctor about the high residual gastric contents.

When you're ready to deliver the feeding, wash your hands and prepare the formula in the proper manner. For a *bolus feeding*, draw the formula into a syringe, attach the syringe to the end of the tube, and slowly inject the formula through the tube. For an *intermittent* or *continuous feeding*, prepare the formula and place it in a container or bag. Remove all air from the feeding bag tubing. Hang the bag on a door hook or prepare the administration pump. Attach the feeding tubing to the end of the NG tube and tape the connection. Then either manually regulate the feeding flow or set the pump to administer the prescribed amount. Be sure to clamp the tubing before the container empties to keep air from entering the patient's stomach.

When you complete the feeding, remove the syringe or feeding tubing and flush the NG tube with 50 ml of water (as shown below). Keep the patient in an upright position for 45 to 60 minutes to reduce the risk of aspiration. Examine his nares for any

FLUSHING THE FEEDING TUBE

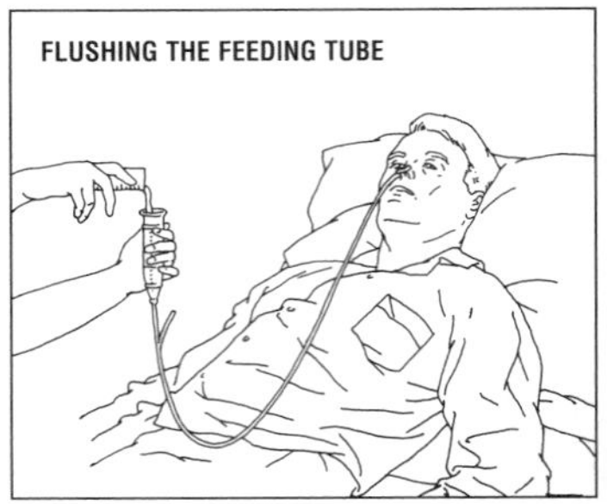

signs of skin breakdown, necrosis, or bleeding.

If the feeding equipment is disposable, discard it when you're finished with the feeding. If not, flush it and store it in a clean place. Check your agency's policy to see how long you can use the equipment. Finally, clean up and discard all used items in a plastic trash bag. Remove your gloves and wash your hands.

Gastrostomy tube

To deliver a gastrostomy tube feeding, you'll follow basically the same procedure used for an NG tube feeding, with a few modifications. First, you'll need to expose the gastrostomy tube. Place a small basin on the patient's abdomen, and uncap the tube or remove the tube's plug. Assess to make sure the tube is still placed properly; then aspirate and reinsert the residual gastric contents. Contact the patient's doctor if you encounter high gastric residual contents, if you don't hear bowel sounds, or if the patient complains of abdominal discomfort before the feeding.

Draw up about 50 ml of warm water in a syringe, and gently irrigate the tube. If the patient begins to cough or choke, don't administer the feeding. Instead, withdraw the syringe, cap the gastrostomy tube, and contact the patient's doctor.

If the doctor ordered a *bolus feeding*, allow it to drain into the tube at a rate of 200 to 300 ml over 10 to 15 minutes. Then flush the tube with about 50 ml of warm water. For an *intermittent* or *continuous feeding*, follow the same procedure as for an NG tube feeding. When you finish, add about 50 ml of warm water to the feeding container to flush the gastrostomy tube.

Gastrostomy button

To deliver a gastrostomy button feeding, you'll basically follow the same procedure used for a gastrostomy tube feeding, with a few modifications. After exposing the gastrostomy button, open the safety plug and attach the adapter and feeding tubing to the button (as shown below).

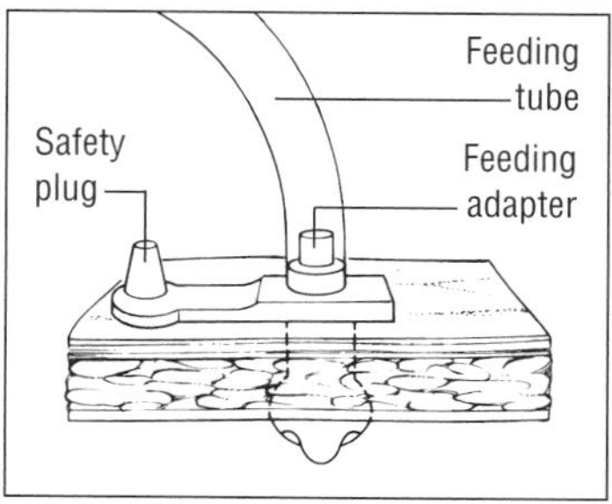

If the doctor ordered a *gravity feeding*, raise the syringe or feeding container above the level of the patient's stomach, and instill the formula over 15 to 30 minutes. For an *intermittent* or *continuous pump feeding*, attach the feeding tubing to the button, and set the pump to administer the prescribed amount of formula.

When you've completed the feeding, lower the syringe or feeding tubing below the patient's stomach level to allow "burping" before you remove the feeding apparatus from the button. Gastrostomy buttons have an antireflux valve to prevent gastric reflux.

Finally, flush the button with about 10 ml of water, and clean the inside of the catheter with a cotton-tipped applicator. Snap the safety cap back into place. If the patient feels nauseated or vomits, vent the button with the adapter and feeding catheter to control emesis.

Special considerations

No matter what kind of feeding your patient will be receiving, don't give him medications along with the feeding. Instead, crush the drugs or have them prepared as an elixir. Give them

How to reinsert a gastrostomy button

If your patient's gastrostomy feeding button pops out (during coughing, for instance), either you or he will need to reinsert the device. Here are some steps to follow.

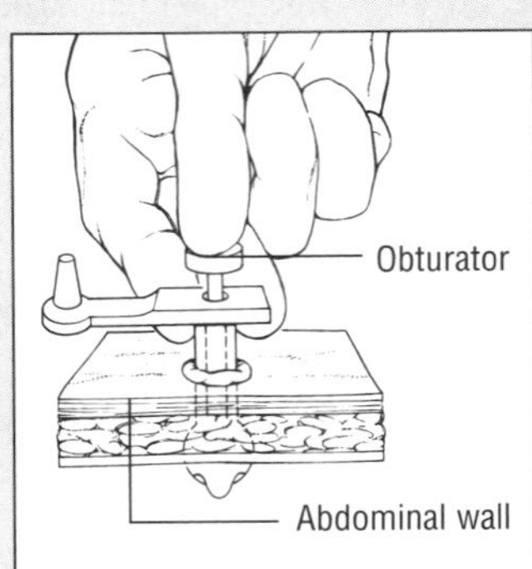

Preparing the equipment
Collect the feeding button, an obturator, and water-soluble lubricant. If the button will be reinserted, wash it with soap and water and rinse it thoroughly.

Inserting the button
◆ Check the depth of the patient's stoma to make sure you have a feeding button that's the correct size. Then clean around the stoma.
◆ Lubricate the obturator with the water-soluble lubricant, and distend the button several times to make sure the antireflux valve is patent.
◆ Lubricate the mushroom dome and the stoma. Gently push the button through the stoma into the stomach (as shown above right).
◆ Then remove the obturator by gently rotating it to keep the antireflux valve from adhering to it. If the valve sticks anyway, gently push the obturator back into the button until the valve closes.
◆ After removing the obturator, check the valve to make sure it's closed. Then close the flexible safety plug, which should be relatively flush with the skin surface (as shown below).

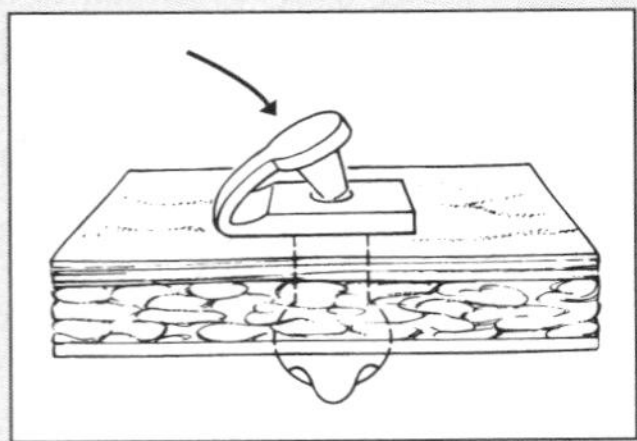

◆ If you need to administer a feeding right away, open the safety plug and attach the feeding adapter and feeding tube. Deliver the feeding as ordered.

with about 5 ml water; then flush the tubing to prevent blockage.

Make sure all feeding formulas are within their freshness dates and delivered at room temperature. Store open formula containers in the refrigerator, and don't administer formula that's been open too long (more than 8 hours for intermittent or continuous feedings, 24 hours for bolus feedings). Don't mix old and new feeding solutions.

If the patient has an NG tube, tell his caregivers to check the tube placement regularly and to notify his doctor if the tube moves or comes out or the patient begins to choke during a feeding. Emphasize the importance of the patient sitting up at a 45-degree angle (or more) for at least 60 minutes after each feeding.

If the patient has a gastrostomy tube, remember that the hypertonic feeding solution might cause diarrhea. If it does, try decreasing the solution's concentration or slowing the infusion rate. Check with the patient's doctor about antidiarrhea medication.

To clean a gastrostomy tube insertion site, remove any gauze dressing and discard it in a plastic trash bag. After putting on gloves, wash around the site with soap and warm water. Use a cotton-tipped applicator to clean hard-to-reach areas. Rinse the skin well and pat it dry. Apply a topical antiseptic (if ordered) with a cotton-tipped applicator. Then apply a gauze dressing, tape it, and secure the gastrostomy tube to the dressing with tape.

To clean a gastrostomy button site, wash the skin around the button with soap and warm water. Apply a topical antiseptic ointment as prescribed, and keep the button open to air.

Teach the patient and home caregivers how to insert and care for the button. Remind the patient to notify the doctor if the button's appearance or location changes. And make sure a spare button is available at all times, in case the original one becomes dislodged. (See *How to reinsert a gastrostomy button*.)

If the patient begins to experience gastric reflux, contact the doctor and arrange for the button to be replaced. Antireflux valves commonly wear out after 3 or 4 months of use.

◆ INFECTION CONTROL

The procedures you use to reduce the risk of disease transmission both inside and outside patients' homes are as important as any of the procedures you use to treat patients' illnesses. Infection-control procedures, collectively defined as *standard precautions* by the Centers for Disease Control and Prevention (CDC), are mandated by the Occupational Safety and Health Administration.

Standard precautions take as their premise the notion that all body fluids could be infectious. Consequently, the procedures required to uphold standard precautions are designed to prevent infection caused by exposure to body fluids.

Equipment and preparation

Central to the concept of standard precautions are personal protective devices that create barriers between you and potentially contaminated substances. These devices include gloves, gowns, shoe coverings, caps, masks, goggles, disposable cardiopulmonary resuscitation (CPR) masks, air-purifying respirators, sharps containers, and disinfectant or phenolic solution used to clean an area contaminated with blood.

Gloves

Wear clean (nonsterile) gloves any time you may come into contact with a patient's body fluids or broken skin. Change your gloves between each procedure. For aseptic procedures, such as dressing changes or insertion of an indwelling urinary catheter, wear sterile gloves.

Gowns, shoe covers, caps

Wear a waterproof disposable gown or apron, shoe covers, and a cap if your clothing, shoes, or hair could become contaminated with body fluids. Remove disposable protective clothing after use, and place it in a plastic trash bag.

Masks

Wear a disposable face mask if you'll be around aerosolized or splattering fluids. Discard the mask after use in a plastic trash bag in the patient's home.

Goggles
Wear goggles or safety glasses with side shields when droplets or fluids could splatter into your eyes. Wash the goggles with soap and water after each use so that you can wear them again. If they become cracked or heavily contaminated, discard them in a plastic trash bag in the patient's home.

CPR masks
If a patient requires CPR, use a disposable mask until the emergency medical team arrives.

Respirators
Air-purifying respirator masks filter particles down to 1 micron in size with a filter efficiency of more than 95%. Wear one when caring for a patient who has tuberculosis.

Sharps and containers
Don't bend, shear, recap, or remove a needle from a syringe after use. Instead, place all sharp objects and needles in a disposable sharps container. Sharps containers should be punctureproof, leakproof, red in color, and labeled with a biohazard sign. Never fill sharps containers more than two-thirds full. In the home, sharps containers should be stored out of the reach of children and discarded according to local and state ordinances.

Specimen collection
Place all specimens in leakproof bags and punctureproof containers during transport. Handle all specimens carefully to reduce the risk of spilling. Secure the container on the floor of your vehicle's trunk during transport.

Implementation
Some of the procedures associated with standard precautions in the home environment include hand washing, glove handling, protecting your bag from contamination, managing soiled linens, disposing of soiled dressings properly, and cleaning equipment.

Handwashing
As you know, hand washing is the best-known method for reducing the risk of cross-contamination between patients and caregivers. To be safe, you should carry hand-washing equipment with you in your bag, including paper towels, liquid soap, betadine scrub (depending on agency policy), hand lotion, and antiseptic hand cleaner or wipes.

As soon as you arrive at a patient's home, wash your hands for a full minute or more. If the patient does not have running water or clean facilities, use an antiseptic hand cleaner before you provide care. Then wash your hands with soap and running water as soon as clean facilities are available.

Handling gloves
If you need to wear sterile gloves to perform an aseptic procedure in your patient's home, you'll need to know how to put them on properly to maintain their sterility. Whether you wear sterile gloves or simply clean examination gloves, make sure you know how to take them off and discard them properly. (See *How to put on and remove gloves*.)

Protecting your bag
Besides protecting yourself from contamination in a patient's home, you'll need to protect your bag as well. You can do so by carrying with you to each visit a supply of paper towels, newspaper or other material suitable

How to put on and remove gloves

When putting on sterile gloves, don't let the outer surface of either glove touch any nonsterile surface, including your hands, as you put them on. When removing contaminated gloves, don't let the surface of either glove touch your skin. Here's how to accomplish both goals.

Putting on sterile gloves

◆ Make sure the opening of each glove is cuffed, allowing you to handle the nonsterile inside of the glove rather than the sterile outside.

◆ Using your nondominant hand, pick up the glove for the dominant hand by grasping the cuff (as shown below).

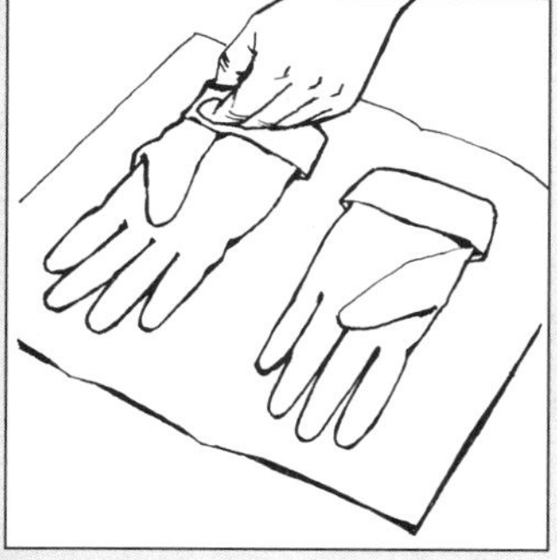

◆ Pull the glove onto your dominant hand. Be sure to keep your dominant thumb folded in against your palm (as shown above right) to avoid touching the sterile outside of the glove as you pull it on.

◆ Allow the glove to come uncuffed as you finish inserting your hand, but don't touch the outside of the glove with your nondominant hand.

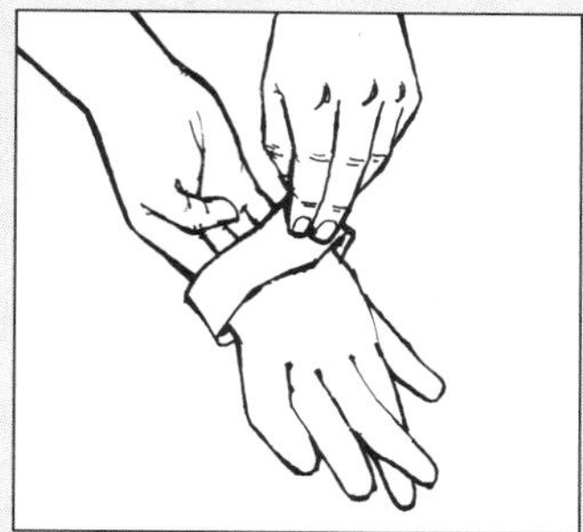

◆ Slip your gloved dominant fingers under the other glove's cuff to pick it up (as shown below).

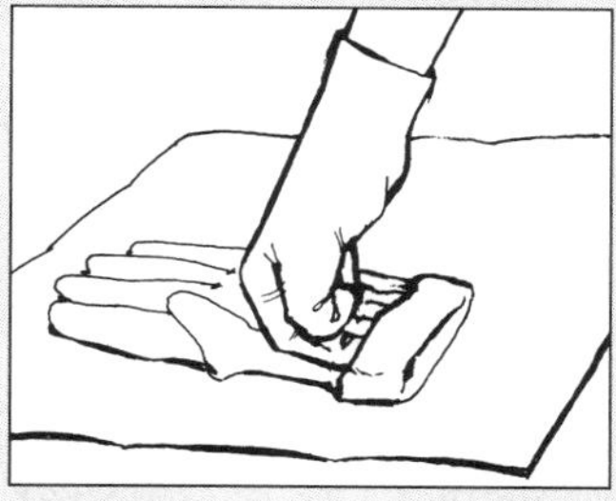

This way, your sterile dominant fingers touch only the sterile outside of the nondominant glove.

◆ Allow the glove to come uncuffed as you finish putting it on, but don't touch the skin side of the cuff with your sterile dominant hand (as shown below).

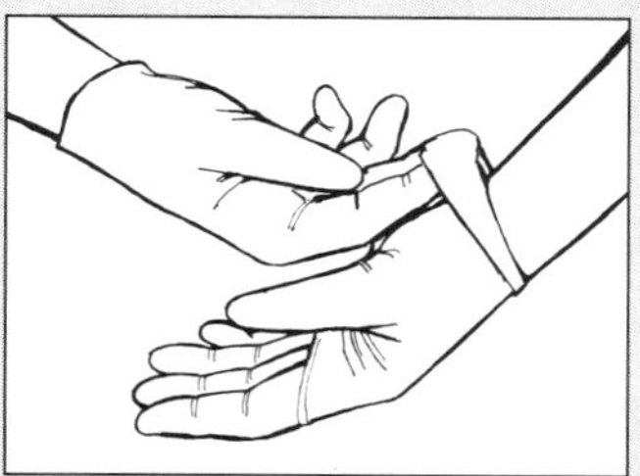

(continued)

How to put on and remove gloves *(continued)*

Removing contaminated gloves

◆ Using your nondominant hand, pinch the glove of the dominant hand near the top (as shown below). Avoid allowing the glove's outer surface to buckle inward against your skin.

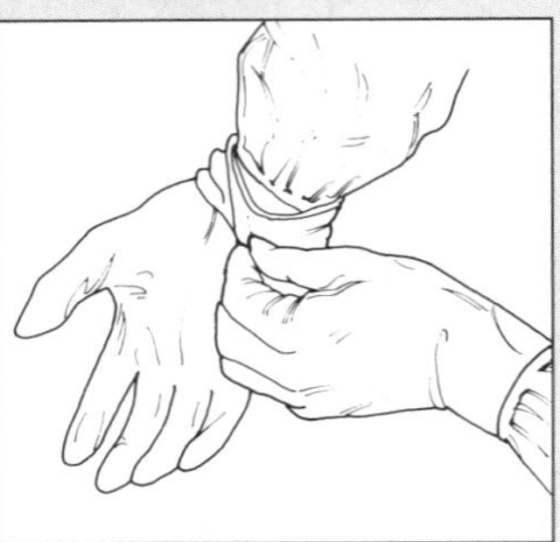

◆ Pull downward, allowing the glove to turn inside out as it comes off (as shown below). Keep the glove from your dominant hand in your nondominant hand after removing it.

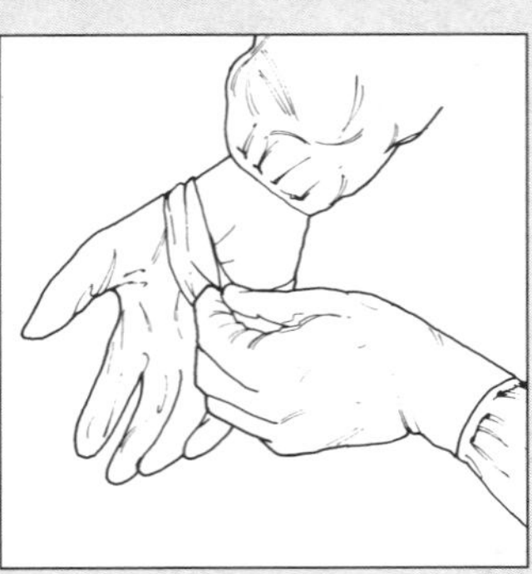

◆ Now insert the first two fingers of your ungloved dominant hand under the edge of the nondominant glove and use the fingers to begin turning the glove inside out as you remove it from your hand (as shown below). Avoid touching the glove's outer surface or folding it against the wrist of your nondominant hand.

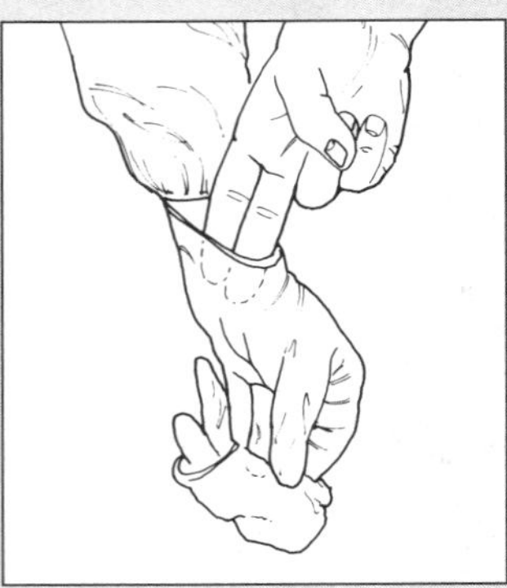

◆ Pull downward so that the glove turns inside out as it comes off (as shown below). Continue pulling until the glove completely encloses the glove from your dominant hand and has its uncontaminated inner surface facing out.

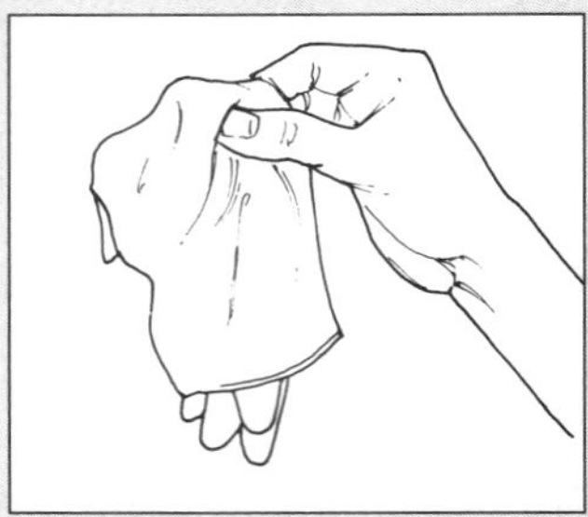

◆ Discard your gloves in the appropriate trash bag or container.

for a barrier, and a cardboard box for storing your bag in your car.

When you arrive at a patient's home, remove your bag from the cardboard box in your car and carry it into the house. Don't put it down on the furniture or the floor. Instead, find a clean spot on which to spread your newspaper or other barrier material, and place your bag on top of that.

Keep your hand-washing supplies at the top of your bag so you can open the bag and wash your hands first. Then remove whatever items you need for your visit. Remember to apply whatever personal protective devices you need. Then close the bag for the rest of the visit. Consider the inside of your bag clean.

At the end of your visit, disinfect all reusable items before returning them to your bag. Pick up and hold your bag, then gather used paper towels, the newspaper your bag sat on, and any other used supplies into a separate plastic bag. Secure the plastic bag and place it with the patient's trash for disposal. Wash your hands, and replace your hand-washing supplies in the top of your bag.

Linen management

If you must handle heavily soiled linens, wash your hands and put on gloves. Place the soiled linens in a pillow case; then place the pillow case in a plastic bag to prevent leakage.

Instruct family members to wash soiled linens as soon as possible to reduce the growth and spread of bacteria. Tell them to wash soiled linens separate from other family clothing and then clean the contaminated washing machine by putting commercial disinfectant or a cup of full-strength bleach in the machine and running it through a wash cycle empty.

Dressing disposal

Place soiled dressings in a plastic trash bag and seal the bag. If the dressing is heavily soiled or may leak, double-bag it. Then place the plastic bag with the patient's other trash for disposal.

Equipment cleaning

To help prevent contamination, try to use disposable equipment whenever possible. When that's not possible, try to leave equipment in the patient's home so you can use it for only one patient. That includes scissors, forceps, and thermometers. Remember that any equipment you carry from house to house must be disinfected before you put it back into your nursing bag or car. Your agency will probably have a preferred disinfectant (spray or towelette) for you to use.

Special considerations

Be sure to teach your patients how to reduce the risk of infection in the home. (See *Controlling infection in the home,* page 252.) If you encounter a blood spill, clean the area with a disinfectant solution; then apply a phenolic solution to the area for 10 minutes.

If a patient's body fluid gets on your skin or in your eyes, irrigate the area with plenty of running water. For your eye, try to irrigate with sterile water. Run the stream from the inner corner to the outer corner to avoid contaminating the other eye. For skin contact, use soap and running water. Then change your clothes for a spare set carried in your car, and call your agency supervisor for follow-up procedures.

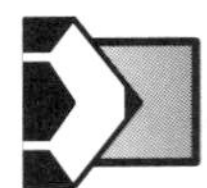

TEACHING POINTS

Controlling infection in the home

Help your patients and their families avoid transmitting infections in the home by giving them these basic instructions.

◆ Maintain good personal hygiene by bathing every day, washing your hair at least weekly, brushing your teeth after every meal and at bedtime, trimming your fingernails and toenails every week, wearing clean clothes, and changing dirty clothes as soon as you notice they're soiled.

◆ Wash your hands frequently, including before you prepare meals, eat, or serve food; after you use the toilet or touch your own or another person's body fluids; after you blow or wipe your nose; and after you take part in outdoor activities.

◆ Clean your home frequently, including dusting and vacuuming each week, mopping kitchen and bathroom floors each week, and cleaning kitchen surfaces with disinfectant. Use separate implements to clean the bathroom and the kitchen, and don't pour water used to mop the floor down the sink. Don't clean urinals or bedpans in the kitchen sink. Clean the inside of the refrigerator each week. Also, keep household clutter to a minimum. Ventilate your home with fresh air. Wear gloves when cleaning up after pets. Don't share towels, washcloths, and other personal care items with the patient.

◆ Disinfect reusable medical supplies frequently and thoroughly, according to the manufacturer's instructions. Call your equipment supplier for replacement parts as needed.

◆ Minimize exposure to people who are sick or infected. Specifically, avoid people diagnosed with bacterial infections and those with colds, cold sores, shingles, or the flu. Avoid crowds and people who recently received vaccinations. Always cover your mouth with a tissue or your hand when you sneeze or cough, and then wash your hands as soon as possible. Don't share eating utensils, and don't drink from another person's glass.

◆ MEDICATION ADMINISTRATION

Which medications you administer in the home and how depend largely on your agency's policies, your state's nurse practice act, and the policies of the patient's insurer. Familiarize yourself with all applicable policies before you begin.

Typically, payers will not reimburse nursing visits made simply to administer oral, topical, or subcutaneous (S.C.) medications in the home because they feel that these modes of delivery don't require a nurse's skill. You may give these medications as part of a visit prompted for another reason. But most payers reimburse only for I.M. and I.V. administration.

Make sure the medication isn't the patient's first dose of a new prescription; usually, such a dose must be given in a more controlled environment.

No matter which medication route you use, you still are responsible for ensuring that your patient understands his medications, their expected effects, possible adverse effects, and any contraindications. You also may need to teach the patient or an appropriate in-home caregiver how to administer the medication properly.

Equipment and preparation

One of the best ways to prepare yourself for administering medications in the home and teaching patients about them is to obtain and study a list of the patient's other medications. The equipment you'll need will depend on the medication, prescribed route, dosage, and frequency.

To administer injectable medications, take the following: ◆ needles and syringes of appropriate size ◆ sharps container ◆ gloves ◆ alcohol or other topical disinfectant ◆ hand-washing supplies ◆ teaching material.

Implementation

Complete the patient's medication record, including the patient's name, medications, dose, administration route and frequency, allergies, and start and stop dates. Double-check yourself by reviewing the five rights of medication administration: right medication, right patient, right time, right route, and right dose. Ask the patient to make a list or gather the containers of all medications he takes routinely, including over-the-counter preparations. Review the purpose, action, and possible effectiveness of each medication with the patient.

Oral medications

Ask the patient to describe or demonstrate how he takes each of his oral medications. Provide instructional medication sheets as needed. If necessary, help the patient and his family establish an administration schedule to remind the patient which medications to take when. Offer to organize the patient's medications in multichambered pill holders, an egg crate, or another container.

At each visit, review the medications and evaluate their effectiveness, possible adverse effects, and the patient's compliance.

S.C. injections

Assemble the equipment for the injection, and wash your hands. Put on gloves and prepare the syringe. Change the needle if necessary before administering the drug. Expose the appropriate body area, and prepare the skin with a topical antiseptic swab. The best sites are the upper arms, abdomen, and anterior thighs.

Remove the needle cap, express any air bubbles, and pinch the skin between your thumb and forefinger. Insert the needle at a 45-degree angle through the skin to the S.C. layer. Inject the medication, remove the needle, and massage the area with an antiseptic swab. (Don't massage the site if you're using heparin.)

Place the used needle and syringe in the sharps container. Make the patient comfortable. Then discard all used items in a plastic trash bag, remove your gloves, and wash your hands. If the patient or a family member will be taking over the S.C. injections, carefully teach the appropriate person how to perform the injection and provide written instructions. Review appropriate injection locations, the need to rotate sites, and how to prepare the medication.

Performing a Z-track injection

By blocking the needle pathway after injection, this technique allows I.M. injection while minimizing the risk of subcutaneous irritation and staining from such drugs as iron dextran. The illustrations below show how to perform a Z-track injection.

Before the procedure begins, the skin, subcutaneous fat, and muscle lie in their normal positions (as shown below).

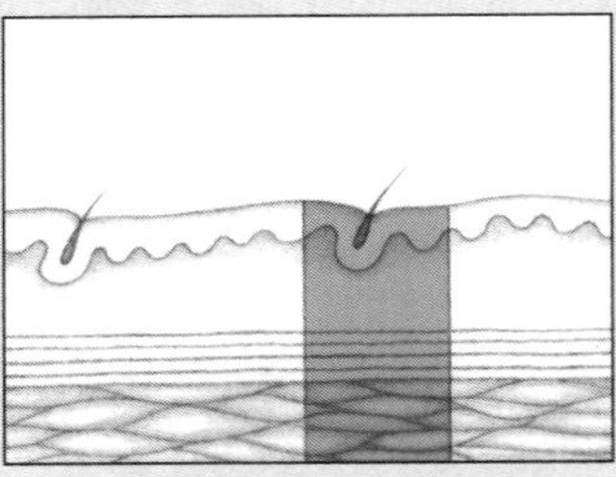

To begin, draw up 0.2 to 0.5 cc of air in the prepared syringe to create an airlock; then replace the needle with another sterile needle. Place your finger on the upper outer quadrant of the patient's buttocks and pull the skin about 1″ (2 cm) laterally away from the injection site (as shown below). Maintain this position.

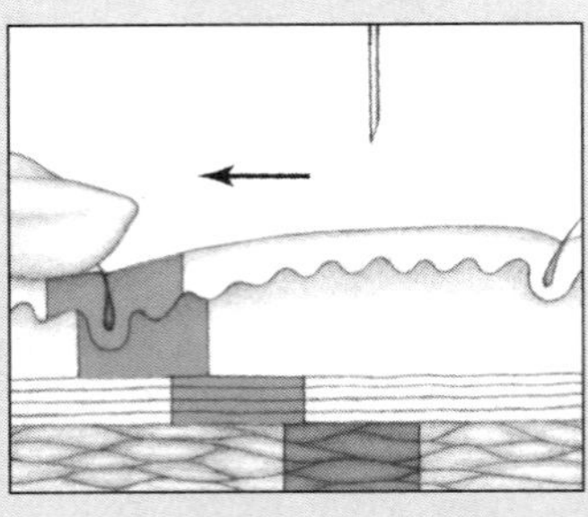

Insert the needle at a 90-degree angle deep into the muscle in the site where you first placed your finger (as shown below). Pull back on the plunger to make sure the needle isn't in a blood vessel. Then slowly inject the medication.

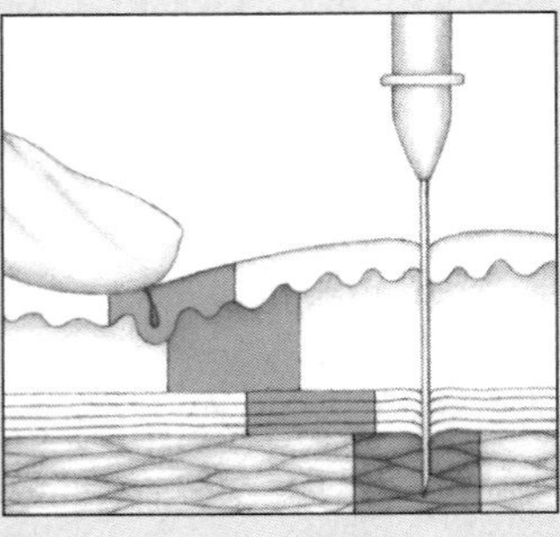

Wait about 10 seconds before withdrawing the needle. Then, as you do, release the displaced tissue. Don't massage the injection site. The needle track (shown by the dotted line below) is now broken at the junction of each tissue layer, trapping the drug in the muscle.

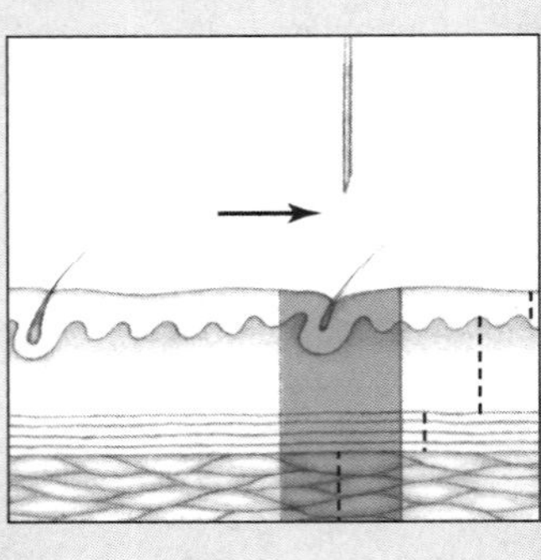

I.M. injections

Before giving an I.M. medication, assemble your equipment in a convenient location, wash your hands, put on gloves, and prepare the syringe. Change the needle, if necessary, before administering the drug.

Choose the best injection site by considering the amount of drug to be given and the medication itself. Expose the appropriate body area, and prepare the skin with a topical antiseptic swab. Remove the needle cap and insert the needle at a 90-degree angle through the skin and into the muscle. Aspirate for blood by pulling back on the plunger. If blood appears, remove the syringe, discard it, and prepare a new injection.

If no blood appears, inject the medication slowly, remove the needle, and apply an antiseptic swab over the injection site. Unless contraindicated, gently massage the injection site to distribute the medication. Keep in mind that, for some medications, you may want to use the Z-track injection method. (See *Performing a Z-track injection.*)

Place the used needle and syringe in the sharps container. Make the patient comfortable. Then discard all used items in a plastic trash bag, remove your gloves, and wash your hands. If the patient or a family member will be taking over the patient's I.M. injections, carefully teach the appropriate person how to perform the injection and provide written instructions. Review appropriate injection locations and methods to prepare the medication.

Special considerations

If you're caring for an elderly patient, watch carefully for medication errors and interactions common in this population. Typical problems include taking a medication at the wrong time, taking an outdated medication, and not taking a medication at all. If you detect a medication error, follow your agency's policy about reporting and following up on it. You'll need to provide thorough documentation about your medication teaching and the patient's response to teaching.

◆ OSTOMY CARE

As you know, an ostomy is an opening surgically created to replace a normal physiologic function. Ostomies typically are created for elimination of feces, urine, or both. (A tracheostomy provides a patent airway. For more information, see "Tracheal suctioning" later in this chapter.)

Depending on where the stoma is located, the patient may or may not have to wear an appliance to collect urine or stool. For example, a patient with an ileal conduit or ureterostomy typically wears an appliance. A patient with a continent urinary diversion may be able to catheterize the stoma rather than wear an appliance.

Likewise, a patient with an ileostomy or an ascending or transverse colostomy will wear an appliance to collect fecal material, whereas a patient with a descending or sigmoid colostomy may be able to learn bowel evacuation, thus reducing the need to wear and care for an appliance.

Equipment and preparation

When preparing to care for a patient with a urinary diversion, gather the following equipment: ◆ pouching system ◆ stoma measuring guide ◆ stoma adhesive ◆ pouch cleaning solution (optional) ◆ pouch deodorant (optional) ◆ gauze pads ◆ soap and paper towels ◆ gloves ◆ scissors ◆ plastic trash bag ◆ printed ostomy instructions.

When preparing to care for a patient with an ileostomy or an ascending or transverse colostomy, gather the following equipment: ◆ pouching system (either a one- or two-piece system, with or without an attached skin barrier) ◆ stoma measuring guide ◆ stoma adhesive ◆ skin barrier ◆ pouch cleaning solution (optional) ◆ pouch deodorant (optional) ◆ soap and paper towels ◆ gloves ◆ scissors ◆ plastic trash bag ◆ printed ostomy instructions.

When preparing to irrigate a descending or sigmoid colostomy, gather the following equipment: ◆ irrigation bag with tubing ◆ irrigation sleeve with belt (optional) ◆ water-soluble lubricant ◆ plastic trash bag ◆ pouch system (optional) ◆ soap and paper towels ◆ gloves.

Start by selecting an appropriate location in the patient's home to perform the procedure — preferably the bathroom. If you'll be performing an irrigation and the patient's home has only one bathroom, alert other family members before you start, and tell them that the procedure will take at least 30 minutes.

Implementation

Appropriate procedures vary somewhat depending on the location and function of the stoma, as described below. For all procedures, start by explaining to the patient what you'll be doing. Then arrange your equipment in a convenient location.

Urinary diversion

- Measure the size of the stoma before preparing the skin barrier.
- Prepare gauze pads to place over the stoma once you remove the appliance. Remember that urine will continue to drain.
- Put on gloves; then either remove the appliance and discard it or place it in the disinfecting container.
- Perform skin and ostomy care. Remove any drainage on the stoma with a tissue.
- Clean the peristomal skin with soap and water while holding the end of a piece of rolled gauze in the stoma to wick urine away. Pat the skin dry.
- Apply a skin barrier or adhesive. Then press the pouch to the stoma. Continue applying gentle pressure for 3 to 5 minutes.
- Make the patient comfortable.
- Clean the work area and discard supplies according to standard precautions.

Ileostomy or ascending colostomy

- Help the patient to a comfortable position with easy access to the stoma and appliance.
- Wash your hands and put on gloves. Then assess the patient's abdomen, bowel sounds, and the amount and characteristics of the ostomy drainage.
- Remove the appliance and drain fecal material into the toilet.
- If the pouching system is reusable, put the pouch aside.
- Gently remove and discard the pouch adhesive (either a large square or a smaller ring); then change your gloves.
- Clean the skin around the stoma with soap and warm water. Gently swab away any fecal material from the stoma; don't scrub vigorously. Then pat the surrounding skin dry.
- Examine the skin and stoma for increased redness, dark discoloration, or areas of breakdown. A normal stoma is pink-red and moist and excretes mucus.
- Measure the stoma and prepare a new skin barrier (if a two-piece system) or a new pouch.

◆ If applicable, dust or paint the skin around the stoma with a liquid or powder adhesive before applying the skin barrier.
◆ If you're using a two-piece system, apply the skin barrier, avoiding wrinkles or gaps. Be alert to the patient's natural skin folds surrounding the stoma.
◆ Select the new pouch, insert deodorant drops or tablets if desired, and apply it to the skin barrier.
◆ Gently press the pouch into place with your fingers to enhance its adhesion to the skin.
◆ Make sure the appliance is fastened securely to the skin barrier and the closure clasp is fastened. Leave a small amount of air in the pouch before fastening the clasp to facilitate drainage to the bottom of the pouch.
◆ Reinforce the skin barrier on all four sides with tape. Apply an appliance belt, if desired, to further secure the pouch. Make the patient comfortable.
◆ Clean the work area using standard precautions and, if necessary, place the reusable pouching system in a disinfectant container.

Descending colostomy

When a descending or sigmoid colostomy that requires irrigation needs changing, supplement the standard procedure with the following steps:
◆ Fill the irrigation bag with 500 to 1,000 ml of warm water, and flush the tubing to remove air.
◆ Hang the bag on a door or shower hook.
◆ Put on gloves to remove the patient's appliance (if applicable).
◆ If necessary, clean the stoma with warm water to remove any fecal material.
◆ Place the irrigation sleeve over the stoma, directing its end into the toilet. If the sleeve doesn't have adhesive backing, secure it with an ostomy belt.
◆ Attach the cone tip to the irrigation tubing. Lubricate with water-soluble lubricant, and gently insert the cone into the stoma for a snug fit.
◆ Never force the cone tip into the stoma. If you meet resistance, lubricate your gloved little finger and insert it into the stoma to remove surface fecal material; then try again.
◆ Open the clamp on the irrigation tubing, and allow the solution to flow over 15 minutes. Apply steady pressure on the cone to ensure a snug fit and to keep the solution from leaking around the cone.
◆ If the patient experiences cramps, stop the irrigation and wait until the pain subsides. If you're feeding the solution manually, drop the bag to the height of the stoma to stop the flow.
◆ When you finish the irrigation, remove the cone and either set it aside for later cleaning or discard it in the plastic trash bag.
◆ Clamp the bottom of the sleeve once most of the solution has drained.
◆ Help the patient to a comfortable position, and tell him that it will take about 30 more minutes for the bowel to empty completely. Once it's empty, you can complete the ostomy care.

Special considerations

When caring for a patient with a stoma, especially a new one, one of your most important duties will be helping him adapt to the appliance and the changes in his body. (See *Adapting to an ostomy*, pages 258 and 259.)

When providing ostomy care, note the size and appearance of the stoma and the condition of surrounding skin. As appropriate, document the characteristics of the patient's urine or fecal material.

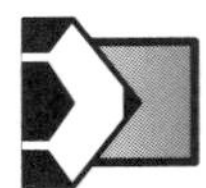

TEACHING POINTS

Adapting to an ostomy

If your patient has an ostomy and an appliance, offer these suggestions to help him maximize his independence.

◆ If the appliance leaks, change it. Don't simply tape a leaking appliance to your skin.
◆ Tell your doctor about any burning or itching around the stoma.
◆ For an ileostomy or colostomy, empty the pouch when it's half full to keep the seal from breaking.
◆ Use mild soap; avoid soaps that contain lotion, creams, or oils.
◆ Bathe or shower without the appliance.
◆ Remove body hair around the appliance with an electric razor or blunt scissors to keep the adhesive from pulling your hair.
◆ To help prevent skin irritation, avoid tight clothing or belts.
◆ Muffle the sound of flatus by gently pressing over the stoma during evacuation.
◆ Periodically release built-up gas in the pouch.
◆ Try various foods to reduce unpleasant effects, such as diarrhea or excessive flatus.
◆ Try various pouch deodorants for odor control.
◆ Measure the stoma before ordering additional supplies.
◆ Always carry appliance equipment with you.

If the patient has an ileostomy, give him these additional instructions:

◆ Expect frequent drainage 30 to 60 minutes after eating.
◆ Plan to change your appliance when the stoma isn't draining.
◆ Avoid foods high in fiber (such as corn, popcorn, nuts, mushrooms, celery, and fruit skins) because they can block your stoma.
◆ If the stoma swells or becomes discolored, contact your doctor immediately.
◆ If you experience sudden cramps and vomiting, or if the drainage stops or changes from semiformed to liquid, contact your doctor immediately.
◆ Never use laxatives or stool softeners. If you have very watery drainage for more than 48 hours, contact your doctor.

If the patient performs irrigation routinely, give him these additional instructions:

◆ Irrigate on a planned schedule (daily or every other day) at about the same time of day.
◆ Don't try to hurry the irrigation.
◆ Drinking a warm liquid, such as coffee or tea, before the irrigation may help in evacuating stool.
◆ Gently rubbing your abdomen during irrigation will help expel irrigant and stools.
◆ If no irrigant drains out of the stoma, don't repeat the irrigation. Contact your doctor.
◆ Don't irrigate if you're experiencing loose stools or diarrhea. Contact your doctor.
◆ Don't irrigate if the stoma shrinks or becomes enlarged or if an abnormal bulge appears under the skin around the stoma. Contact your doctor.

Adapting to an ostomy *(continued)*

If the patient has a urinary ostomy, give the following instructions:

◆ If your urine becomes dark or cloudy from mucus, increase your fluid intake.

◆ During appliance changes, roll a gauze sponge and hold a rolled end in the stoma to wick urine.

◆ Connect a continent pouch to a drainage bag at night.

◆ Contact your doctor if you develop skin breakdown, a foul urine odor, a fever, bloody urine, or pain in your side or back.

◆ OXYGEN DELIVERY

Medicare will reimburse the patient for home oxygen therapy if PaO_2 is ≤55 mm Hg and SaO_2 is ≤85%.

A supplier of durable medical equipment will bring the oxygen to the patient's home, set it up, educate the patient about it, and maintain the system. (See *How to handle oxygen at home,* page 260.) You are responsible for ensuring that the oxygen is administered as prescribed and for evaluating the patient's response to therapy.

The type of system used depends on the patient's condition, the length of time he may need the oxygen, and the cost. Home oxygen therapy can be provided in three ways:

◆ oxygen tank — A metal cylinder filled with compressed gas is used for patients who need oxygen on an intermittent or standby basis.

◆ oxygen concentrator — This electrical device extracts oxygen from room air, so it doesn't need to be refilled with compressed gas. It can be used for low oxygen flow (less than 4 L/minute).

◆ liquid oxygen — Patients who are oxygen-dependent but still mobile may use a large liquid reservoir containing oxygen. For leaving the home, a smaller, portable unit is filled.

Equipment and preparation

You'll need the following equipment for home oxygen therapy: ◆ source of oxygen supply (cylinder, concentrator, liquid oxygen reservoir) ◆ regulator flow meter ◆ appropriate oxygen delivery system (nasal cannula, face mask, tracheostomy collar, other mask) ◆ tubing (large- or small-bore depending on delivery system) ◆ humidifier ◆ sterile or distilled water (depending on oxygen system).

Coordinate with the equipment supplier when the oxygen system will be delivered to the patient's home. Review the doctor's order to ensure delivery of all appropriate materials. Make sure that all appropriate laboratory tests have been done as well, including arterial blood gas analysis.

Evaluate the patient's home for an appropriate site in which to install a liquid oxygen reservoir or concentrator. Make sure the site has a grounded electrical outlet for an oxygen concentrator.

Implementation

Review the doctor's order for the type of oxygen therapy needed, the source

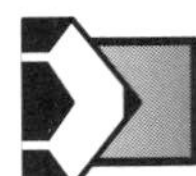

TEACHING POINTS

How to handle oxygen at home

If your patient is on home oxygen therapy, give him these instructions:

- ◆ Do not smoke near oxygen. Place "no smoking" signs where oxygen is used or stored.
- ◆ Do not place or store oxygen near a stove, space heater, or other heat source.
- ◆ Keep oxygen at least 5′ (1.5 m) away from electrical outlets and appliances.
- ◆ Do not use an electric blanket or heating pad near oxygen.
- ◆ Prevent static electricity from building up by using all-cotton bed linens and clothing. Polyester and nylon encourage static electricity, increasing the risk of oxygen combustion.
- ◆ Avoid skin care products that contain oil or alcohol for at least 6 hours after using oxygen. Oil and alcohol are flammable, and oxygen can remain in clothing for up to 6 hours after being turned off.
- ◆ Do not run oxygen tubing under your clothes, bed linens, furniture, or carpeting. You need to be able to see the tubing clearly at all times.
- ◆ Maintain the oxygen container in an upright position.
- ◆ Turn off the oxygen when it is not being used.
- ◆ Regularly check the oxygen level remaining in the system.
- ◆ Keep a fire extinguisher near the room where oxygen is being used.
- ◆ Inform the electric company, local fire department, and ambulance company that oxygen is being used in your home. List emergency telephone numbers, along with the number of the oxygen supplier, near the telephone.
- ◆ Consult your doctor before altering the oxygen flow rate.

If your patient uses an oxygen compressor, give him these additional instructions:

- ◆ Keep the compressor in a traffic-free area in the home.
- ◆ Keep at least a 3-day supply of oxygen in the home.
- ◆ If the tank seems to be emptying too quickly, especially if it's making a hissing sound, open the windows and call the supplier.

If your patient uses an oxygen concentrator, give him these additional instructions:

- ◆ Do not use an extension cord with the concentrator.
- ◆ Clean the filter at least twice each week.
- ◆ If the power fails, turn off the concentrator and use a back-up oxygen tank until the power is restored.
- ◆ If the alert buzzer doesn't come on when you push the power switch, turn the concentrator off, use a back-up tank, and call the supplier.

If your patient uses liquid oxygen, give him these additional instructions:

- ◆ Always keep the unit upright in a well-ventilated area.
- ◆ Don't touch the unit's metal parts with bare hands because they're extremely cold and could cause frostbite.

of oxygen supply, and the mode of delivery. Explain the need for oxygen therapy to the patient, family members, and other caregivers.

Assess the patient's cognitive and cardiopulmonary status for signs and symptoms of early hypoxia, including dyspnea, headache, hypertension, hyperventilation, restlessness, slight confusion, tachycardia, and visual disturbances. Signs and symptoms of chronic hypoxia include clubbing of the fingers, pallor, polycythemia, and thrombosis. Signs and symptoms of advanced hypoxia include bradycardia, hypotension, metabolic acidosis, and profound changes in mental status (such as combativeness).

If the patient has chronic obstructive pulmonary disease, assess for signs and symptoms of carbon dioxide retention, such as elevated blood pressure, bounding pulse, clammy skin, and headache.

Document the patient's vital signs, skin color, respiratory effort, and lung sounds. Also note how the patient is tolerating the oxygen therapy and if there's any improvement in his overall condition.

Teach the patient about oxygen in general and the specific mode of delivery ordered.

Special considerations

Home oxygen therapy requires extensive patient teaching. Reinforce and enhance the instructions the equipment supplier provided to the patient and home caregivers on the delivery system.

Never administer oxygen at more than 2 L/minute by nasal cannula to a patient with chronic lung disease unless you have a specific order to do so. Some patients with chronic lung disease have become dependent on a state of hypercapnia and hypoxia to stimulate respirations; supplemental oxygen could cause them to stop breathing. Explain this to the patient and, as appropriate, family members.

◆ TOTAL PARENTERAL NUTRITION

Used to provide nutritional support for patients who are significantly malnourished and unable to eat or swallow properly, total parenteral nutrition (TPN) has become more widely used in the home care environment. However, the initial TPN infusion is usually given in the acute care setting in case an adverse reaction occurs. Usually, you'll deliver TPN by a central venous line or an implanted vascular access device.

Equipment and preparation

Before you can provide home TPN, you'll need special training and expertise in I.V. therapy, medication administration, and methods to care for a central venous line or an implanted vascular access device.

When you prepare to deliver home TPN, gather the following equipment: ◆ nutrition solution (intralipids may be mixed in the solution or can be administered separately) ◆ sterile normal saline solution ◆ heparin (100-units/ml solution for irrigation and flush, as needed) ◆ I.V. tubing with a 1.2-micron filter ◆ external occlusion clamp, if needed ◆ infusion pump ◆ refrigerator for storing nutrition solution ◆ 12-ml syringe with 1″ needle ◆ 3-ml syringes with 23G 1″ needles ◆ topical antiseptic swabs (alcohol, povidone-iodine) ◆ gloves ◆ sharps container ◆ hand-washing supplies.

Make arrangements for the TPN solution, administration pump, and other supplies to be delivered directly to the patient's home. Also assemble all of the patient-education materials and nutrition literature that you'll need.

Keep in mind that your first visit for home TPN will be lengthy.

Implementation

Begin your first visit by explaining the procedures associated with TPN: ensuring a patent access site, preparing the solution and pump, securing the infusion, and evaluating the patient's response. Provide educational materials about TPN, what the doctor wants the patient to receive, what the patient might expect during and after an infusion, and what the patient needs to learn to manage his own TPN.

At subsequent visits, assess the patient's nutritional status, including weight and intake and output. Monitor for adverse effects, including electrolyte imbalances and elevated blood glucose level. Urge the patient to monitor his blood glucose level at least once daily with a fingerstick sample. Review his results and report any elevations to his doctor.

To deliver a feeding, start by assembling all needed equipment in a convenient area. Help the patient into a comfortable position that gives you easy access to the infusion site. Because the TPN solution is high in glucose, electrolytes, and vitamins, the patient's doctor may order preinfusion laboratory studies. If so, perform them before you begin the infusion.

After completing laboratory testing and removing used items, wash your hands and examine the TPN bag for leaks. Check the expiration date. Make sure the mixture includes all elements specified in the doctor's order.

Remember that multivitamins and other additives may not be premixed because they aren't stable in a mixture over time. So you may have to inject multivitamins into the mixture before administering it. If so, draw up the vitamins and other additives with the 12-ml syringe using aseptic technique. Then inject the contents through the medication port on the bag. Invert the bag several times to mix the additives with the solution.

Prepare the solution for administration by priming the tubing and attaching it to the administration pump according to the manufacturer's directions. Prime the pump's cassette and all tubing, eliminating micro air bubbles as necessary. Set the pump to infuse at the ordered rate. Remove all items used to prepare the solution and pump for administration, and wash your hands.

Assess the catheter insertion site for redness, drainage, or signs of thrombophlebitis or infection. Prepare the site by first putting on a new pair of gloves and then drawing up 3 ml of sterile normal saline solution in a syringe. Clean the injection cap site with a topical antiseptic (povidone-iodine) and then with an alcohol swab. Irrigate the lumen with 2.5 ml of normal saline solution. Remove the syringe and attach the infusion tubing. Turn on the pump and begin the infusion. Tape all connections securely, and loop a section of tubing near the infusion site and secure it with tape.

When the infusion is finished, turn off the pump and disconnect the tubing from the access site. Then wash your hands, put on gloves, and draw up sterile normal saline solution and heparin in separate syringes. Disinfect the access site with povidone-iodine and alcohol swabs. Inject 2.5 ml of sterile normal saline solution followed by slow injection of 2.5 ml of heparin. Discard used items in the sharps container and plastic trash bag, remove your gloves, and wash your hands.

Examine the access site for signs and symptoms of inflammation, including drainage, pain, redness, warmth, and swelling. Document the condition of the access site both before and after the infusion. Provide care for the access site, as needed.

Special considerations

On your first visit to the patient's home, you may need to set up the infusion and then come back later in the day to discontinue it. Or, if the patient's doctor ordered a continuous infusion, you might need someone else in the home to help the patient with TPN procedures.

During your first visit, assess the patient's ability to perform the procedures independently. Also consider who else in the home might be able to help. Begin instructing all potential helpers in TPN procedures early in the process. Doing so will help the patient and other caregivers understand right away what's involved with TPN.

As you teach the patient and other caregivers, keep your sessions short and focus on one skill at a time. Don't expect them to learn home infusion in one or two sessions; instead, have them practice selected skills while you're in the home. Watch them and offer suggestions. Provide positive reinforcement in all teaching sessions.

Make sure the patient and his caregivers know which signs and symptoms may offer a warning, including fluid retention, circulatory overload, elevated blood glucose level, and catheter site inflammation.

Remind the patient and his family to refrigerate any TPN solution delivered to the home. Ask them to remove one solution bag from the refrigerator at least 1 hour before you're scheduled to arrive.

Keep an extra infusion pump in the patient's home in case the original one malfunctions. Make sure the pump has a built-in, battery-operated back-up system so that TPN can continue, even if the power fails. Also ask the pharmacy to provide at least one extra solution bag in case one leaks or delivery of the solution is delayed.

If the patient's condition changes or the access site develops complications, contact the patient's doctor. Expect the doctor to phone in solution changes in concert with the patient's laboratory data.

◆ TRACHEAL SUCTIONING

In tracheal suctioning, a catheter is inserted through the mouth, nose, tracheal stoma, or tracheostomy tube to remove mucus or secretions from the patient's trachea or bronchi. In acute care facilities, it's a sterile procedure. In the home environment, however, it's performed as a clean procedure under certain circumstances. If necessary, be prepared to teach the patient or a caregiver how to suction. (See *Suctioning at home,* page 264.)

Equipment and preparation

For a patient who requires suctioning at home, contact a supplier of durable medical equipment and ask that they deliver suction apparatus to the home. Make sure a back-up system will be available in case of malfunction. Also make sure you'll have the following equipment at the patient's home: ◆ suction tubing ◆ suction catheters (14 or 16 French) ◆ water-soluble lubricant ◆ disinfecting container ◆ sterile water ◆ sterile normal saline solution (if ordered by the doctor for tracheal instillation) ◆ sterile and clean gloves ◆ handwashing supplies ◆ plastic trash bag ◆ patient-education materials.

Implementation

Explain the procedure to the patient, and assemble your equipment in a convenient work area. Make sure the

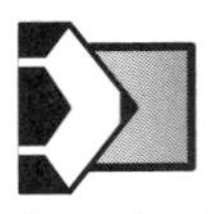

TEACHING POINTS

Suctioning at home

If family members will be suctioning the patient at home, provide plenty of teaching and ongoing support to ensure success. You'll need to teach the purpose of the procedure, the equipment to be used (including the suction machine), and the procedure itself. Also, teach that the suction tubing must be changed every 24 hours.

If suction catheters will be reused, teach how to clean them. Tell caregivers to soak the tubing and catheters in disinfectant solution (50% hydrogen peroxide and 50% sterile water or sterile normal saline solution) and then boil them for at least 10 minutes. Hanging the tubing over a bathroom shower rod is one way to make sure the tubing drains and dries completely. The catheters can be air-dried and placed in new plastic bags until needed.

Also teach home caregivers how to empty the suction collection bottle. Urge them to clean it every 24 hours with soap and hot water.

suction machine is working properly, fill appropriate containers with water before use, and set the suction between 5 and 10 mm Hg.

After washing your hands, assess the patient's respiratory status and measure his vital signs. Remember that heart rate and blood pressure will increase during and just after suctioning.

Help the patient into a comfortable position — semi-reclining for a bedbound patient. Gently move the patient's head toward you. If possible, have him take several deep breaths before you start (with supplemental oxygen, if available) to reduce the risk of hypoxia while you suction.

Follow aseptic technique for any patient who is immunosuppressed or intubated, requires deep suctioning, or has a new tracheostomy. Usually, you can use clean technique in the home environment for a patient who will be suctioned by nose or mouth or who has had a tracheostomy for many years.

Open the catheter kit, find the water container in it, and fill it with sterile water (tap water if you're using clean technique). If gloves are included in the kit, put them on now before handling the catheter. If the catheter is packaged separately, open the catheter following sterile technique, put on gloves, and then handle the catheter.

Attach the suction catheter to the suction tubing on the machine. Test the suction machine by lightly dipping the tip of the catheter in the sterile water and applying suction. Continue to suction all water out of the catheter.

If preparing to suction through the nares, estimate the length of catheter you'll need to advance before applying suction. Do so by measuring the length of catheter needed to reach from the tip of the patient's nose to the end of his earlobe.

Lubricate the tip of the catheter with water-soluble lubricant; then begin to insert the catheter. The patient may cough and choke while you're advancing it. However, if he begins to swallow, you'll need to withdraw the catheter and start again because the catheter entered the esophagus instead of the trachea.

Once you've advanced your estimated length of tubing, apply suction by covering the port with your thumb as you gently rotate and withdraw the catheter. Suction for 5 to 10 seconds; then withdraw the catheter and flush it with sterile water. Wait a few minutes for the patient's respirations to recover; then suction again. Repeat the suctioning procedure until the patient's secretions have cleared, auscultating for breath sounds periodically to assess the procedure's effectiveness. Analyze the amount, color, and tenacity of suctioned secretions.

If you're suctioning by a tracheostomy or endotracheal tube, insert the catheter only until you feel resistance (usually 4″ to 6″ [10 to 15 cm]). If the patient experiences severe choking and coughing, stop suctioning, wait for him to recover, and try again. Irritation of the trachea causes an involuntary cough reflex.

When you complete the procedure, flush the catheter with sterile water and either discard it or place it in the disinfecting container. Remove your gloves and make the patient comfortable. Readjust the patient's head and provide oral hygiene. Discard all used disposable equipment in a plastic trash bag, and wash your hands thoroughly.

Document the patient's response to suctioning, his vital signs before and after suctioning, and the amount, color, and tenacity of secretions.

Special considerations

Because the right mainstem bronchus is shorter, wider, and more vertical than the left, the suction catheter may tend to enter this bronchus. If the patient appears to gasp during your suctioning procedure, remove the catheter and allow the patient to recover before you continue. Then, advance a shorter length of catheter.

If the patient produces excessive oral secretions while you're suctioning, consider using a Yankauer catheter to remove them. This oral catheter is plastic and rod-shaped, with holes in the end. It has no port to adjust suction pressure, so suction is constant. If you use this catheter, clean it using the same method as you do for the tracheal catheter and suction tubing.

To change a tracheostomy tube, start by explaining the procedure to the patient. Then wash your hands and put on gloves. Prepare the new tracheostomy tube by placing new ties on it, then lubricating the outer surface of the tube. Insert the obturator through the tube to protect the mucosa during insertion. Next, cut the old tracheostomy ties and remove the tube from the patient's neck by pulling downward and outward. If the patient begins to cough, stop and allow him to recover before you continue. Insert the new tube gently through the stoma; then remove the obturator and fasten the ties. Make the patient comfortable, and either discard or disinfect all used items.

Keep in mind that if your patient depends on a tracheostomy tube for ventilation, it's prudent to teach him how to change and reinsert the tube. Tell the patient that he'll need to change the tube regularly because adherent secretions can reduce the lumen size and raise the risk of infection. (See *Replacing a tracheostomy tube,* page 266.)

Replacing a tracheostomy tube

Act fast to replace a removed or dislodged tracheostomy tube. Follow these steps:
◆ Wait until the patient stops coughing before trying to reinsert the tube.
◆ If possible, tilt the patient's head back slightly.
◆ Apply a water-soluble lubricant to a new tube and insert the stylet.
◆ Attempt to reinsert the tube. If you meet resistance, don't force the tube.
◆ If necessary, try to reinsert the old tube. Don't force it if you meet resistance.
◆ Insert a suctioning catheter and cut it about 6" (15 cm) out from the stoma. Hold the catheter in place. Don't let go.
◆ Contact the emergency medical system for transport to the nearest emergency department. Stay with the patient until transportation has arrived, the airway is secure, and ventilation has been reestablished.

◆ URINARY CATHETER CARE

If your patient has urine retention or obstructed urine flow, he'll need a urinary catheter. The doctor may order an external catheter, intermittent catheterization, or an indwelling urinary catheter. Intermittent catheterization and changing an indwelling urinary catheter are usually reimbursable, for a limited period of time, because they're both considered reasonable and necessary skills.

Intermittent catheterization is considered a skill that either the patient or another home caregiver can be taught to perform. Care of an external catheter might be questioned as a reimbursable skill unless accompanied by other skilled services.

Equipment and preparation

If you'll be inserting a urinary catheter, gather the following equipment: ◆ sterile urinary catheter kit ◆ perineal washing supplies ◆ hand-washing supplies ◆ clean gloves ◆ adhesive tape ◆ plastic trash bag.

Before performing intermittent catheterization or changing an indwelling catheter, contact the patient's doctor for any specific instructions, such as changing the size of the catheter or collecting a urine specimen. Ask whether the procedure will be done sporadically or routinely or if the patient will need to learn how to perform the procedure independently. Also check to see whether there's an amount of residual urine for which the doctor would order an indwelling catheter. Determine if the equipment needs to be sterile or if the clean technique is acceptable.

If the patient needs intermittent catheterization, prepare materials you can use to teach the patient or a caregiver how to perform the procedure. Plan to begin teaching with the first catheterization. If the patient is ambulatory and has an indwelling catheter, take a leg bag with you so you can teach him how to use it. (See *Using a leg bag*.)

If you'll be applying or changing an external catheter, gather the following equipment: ◆ external catheter (includes double-sided adhesive tape) ◆ urinary collection tubing ◆ perineal washing supplies ◆ hand-wash-

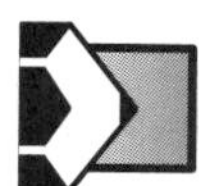

TEACHING POINTS

Using a leg bag

A urine drainage bag attached to the leg provides the catheterized patient with greater mobility. Leg bags usually are worn during the day and replaced with standard collection devices at night.

Attaching the leg bag

◆ Provide privacy and explain the procedure. Caution the patient that a leg bag is smaller than a standard collection device and may need to be emptied more often.

◆ Remove the protective covering from the tip of the drainage tube. Then show the patient how to clean the tip with an alcohol sponge, wiping away from the opening to avoid contaminating the tube. Show him how to attach the tube to the catheter.

◆ Place the drainage bag on the patient's calf or thigh, and fasten the straps securely (as shown below). Then show him how to tape the catheter to his leg. Emphasize that he must leave slack in the catheter to minimize pressure on the bladder, urethra, and related structures.

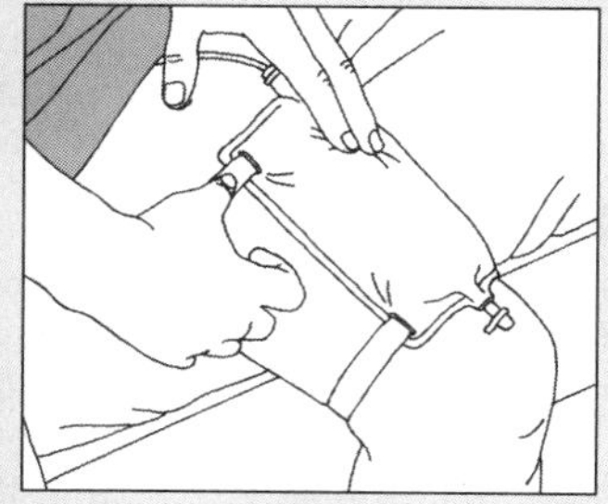

Avoiding complications

◆ Explain that excessive pressure or tension on the catheter can lead to tissue breakdown. Also tell the patient not to fasten the leg bag's straps too tightly to avoid interfering with circulation.

◆ To prevent a full leg bag from damaging his bladder wall and urethra, encourage the patient to empty the bag when it's only half full. He also should inspect the catheter and drainage tubing periodically for compression or kinks, which could obstruct flow and cause bladder distention.

◆ Although most leg bags have a valve in the drainage tube that prevents urine reflux into the bladder, urge the patient to keep the drainage bag lower than his bladder at all times because urine in the bag is a perfect growth medium for bacteria. Also caution him not to go to bed or take long naps wearing the bag.

◆ Tell the patient to wash the leg bag with soap and water or a bacteriostatic solution before each use to prevent infection.

ing supplies ◆ clean gloves ◆ adhesive tape ◆ plastic trash bag.

Before going to the patient's home, contact his doctor to see if you need to collect urine specimens. Take several external catheters with you on the first visit, and tell the patient to change the catheter when he bathes each day. Be prepared to teach the patient or caregivers how to apply an external urinary catheter. If the patient is ambulatory, take a leg bag.

Implementation

Depending on the patient's condition and abilities, you'll either catheterize the patient yourself or teach him to perform the procedure on his own.

Urinary catheterization

Explain the procedure to the patient, and assemble the equipment at a convenient and private work area. Wash your hands before helping the patient into a comfortable position. Place a male patient in the supine position, with his legs slightly abducted and separated. Place a female patient in the supine position, with her knees flexed and separated.

Assess the patient for bladder distention, pain, urgency, and time of the last voiding. Prepare a basin or container of warm water. Put on gloves. With soap and a washcloth, begin washing the perineal area. For a man, begin cleaning in a circular motion from the tip of the penis. For a woman, use downward strokes to clean the perineum. Rinse the perineum well and dry it. Discard the used water, remove the cleaning items, remove your gloves, and wash your hands.

Return to the patient and take the plastic wrapper off of the catheter kit. Carefully remove the kit and gently begin to peal back the paper wrapper surrounding the inner tray. This paper will become the sterile field. On top of the tray will be a pair of sterile gloves; put them on using sterile technique.

Once you've put on the gloves, take the smaller tray out of the package. Place the fenestrated drape over the patient for privacy. Open the bottle of povidone-iodine solution, and saturate the cotton balls with the solution. Now pick up the catheter, open the water-soluble lubricant, and place the catheter tip inside the lubricant package.

For an indwelling catheter, pick up the sterile empty syringe and attach it to the balloon port of the catheter. Inject 10 cc of air into the port, and watch to make sure the balloon inflates. (If it doesn't, don't use that catheter.) Then deflate the balloon, remove the syringe, and put the catheter down on the sterile field. Attach the collection tubing to the catheter's drainage port, and make sure the bag's clamp is closed.

For a male patient, hold the penis with your nondominant hand. For a female patient, separate the labia minora outward and upward with your nondominant hand. With your dominant hand, use forceps to pick up an antiseptic-soaked cotton ball. For a man, begin at the tip of the penis and go around in a circular motion. For a woman, begin at the top of the urethral meatus and move down toward the vagina. Use one cotton ball for every motion. Drop each contaminated cotton ball on a section of the sterile field, away from the sterile catheter. Continue cleaning until you've used all the saturated cotton balls. Then place the forceps near the used cotton balls. Continuing with your dominant hand, pick up the catheter and slip the water-soluble lubricant package off of the tip.

To catheterize a man, hold the penis at a 90-degree angle and insert the catheter into the urinary meatus. Advance the catheter until the urine begins to flow (usually 6″ to 10″ [15 to 25 cm]). If you meet resistance, twist the catheter slightly from side to side or reduce the angle of the penis to about 70 degrees to help move the catheter past the external sphincter. Have the patient take slow, deep breaths to help relax his muscles.

To catheterize a woman, gently insert the catheter into the urinary meatus until urine begins to flow (usually 2″ to 3″ [5 to 7.5 cm]). If you meet resistance, have the patient take slow, deep breaths to relax her muscles.

If you're performing an intermittent catheterization, hold the catheter in position until the flow of urine stops. Pay attention to how much urine drains. Most home care instructions recommend draining only 800 ml of urine for each intermittent catheterization. When the flow of urine stops, pinch the catheter and gently withdraw it. Place the used catheter within the sterile field.

If you're inserting an indwelling catheter, attach the 10-ml syringe prefilled with sterile normal saline solution to the balloon port. While holding the catheter firmly in place, inject at least 5 ml of saline solution through the port to inflate the balloon. If the patient has been catheterized many times, you might need to inject the full 10 ml to keep the balloon in place in the bladder. Tug gently on the catheter to make sure the balloon is inflated and will hold the catheter in place.

Secure the catheter tubing to the patient's inner or upper thigh, leaving a few inches of slack to allow for position changes. Use enough adhesive tape to make sure the tubing is attached securely, but don't tape around the circumference of the leg. Catheter straps are also available to secure the catheter without tape.

Remove the drape and make the patient comfortable. Bundle all used catheter items, and discard them in a plastic trash bag. Remove your gloves and wash your hands. Make sure the collection bag stays below the level of the patient's bladder.

If the patient has an indwelling catheter, tell him not to pull on the tubing. Also tell him or a caregiver to clean the perineal skin around the catheter every day with soap and water and then pat it dry. Daily, he should remove the tape that secures the catheter, clean the underlying skin with soap and water and pat it dry, and then reapply the tape, leaving enough slack to allow for position changes. He should clean the urine collection bag by washing it with soap and water, then soaking it in one part white vinegar to three parts tap water for about 30 minutes. Then he should empty the bag and allow it to air-dry. Once dry, he can store it in a clean plastic bag until he needs it again.

Intermittent self-catheterization

Many patients can perform intermittent catheterization on their own once you teach them how to do it. Start by explaining the needed equipment as you assemble it in a convenient area. Then have the patient wash his hands and assume a comfortable position. Many men prefer to sit on or near the toilet. Women can try lying or sitting down with knees flexed, standing with one foot on the toilet, or sitting on the toilet. Use a mirror to help the female patient find her urinary meatus.

Show the patient how to clean the perineum and lubricate the catheter tip. Then walk the patient through the steps of self-catheterization. (See *Performing self-catheterization,* page 270.) Make sure the drainage end of the catheter is in the toilet or, if you need to track output, in a suitable container. When urine stops flowing, instruct the patient to gently pinch the catheter and slowly withdraw it from the meatus. Discard the urine and make the patient comfortable.

Instruct the patient to clean the catheter with soap and warm water and then boil it for at least 20 minutes. After removing it from the boiling water, the patient should place

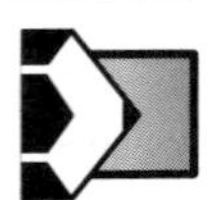

TEACHING POINTS

Performing self-catheterization

Teach a female patient to hold the lubricated catheter in her dominant hand about ½″ (1 cm) from its tip, as if it were a pencil or a dart. Tell her to use her nondominant hand to keep her labial folds separated and slowly insert

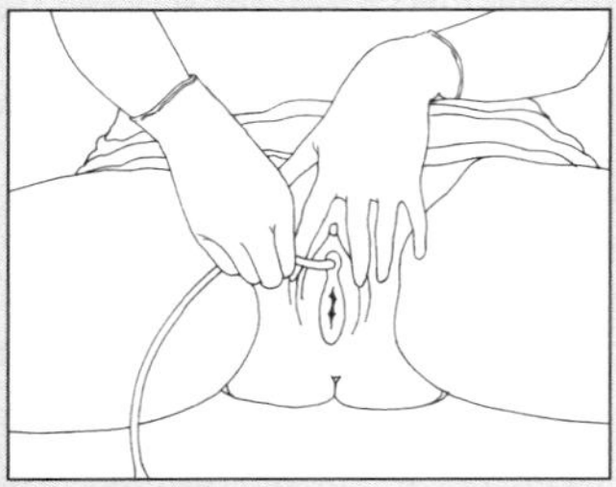

the lubricated catheter tip into her urinary meatus until urine begins to flow (about 3″ [7.6 cm]). Tell her to press down with her abdominal muscles to encourage all urine to drain from her bladder.

Teach a male patient to hold his penis at a right angle from his body in his nondominant hand. He should hold the lubricated catheter in his dominant hand as if it were a pencil or a dart and slowly insert it into the urinary meatus until urine begins to flow (about 7″ to 10″ [18 to 25 cm]). Then he should gently advance the catheter about 1″ (2.5 cm) farther, allowing all urine to drain.

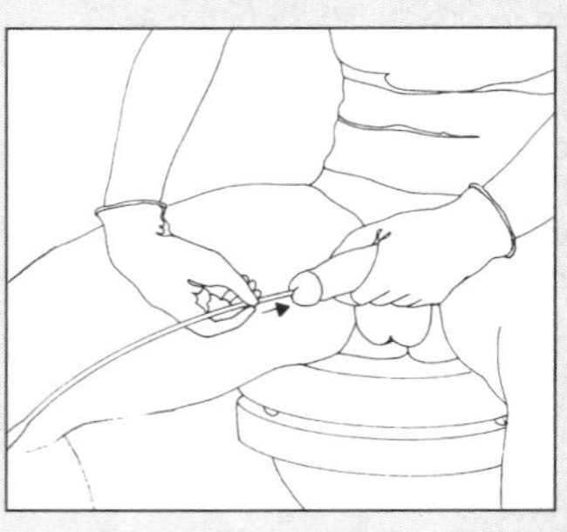

the catheter on paper towels, let it air-dry, and then store the clean catheter in a clean plastic bag for future use. Tell him not to use a catheter that's torn, hardened, or cracked because it will injure the urinary mucosa and might lead to infection.

Special considerations

Tell the patient to report any signs of infection, including a change in urine color, blood in the urine, a burning sensation, a foul odor, abdominal pain, or fever. Severe abdominal pain warrants a trip to the emergency department.

If the patient has an indwelling catheter, tell him to notify you right away if the catheter comes out, if it begins to leak urine around the meatus, if no urine has drained from the catheter in 6 hours or more, or if he needs more catheter supplies.

If the patient performs intermittent catheterization, tell him to do so at least four times daily and before bed.

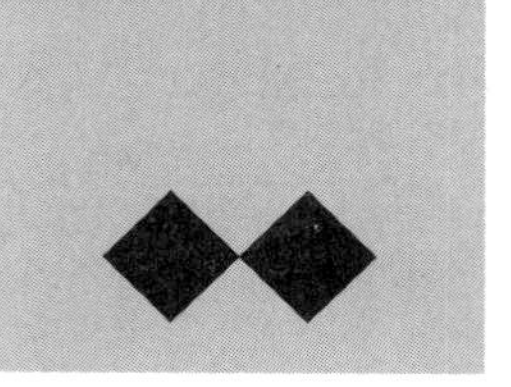

CHAPTER 9

Detecting danger signs and symptoms

As you know, certain key signs and symptoms can warn that your patient has a serious — possibly ominous — health problem. Especially when you're on your own in a patient's home, you'll need to be able to differentiate quickly and accurately between benign signs and those that represent a threat to your patient's health or life.

This chapter offers important clues to help you succeed. It presents a collection of hallmark danger signs and symptoms and provides assessment tools that can help you decide on the most prudent response to your patient's condition.

◆ ABDOMINAL PAIN

A common complaint, abdominal pain can result from nothing more than passing indigestion, or it can warn of something as ominous as a dissecting aneurysm. Clearly, you must be well equipped to assess for its varied causes.

Abdominal pain may originate in the abdominopelvic viscera, the parietal peritoneum, or the capsules of the liver, kidneys, or spleen. It may involve capsular stretching (as in liver distention), irritation of the mucosa (as in acute gastritis), severe smooth muscle spasm (as in acute enterocolitis), peritoneal inflammation (as in acute appendicitis), or direct splanchnic nerve stimulation (as in pancreatic cancer). Abdominal pain may be acute or chronic, diffuse or localized. Even mild or nonspecific pain can herald a potentially life-threatening problem.

Usually, a direct, concise history and a thorough physical examination will provide much of what you need to investigate abdominal pain. If necessary, the patient's doctor may order laboratory, radiologic, or endoscopic testing as well. (See *Evaluating abdominal pain*, pages 272 and 273.)

Health history

During the history, ask the patient to describe what the pain feels like, how it started, how long it lasts, and what factors make it better or worse. Ask if the patient has ever had this pain before. Have him point to where it hurts. Ask if the pain radiates to another place, such as his chest or back, or if it gets better or worse when he changes positions, exerts himself, coughs, or has a bowel movement.

Find out if the patient has additional abdominal signs and symptoms, such as appetite changes, constipation, diarrhea, nausea, vomiting, pain with urination, pink or cloudy urine, or urinary frequency or urgency. Ask if he has had a fever with the pain.

CRITICAL DECISIONS

Evaluating abdominal pain

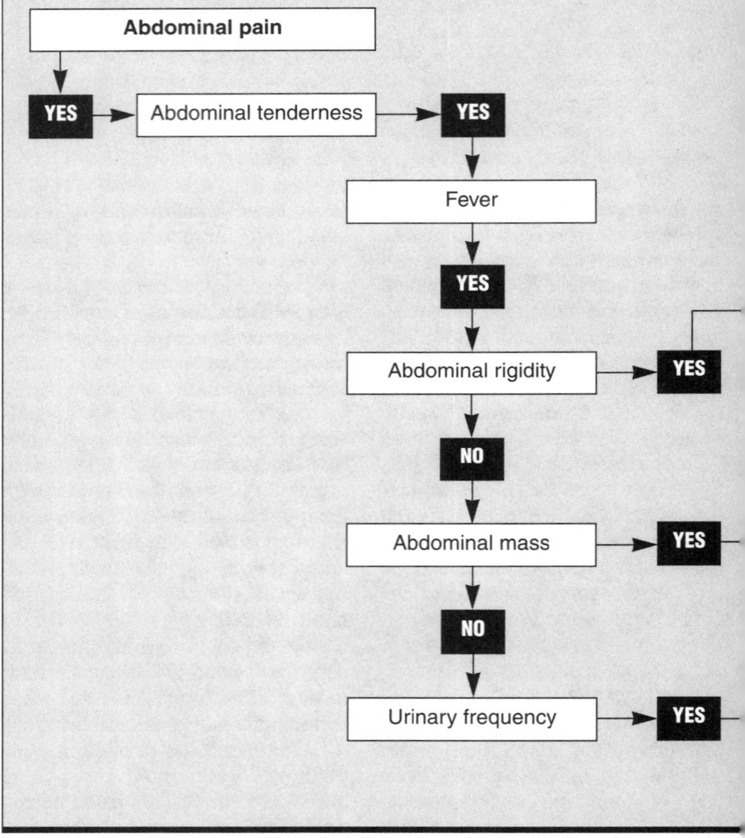

Abdominal pain

YES → Abdominal tenderness → YES

Fever

YES

Abdominal rigidity → YES

NO

Abdominal mass → YES

NO

Urinary frequency → YES

Investigate whether the patient has a history of disorders that could influence abdominal pain, such as adrenal disease, heart disease, recent infection, or recent blunt trauma to the abdomen, flank, or chest. Ask about conditions that could predispose him to emboli or atherosclerosis. See if he has recently had a urinary tract procedure or surgery. Find out if he has been to a foreign country recently. Finally, ask if he has ever used I.V. drugs, how much alcohol he drinks (or drank), and which prescription and over-the-counter drugs he takes.

If the patient is a woman of childbearing age, also ask for the date of her last menses. Find out if her men-

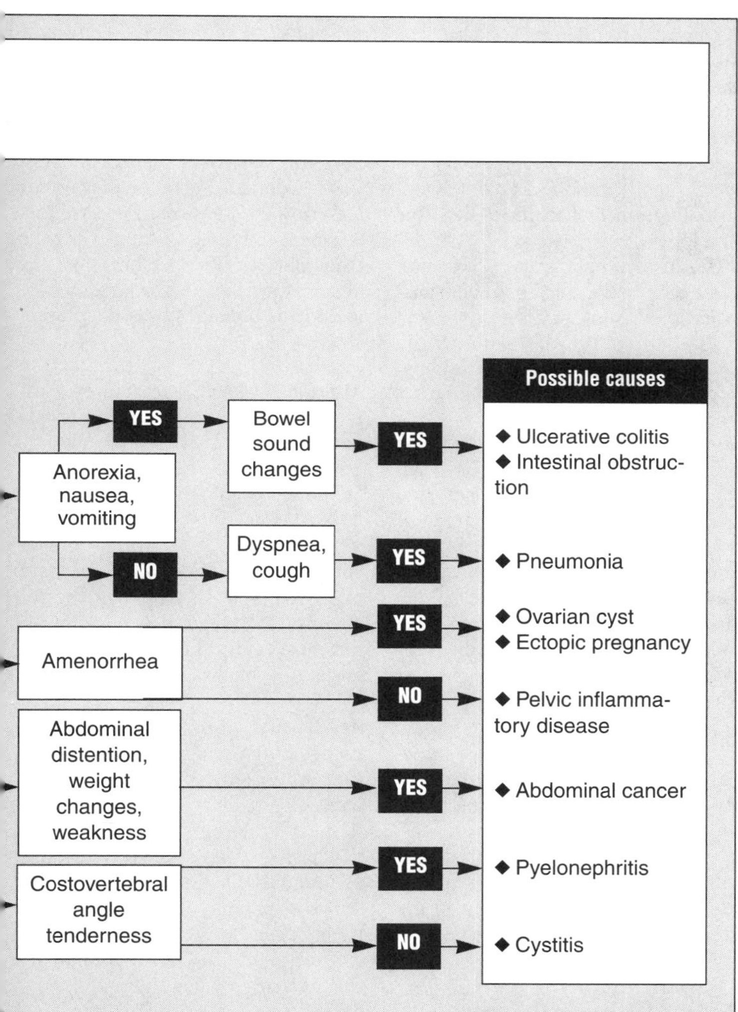

strual pattern has changed recently. Also ask if she could be pregnant.

Physical examination

While completing the history, assess the patient's level of consciousness, and observe his skin for diaphoresis and jaundice. Observe the way he's positioned and his general appearance. Inspect for neck vein distention, and monitor the rate and depth of his respirations. Ask for a urine specimen so you can observe its color and odor.

During the physical examination, check blood pressure, respirations, and pulse. Assess peripheral pulses for rate, rhythm, and intensity. Listen to the patient's heart and breath sounds.

Inspect the abdomen and chest for signs of trauma, including a bluish discoloration around the umbilicus (Cullen's sign) or flank area (Turner's sign). Obtain and record a baseline measurement of abdominal girth at the umbilicus. Check for coolness, discoloration, and edema of the arms and legs.

Because palpation and percussion can alter bowel sounds, start with auscultation. Listen for bowel sounds in each quadrant, noting whether the sounds are high-pitched and tinkling, hyperactive, or absent. Listen for rubs, hums, and bruits.

Percuss the abdomen for organ size, masses, and tympany. Percuss each quadrant, noting tenderness, increased pain, and percussion sounds. Dull sounds indicate free fluid; hollow sounds indicate air. Then systematically palpate the abdominal, pelvic, flank, and epigastric areas, noting any enlarged organs, masses, rigidity, tenderness, rebound tenderness, or guarding.

You may need to examine a male patient for hernia and testicular masses. For a woman, you may need to perform a pelvic examination to assess for tenderness, discharge, and masses. If indicated, perform a rectal examination to check for sphincter tone, masses, and blood in the stool.

Possible causes

Abdominal pain most often results from GI disorders, but it can also stem from reproductive, genitourinary, musculoskeletal, cardiac, or vascular disorders as well as drug use or the effects of toxins. Your response to abdominal pain depends entirely on the cause of the problem. The following conditions may cause abdominal pain.

Abdominal aortic aneurysm. Constant, dull upper abdominal pain that radiates to the lower back may herald rupture of a rapidly enlarging aneurysm. If it's dissecting slowly, the patient may complain of a "tearing" feeling in his abdomen. Palpation may reveal a pulsating epigastric mass. Auscultation may reveal a systolic bruit over the aneurysm. You also may note abdominal rigidity, increasing abdominal girth, and signs of hypovolemic shock.

Abdominal trauma. After traumatic injury, the patient may have generalized or localized abdominal pain, ecchymosis, tenderness, or vomiting. Hemorrhage into the peritoneal cavity will cause increasing abdominal girth. You may hear hollow bowel sounds from a perforated abdominal organ, or you may hear no bowel sounds. If you hear bowel sounds in the chest cavity, the patient probably has a torn diaphragm.

Appendicitis. Typically, appendicitis causes epigastric or umbilical pain that increases over a few hours or days, localizing at McBurney's point in the right lower quadrant. The patient also may have flulike symptoms, abdominal rigidity, and rebound tenderness. He may report that symptoms began before the pain did, including anorexia, constipation, diarrhea, nausea, or vomiting.

Ectopic pregnancy. The patient will have pain in the lower abdomen that can be sharp, dull, or cramping. It may be constant or intermittent. The pain may be accompanied by breast tenderness, nausea, vaginal bleeding, vomiting, and urinary frequency. The patient typically has a 1- to 2-month history of amenorrhea. Rupture of the fallopian tube produces sharp lower abdominal pain that may radiate to the shoulders and neck and may become severe with cervical or adnexal palpation.

Hepatitis. Liver enlargement from any type of hepatitis causes discomfort or dull pain and tenderness in the right upper quadrant.

Intestinal obstruction. The patient will experience short episodes of intense, colicky, cramping pain alternating with pain-free periods.

Pancreatitis. The characteristic symptom is fulminating, continuous, upper epigastric pain that may radiate to both flanks and to the back.

Renal calculi. Depending on the location of the calculi, the patient may feel severe abdominal or back pain. The classic picture is colicky pain from the costovertebral angle to the flank, suprapubic region, and external genitalia.

Other causes. Abdominal cancer, adrenal crisis, cholecystitis, constipation, cystitis, diabetic ketoacidosis, diverticulitis, gallbladder disease, gastroenteritis, genitourinary tract infection, heart failure, hepatic abscess, incarcerated inguinal hernia, inflammatory bowel disease, mesenteric artery ischemia, myocardial infarction, ovarian cyst, pancreatitis, pelvic inflammatory disease, peptic ulcer disease, perforated ulcer, peritonitis, pneumonia, pneumothorax, pyelonephritis, renal infarction, splenic infarction, ulcerative colitis, volvulus; also salicylate and nonsteroidal anti-inflammatory drugs.

Implications

If indicated, report the abdominal pain and associated findings to the patient's doctor. Then carry out diagnostic procedures, interventions, and treatments as ordered. Provide patient and family teaching as needed. Continue to monitor the course of the abdominal pain and related findings in subsequent visits until the pain resolves.

◆ BOWEL SOUNDS, ABSENT

Absent bowel sounds almost always suggest intestinal obstruction, especially if the patient can't pass flatus. Assess carefully to determine if the patient indeed has no bowel sounds or if they're diminished but present.

Health history

Ask the patient when he last passed gas and when he had his last bowel movement. Ask him to describe the stools. Ask if he has abdominal pain and, if so, to describe its location and character. Find out when the pain started; if it's constant, episodic, or cramping; and if anything relieves it. Finally, find out if the patient has been vomiting. Ask when it started, how much he vomited, and if he can keep any foods down.

Physical examination

It's imperative that you carefully validate a finding of absent bowel sounds. Listen for 2 full minutes to each of the four abdominal quadrants. Examine the patient's abdomen for signs of distention, and measure his abdominal girth. Finally, assess vital signs, including temperature, pulse, and blood pressure. Check for adequate tissue perfusion, and examine the skin and mucous membranes for turgor and signs of dehydration.

Possible causes

The following conditions may cause absent bowel sounds.

Bowel obstruction. Obstruction usually forms in the small intestine. It may result from various causes, including cancer. Large-bowel obstruction typically stems from cancer as well.

Paralytic ileus. If peristalsis stops, bowel sounds will too, and signs and symptoms of intestinal obstruction will develop. Ileus is most common after a surgical procedure.

Peritonitis. This inflammation of the peritoneum or abdominal lining may result from a number of causes, including a ruptured appendix, a perforated bowel, trauma, and continuous ambulatory peritoneal dialysis.

Implications

After careful assessment, notify the patient's doctor about your findings. Provide comfort and pain relief measures as indicated until the patient can be taken to the doctor's office or the emergency department. If the patient develops hypothermia, hypotension, or both, he may be developing septic shock from a bowel perforation. Monitor him for high fever, which may indicate infection.

◆ BREATH SOUNDS, ABSENT OR DIMINISHED

Absent or diminished breath sounds are always an abnormal finding, but they don't necessarily indicate a life-threatening problem. Careful assessment can help you determine the cause and your best course of action. (See *Assessing breath sounds*.)

Health history

Ask the patient if he's coughing and, if so, whether it's productive or not. Also ask if he has chest pain or has had a recent accident, respiratory tract infection, or lung surgery. Find out if he smokes (or smoked), for how long, and how much. Ask if he has been exposed to allergens or been short of breath recently.

Physical examination

Observe the patient's respiratory efforts and chest movements. Watch the symmetry of chest expansion and the activity of his abdominal wall and intercostal muscles. Check to see if his trachea is at midline. Assess respiratory rate and depth. If the problem stems from an accident, examine his chest for a puncture wound or painful area. Assess the patient's neurologic status, including level of consciousness, orientation, and mental status. Also check skin color and temperature to assess circulatory perfusion. Auscultate for heart rate and rhythm, and measure blood pressure.

Possible causes

The following conditions may cause absent or diminished breath sounds.

Atelectasis. Consolidation of pleural secretions will diminish your ability to hear breath sounds. You also may notice a tracheal shift toward the side with diminished sounds, plus decreased chest movement on that side.

Hemothorax. Traumatic injuries may allow blood to accumulate in the pleural cavity, possibly causing partial or total atelectasis with a mediastinal shift.

Pleural fluid or thickening. Although fluid or thickening of pleural membranes will inhibit auscultation of breath sounds, it usually is not an acute symptom.

Pneumothorax. If your patient has a pneumothorax, you'll observe tracheal deviation or a mediastinal shift away from the affected side. You also may observe subcutaneous emphysema.

Assessing breath sounds

Use these illustrations as a key when assessing breath sounds. Remember that tracheal sounds result from air passing through the glottis. They're harsh and discontinuous. The inspiration to expiration ratio is 1:1.

Bronchial sounds result from high rates of turbulent air flowing through large bronchi. They're loud, high-pitched, hollow, and harsh or coarse. The inspiration to expiration ratio is 2:3.

Bronchovesicular sounds result from transitional airflow moving through the branches and convergences of the smaller bronchi and bronchioles. They're soft, breezy sounds pitched about two notes lower than bronchial sounds. The inspiration to expiration ratio is 1:1.

Vesicular sounds result from laminar airflow moving through the alveolar ducts and alveoli at low flow rates. They're soft, swishy, breezy sounds pitched about two notes lower than bronchovesicular sounds. The inspiration to expiration ratio is 3:1.

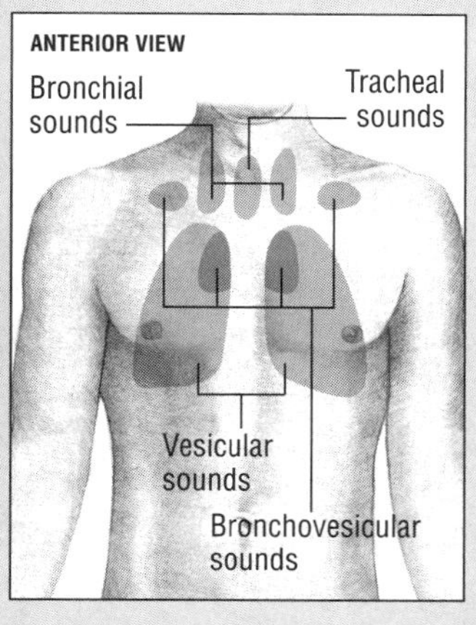

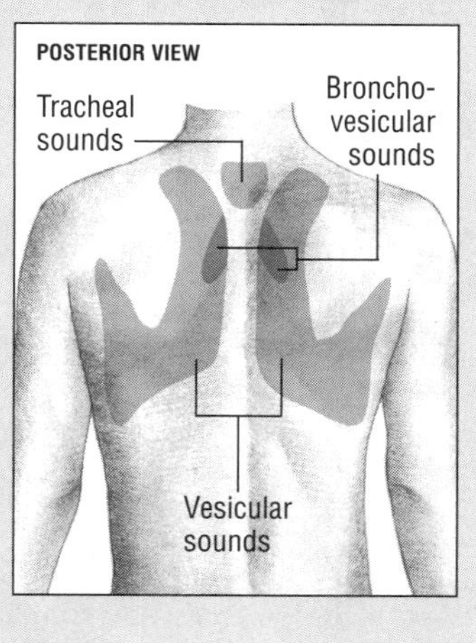

Other causes. Acute respiratory failure, chemical inhalation, drug overdose, postoperative lobectomy.

Implications

After careful assessment, notify the patient's doctor of your findings. If the patient has severe respiratory impairment, cyanosis, and tachypnea, you'll most likely need to arrange transport to the nearest emergency department. Until the emergency team arrives, provide comfort and relief measures, and keep the patient's head and chest elevated at least 30 degrees to assist his respiratory effort.

If the patient has a chest wound, cover it as appropriate. If it's a sucking wound, cover it with petroleum gauze, if available, until assistance arrives.

◆ CHEST PAIN

Chest pain typically stems from the thoracic wall and can be related to various conditions of the muscles, nerves, and bones. It also can result from hematologic and musculoskeletal disorders. It may signal cardiovascular disaster.

Health history

Ask the patient when the pain began and what it feels like (sharp, stabbing, crushing, dull, aching). Ask if it started suddenly or gradually, if it's constant or intermittent, and if it feels localized or diffuse. Find out if it radiates to the neck, arms, jaw, or back. Inquire if anything makes the pain better or worse, such as changing positions, breathing differently, or stopping activity.

Find out if the patient has other symptoms, such as coughing, shortness of breath, headache, nausea, palpitations, vomiting, or weakness. Ask if he has ever had cardiac or respiratory disease, cardiac surgery, chest trauma, or intestinal disease. Find out if he has a family history of cardiac disease and if he smokes, drinks alcohol, or uses illicit drugs. Ask for a list of his medications.

Physical examination

Assess the temperature, color, and general appearance of the patient's skin. Note coolness, cyanosis, diaphoresis, mottling below the waist, pallor, peripheral edema, and prolonged capillary refill time. Also assess for facial edema, jugular vein distention, and tracheal deviation. Evaluate for any signs of altered level of consciousness, anxiety, dizziness, or restlessness.

Observe the rate and depth of the patient's respirations. Note any abnormal patterns or difficulty. If he has a productive cough, examine the sputum. Palpate the neck, chest, and abdomen. Note any abnormalities, masses, subcutaneous emphysema, tenderness, or tracheal deviation.

Percuss the chest and note any dullness. Auscultate the lungs to identify adventitious, diminished, or absent breath sounds; pleural friction rubs; crackles; or wheezing. Auscultate the heart for clicks, gallops, murmurs, or pericardial friction rub. Auscultate the abdominal aorta for bruits. Evaluate the patient's blood pressure.

Possible causes

The following conditions may cause chest pain.

Angina. Usually arising in the retrosternal region, angina may radiate to the neck, jaw, or arm. The pain may last 2 to 10 minutes and responds to sublingual nitroglycerin. Angina may induce diaphoresis, dyspnea, nausea, vomiting, palpitations, and tachycardia. Typically, it results from exertion, emotional stress, or a heavy meal. Auscultation may reveal an atrial gallop, an extra S_4 heart sound, or a murmur.

Aortic aneurysm. A dissecting aortic aneurysm causes sudden, excruciating, "tearing" pain in the chest and neck, radiating to the upper back, lower back, and abdomen. Other signs and symptoms include abdominal tenderness, heart murmurs, jugular vein distention, systolic bruit, tachycardia, weak or absent femoral or pedal pulses, and pale, cool, diaphoretic, mottled skin below the waist.

Cholecystitis. The patient will complain of sudden pain in the epigastric or right upper quadrant region. It may be steady or intermittent, sharp or intense. It may radiate to the back. Other symptoms are chills, diaphoresis, nausea, and vomiting. Palpation of the right upper quadrant may reveal rigidity, tenderness, and a mass.

Esophagitis. Inflammation of the esophagus tends to cause GI symptoms, such as painful swallowing relieved by antacids, in addition to chest pain.

Musculoskeletal strain. Strain or spasm of thoracic muscles (and fractured ribs) will cause pain that increases with inspiratory effort. Pain relief measures include positioning, local application of heat or cold, and anti-inflammatory and analgesic agents.

Myocardial infarction. Typically, the patient will have crushing substernal pain that may radiate. Related signs may include diaphoresis, anxiety, clammy skin, dyspnea, nausea, vomiting, pallor, or restlessness.

Peptic ulcer. Sharp, burning pain in the epigastric region may be eased or aggravated by eating. Other symptoms may include epigastric tenderness, nausea, and vomiting. Antacids may relieve the pain.

Pneumothorax. A collapsed lung produces dyspnea and sudden, severe, unilateral chest pain that increases with movement. Diminished or absent breath sounds may also occur.

Other causes. Acute bronchitis, anxiety, lung abscess, pancreatitis, pneumonia, pulmonary embolism, rib fracture, tuberculosis, withdrawal from beta blockers.

Implications

Evaluate the patient carefully and report his signs and symptoms to his doctor. Teach the patient with angina how to use sublingual nitroglycerin and rest to stop the pain. (See *Responding to chest pain.*) If the pain

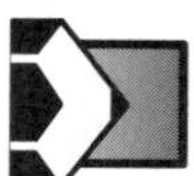

TEACHING POINTS

Responding to chest pain

If your patient has chest pain caused by angina, give him these instructions:

- ◆ At the first sign of chest pain, stop what you're doing. Sit down and rest.
- ◆ Make note of the time.
- ◆ Place a nitroglycerin pill under your tongue and let it dissolve.
- ◆ If you still have chest pain after 5 minutes, take another pill.
- ◆ If you still have chest pain after 5 more minutes, take a third pill.
- ◆ If you still have chest pain 15 to 20 minutes after it started, call your doctor or arrange to be taken to an emergency department. Do not drive yourself.
- ◆ Call your doctor if your episodes of chest pain become more frequent or if they occur at rest or with less activity. Also call if the pain worsens or changes character. And call if the chest pain is accompanied by shortness of breath, fainting, or an irregular pulse or heart rate that's below 60 or above 100 beats per minute.
- ◆ Keep emergency numbers posted by every phone.
- ◆ Always carry medical identification.

doesn't stop or symptoms progress, contact an emergency service.

◆ COUGH, PRODUCTIVE

Usually caused by a cardiopulmonary disorder, productive coughing typically stems from an acute or chronic infection that causes inflammation, edema, and increased mucus production in the airways. Such coughing can also result from inhaling antigenic or irritating substances; the most common cause is cigarette smoking.

Health history

Ask the patient when the cough started, if he has had a productive cough before, and how much sputum he thinks he coughs up in a day. Have him describe what the cough sounds and feels like. Ask if sputum production is associated with certain times of day, activities, meals, or environments. Have him describe the color, odor, and consistency of the sputum, and ask if it has increased in volume since the coughing began.

Find out if the patient has noticed recent changes in appetite or weight. Ask about recent surgeries and allergies and if the patient works around chemicals or respiratory irritants. Finally, ask if the patient drinks alcohol or smokes and how much.

Physical examination

Examine the patient's mouth and nose for congestion, drainage, and inflammation. Inspect his neck for vein distention. Observe his respiratory effort for accessory muscle use or uneven expansion. Palpate for cervical lymph node enlargement. Auscultate for abnormal breath sounds, pleural friction rubs, crackles, and wheezing.

Possible causes

The following conditions may cause a productive cough.

Bacterial pneumonitis. Infectious processes may begin as a dry cough and progress into sputum production. Purulent sputum suggests staphylococcal or streptococcal pneumonia.

Bronchitis. Bronchial infection may be acute or chronic. Yellow- or green-tinged sputum suggests an acute infective state.

Cancer of the lung. Patients with lung cancer commonly have a productive cough. Sputum may appear rust-colored.

Chronic obstructive pulmonary disease (COPD). Patients with COPD commonly have a chronic productive cough with white or gray sputum. Acute infection added to COPD may produce yellow- or green-tinged sputum.

Human immunodeficiency virus (HIV). A patient infected with HIV is at risk for a number of cough-producing disorders, including tuberculosis and bacterial, fungal, and parasitic lung infections (such as *Pneumocystis carinii* pneumonia).

Tuberculosis. A disease increasing in prevalence in the United States, active tuberculosis causes a mild to severe productive cough, with white or blood-tinged sputum and malaise, dyspnea, and pleuritic chest pain.

Upper respiratory infection. Acute upper respiratory and sinus infections may produce a productive cough with white or yellow-tinged sputum.

Implications

If your patient has a fever, his cough probably relates to an infectious process. Be sure to describe your findings carefully to the patient's doctor; then carry out any ordered diagnostic tests, interventions, or treatments. If the patient has tuberculosis, you'll need to help ensure compliance with what will likely be weeks or months of antibiotic therapy.

◆ CYANOSIS

A bluish discoloration of the skin and mucous membranes, cyanosis results from an increase in the absolute amount of reduced hemoglobin. Central cyanosis may signal respiratory insufficiency; peripheral cyanosis may suggest reduced venous saturation.

Health history

Ask the patient or a family member how long he has noticed the bluish discoloration. Ask if he has been short of breath while resting or exerting himself. Find out if any activities have an effect on his condition. Ask if he has a productive cough and what his sputum looks like.

Also ask the patient if he smokes (or smoked), and how much. Find out what medications he takes and if he has allergies or has recently been exposed to chemical irritants. Finally, ask if he has ever been diagnosed with a vascular disorder or has a history of Raynaud's phenomenon or systemic lupus erythematosus.

Physical examination

The appropriate physical examination differs depending on whether the patient has central or peripheral cyanosis.

Central cyanosis

Note the patient's respirations. Observe their rate and depth and any breathing difficulties or abnormal respiratory patterns. Check for flaring nostrils, grunting respirations, inspiratory stridor, intercostal retractions during inspiration, and pursed-lip expirations. Examine the patient for barrel chest, diaphoresis, neck vein distention, peripheral edema, and finger clubbing. (See *Assessing for clubbed fingers*, page 282.) Note the color, consistency, and odor of any sputum.

Palpate the patient's chest for asymmetrical expansion, decreased diaphragmatic excursion, tactile fremitus, and subcutaneous crepitation. Check the rate, rhythm, and intensity of peripheral pulses. Auscultate the lungs for decreased or absent breath sounds, crackles, pleural friction rubs, or wheezing. Auscultate for abnormal heart sounds and rhythms, pericardial friction rubs, and tachycardia. Assess blood pressure. If available, perform pulse oximetry.

Peripheral cyanosis

Assess peripheral pulses. Examine the nail beds for color and capillary refill time. Also check skin temperature on the affected limb or limbs.

Possible causes

The following conditions may cause cyanosis.

Airway obstruction. Mechanical airway obstruction reduces airflow and causes respiratory distress and central cyanosis. Related symptoms may include inspiratory stridor and dyspnea. Other signs include accessory muscle use, anxiety, asymmetrical chest expansion, decreased or absent breath sounds, diaphoresis, hypotension, and tachypnea.

Arterial occlusion. Arterial occlusion in a limb, from vascular disease or a blood clot, can cause peripheral cyanosis and requires emergency treatment to restore blood flow to the area. Evaluate peripheral pulses carefully. Arterial occlusion may also result from respiratory depressant

Assessing for clubbed fingers

To assess for chronic tissue hypoxia, check the patient's fingers for clubbing. Normally, the angle between the fingernail and the point where the nail enters the skin is about 160 degrees. In clubbing, that angle increases to 180 degrees or more, as shown in the illustration on the right.

To verify your suspicion of clubbing, ask the patient to place the first phalange of each finger together, nail to nail. Normal concave nail bases create a small space between the forefingers at the nail bases. Clubbed fingers are convex at the nail bases and touch without leaving a space between them.

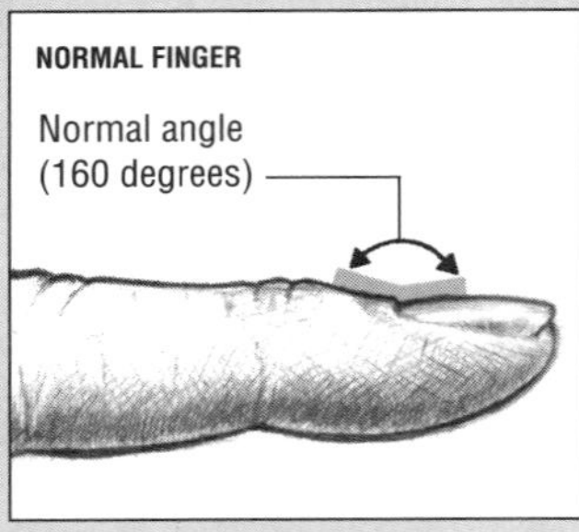

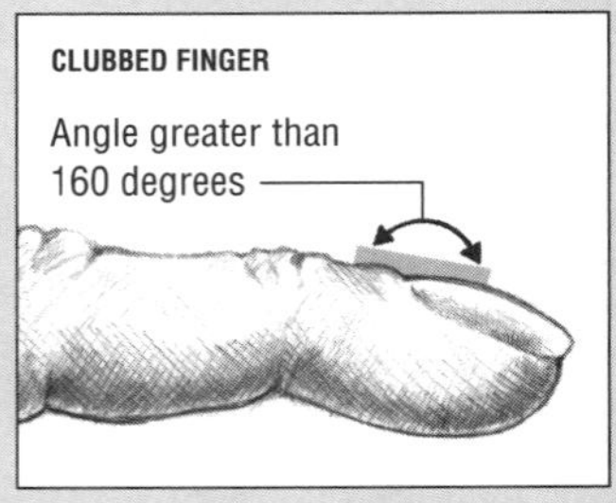

drugs, weakness or paralysis of respiratory muscles, chest trauma, or vascular diseases (Raynaud's phenomenon, systemic lupus erythematosus).

Chronic obstructive pulmonary disease (COPD). Chronic bronchitis, pulmonary emphysema, and bronchial asthma are the three most common pulmonary disorders associated with central cyanosis. Increased resistance to air flow results in poor perfusion and reduced oxygen saturation of the tissues.

Head injury. Cerebral trauma and the resulting edema may depress respiratory efforts, causing central cyanosis. Be sure to assess the patient's level of consciousness and other neurologic parameters if you suspect head injury.

Implications

Acute cyanosis requires an emergency response whether it's central or peripheral. If the patient is in respiratory distress, airway management is your first priority. Have the patient sit upright to ease his respiratory effort; then activate emergency medical services, as indicated.

Chronic central cyanosis develops in patients who have COPD. Explain your assessment findings to the patient's doctor, and implement home oxygen therapy or home pulmonary treatments and medications, as ordered. If your patient has chronic peripheral cyanosis, assess pulses and notify the doctor of your findings.

◆ DIARRHEA, PERSISTENT

Diarrhea is defined as an abnormal increase in stool liquidity, frequency, and daily weight (more than 300 g in 24 hours). Several acute and chronic conditions can cause persistent diarrhea, a condition that can lead to dehydration and malnutrition in addition to reducing the patient's quality of life. (See *Dealing with diarrhea.*)

TEACHING POINTS

Dealing with diarrhea

If your patient has persistent diarrhea, try giving him these suggestions.

- ◆ Eat a diet low in residue, high in protein, and high in calories.
- ◆ Try foods in the BRAT diet (bananas, rice, applesauce, toast, and tea) because they're less disruptive to the GI system.
- ◆ Avoid whole grains, nuts, raw vegetables, fried foods, gas-producing foods, spicy foods, milk products, caffeine, and alcohol.
- ◆ Eat small, frequent meals.
- ◆ Maintain hydration with water, sports drinks, and diluted fruit juices.
- ◆ Perform meticulous skin care in the perianal area.
- ◆ Use antidiarrheal agents, as prescribed.

Health history

Ask the patient to describe the pattern of his diarrhea, including when it started, how long it has been happening, how often it occurs, and what the stool looks like. Have the patient estimate the amount of diarrhea he produces in a day. Find out if he has associated symptoms, such as cramping, flatus, abdominal distention, or blood in the stool. Ask to what extent the condition interferes with his quality of life and ability to accomplish activities of daily living.

Investigate possible stress factors, anxiety, and recent travel. Also investigate the patient's nutritional intake and food habits. Find out how he obtains food, what types of foods he likes and dislikes, who prepares his food, and how it's prepared. Ask him which medications he takes. Finally, ask if he has lost weight along with having diarrhea.

Physical examination

Take the patient's temperature and assess his skin turgor. Auscultate for bowel sounds in all four quadrants, and palpate the abdomen for tenderness. Check for altered tissue perfusion or significant loss of muscle mass. Assess skin integrity, especially in the perineal area, for redness or skin breakdown.

Possible causes

The following conditions may cause persistent diarrhea.

Amoebic infection. If the patient has traveled outside the United States and Canada, consider amebiasis as a possible cause of persistent diarrhea.

Bacterial infection. Many pathogens can cause diarrhea if introduced into the GI system. Also, antibiotic use can reduce numbers of helpful bacteria normally found in the bowel, allowing others to overgrow.

Viral or fungal pathogens. Viruses and fungi may grow in the bowel, especially if the patient is immunocompromised, as in chronic renal failure, HIV infection, and organ transplant. Cryptosporidium may be a factor as well.

Other causes. Chronic colitis, lactose intolerance, malabsorption syndrome.

Implications

Tell the patient how important it is to rehydrate and to maintain an adequate fluid balance. Also teach him about dietary interventions to help reduce the diarrhea. Explain your findings to the patient's doctor and implement diagnostic tests, interventions, and treatments, as ordered.

◆ DYSPNEA

Also known as shortness of breath, dyspnea may be acute or chronic, and it may vary greatly in severity. It always warrants a careful assessment and response.

Health history

Ask the patient when he began feeling short of breath, if it began suddenly or gradually, and if he has ever had it before. Ask if it's constant or intermittent and if it occurs at rest or only during activities. Find out if anything makes it better or worse.

Also ask if the patient has a productive cough, chest pain, a recent upper respiratory tract infection, or recent traumatic injury. Find out if he smokes (or smoked), how much, and for how long. Ask if he has any allergies and if he could have been exposed to allergens. Finally, ask what medications he takes.

Physical examination

Observe the patient's respirations, noting rate, depth, and any breathing difficulties or abnormal respiratory patterns. Check for flaring nostrils, grunting respirations, inspiratory stridor, intercostal retractions during inspiration, and pursed-lip expirations. Look for barrel chest, diaphoresis, neck vein distention, finger clubbing, and peripheral edema. Note the color, consistency, and odor of sputum.

Palpate the patient's chest for asymmetrical expansion, decreased diaphragmatic excursion, tactile fremitus, and subcutaneous crepitation. Check the rate, rhythm, and intensity of peripheral pulses. Percuss the lung fields, noting percussion sounds. Auscultate the lungs for crackles, decreased or absent breath sounds, pleural friction rubs, or wheezing. Auscultate for abnormal heart sounds, pericardial friction rubs, gallops, or tachycardia. Assess blood pressure.

Investigate the patient's medication regimen for drugs that can precipitate heart failure and dyspnea, such as certain beta blockers and corticosteroids.

Possible causes

The following conditions may cause dyspnea.

Heart failure and pulmonary edema. Pump failure causes fluid to accumulate in the pulmonary system, which leads to dyspnea. Onset may be gradual or acute.

Pneumonia. Acute pneumonitis usually is accompanied by fever, chills, and a sudden onset of dyspnea. Sputum may be discolored and malodorous.

Pulmonary embolism. Severe dyspnea accompanies intense pleuritic pain that may worsen with deep breathing and thoracic movement. The patient's history may include myocardial infarction, heart failure, hip or leg fracture, oral contraceptive use, pregnancy, thrombophlebitis, or varicose veins.

Other causes. Adult respiratory distress syndrome, anemia, anxiety, asthma, cardiac arrhythmias, inhalation injury, lung cancer, myocardial infarction, pleural effusion, pneumothorax.

Implications

Notify the patient's doctor about episodes of acute dyspnea or, if necessary, contact an emergency medical service. Elevate the patient's head or help him to a sitting position. Loosen tight clothing and open a nearby window, if possible.

◆ EDEMA, GENERALIZED

Also called idiopathic edema, this condition is a symptom of an underlying process that must be determined and addressed. You'll need to consider a wide-ranging group of possible causes while performing your assessment.

Health history

Ask the patient when he first noticed the swelling and where it began. (If it developed over hours or days, suspect an acute cause; if over weeks or months, suspect a chronic cause.) Find out if the patient has any other symptoms. Ask for a complete list of his medications; ask specifically about hormones, diuretics, and antihypertensives.

Physical examination

Perform a head-to-toe assessment, paying special attention to the cardiovascular system, respiratory system, and abdomen. Note any superficial dilated or tortuous veins on the patient's abdomen. Grade the edema by pressing the swollen flesh with your thumb. Record the results using a scale from 1+ to 4+, as described below:

- 1+: slight pit, normal limb contours
- 2+: deeper pit, fairly normal limb contours
- 3+: deep pit, puffy limb
- 4+: deep pit, frankly swollen limb.

When examining the feet, exert pressure over the medial malleolus or pretibial area. Measure the circumference of the swollen limb a specified distance from the malleolus; record your measurement at this distance during each visit.

Carefully note the distribution of the patient's edema. Check to see if it's equal bilaterally. Assess if it changes with the patient's position changes. Also note any changes in the skin (dimpling, breakdown, thickening, pigmentation).

Possible causes

The following conditions may cause generalized edema.

Decreased oncotic pressure. Decreased pressure in the vascular space may result from hypoproteinemia related to nephrotic syndrome, starvation, or protein-wasting enteropathy.

Increased hydrostatic pressure. Increased pressure in the vascular space may result from increased volume, as from heart failure, renal failure, hormones, or certain drugs. It also may result from increased mechanical pressure (with normal or low volume), as from venous thrombosis, a tumor, scarring, fibrosis, gravid uterus, pericardial constriction, or portal hypertension.

Medications. Antihypertensives, diuretics, and hormones are known to increase the risk of edema.

Tissue or vascular damage. Damage may result from vasculitis, allergy, trauma, burns, ischemia, or infection.

Other causes. Abscess, chronic venous insufficiency, compartment syndrome after arterial bypass, deep vein thrombosis, heart failure, hepatic cirrhosis, infection, lymphedema, malnutrition, myxedema, Graves' disease, nephrotic syndrome, orthostatic sodium retention, overactive renin-angiotensin-aldosterone system, tumors in the pelvis, abdomen, or retroperitoneal space.

Implications

Monitor the patient's edema and skin integrity on a regular basis, and teach the patient and family members how to do so as well. Tell them what kind of changes to report to the doctor. As needed, report your own findings to the doctor. Then carry out diagnostic tests, interventions, and treatments, as ordered.

◆ FEVER

Body temperature elevated above 98.6° F (37° C) is a common sign that can arise from disorders in almost any body system. A highly useful indicator of abnormality, fever results from an increased metabolic rate and is accompanied by increased heart and respiratory rates and increased oxygen consumption.

Health history

Ask the patient when his fever started and how high it went. Find out if it's constant or if it disappears, only to reappear later. Ask if the patient has other symptoms associated with the fever, such as chills, fatigue, or pain. Ask if he has had a recent immunodeficiency disorder, infection, traumatic injury, surgery or anesthesia, diagnostic test (especially with contrast medium), or invasive procedure. Find out if other family members have been ill recently or if the patient has traveled recently.

Physical examination

Perform a head-to-toe assessment, paying special attention to any signs or symptoms of genitourinary and respiratory problems. Assess all skin carefully. Complete additional assessments based on the patient's age.

Keep in mind that many adults have a normal temperature up to 99.4° F (37.4° C) caused by activity or a hot environment. Most older adults have a baseline temperature 0.5° to 1° F (0.28° to 0.6° C) below the 98.6° F (37° C) that's considered normal. Therefore, it's essential to have a baseline temperature for older adults. A temperature classified as a low or mild fever in children and adults could be a significant fever in older adults.

Possible causes

Any factor that increases the body's metabolic rate will increase the body's temperature. For example, fever can result from contrast media, drug hypersensitivity, illness, immunosuppression, injury, invasive devices, reactions to blood transfusions, and surgery. In addition, the following conditions may cause fever.

Immune complex dysfunction. When present, fever remains low, although moderate elevations may accompany erythema multiforme. Fever may be remittent or intermittent, as in acquired immunodeficiency syndrome or systemic lupus erythematosus, or sustained, as in polyarteritis.

Infectious and inflammatory disorders. Among adults, the most common infectious causes of fever are urinary and respiratory tract infections. Depending on the disorder involved, fever can range from low (as in Crohn's disease) to extremely high (as in bacterial pneumonia or Ebola virus). It may be remittent (as in otitis media), hectic (as in lung abscess), or relapsing (as in malaria). It may arise abruptly or insidiously. Associated signs and symptoms involve all body systems and include weakness, anorexia, malaise, chills, and diaphoresis.

Neoplasms. Primary neoplasms and metastases can produce prolonged fever of varying elevations.

Thermoregulatory dysfunction. Sudden onset of a fever as high as 107° F (41.7° C) occurs in life-threatening disorders. Low or moderate fever appears with dehydration.

Implications

Monitor your patient's temperature on a regular basis and act on standing orders or describe abnormal findings to the patient's doctor. (See *Classifying fever.*) Carry out diagnostic tests, interventions, and treatments as ordered. Teach the patient or a family member how to monitor his temperature between your visits and when to report a fever to the doctor. Monitor the patient for compliance.

Classifying fever

When assessing your patient's fever, remember the ranges shown on the illustration below. Also remember that a "normal" temperature varies with age. The ranges shown below refer to oral temperature readings; rectal temperatures typically run 0.5° to 1° F (0.28° to 0.6° C) higher.

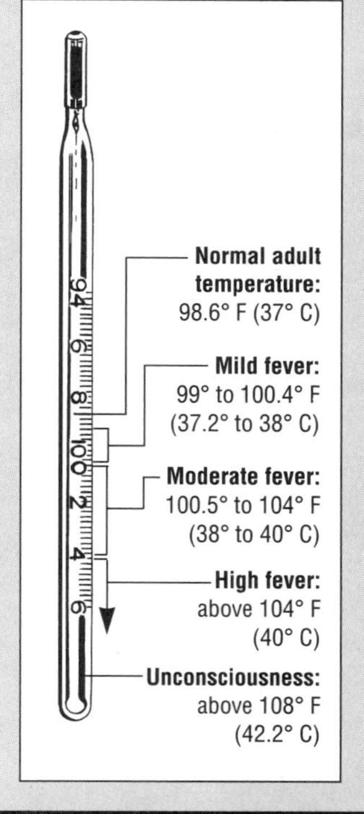

◆ HEADACHE

One of the most common of all health complaints, headaches usually result from tension or another relatively benign condition. Only rarely do they warn of a truly threatening problem. Even so, you'll need to be ready to assess the patient carefully and to respond appropriately. Common headache types include cluster, tension, and migraine. (See *Clinical features of migraine headaches*, page 288.) Headaches may involve vascular changes, muscle contractions, or both.

Clinical features of migraine headaches

Migraine form	Features
Common	◆ The most prevalent form ◆ Commonly occurs on weekends and holidays ◆ Prodromal symptoms that precede headache by about a day and include fatigue, nausea, vomiting, and fluid imbalance ◆ Causes sensitivity to light and noise ◆ Pain that's unilateral or bilateral, aching or throbbing, and longer-lasting than classic migraine
Classic	◆ Usually occurs in compulsive personalities and within families ◆ Prodromal symptoms, including visual disturbances (flashing or zigzag lights), sensory disturbances (tingling of face, lips, hands), or motor disturbances (staggering) ◆ Recurrent
Hemiplegic and ophthalmoplegic	◆ Rare ◆ Severe unilateral pain ◆ Extraocular muscle palsies (cranial nerve III) and ptosis ◆ Possible permanent injury to cranial nerve III with repeated headaches ◆ Neurologic deficits (hemiparesis, hemiplegia) that may persist after hemiplegic migraine ends
Basilar artery	◆ Occurs in young women before menstrual periods ◆ Prodromal symptoms, including partial vision loss followed by vertigo, ataxia, dysarthria, tinnitus, and possibly tingling of fingers and toes, lasting several minutes to almost an hour ◆ Severe occipital throbbing and vomiting

Health history

Ask the patient when his headache began, what it feels like, and if it's different from headaches he has had in the past. Ask him if it's localized or generalized, constant or intermittent. Have him describe the pain (throbbing, stabbing, dull, viselike). Ask if it tends to occur at a certain time of day or if anything seems to trigger it. Find out if anything makes it better or worse.

Ask the patient if he has been under unusual stress recently. Also ask him if he has any associated symptoms, such as confusion, dizziness, drowsiness, eye pain, fever, muscle twitching, nausea, photophobia, seizures, difficulty speaking or walking, neck stiffness, visual disturbances, vomiting, or weakness.

Find out what medications the patient takes. Ask if he has fallen, been injured, or had blackouts or periods of unconsciousness recently. Ask if he has recently had dental work or sinus, ear, or other infections.

Investigate the patient's diet over the previous few days. Find out if he has consumed foods, drinks, or chemicals known to cause headaches, such as chocolate, cheese, alcohol, and monosodium glutamate. Find out if he stopped smoking or drinking caffeine-containing beverages recently. Finally, ask the patient or a family member if there has recently been a change in the patient's behavior or personality. Also find out if the patient has a history of blood dyscrasia, cardiovascular disease, glaucoma, hemorrhagic disorders, hypertension, poor vision, or seizures.

Physical examination

Perform a head-to-toe assessment, paying special attention to the respiratory and neurologic systems. Observe the rate and depth of the patient's respirations. Note any difficulty breathing or abnormal breathing patterns.

Check the patient's level of consciousness (LOC) carefully. Examine his eyes, noting pupil size, equality, and response to light. With the patient both at rest and active, note any tremors. Gently palpate his skull and sinuses for tenderness. Inspect his head for bruising, swelling, and sinus bleeding.

Check for extravasation of blood into the soft tissue behind the patient's ears. Called Battle's sign, this finding warns of skull fracture. Also check for cerebrospinal fluid draining from the patient's ears or nose and for a painful or stiff neck (a sign of possible meningeal irritation).

Assess motor strength and palpate the patient's peripheral pulses, noting their rate, rhythm, and intensity. Check the patient's reflexes, including Babinski's reflex. Then auscultate over the temporal artery, listening for bruits. Be sure to monitor the patient's blood pressure and pulse pressure.

Possible causes

The following conditions may cause a headache.

Brain abscess. The headache that results from a brain abscess typically intensifies over a few days, localizes to a particular spot, and worsens with straining. The patient also may have a decreased LOC, focal or generalized seizures, nausea, vomiting, aphasia, ataxia, impaired visual acuity, hemiparesis, personality changes, or tremors. His history may include osteomyelitis or a compound fracture of the skull, a penetrating head wound, or a systemic, chronic infection of the middle ear, mastoid, or sinuses.

Brain tumor. Initially, the headache develops near the tumor site and becomes more generalized as the tumor grows. Pain usually is intermittent, deep, dull, and most intense in the morning. It's aggravated by coughing, stooping, Valsalva's maneuver, and changes in head position.

Cerebral aneurysm. A ruptured cerebral aneurysm causes a sudden, excruciating headache. It may be unilateral and usually peaks within minutes. It may be accompanied by nausea, vomiting, and signs of meningeal irritation. The patient may lose consciousness. His history may include hypertension or other cardiovascular disorders, a stressful lifestyle, or smoking.

Encephalitis. The patient will have a severe, generalized headache and an LOC that declines over a 48-hour period. Fever, focal neurologic deficits, irritability, nausea, nuchal rigidity, photophobia, seizures, and vomiting also may develop. The history may reveal exposure to viruses that commonly cause encephalitis, such as mumps or herpes simplex.

Epidural hemorrhage. Acute hemorrhage causes a brief loss of consciousness followed by a progressively severe headache. LOC declines rapidly and steadily. Accompanying signs and symptoms include increasing intracranial pressure, ipsilateral pupil dilation, nausea, and vomiting. The history usually reveals head trauma within the past 24 hours.

Glaucoma. An ophthalmic emergency, acute angle-closure glaucoma may cause an excruciating headache. Other signs and symptoms include blurred vision, a cloudy cornea, halo vision, a moderately dilated and fixed pupil, photophobia, nausea, and vomiting.

Hypertension. The patient may have a slightly throbbing occipital headache on awakening that improves during the day. If his diastolic pressure exceeds 120 mm Hg, the headache will remain constant, and he may have blurred vision and nausea.

Meningitis. This severe, constant, generalized headache starts suddenly and worsens with movement. The patient may have chills, fever, hyperreflexia, nuchal rigidity, photophobia, and positive Kernig's and Brudzinski's signs. The history may include recent systemic or sinus infection, dental work, or exposure to meningitis-causing bacteria or viruses, including *Haemophilus influenzae*, *Streptococcus pneumoniae*, enteroviruses, and mumps.

Sinusitis. Patients with acute sinusitis have a dull, periorbital headache that's typically aggravated by bending over or touching the face. They also may have fever, malaise, nasal discharge (yellow or green), nasal turbinate edema, sinus tenderness, and sore throat. Sinusitis is relieved by sinus drainage.

Subarachnoid hemorrhage. The hallmarks of this disorder are a sudden, violent headache along with dizziness, hypertension, ipsilateral pupil dilation, nausea, nuchal rigidity, seizures, vomiting, and an altered LOC that may rapidly progress to coma. The history may include congenital vascular defects, arteriovenous malformation, cardiovascular disease, smoking, or excessive stress.

Subdural hematoma. Although half of the patients with this disorder have no history of head trauma, subdural hematoma is typically attributed to head trauma, particularly that which causes loss of consciousness, a latent period of drowsiness, confusion or personality changes, agitation, and possibly seizures. Along with these manifestations comes a severe and gradually intensifying localized headache. Later, signs of increased intracranial pressure may develop.

Temporal arteritis. A unilateral throbbing headache in the temporal or front temporal region is typical. It may be accompanied by vision loss, hearing loss, confusion, and fever. The temporal arteries are tender, swollen, nodular and, sometimes, erythematous.

Other causes. Embolic or thrombotic stroke; lifestyle factors; psychogenic factors; traction, distortion, or pressure on blood vessels, meninges, or other extracranial structures, including the skull, paranasal sinuses, scalp, ears, eyes, nose, mouth, and neck muscles; vascular malformations (aneurysms or angiomas); the effects of drugs (such as nifedipine, nitrates, estrogens, and histamine-2 blockers), tests, and treatments.

Implications

Although common and usually harmless, headaches can be disabling and, at times, threatening. Your goal is to quickly distinguish between the harmless and the threatening. Pay close attention when a patient describes a headache as being different from those he has had in the past.

As needed, report your findings to the patient's doctor. Then carry out diagnostic tests, interventions, and treatments as ordered. Early diagnosis and appropriate treatment can minimize the mortality and morbidity associated with the 1 in 10 headaches caused by underlying pathology.

◆ HEMATURIA

The presence of blood in urine is a cardinal sign of renal and urinary tract disorders. Dark or brownish blood indicates renal or upper urinary tract bleeding; bright red blood indicates lower urinary tract bleeding. Remember that many red blood cells must be present before you can see hematuria with the naked eye. Whether trace or gross, however, hematuria requires assessment and treatment.

Health history

Ask the patient when he first noticed blood in his urine and if it was dark or bright red. Ask if it appears every time he urinates and if it includes clots. Find out if he has had blood in his urine before.

Ask the patient if he has pain and, if so, if it occurs only during urination or all the time. Ask if he has bleeding hemorrhoids or has had recent trauma or invasive procedures involving the urethra. Find out if he has performed strenuous exercise recently or if he has a history of renal, urinary, prostatic, or coagulative disorders. If the patient is female, ask if she was menstruating when she saw the blood and what medications she takes.

Physical examination

Inspect the patient's urine for gross hematuria. If he says the problem is intermittent, ask him to urinate into a container and save any blood-tinged samples for you in the refrigerator. Or you can check for trace amounts of blood by using a Hemastix test.

Possible causes

The following conditions may cause hematuria.

Benign prostatic hypertrophy. Encroachment of an enlarged prostate on the bladder neck or urethra may cause bleeding. Other symptoms include difficult or painful urination, hesitancy in starting the urine stream, and postmicturition dribbling.

Kidney or bladder calculi. By irritating membranes lining the urinary system, calculi may spark bleeding.

Renal infarction. Patients with renal infarction usually have gross hematuria. Other signs and symptoms include anorexia, costovertebral angle tenderness, and constant, severe flank and upper abdominal pain. (See *Assessing costovertebral angle tenderness*, page 292.)

Assessing costovertebral angle tenderness

To assess for tenderness at each costovertebral angle, you'll need to perform mediate kidney percussion. Start by asking the patient to sit upright facing away from you. Visualize the location of the costovertebral angle, as shown in the illustration. Then place your nondominant hand over the angle and strike it gently with the ulnar surface of your dominant fist. Repeat over the other kidney. Normally, the patient should feel a thudding sensation, not pain.

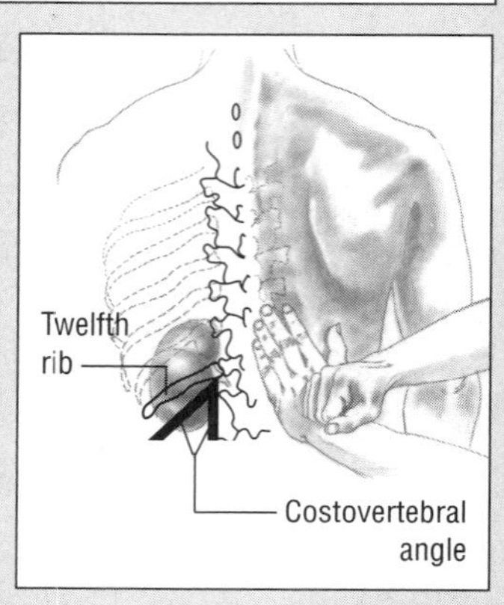

Trauma. Traumatic injury to any part of the urinary system may cause hematuria. Severe trauma may rupture the bladder or urethra or fracture the kidney.

Tumor. A primary cause of gross hematuria in men, bladder cancer may produce pain in the bladder, rectum, pelvis, flank, back, or legs. Any tumor of the urinary system can cause bleeding.

Urinary tract infection. Cystitis and urinary tract infection can cause bleeding that may be accompanied by pus in the urine.

Other causes. Anticoagulant therapy, bone marrow transplant, chemotherapy, kidney transplant.

Implications

Always notify the patient's doctor about hematuria, especially if it's a new development. Then carry out diagnostic tests, interventions, and treatments as ordered. If the patient may have kidney or bladder calculi, teach him to strain his urine and to save any calculi in an appropriate container.

◆ HEMOPTYSIS

The presence of blood in sputum provides an important clinical indicator of active tuberculosis; however, this sign also may warn of a number of other inflammatory conditions or lesions that cause erosion and necrosis of bronchial tissues and blood vessels.

Health history

Ask the patient when he started coughing up blood and how often it happens. Have him describe the amount of blood he's coughing up. Ask if he recently had the flu, an invasive pulmonary procedure, or a traumatic injury. Ask if he smokes (or smoked), and if so, how much and for how long. Ask if he has ever had a human immunodeficiency virus test or tuberculosis skin test or has ever been diagnosed with a cardiac, respiratory, or bleeding disorder. See if his history includes recent fever or night sweats. Finally, find out what medications the patient takes (ask especially about anticoagulants).

Physical examination

Your first priority is to make sure the patient is bleeding from the lower respiratory tract, not from the mouth, throat, nasopharynx, or GI tract. Also auscultate for adventitious or diminished breath sounds. Observe the rate and depth of respirations, noting any abnormal patterns or difficulty breathing. Inspect the skin for central and peripheral cyanosis, diaphoresis, lesions, and pallor. Note the position of the trachea. Palpate the rate, rhythm, and intensity of pulses. Note any edema.

Possible causes

The following conditions may cause hemoptysis.

Active tuberculosis. The bacillus tubercle produces bleeding by damaging lung tissues. Additional symptoms include night sweats, fever, and fatigue.

Bronchogenic carcinoma. Tumors that originate in the bronchi most often stem from smoking. Symptoms may include wheezing, fatigue, clubbed fingers, and weight loss.

Pulmonary edema. The patient may expectorate copious amounts of blood-tinged, pink sputum. Other signs and symptoms include dyspnea, orthopnea, and diffuse crackles in all lung fields.

Pulmonary embolus. Frothy, blood-tinged sputum may be accompanied by dyspnea and other signs of respiratory distress. Similar signs may be attributed to heart failure.

Upper respiratory infection. Active coughing can cause hemoptysis, but the condition shouldn't persist.

Other causes. Fungal or parasitic lung infection, Kaposi's sarcoma, lung abscess, pneumococcal pneumonia, pulmonary infarction.

Implications

If your patient has frank bleeding and a possible pulmonary hemorrhage, contact an emergency medical service. Severe hemoptysis requires emergency endotracheal intubation and suctioning.

For less severe hemoptysis, notify the patient's doctor of your findings and suspected causes. Then carry out diagnostic tests, interventions, and treatments as ordered. If the patient turns out to have active tuberculosis, notify your employer about your exposure to it.

◆ NAUSEA AND VOMITING

Nausea is a vague, unpleasant sensation of being repulsed by food. You must distinguish it from anorexia, which is a decreased or lost appetite. Persistent nausea can make a person weak, light-headed, and dizzy in addition to altering respirations and heart rate. If nausea turns into vomiting, as it commonly does, the patient faces additional hazards.

During vomiting, the heart rate slows to the point of bradycardia, possibly leading to other cardiac arrhythmias. Persistent vomiting can lead to profound nutritional and metabolic abnormalities, including sodium, water, and potassium depletion. In infants and children, it can quickly progress to severe alkalosis and dehydration.

Health history

Ask the patient to describe his condition and when it started. Did it seem connected to an illness, emotion, or ingestion of certain foods or medications? Find out how long it took for the nausea to turn into vomiting, if it did at all. Have the patient describe the vomitus. Ask whether other family members have been sick recently and if the patient has had persistent nausea or vomiting before.

Ask the patient if his nausea is constant or intermittent and if he has any associated symptoms, such as pain, chills, fatigue, or dizziness. If he reports pain, assess it carefully and thoroughly. Ask if he has had a recent illness, infection, traumatic injury, surgery, or diagnostic test. Have him list the medications he takes. Find out if he has traveled lately or been exposed to new chemicals or toxins. Investigate reports of headache, stiff neck, vertigo, focal paresthesia, or weakness.

Spend some time investigating any changes in the patient's activities, diet, bowel habits, and stool. Ask if he has noticed an increased yellow color to his skin. If the patient is female, ask about her menstrual history and possible threatened abortions, tubal pregnancies, and pelvic inflammatory disease.

Physical examination

Complete a total head-to-toe assessment, paying special attention to the abdominal and neurologic examinations. Make note of fever, focal tenderness, guarding, or rebound tenderness.

Possible causes

The following conditions may cause nausea and vomiting.

Abdominal and pelvic organ disorders. Inflammatory involvement of abdominal or pelvic organs may cause anorexia, nausea, and vomiting. Examples include acute appendicitis, pancreatitis, hepatic–biliary tract disease, and peptic ulcer disease.

Cardiac disorders. Acute myocardial infarction and heart failure commonly cause vomiting, with or without abdominal pain.

Drugs and chemicals. In small amounts, some drugs and chemicals can cause anorexia; in larger amounts they may cause nausea, vomiting, or both. Examples include mercury bichloride, ammonium chloride, copper sulfate, amphetamines and their derivatives, aminophylline, large amounts of diuretics, digitalis glycosides, and chemotherapy drugs.

GI disorders. Many abnormalities of the GI tract can cause anorexia, nausea, and vomiting. They include bowel obstruction, gastric surgery, gastric ulcers, and tumors.

Infection. Nausea and vomiting commonly result from febrile infectious diseases caused by bacterial enterotoxins. Urinary tract infection is one example, especially if the patient has urinary tract obstruction and ureteral colic.

Ménière's disease. A disorder that primarily affects people over age 50, Ménière's disease may cause acute episodes of vertigo and tinnitus that are associated with nausea and vomiting.

Migraine headache. Nausea and vomiting may occur in the prodromal stage, as may photophobia and light flashes.

Psychological factors. Fear, depression, severe psychoses, and anorexia nervosa can cause anorexia, nausea, and vomiting by altering activity in the GI tract.

Other causes. Alcohol intoxication, extended fasting, high altitude, malnutrition, motion sickness, pregnancy (early stages); in infants and children, acute infection, bowel obstruction, diabetes mellitus, esophageal atresia, fear or severe anxiety, increased intracranial pressure (possibly resulting from meningitis, hydrocephalus, or a space-occupying intracranial lesion, such as a tumor, hemorrhage, or abscess), pain, pyloric stenosis.

Implications

Evaluate the patient's signs and symptoms carefully and, as needed, report them to his doctor. Then carry out diagnostic tests, interventions, and treatments as ordered. For example, you'll most likely need to monitor the patient's hydration status and possibly his electrolyte levels. Teach the patient or a family member how to measure fluid intake and output. Urge them to report increased vomiting immediately.

Encourage the patient to ingest clear liquids, such as tea, broth, flavored gelatin, and carbonated beverages. Also encourage him to eat small amounts of dry foods, such as salted crackers.

◆ PULSE, ABSENT

Although an absent dorsalis pedal pulse is considered a normal variation, you should be able to detect all other peripheral pulses. If you can't palpate one or more of your patient's peripheral pulses — brachial, radial, ulnar, temporal, carotid, posterior tibial, popliteal, and femoral — you'll need to follow up with a detailed assessment and response.

If the patient has an absent apical pulse, he's in cardiac arrest. Unless he has a do-not-resuscitate order, start cardiopulmonary resuscitation immediately and initiate an emergency medical response. Try to determine what happened from family members.

Health history

Ask the patient if he has noticed a change in the color of the affected limb. Also ask if the limb feels cold and when that feeling began.

Physical examination

Assess temperature, pallor, and mottling in the affected limb. Palpate all other pulses. Evaluate all limbs for capillary refill time and perfusion. Measure the patient's blood pressure, but don't use the affected limb to do it. (See *Dealing with a diminished or absent pulse*, pages 296 and 297.)

Possible causes

The following conditions may cause an absent peripheral pulse: arterial insufficiency, atherosclerosis, embolism, occlusive arterial disease, shock (hypovolemic or cardiogenic). An absent apical pulse may result from cardiac disease, drug overdose, electrocution, or sudden cardiac arrest from other causes.

Implications

If your patient has an absent peripheral pulse, notify his doctor. Then carry out diagnostic tests, interventions, and treatments as ordered. Teach the patient how to avoid injuring the affected limb.

(Text continues on page 298.)

CRITICAL DECISIONS

Dealing with a diminished or absent pulse

A diminished or absent pulse can result from several life-threatening disorders. Your assessment and interventions will vary, depending on whether the diminished or absent pulse is localized to one extremity or

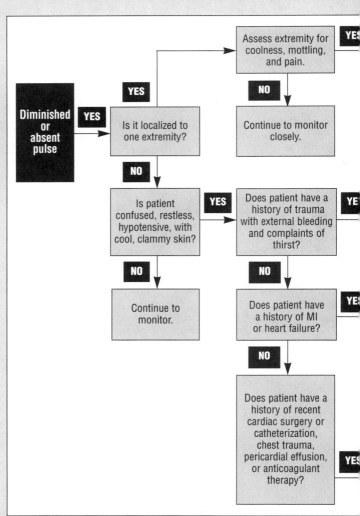

Diminished or absent pulse — YES → Is it localized to one extremity?

Is it localized to one extremity?
- YES → Assess extremity for coolness, mottling, and pain.
  - YES →
  - NO → Continue to monitor closely.
- NO → Is patient confused, restless, hypotensive, with cool, clammy skin?
  - NO → Continue to monitor.
  - YES → Does patient have a history of trauma with external bleeding and complaints of thirst?
    - YES →
    - NO → Does patient have a history of MI or heart failure?
      - YES →
      - NO → Does patient have a history of recent cardiac surgery or catheterization, chest trauma, pericardial effusion, or anticoagulant therapy?
        - YES →

generalized. They will also depend on associated signs and symptoms. Use the flow chart below to help you establish priorities for managing this problem.

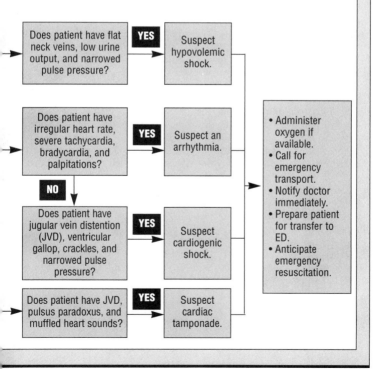

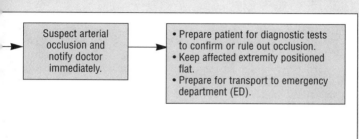

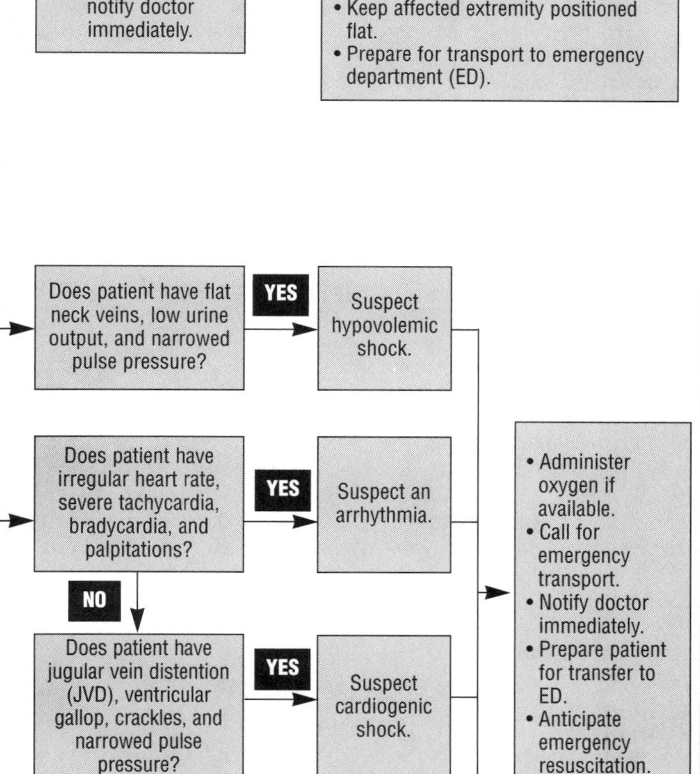

◆ PULSE, IRREGULAR

Although an irregular heart rate does not necessarily signal a life-threatening condition, it does need careful assessment and an appropriate response.

Health history

Ask the patient if he can feel an irregularity in his heartbeat. If he can, ask him to describe it to you (fluttering, missing beats, skipping beats). Ask him when he first noticed the irregularity and if he feels it all the time or only sometimes. Also ask if he has chest pain or feels weak or dizzy. Find out if he has a history of heart disease or an irregular pulse. Ask if he's currently under unusual levels of stress. Ask him to list his medications (including over-the-counter) and to estimate his level of caffeine intake. Finally, ask if he smokes, drinks, or has been recently heat-stressed.

Physical examination

Assess the patient's level of consciousness, making special note of his anxiety level. Note the rate and depth of his respirations. Check for abnormal patterns and breathing difficulty. Inspect his skin for pallor and diaphoresis. Take his blood pressure. Auscultate for heart sounds, listening closely for extra sounds, such as murmurs or gallops. Count his apical pulse for a full minute. Assess peripheral pulses and check his nail beds for capillary refill time.

Possible causes

The following conditions may cause an irregular pulse.

Atrial fibrillation. Characterized by disorganized electrical activity in the atria, this condition may be acute or chronic.

Cardiomyopathy. Cardiac dysfunction results because enlargement of the heart muscle decreases contractility and efficient function. Electrical conduction may be impeded as well.

Dehydration. Electrolyte imbalance alters rhythm and conduction. Correcting the imbalance also can affect the heart rate.

Medications. Some medications (or inappropriate use of medications) can contribute to cardiac irregularities. Examples include antihypertensives, cardiac drugs, and diuretics. Caffeine may affect the heart's rhythm as well.

Pacemaker malfunction. Noncapture of pacer signals may result in an irregular heart rate. Assess pacemaker function and determine the last date of maintenance.

Other causes. Anemia, exercise, fear and anxiety, hypertension, hyperthyroidism, severe lung disease.

Implications

Notify the patient's doctor of an irregular pulse or a change from the patient's previous status. Then carry out diagnostic tests, interventions, and treatments as ordered. Teach the patient how to take and record his own pulse. Also tell him what to do if his condition worsens or he experiences dizziness or syncope.

◆ RASH, PAPULAR

Papules are small, localized, possibly discolored lesions that have substance or mass, are palpable, and usually are elevated above the skin surface. They result either from proliferation of skin cells (inflammatory, metastatic, and leukemic), from fluid accumulation in the skin, or both.

A papular rash can erupt anywhere on the body in virtually any pattern.

Health history

Ask the patient when and where his rash erupted and what it looked like initially. Find out if it has spread or changed in any way. Ask if it itches or burns and if it's tender or painful. Ask if he has ever had a rash like this one before. If so, have him describe the situation. Ask if he has had other symptoms with the rash, such as a fever, stomach upset, or headache.

Investigate if the patient is allergic to any foods, cosmetics, or medications. Ask if he has used new soaps, lotions, or cosmetics recently. Ask if he has recently been exposed to someone with an infectious disease or been bitten by an insect or a rodent. Find out whether he has been outdoors or in the country recently for extended periods.

Find out if he has ever had a sexually transmitted disease, another infectious disease, or a tumor. Ask which childhood diseases the patient has had. Finally, ask if the patient has used a topical medication on the rash, which one, when he last applied it, and what happened as a result.

Physical examination

Perform a head-to-toe physical examination. Note any unusual findings that might be related to the rash. When examining the skin, observe the color, configuration, and location of the rash. (See *Assessing lesions by configuration,* page 300.) Palpate the papules in several different areas, noting their firmness under the skin and any drainage.

Possible causes

A papular rash may result from acne vulgaris, allergies, infectious mononucleosis, insect bite, Kaposi's sarcoma, psoriasis, sarcoidosis, and other infectious and systemic disorders. It also could result from a hypersensitivity reaction to a topical agent or drug, such as a nonsteroidal anti-inflammatory drug, succimer (Chemet), or interferon.

Implications

As needed, report your findings to the patient's doctor after completing a thorough history and physical examination. Then carry out diagnostic tests, interventions, and treatments as ordered. Teach the patient and family how to monitor and care for the rash and any associated or underlying conditions. Continue to monitor the course of the rash and related findings in subsequent visits until it's controlled or gone.

◆ TACHYPNEA

Rapid, shallow breathing (greater than 40 breaths/minute or greater than the patient's baseline rate) may occur with a variety of respiratory diagnoses and deserves a thorough investigation.

Health history

Question the patient about possible precipitating factors and any relief measures he has used to control the tachypnea.

Physical examination

Evaluate the patient's respiratory status, including breath sounds and the rate, rhythm, and depth of respirations. Also evaluate his cardiovascular status, including perfusion and blood pressure. If possible, check his oxygen saturation with pulse oximetry. Assess his level of consciousness and orientation, and watch for signs of confusion.

Possible causes

The following conditions may cause tachypnea.

Assessing lesions by configuration

Document lesion configuration by one of the patterns illustrated below.

Discrete
Separate, distinct lesions

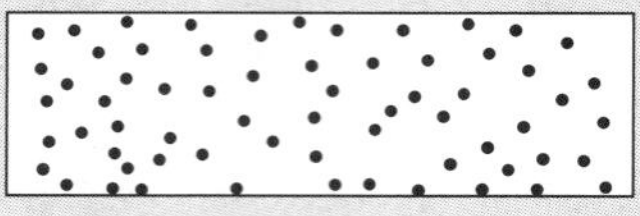

Annular
Lesions forming a circle

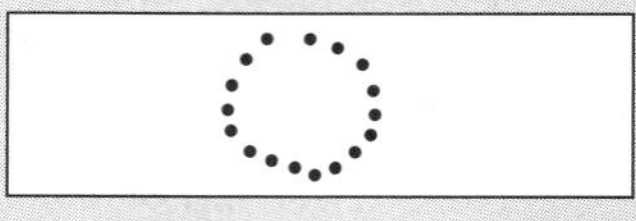

Grouped
Clusters of lesions

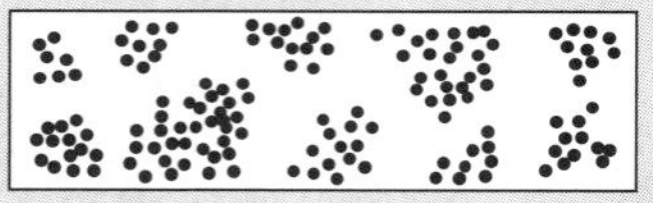

Polycyclic
Two or more rings or circles

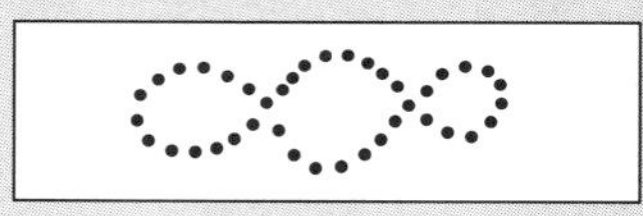

Confluent
Lesions merging together

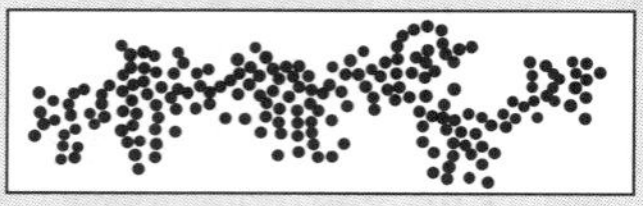

Arciform
Lesions forming arcs or curves

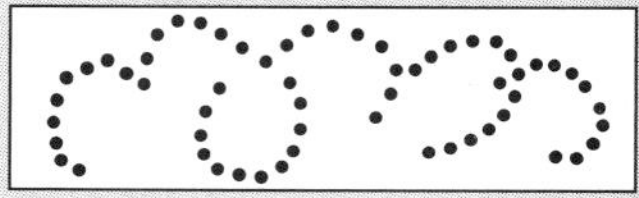

Linear
Lesions forming a line

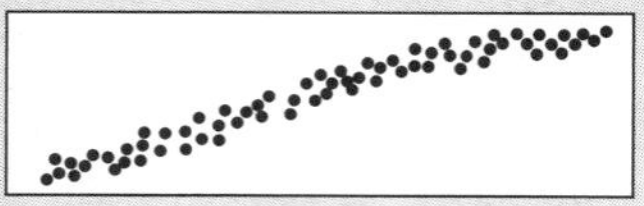

Reticular
A meshlike network

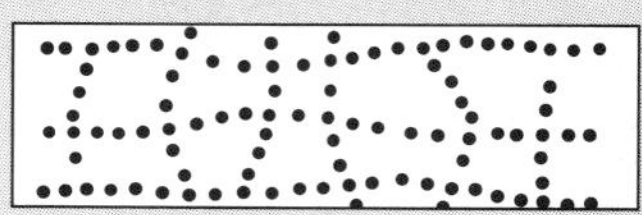

Acute respiratory failure. In this functional disorder, gas exchange is not adequate to meet the body's metabolic needs, so the body responds by speeding the patient's breathing. It can result from neurologic, neuromuscular, cardiovascular, and respiratory disorders.

Adult respiratory distress syndrome. Also associated with a wide variety of clinical disorders, this syndrome is known by a sudden onset of severe, life-threatening respiratory distress in patients who have no major underlying lung disease.

Pneumonia. Lung consolidation diminishes available surface for gas exchange; the patient breathes faster to make up for that reduction. The patient also may have fever and pleuritic chest pain.

Pneumothorax. Sudden lung collapse increases the respiratory drive.

Restrictive pulmonary diseases. These diseases diminish air flow and lung capacity, thus boosting respiratory drive.

Other causes. Acute anxiety attacks, obesity, pleurisy.

Implications

Evaluate the patient for signs and symptoms of possible causes, and notify his doctor of your findings. If the patient uses home respiratory equipment, assess its function and appropriateness. Reinstruct him as necessary. For acute and severe tachypnea, call an emergency medical service.

◆ WEIGHT LOSS

Weight loss may reflect decreased food intake, increased metabolic requirements, a disease state, or some combination of the three. Unintentional weight loss is associated with an increased likelihood of sickness and death, especially among elderly patients.

Health history

Ask the patient to describe his weight in general terms over the course of his life. Ask if he has been ill or diagnosed with a thyroid condition recently. Have him estimate how much weight he has lost, if it was intentional or not and, if not, when he first started noticing the loss. Ask if he can think of any reason for the loss. Find out if he has traveled outside the country recently.

Investigate the patient's diet by asking him what he usually eats in a day. Have him list what he ate the previous day. Ask if his eating habits have changed recently and, if so, how and why. Find out if he has noticed changes in his stools. Ask if he has had diarrhea or noticed bulky, floating stools.

Find out if the patient has had abdominal pain, excessive thirst or urination, increased hunger, altered heat tolerance, nausea, vomiting, increased fatigue, or changes in sleep pattern. Ask about his sex life, including if he has unprotected sex and more than one sex partner.

Ask the patient if he has experienced major changes recently, such as a divorce, change in job, death of a loved one, or a child leaving home. Ask if he feels anxious, depressed, or stressed. Have him list the prescription and over-the-counter medications he takes. Ask specifically about diet pills and laxatives.

Physical examination

Perform a head-to-toe physical examination. Record the patient's height and weight. As you take his vital signs, note his general appearance. Does he appear well-nourished? Do his clothes fit? Can you detect muscle wasting? Does he have jaundice or pallor?

When examining the skin, check turgor and pigmentation, especially around the joints. Examine the condition of his teeth, gums, and dentures. Check his eyes for exophthalmos and his neck for swelling. When palpating the abdomen, check carefully for liver enlargement, masses, and tenderness.

Possible causes

The following conditions may cause weight loss.

Anorexia nervosa. This psychogenic disorder is most common in young women and is characterized by severe, self-imposed weight loss. It may be accompanied by amenorrhea, blotchy or sallow skin, cold intolerance, constipation, frequent infections, loss of fatty tissue, loss of scalp hair, and skeletal muscle atrophy.

Cancer. A common cause of unintentional weight loss, cancer's associated signs and symptoms reflect the type, location, and stage of the tumor and may include abnormal bleeding, anorexia, fatigue, nausea, pain, a palpable mass, and vomiting.

Crohn's disease. Weight loss occurs with abdominal pain, anorexia, and chronic cramping. Other findings include diarrhea, hyperactive bowel sounds, tachycardia, and abdominal distention, tenderness, and guarding.

Depression. In severe depression, weight loss may occur along with anorexia, apathy, fatigue, feelings of worthlessness, and insomnia or hypersomnia.

Leukemia. Acute leukemia causes a progressive weight loss accompanied by bleeding tendencies, high fever, and severe prostration. Chronic leukemia causes a progressive weight loss with anemia, anorexia, bleeding tendencies, an enlarged spleen, fatigue, fever, pallor, and skin eruptions.

Medications. Many drugs interfere with appetite by causing abdominal discomfort, anorexia, nausea, diarrhea, inhibition of gastric emptying, or other symptoms. Examples include amphetamines, chemotherapeutic agents, laxatives, and thyroid preparations.

Other causes. Acquired immunodeficiency syndrome; adrenal insufficiency; chronic heart, lung, or renal disease; diabetes mellitus; endocrine disorders; GI disorders; infection; lymphoma; neurologic lesions that cause paralysis or dysphasia; nutritional deficiencies; poverty; psychological disorders; rheumatoid arthritis; systemic lupus erythematosus; thyroid disorders; ulcerative colitis; in children, abuse (emotional or physical), chronic illness, defects in assimilation of food (cystic fibrosis, malabsorption syndrome), hypopituitarism, hypothyroidism, impairment of organ function (such as heart failure), infection, malnutrition; in the elderly, altered perception of satiety; altered perception of taste and smell; bereavement; cancer; cerebrovascular accident; conditions that prevent sufficient food intake, such as painful oral lesions, ill-fitting dentures, and the loss of teeth; dementia; depression; isolation; loss of appetite; Parkinson's disease; polypharmacy.

Implications

A physical cause for weight loss can be found about 65% of the time, and it's critical that you assess the patient carefully. After completing a thorough history and physical examination, report the patient's weight loss and associated findings to his doctor, as indicated. Then carry out diagnostic tests, interventions, and treatments as ordered. Continue to monitor the patient's weight during subsequent visits as indicated. Be sure to always weigh the patient using the same scale, in similar clothing, and at about the same time of day.

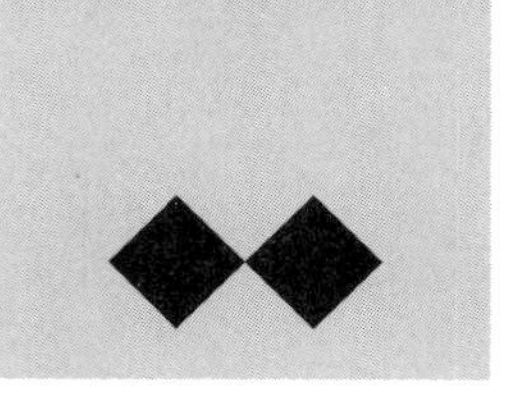

CHAPTER 10

Adapting care, equipment, and teaching to the home

As a visiting nurse, your ability to adapt your care effectively to the home setting may be as important as your ability to perform fundamental nursing skills. In the patient's home, you're likely to encounter limitations of both time and available resources. For instance, you may be able to make only a few visits. Many patients can't afford all the medical supplies or equipment they need to maintain health or an adequate level of functioning — and some items may not be covered or reimbursed by insurance.

However, through careful planning and creativity, you can overcome these challenges and help your patient achieve a maximal level of wellness and independence. In fact, by making the most of available resources, you can ensure adequate care, even for the patient with multiple chronic health problems.

This chapter describes how to adapt your nursing care to virtually any home setting. It identifies low-cost alternatives to expensive medical supplies and equipment, and it tells you how to turn ordinary household items into acceptable substitutes for some types of health care equipment. It provides tips and techniques for improving the patient's medication compliance and teaching him how to self-administer injections and I.V. therapy. The chapter also explains how to assess the patient's nutritional status, help him streamline home cleaning and disinfection practices, and ensure that he can get help in an emergency. It concludes by presenting effective teaching strategies for the home patient.

Respecting the patient's autonomy

Keep in mind that, when working in a patient's home, a domineering approach can easily backfire. The patient's home, unlike a health care facility, is *his* territory, not yours. Respect his autonomy at all times, and keep in mind that he has the right to reject your proposed plan of care or even your presence in his home.

Also, you are responsible for informing the patient of additional costs associated with the proposed plan of care. For example, he may refuse to purchase medical supplies and equipment, even if doing so means jeopardizing his well-being. If a patient refuses your visits, remember that you and your home health agency share responsibility for providing him with adequate care until other arrangements can be made.

◆ MEDICATION ADMINISTRATION

A home care patient may be prescribed medication to take by the oral,

Home visits to administer drugs: Federal guidelines

Will the federal government reimburse the patient for home nursing visits you make *solely* to administer drugs? That depends on the prescribed administration route. Here are some general guidelines:

◆ Oral, topical, and otic administration is not covered or reimbursed because the government considers the patient capable of self-administration by these routes.

◆ Subcutaneous administration is covered or reimbursed if the patient can't self-administer the medication and no one else is available to give it.

◆ I.M. administration is covered or reimbursed for selected drugs if the medication is deemed necessary and can't be given orally.

◆ Intermittent I.V. administration is covered or reimbursed if the medication can't be provided in another form. However, a patient who's receiving long-term antibiotics may be expected to learn self-administration or to travel to an outpatient facility for this therapy.

sublingual, topical, otic, subcutaneous, I.M., or I.V. route. The routes most commonly prescribed for home administration are oral, topical, and otic. (See *Home visits to administer drugs: Federal guidelines*.)

Oral medications

In acute care settings, where nurses administer oral medications, monitoring the patient's compliance with drug therapy is relatively easy. With the home patient, however, gauging compliance isn't as easy.

If you suspect that your patient is not taking his medications, perform a physical evaluation to help detect signs and symptoms of his underlying condition. Then try to find out the cause of his noncompliance. For instance, does he have a visual, physical, or mental limitation that makes it hard for him to see or handle the medication or to remember when to take it? Is the medication expensive? If so, perhaps the patient has decided to take it only in an emergency.

Improving compliance

Spend extra time teaching the noncompliant patient about the importance of taking his prescribed medication. Be sure to cover the purpose of each medication, and list the health problems that could occur if he fails to comply.

If your patient has trouble remembering when to take oral medications, try using visual or audio reminders, such as taping a sample of the tablet or capsule to a written medication schedule or setting an alarm clock for the time of his next dose.

If the patient is using a written medication schedule, make sure it's clear and large. For an easy-to-follow written schedule, divide a sheet of plain white paper into columns. In one column, list each medication by name, and tape a tablet or capsule of that medication next to its name. In the second column, write the times that the patient should take each dose.

If the patient can't follow a written medication schedule, draw medication clocks to help him remember to take his medication. Use two clocks for each medication; write "A.M." in the center of one clock and "P.M." in the center of the other. Use a different color to label each clock so the patient can easily tell them apart. Then write the names of the medications he's supposed to take in the spaces for the hours when he's supposed to take them. Tell the patient to check the clock often during the day so he doesn't miss any doses.

Here are some other techniques that may promote medication compliance.

◆ Group medications that the patient is supposed to take at the same time.

◆ If your patient watches much television, advise him to take medication when a certain television program comes on (depending, of course, on the administration schedule).

◆ Place the patient's morning medications in the kitchen and nighttime medications in the bedroom.

◆ Put medications to be taken at different times in containers of different colors.

Using medication containers

Pharmacies, groceries, and other stores sell medication containers made of hard plastic, with separate chambers for each medication. The best containers have chambers labeled for each day of the week and for various times of day, such as breakfast, lunch, dinner, and bedtime. (See *Using compliance aids,* page 306.)

If desirable, you can fill the patient's medication containers for him. However, be aware that this task isn't reimbursed or covered under federal reimbursement guidelines.

Substituting household items. If the patient can't afford to buy plastic medication containers with separate chambers, suggest that he store medications in clean, empty, clearly labeled jars; extra prescription bottles (obtainable from the pharmacist); or envelopes labeled with the name of the medication and times of day to take doses. Recommend that he fill the jar, bottle, or envelope every morning with the correct number of tablets or capsules.

If the patient lacks the manual dexterity or strength to open a prescription bottle or a jar, suggest that he store medications in an egg carton, which is easy to open and close. He simply fills each egg well with a different medication and labels each well clearly with the name of the medication. If he takes only a few medications, he can cut the carton to size.

If the patient is taking a single, short-term medication — for example, a 7-day course of antibiotic therapy — advise him to place the doses for each day in seven separate egg wells and then label each well with the appropriate day.

A muffin baking tin is another alternative for storing medications. The 6 or 12 muffin wells in these tins are large enough that even a patient with limited dexterity can easily remove a tablet or capsule from the well.

Other household items that the patient can use to store medications include breath mint, film, and paper clip containers. Instruct him to thoroughly wash and dry the container before placing medications in it and, once filled, to store it out of direct sunlight to avoid loss of medication strength.

Topical and otic medications

If the patient is supposed to apply a topical medication after bathing, advise him to keep the medication in the bathroom (unlike other medications, which you should advise him *not* to keep in the bathroom). That way, the medication tube will serve as a visual reminder to apply the medication after a shower or bath.

To promote compliance, make a written schedule or a medication

Using compliance aids

To help your patient comply with oral or injectable drug therapy, you or a caregiver may premeasure doses for him, using compliance aids such as those shown below or ones you create yourself. Most pharmacies and community service agencies can supply similar aids.

One-day pill pack
A plastic box with four lidded medication compartments marked "breakfast," "lunch," "dinner," and "bedtime" helps the patient see whether he has taken all medications prescribed for the day. If needed, the lids can be embossed with Braille characters.

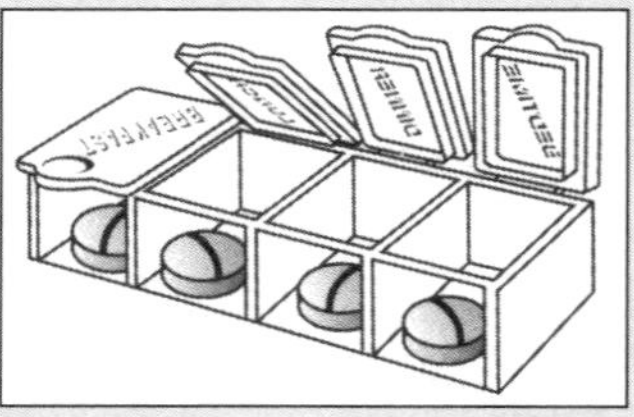

You, the patient, or a caregiver must remember to fill the device each day because it doesn't hold many tablets or capsules.

Seven-day pill reminder
The boxes shown below will help your patient remember whether he has taken all the tablets and capsules prescribed for each day of the week. Each box has seven medication compartments marked with the initials for each day of the week (in both Braille characters and printed letters).

Like the 1-day pill pack, these devices are inappropriate for large numbers of tablets or capsules or for tablets and capsules that must be taken at different times each day.

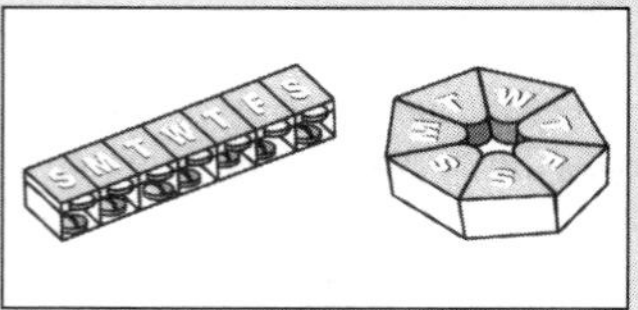

clock for a topical or otic medication, just as you would for an oral medication. Although you can't tape a medication tube or bottle directly to the medication schedule, you can use color-coding to help your patient stay on track. Simply place a self-adhesive colored dot (sold in office supply stores) on the medication schedule, or draw in a dot or bar of color using a permanent marker; then place the same color on the tube or bottle of the corresponding medication.

Injectable medications

Many patients fear injecting themselves with needles, so noncompliance can be a real problem for the patient who's prescribed an injectable medication. Poor skills may also pose a challenge in effective self-injection.

Before teaching your patient how to inject medications, evaluate his ability for self-administration so you can adapt your teaching accordingly. For instance, an elderly, debilitated patient with impaired vision or mobility will need additional time and support to learn how to manipulate a syringe — and to overcome the fear of injecting himself.

If your patient must inject I.M. drugs, teach him about appropriate needle lengths, injection sites, the amount of medication to draw into the syringe, and the injection schedule.

Handling the syringe

With most patients, you'll need to maintain a fairly slow pace when teaching how to handle a syringe and spike a vial. After demonstrating the proper injection technique, leave a spare syringe (without a needle) at the patient's home so he can practice pulling and pushing on the plunger. On your next visit, observe his ability to use a syringe before teaching him the next step of the injection procedure.

Spiking the vial

Spiking the medication vial with the needle can be especially difficult for a patient with poor vision, hand tremors, or arthritis. Particularly if the medication vial is small, you may need to demonstrate alternative ways to steady the vial while inserting the needle. Make sure you or another caregiver is present when the patient first attempts to spike the vial because he could accidentally injure himself.

Drawing up medication

Once your patient masters handling the syringe and spiking the vial, teach him how to draw up medication in the syringe. If he's a diabetic with impaired vision, he may have trouble seeing the small increment markings on the traditional insulin syringe; ask your home care pharmacy or a medical supply company to order special insulin syringes with larger markings. (See *Syringe-filling aids,* page 308.) Or provide the patient with a magnifying glass.

If your patient must inject more than one medication, he may be able to administer certain medications together to reduce the number of needle sticks. For example, a diabetic patient may combine several types of insulin in one syringe.

Prefilling syringes

If your patient can't draw up his own subcutaneous medication, even after adequate instruction and demonstration, you can prefill his syringes for him. After explaining the procedure, assemble all of the equipment in a convenient work area, verify the prescribed dosage, and wash your hands. Draw up the prescribed amount of medication in the syringe; place a small piece of tape on the syringe, and label it with the date and time the medication was drawn up and the date and time the patient should take the injection. Then put the prefilled syringe in the patient's refrigerator.

When prefilling two different syringes, place each in a separate spot in the refrigerator. If children or mentally challenged adults live in the home, place prefilled syringes in a covered container or an out-of-the-way area of the refrigerator.

Instruct the patient to administer prefilled syringes within 21 days of filling them and to store the syringes flat, not suspended with the needle facing down. Tell him to take the syringe out of the refrigerator at least 1 hour before injecting the medication. Just before injection, he should gently roll the syringe between his hands to mix the medication and warm it. After injection, tell him to place the used syringe and needle in the household sharps container.

Be aware that under federal guidelines, home nursing visits made solely to prefill medication syringes aren't reimbursed. (Daily visits to *administer* insulin are reimbursed if your

Syringe-filling aids

If your home care patient needs to take insulin but is visually impaired, you can obtain special aids to help him fill the syringe accurately.

Syringe-filling device
The syringe-filling device (shown at right) precisely measures insulin doses for a visually impaired diabetic. Designed for use with a disposable U-100 syringe and an insulin bottle, it's set by the caregiver to accommodate the syringe's width. After setting the syringe, the caregiver positions the plunger at the point determined by the dose and tightens the stop. When the device is set, the patient can draw up the precise dose ordered for each injection.

Like any device, the syringe-filling device has certain drawbacks:

◆ It can't be used if insulin needs to be mixed or if doses vary.

◆ Settings must be checked and adjusted whenever the syringe size or type changes.

◆ Screws must be checked regularly because they loosen with repeated use.

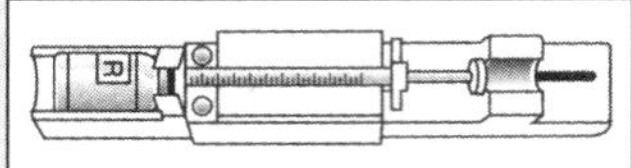

Syringe scale magnifier
The syringe scale magnifier (shown below) helps a visually impaired diabetic read syringe markings, thereby enabling him to fill his own syringe. The plastic magnifier snaps onto the syringe barrel. This device may be impractical for a patient with arthritis who can't easily attach the magnifier to the syringe.

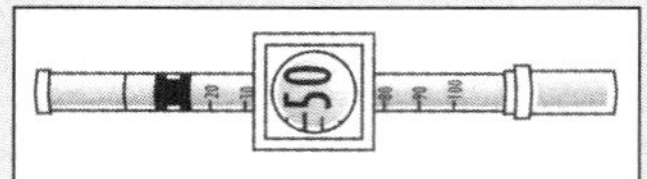

documentation shows that the patient isn't capable of self-administration and no one else is available to administer the insulin.) However, keep in mind that you can prefill syringes during the course of another visit or you can request that the patient's pharmacy supply the medication in prefilled syringes.

Reusing needles and syringes

Depending on the type of medication needed and the frequency with which your patient requires injections, he may be able to reuse needles and syringes rather than using a sterile syringe and needle for each injection. This is especially likely if he's taking insulin.

Be sure to check with the patient's doctor before advising him to reuse needles. If reuse is permitted, teach the patient how to recap the needle correctly. Instruct him to place the cap on a firm, flat surface, stabilize it with his finger, guide the needle back into the cap, and close it securely. Warn him not to try to recap the needle while holding the cap.

I.V. therapy

The patient or caregiver who must administer I.V. therapy at home must master a host of skills, including inspecting the indwelling catheter site, changing the dressing, flushing the catheter, preparing the medication, priming the tubing, discarding used equipment, and troubleshooting problems.

After demonstrating the proper technique for performing these skills, provide ample opportunity for return demonstrations. Include other caregivers in all teaching sessions, and reinforce your instructions with written handouts that were used in the hospital for the patient receiving I.V. therapy.

If the patient can't afford special I.V. equipment, suggest that he substitute items found in the home. For instance, instead of buying an I.V. pole, he can hang the I.V. bag from a door hook. Here are some other suggestions:

- ◆ Use a cotton ball saturated with alcohol solution in place of an alcohol sponge.
- ◆ Reuse syringes and needles used to flush tubing.
- ◆ Use multidose heparin vials and sterile saline solution vials.
- ◆ Draw up catheter flushes instead of buying prefilled cartridges.
- ◆ Place waterproof plastic wrap over the indwelling catheter before taking a shower.

Special considerations

- ◆ If your patient isn't complying with his prescribed medication regimen, assess him for a physical condition or an adverse medication effect that could be causing mental impairment or confusion.
- ◆ Include family members or other home caregivers in medication teaching whenever possible.
- ◆ If the patient lives alone, make sure he has assistive devices to help him take his medication.
- ◆ Instruct the patient to store medications separately from other household items, such as on a different cabinet shelf.

◆ HOME REMEDIES

Home remedies have been used to treat everything from the common cold to terminal cancer. Some patients use a home remedy because it's cheaper than prescribed medical treatments or because they think the remedy is safer or more effective. With others, using the remedy may be a family, cultural, or ethnic tradition.

To find out if your patient is using a home remedy, identify and evaluate *every* preparation he uses, not just prescribed medications. (See *Is your patient using a home remedy?* page 310.) If you discover that he is using one, ask what its purpose is, how often he uses it, and whether he's using it instead of or in addition to a prescribed medication or other treatment. Also, try to determine how he's responding to the remedy by performing a thorough physical assessment.

Be sure to inform the doctor that the patient is using the home remedy. If necessary, arrange to have its contents analyzed to find out if it's potentially harmful or incompatible with prescribed medications or if any of its ingredients are contraindicated for the patient's medical condition.

Incorporating home remedies

If the patient's home remedy is harmless, work with him to create a sensible dosing schedule that doesn't interfere with the prescribed medication regimen. Provide appropriate precautions based on the contents of the home remedy. Watch him or a caregiver prepare the remedy, and observe for effects.

Finally, advise the patient how to store the home remedy (some prepa-

Is your patient using a home remedy?

Would you know a home remedy if you saw one in your patient's home? Review this list of common home remedies to help determine which ones your patient may be using:
◆ alcoholic beverages (to promote sleep at bedtime)
◆ black cherry or cranberry extract (for urinary tract infections, kidney stones, or bladder cancer)
◆ bleach solution (as a foot soak to treat calluses)
◆ butter (to soothe a burn)
◆ celery (for hypertension)
◆ cola, warmed (for indigestion, nausea, or vomiting)
◆ dandelion root (for kidney or bladder problems)
◆ Epsom salts (for psoriasis)
◆ garlic capsules (for hypertension)
◆ mineral oil or cooking oil (for an ear obstruction)
◆ mustard plaster (for chest congestion)
◆ sodium bicarbonate (for indigestion)
◆ vinegar poultice (for an insect sting)
◆ wine or whiskey, warmed and sweetened (to ease sore throat or cough).

rations must be refrigerated) and how to check for spoilage.

Special considerations

◆ Remain nonjudgmental if your patient insists on using a home remedy instead of taking a higher-priced prescription drug. Unless it's harmful, don't try to talk him out of using it.

◆ Be sure to document the patient's use of the remedy and its effects.

◆ DIETARY SUPPLEMENTS AND NUTRITION THERAPY

A patient with nutritional deficits resulting from disease, debilitating illness, or an inability to buy food or prepare meals will probably need to take prescribed dietary supplements. To help determine if your patient is receiving adequate nutrition, weigh him during every visit. Ask him or a caregiver to keep a diary or log of everything he eats and drinks. A thorough dietary assessment can help determine if a dietary consultation is indicated or if the patient needs dietary supplements or nutrition therapy.

During the dietary assessment, identify the following:
◆ the patient's normal meal pattern
◆ types of foods and beverages he usually eats
◆ amounts of foods and beverages he typically consumes in one sitting
◆ types and amounts of snack foods he eats
◆ use of alcoholic beverages.

A dietary questionnaire can help you determine the patient's actual daily nutritional intake.

Oral supplements

Many commercially prepared dietary supplements are available. For example, Ensure, taken by mouth, is a high-calorie, carbohydrate-based solution containing vitamins and minerals. Available in grocery stores, it comes in a wide assortment of flavors, plus a low-sugar version for diabetics, a low-fat version for those who must limit their fat intake, and a double-strength formula for patients with fluid restrictions.

If the doctor prescribes Ensure, keep in mind that the manufacturer offers discounts to patients who need but can't afford the supplement. A representative of the local Ensure vendor can provide teaching programs on the various Ensure products, supply free samples for the patient to try, and offer discount coupons and rebates. Or a social services organization may be able to obtain supplies of Ensure from the manufacturer.

Enteral nutrition therapy

For a debilitated patient who can't ingest adequate nutrients orally but whose GI system is still functioning, enteral tube feeding is the preferred nutritional therapy. Enteral feedings are given through a nasogastric (NG) or gastrostomy tube. Be aware that home use of an NG tube is temporary; most home care patients receiving nutrition through an NG tube will eventually need a more permanent device.

A gastrostomy tube is surgically inserted to bypass the uppermost portion of the alimentary canal. A preparation such as Oscal or Jevity can then be administered through the tube.

Enteral nutrition solutions come in various osmolarities — hypotonic, isotonic, and hypertonic — to meet the needs of a wide range of patients. These solutions provide carbohydrates, proteins, and fats. Some also contain vitamins, minerals, and iron.

Alternative preparations

Commercially available oral dietary supplements can be costly. If your patient can't afford them, he can still receive a diet adequate in protein, calories, vitamins, and minerals by using cheaper products, such as Sustacal, that are available in grocery stores. Originally intended as a meal substitute for individuals trying to lose weight, Sustacal provides a balance of calories, vitamins, and minerals to fit the nutritional needs of most patients.

Carnation Instant Breakfast is another alternative. A powder packaged in single-use pouches, this product is added to a glass of milk. It comes in a variety of flavors and consistencies. Averaging 130 calories before milk is added, it provides 25% to 50% of the recommended daily allowance of protein, iron, vitamin C, and B complex vitamins in addition to 27 g of carbohydrates, 4 g of protein, and 1 g of fat. When mixed with whole milk, it provides 250 calories and 6 g of fat. Patients who need to limit their fat intake can mix it with skim milk instead of whole milk.

Special considerations

- ◆ If appropriate, consult a dietitian, who can perform a calorie count and offer suggestions to help your patient meet his nutritional requirements.
- ◆ If your patient can eat and drink normally but needs additional calories for healing and energy, encourage him to use over-the-counter oral dietary supplements. If he finds these unpalatable, recommend puddings and fortified milkshakes.
- ◆ Provide a list of alternative foods if your patient has special dietary needs. Remind him that many food products are now available to suit the needs of people with various health conditions.
- ◆ If the patient can't afford to buy recommended or prescribed dietary supplements, tell him about programs and organizations that can provide financial support. Inform him that the cost of dietary supplements that serve as his sole source of nutrition may be reimbursed by Medicare or some private insurers. Dietary supplements administered by non-oral routes may also be reimbursed.

◆ If enteral therapy causes diarrhea, advise the patient to dilute the feeding solution.

◆ WOUND-IRRIGATING SOLUTIONS

For convenience or economy, your patient or his caregiver may be able to make a wound-irrigating solution, such as sterile normal saline solution or sterile water, at home.

Making sterile normal saline solution

To make sterile normal (0.9%) saline solution, instruct the patient or caregiver to gather the following items in the kitchen:

◆ glass jar with tight-fitting, screw-on lid
◆ saucepan with lid
◆ teaspoon
◆ measuring cup
◆ noniodized table salt
◆ liquid dish detergent.

Tell the patient to wash the jar, saucepan, lids, teaspoon, and measuring cup in hot, soapy water and then rinse with warm water and dry.

Next, instruct him to boil at least 6 cups of tap water. After pouring 4 cups of the boiled water into the clean jar, he should use the clean teaspoon to add 2 tsp of salt. Tell him to screw the lid on the jar, shake well to mix, and store the solution in a clean, dry place away from direct sunlight.

Making sterile water

To make sterile water, advise the patient or caregiver to gather the following items in the kitchen:

◆ glass jar with tight-fitting, screw-on lid
◆ saucepan with lid
◆ measuring cup
◆ liquid dish detergent.

Instruct the patient to wash the jar, saucepan, lids, and measuring cup in hot, soapy water and then rinse with warm water and dry. Have him place 2 cups of tap water in the clean jar and then loosely screw on the lid. Next, instruct him to place the jar in the saucepan and fill the saucepan with water until it reaches three-quarters of the way up the jar. After placing the lid over the saucepan, he should boil the water for approximately 25 minutes.

Next, he should remove the saucepan from the stove. After the water in the pan cools, he should remove the jar, tighten the lid, and store the jar in a clean, dry place away from direct sunlight.

Special considerations

Irrigating solutions prepared in the home are stable for only 1 week. Help the patient estimate the amount of solution he'll need per week, and advise him to prepare only that amount and discard any he hasn't used after 1 week.

◆ Closely monitor the patient's use of homemade solutions, and regularly examine the wound site for signs of infection, inflammation, and slow healing. If the wound isn't healing adequately, instruct him to try a commercially prepared irrigating solution for a short time; if healing improves with this solution, reinstruct him in proper preparation of the solution.

◆ Instruct the patient to inspect the irrigating solution for particulates before using it and to throw out any solution that's discolored or cloudy.

◆ Tell the patient not to use the irrigating solution if the jar has been opened, if it's cracked or leaking, or if he doesn't know how old the solution is.

◆ Make sure the patient or caregiver can safely operate the stove.

◆ Tell the patient not to heat or boil the solution in a microwave oven.

◆ Caution the patient not to use a plastic or metal container for the irrigating solution. Metal can't be disinfected thoroughly by boiling, and plastic will crack or melt at high boiling temperatures.

◆ Stress that, before reusing a jar that has stored irrigating solution, the patient must boil it empty for 20 minutes and then let it cool before storing more solution in it.

◆ Warn the patient never to use home-prepared solutions for eye irrigation. If eye irrigation is ordered, he must use a sterile ophthalmic solution.

◆ Advise the patient to store equipment used for sterilizing solutions separately from other household items and to reserve these items solely for solution preparation.

◆ DISINFECTION PROCEDURES

Depending on your patient's medical condition and prescribed treatment, he may need to disinfect equipment used for NG or gastrostomy tube feedings, ostomy care, respiratory care, oxygen administration, or urinary catheterization, as well as bedpans, urinals, reusable patient care instruments, equipment, and soiled linens. If he can't afford commercial cleaning agents and disinfectants, inform him that he may be able to substitute cleaners he already has at home. Provide the instructions below on disinfecting medical equipment and performing routine household cleaning and disinfection.

First, help the patient identify appropriate areas in the home where equipment can be disinfected and dried. If possible, he should reserve one tub or sink solely for this purpose.

If the home lacks sufficient sink space or other cleaning areas for disinfection, suggest that he use a large wash basin or tub and reserve it solely for disinfection. Point out that he can also use the basin or tub to transport the item to the appropriate drying area.

Disinfecting NG and gastrostomy tube equipment

Equipment used with NG and gastrostomy tubes — feeding bags and tubing, irrigation trays, feeding containers, and 30- or 60-ml syringes — can be reused after disinfection. Instruct the patient to disinfect these items by soaking them in warm, soapy water for about 20 minutes, rinsing them with warm water, and allowing them to air-dry.

Disinfecting ostomy equipment

Reusable ostomy care items include certain pouches, irrigation solution bags and tubing, and drainage pouches for ileostomies and urostomies. Advise the patient to disinfect these items by rinsing them first in warm water and then soaking them in warm, soapy water for 20 minutes, rinsing them thoroughly, and hanging them to air-dry. To aid drying, instruct him to turn ostomy pouches and bags inside out. Caution him not to reuse these items until all moisture has been removed from the surfaces.

Disinfecting respiratory equipment

Many items used for respiratory care can be disinfected and reused. However, advise the patient not to use bleach or other strong disinfectants to clean items that he will wear or introduce into his body, such as an oxygen mask, a tracheostomy tube, or a suction catheter.

Oxygen equipment

Instruct the patient to disinfect a nasal cannula, mask, tubing, mouthpiece, cartridge inhaler, or humidifier by first rinsing off all visible particles and then submerging the item in warm, soapy water and letting it soak for 20 minutes. Next, he should rinse the item thoroughly to remove all soap. As it air-dries, he should move it periodically to drain moisture from internal parts.

To disinfect tubing from an incentive spirometer, ultrasonic nebulizer, or oxygen connections to a ventilator, instruct the patient to use a solution of 3 parts water to 1 part white vinegar after soaking the item for 20 minutes in warm, soapy water. The patient should then rinse all parts thoroughly with warm, running water and let them air-dry. After they dry, he should store them in a clean, resealable plastic bag. A patient with copious secretions should clean the tubing daily; other patients, at least two to three times a week.

Suction equipment

To disinfect a suction catheter for reuse, instruct the patient to soak it in a solution of 1 part hydrogen peroxide to 2 parts water for 20 minutes and then to boil it for 10 minutes. Then tell him to remove the catheter from the boiling water, hang it to air-dry, place it in a clean plastic bag, and seal the bag tightly.

If the patient has an oral suction (Yankauer) catheter, tell him to wash it daily in warm, soapy water, letting it soak if necessary to remove accumulated secretions. He can use a small-diameter bottle brush to clean internal parts. After a thorough rinsing, he should let the catheter air-dry.

The collection canister, connection tubing, and basins of a suction machine can also be disinfected and then reused. Instruct the patient to remove all used equipment from the suction machine and to apply new equipment. Then tell him to empty filled reservoirs into the toilet. Next, he should rinse the equipment with warm water; soak it in warm, soapy water for 20 minutes; and rinse it thoroughly. Then instruct the patient to boil the equipment for 15 minutes, remove it from the water, and let it cool. After drying it with clean towels, he should store the clean equipment in clean plastic bags, fresh jars, or freshly laundered towels.

Tracheostomy tubes

Some types of tracheostomy tubes can be disinfected for reuse. (See *Disinfecting a tracheostomy tube.*)

Disinfecting urinary catheterization equipment

To disinfect a catheter used for intermittent urinary catheterization, instruct the patient to wash the inside and outside of the catheter with warm, soapy water, rinse it thoroughly, and shake it gently to dry. Tell him to dry the outside of the catheter with a clean paper towel; to place the catheter in a clean glass jar, paper towel, or plastic bag; and to close the container securely.

Urinary collection bags and tubing can also be disinfected. Advise the patient to change and clean these items every 2 weeks. After emptying the bag, he should clean each item in warm, soapy water and rinse thoroughly with warm water. Next, tell him to soak the items for 30 minutes in a solution of 1 part white vinegar to 3 parts water and then hang them to dry. Tell him to disinfect the cap on the tip of the collection tubing using alcohol and then replace the cap on the tip.

Disinfecting patient care instruments

Scissors, hemostats, clamps, and forceps can easily be disinfected. Instruct the patient to first rinse off all crusted material and then soak the instruments in warm, soapy water for 20 minutes. After rinsing thoroughly, the patient should boil the instruments for 15 minutes; let them cool; dry them with clean, lint-free towels; and store them in tightly sealed containers.

Disinfecting bedpans and urinals

Advise the patient to rinse bedpans and urinals after each use and to disinfect them at least once a week. Instruct the patient or caregiver to empty the contents of the bedpan or urinal; wash the item with warm, soapy water; and rinse it thoroughly. Then he should clean all surfaces with a mixture of 1 part bleach to 10 parts water.

Cleaning soiled linens

Instruct the patient or caregiver to wear utility gloves or nonsterile disposable gloves when handling soiled bed linens. Advise him to place soiled linens in a leakproof plastic bag near the bed and then place this bag in a second leakproof plastic bag.

Emphasize that soiled linens must be washed separately from other household laundry in the hottest water possible, using both laundry detergent and 1 cup of household bleach. The washing machine should be set for at least a 25-minute cycle. Soiled linens should be laundered twice, each time using both laundry detergent and bleach. After the patient or caregiver removes the linens from the washer, he can either hang them to dry or use an electric clothes dryer.

If the linens are soiled with excrement, tell the patient to disinfect the

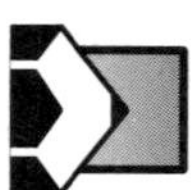

TEACHING POINTS

Disinfecting a tracheostomy tube

The disinfection procedure for a tracheostomy tube varies, depending on whether the tube is metal or plastic.

Metal tracheostomy tube

Instruct the patient to wash a metal tracheostomy tube in warm, soapy water, using a pipe cleaner or small bottle brush to clean the insides. Silver polish can remove tarnish. Then advise him to rinse all parts of the tube thoroughly with warm running water, remove them from the water, and let them cool. Tell him to store the clean metal parts in a clean plastic or glass container with a tight-fitting lid.

Plastic reusable tracheostomy tube

To disinfect a plastic reusable tracheostomy tube, advise the patient to wash it in warm, soapy water, using a pipe cleaner or small bottle brush and, if necessary, a 50% hydrogen peroxide solution to remove crusts. After rinsing all parts of the tube thoroughly with warm running water and a pipe cleaner, he should let them air-dry and store them in a clean plastic or glass container with a tight-fitting lid.

washing machine after laundering the linens by pouring in 1 cup of full-strength bleach and putting the empty machine through a normal wash cycle.

Household cleaning and disinfection

Encourage the patient or caregiver to keep the home as clean as possible. Kitchen counters should be cleaned regularly with scouring powder, the home should be dusted and vacuumed at least weekly, and the kitchen and bathroom floors should be mopped weekly and whenever spills occur. The inside of the refrigerator should be cleaned once a week with warm, soapy water.

Cleaning furniture

If wooden furniture becomes contaminated, instruct the patient or caregiver to disinfect it with a commercially available wood or furniture cleaner. To avoid ruining the finish, caution him not to pour alcohol directly onto the furniture.

Advise the patient or caregiver to consult a local dry cleaner for suggestions on decontaminating drapes or cushions from a sofa or chair. Until the soiled items are cleaned, they should be removed from use.

Dealing with blood spills

Advise the patient or caregiver to contact a laundry facility for advice on the best products for removing blood or body fluids from upholstered furniture and drapes. To clean such spills from other household surfaces, instruct him to put on disposable gloves, wipe up the spill with paper towels, place the used paper towels in a plastic trash bag, and secure the bag tightly. Next, he should remove the gloves, wash his hands, and put on a clean pair of gloves. Then he should pour undiluted bleach over the spill site, wait 10 minutes, and wipe up the bleach with paper towels soaked in disinfectant. He can then discard the paper towels in a plastic trash bag and close the bag securely. Instruct him to wash the spill area a final time — this time using warm, soapy water — and then rinse and dry it.

Special considerations

- Thoroughly instruct the patient or caregiver on safe handling of cleansers and disinfectants. Tell him to clearly label the containers "Poisonous" or "Dangerous if eaten" — particularly if children or mentally impaired persons are in the home. If necessary, help him obtain "poison" or "Mr. Yuk" stickers, which are available free of charge in many pharmacies.
- Warn the patient never to store cleaning agents or disinfectants in containers that resemble juice or food containers to prevent children from confusing them.
- If your patient must disinfect more than one piece of equipment, using a different disinfectant for each, instruct him to clearly label each disinfectant container with the item it's intended for.
- If possible, carry replacement supplies when making home visits in case disinfected equipment becomes damaged.
- If you're not sure how to disinfect a specific piece of equipment, consult your home health agency for instructions. For directions on disinfecting large, intricate pieces of machinery, contact the durable medical equipment or respiratory equipment supplier.
- Tell the patient that he can't disinfect any part of a hemodialysis machine at home. Instruct him to take the machine to a central facility for professional sterilization and disinfection.

◆ IMPROVISED MEDICAL SUPPLIES AND EQUIPMENT

If your patient can't afford the medical supplies or equipment he needs or is awaiting delivery of an item, you can recommend ordinary household objects as substitutes, if appropriate. Easily improvised items include:

- ◆ personal care items to aid routine hygiene and dressing
- ◆ assistive ambulation devices
- ◆ food preparation and eating aids
- ◆ communication aids
- ◆ comfort aids.

Linen protectors

If an incontinent patient can't afford rubber sheets or other costly linen-protection supplies, recommend that he place large plastic trash bags or sheets of plastic under the bottom sheet to protect the mattress. Advise him to stretch the plastic smooth to eliminate bumps and wrinkles, which could injure his skin. Inform him that a local department store may be able to provide large plastic sheets (commonly used to transport furniture), which he can cut to fit his mattress.

Back rest

If your bedbound patient doesn't have a hospital bed, suggest that he simply stack bed pillows behind him when he wants to sit upright. Alternatively, he can angle a small card table against the head of the bed, with the table legs firmly secured to the headboard or bedposts. To cushion the hard table surface, recommend placing pillows or another protective covering over it.

Bed cradle

A small card table can also be used as a bed cradle. Instruct the patient to open the table, place it over his legs, and then arrange the sheets to cover both the table and his lower extremities.

A clean, long cardboard box can serve as a bed cradle. Instruct the patient to remove one side of the box and place the box over his feet and legs. Cardboard boxes can be obtained free of charge from department stores, grocery stores, and liquor stores.

Footboard

The patient who needs a footboard (for example, for footdrop) can improvise one by removing the attachable legs from a card table. Advise him to cover the tabletop with a pillowcase or other soft material and to slip it between the mattress and bed frame at the foot of the bed. Instruct him to secure the tabletop with heavy tape or tie it to the bed frame.

If the bed frame isn't secure, instead of propping the tabletop against the frame, help the patient angle the bed with its foot against the wall. The wall then serves as the footboard.

No matter what object the patient uses as a footboard, make sure he covers any sharp edges with duct or adhesive tape to avoid injury.

Bed table

If your bedbound patient wants a bed table, advise him that a large cardboard box can work just as well as a commercially available bed table, which is expensive, heavy, and cumbersome to carry. Tell him to cut the edges of the box so that one side is completely open and then place the box open-side down. Next, have him cut off two sides of the box, leaving the other two sides for support and carrying. To make handles, he can cut away a small portion near the top of the intact box surface. If the bed table will be carried from room to room, the handles can be taped open with masking tape to provide support for the carrier. Covering the top surface with a tablecloth will make it more attractive.

Other items that can be substituted for a bed table include an ironing board opened and secured at the height of the bed, an oversized book, and a large picture album. Suggest covering the surface of the improvised table with a towel to protect it from spills and soiling.

I.V. pole

To improvise an I.V. pole for a patient receiving home I.V. therapy, advise him to hang the I.V. bag from a door hook or from a metal plant hanger attached to the handle of a high cabinet. He can also slip the I.V. bag through the hook of a wire clothes hanger and place one of the hanger's triangular ends over another supported device to suspend the bag. The hanger works best when hung from a door hook.

I.V. bags can also be hung from a curtain rod, ceiling fan, bookshelf, or closet door to promote gravitational flow of the I.V. solution. Whatever method or item the patient uses, emphasize that the I.V. bag must be fastened securely so it doesn't fall.

Sharps container

If your patient routinely uses needles and syringes for medication administration, make sure he knows how to discard them safely. Instead of buying a hard plastic sharps container from a medical supply company, he can use a household container, such as an empty liquid laundry detergent container or a metal coffee can. Emphasize that whatever container he uses must be made of a rigid, nonpermeable material. Caution him not to use cardboard boxes, paper or plastic bags, or regular household trash bags because sharp instruments can pierce them.

If the patient wants to use a coffee can, advise him to slit its plastic lid to create a slot for used syringes and needles. Remind him to place the sharps container out of the reach of children and to dispose of its contents properly.

Humidifier

The patient who needs humidified air but doesn't have a humidifier can achieve the same effect by placing a bowl of water near a steam heater or placing boiling water in a bowl. Another way for him to breathe humidified air is to go into the bathroom, close the door, and run hot water in the tub or shower.

Ambulation aids

If your patient needs assistance to rise to a standing position, you can make a transfer belt from a pair of suspenders or a regular clothing belt. Before he attempts to rise, make sure the belt is firmly attached. If the belt has integrated suspenders, place these over his shoulders — but make sure the suspenders have some slack.

When using the transfer belt, first help the patient to a semi-sitting position, and then grasp the back of the belt as he rises. Continue to grasp and assist until he achieves a full standing position.

A patient who needs a walker or cane can substitute a household item. A chair placed on wheels, for instance, can serve as walker; the chair moves forward as the patient walks. Advise him to angle the chair so he can grasp the back of it while walking.

Point out that a table leg, a short pole, or a detached, rubber-tipped leg of an ironing board can serve as a cane. A bicycle handle bar can be taped (with heavy tape) to the improvised cane to make a handle. For added support, instruct him to wrap tape around the entire length of the cane.

Feeding devices

If your patient has an unsteady grip, recommend that he use unbreakable plastic dishes instead of glassware; they're lighter and less slippery. If plastic dishes aren't available, the patient can place terry cloth sleeves over glassware for an easier grasp.

A wide variety of special dishes, utensils, and other devices are available to assist at mealtimes. (See *Making eating easier,* page 320.) Specially designed cups include those with two handles or an oversized handle (easier to keep steady), pedestal or T-handle cups (easier to grasp), and cups with weighted bases (to help prevent spills). If the patient has a stiff neck, advise him to use a cup with a V-shaped opening on its rim; he can easily tip it to drink without bending his neck backward.

Some drinking straws are wide enough to use for drinking soups and thick liquids; advise the patient to use a snap-on plastic lid with a slot for the straw.

To keep a plate from sliding, tell the patient to place a damp sponge, washcloth, paper towel, or rubber disk under it, or recommend using a plate with a nonskid base or placemats made of foam or dimpled rubber. Suction cups attached to the bottom of a plate or bowl also help prevent slipping. A plate guard prevents food from falling off the plate and makes it easier to pick up with a fork or spoon. A scooper plate has high sides that provide a built-in surface for pushing food onto the utensil.

Oversized utensils and ordinary flatware with ridged wood, plastic, or cork handles are easier to grasp than smooth metal handles, or the patient can build up the handles with a bicycle handgrip, a foam curler pad, or tape. He can also try strapping the utensil to his hand.

Gastrostomy feeding aids

If your patient has trouble pouring his feeding solution through the barrel of a syringe to administer gastrostomy tube feedings, suggest that he use a funnel. If he doesn't already have one, he can purchase an inexpensive one. Instruct him to place the funnel directly into the tube and to hold it in place with one hand while pouring the solution with the other hand. Afterward, he should wash the funnel with soap and rinse it thoroughly with water.

Bathroom aids

If your patient needs help bathing — for instance, because he's unable to bend forward to wash his feet — tell him how to extend his reach by securing a washcloth or sponge to one end of a large stick or a yardstick. To dry hard-to-reach areas, he can attach a dry towel to another stick.

Although commercially available bathroom rails can help the patient get into and out of the tub or shower or rise from the toilet, these rails aren't federally reimbursed because they're considered a convenience or comfort item. If your patient needs bathroom rails but can't afford them, recommend a footstool to help him get into and out of the shower. Make sure, though, that he has something to hold onto while stepping on and off the footstool.

Alternatively, he can place a lightweight lawn chair in the tub to sit in while bathing. If desired, he can also place the chair in front of the sink so he can sit while brushing his teeth, shaving, or taking a sponge bath. Make sure the stool or chair he uses is in good repair and won't promote falls. Check footstools for rubber or slip-resistant ends.

Making eating easier

If your patient needs help feeding himself, recommend the devices shown here.

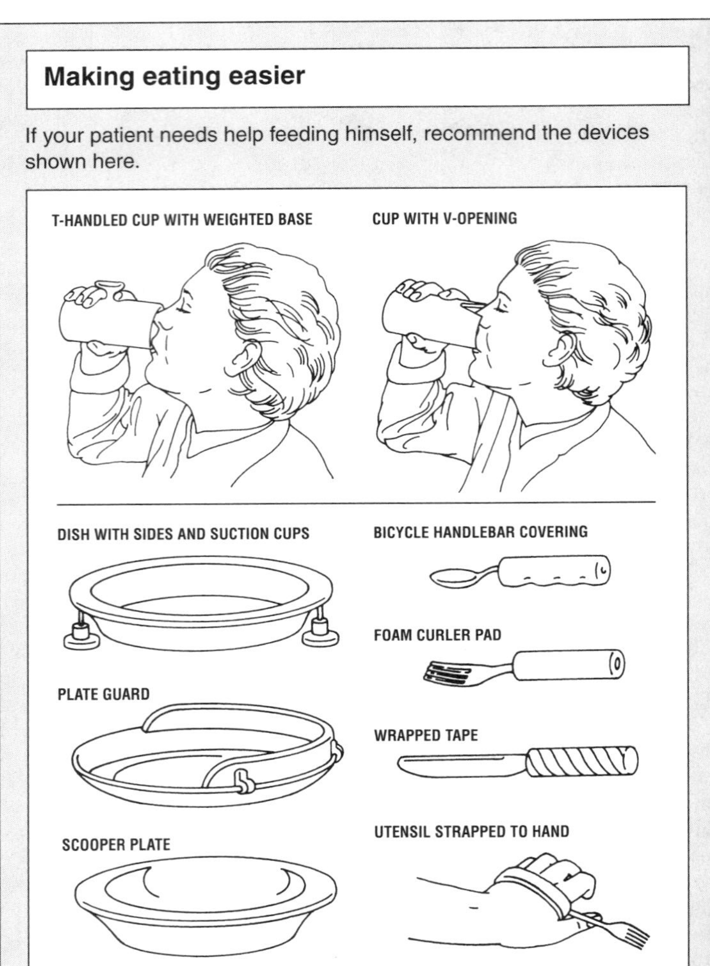

Elimination aids

If your patient can't walk to the bathroom and can't afford a bedside urinal, inform him that he can make one from a coffee can or a plastic, 1-gallon milk container. If he's using a milk container, he simply cuts off the container's top while preserving as much of the handle as possible. After taping the edges to avoid cuts, he should place the container on a firm surface within easy reach. Advise the patient using a plastic container as a urinal to replace it at least twice a week.

A chair with a hole cut out of the seat and a bucket placed under the hole can serve as a bedside commode for a female patient. Covering the edges of the hole prevents injury.

Dressing aids

If your patient can't bend forward to put on shoes or pick up items from the floor, advise him to use a large pair of plastic or metal kitchen tongs as a substitute for a store-bought reacher. He simply opens the tongs and clasps the item. To keep the tongs within reach at all times, instruct him to attach a rope to the tongs and slip the rope over his shoulder. A bent metal clothes hanger can also serve as a reacher in some situations, and an extended shoehorn can help the patient put on his shoes.

If your patient wears heavy peripheral vascular hose such as Teds stockings, suggest that he wear plastic disposable gloves to improve his grasp when pulling them on. Dusting his legs with powder will also ease hose application. If necessary, he can use tongs to help position the hose around his foot, but caution him to be careful not to tear the hose with the tongs.

Flotation devices

The patient who needs a flotation device for his bed or chair needn't purchase a store-bought version. Inform him that he can use a partially inflated pool toy or an air mattress covered with a soft material for flotation.

Carrying aids

For easy transport of medications or other supplies, advise the patient or caregiver to use a carrying case or bowl. He can slip the case over the back of his chair or wear it like a purse. He can place small items together in the bowl for convenient carrying.

Heat therapy supplies

If the doctor prescribes heat therapy or warm soaks, tell your patient about household substitutes for hot packs and other expensive items. For instance, mention that he can fill a hot water bottle with warm water and wrap it in a thin towel.

To warm linens and blankets, suggest that he place them in a metal container placed over a radiator. Caution him not to place a sheet or blanket in a hot oven or microwave. Advise a caregiver to test a heated or warmed item before placing it on the patient's skin. Be aware that a heating pad may be contraindicated for a patient with altered mental or peripheral sensory status.

Cold therapy supplies

If the patient is prescribed cold therapy, evaluate his mental status: A patient with limited mobility, altered mentation, decreased sensation, or an illness affecting blood flow (such as diabetes, peripheral vascular disease, or lower extremity ulcers) shouldn't use cold therapy unattended.

Commercial ice packs and ice holders

Several types of ice packs are commercially available. Your agency's policy may dictate which type or brand you carry in your bag. If you carry chemical ice packs — single-use packs containing a chemical that turns cold when activated — be aware that these are intended mainly for use in emergencies; they're expensive and unnecessary for a home care patient.

Other commercially available ice packs include rigid plastic packs containing a nontoxic gel and malleable, fabric-covered cold compresses; both must be placed in the freezer for several hours before using.

For a patient who needs long-term cold therapy, you may recommend the traditional frozen water method, which uses specially designed ice holders available in various shapes. If the patient will use these holders, make sure his freezer can freeze water within a reasonable time.

TEACHING POINTS

Safety tips for cold therapy

If your patient is prescribed cold therapy, provide the following advice:

◆ If you're using a plastic container to hold the ice, don't fill it all the way. Leave some room at the top for the ice to expand.

◆ Never freeze glass or another container that could crack when frozen.

◆ Don't apply the ice pack directly to your skin because it could cause frostbite. Instead, place it on a thin towel or similar covering.

◆ Don't leave the ice pack on any part of your body for more than 20 minutes. If you accidentally leave it on longer, *don't* use a heat source, such as a hair dryer, to warm the affected body area. Instead, let the area warm slowly to reduce tissue damage.

◆ Wait at least 20 minutes between ice applications.

◆ Stay alert for symptoms of frostbite: pale skin that's cold to the touch, numbness, and tingling. Get medical care at once if these symptoms occur.

Improvised ice packs

If your patient can't afford a commercial ice pack or ice holder, he can make an ice pack by filling various household items with water and freezing them. The most commonly used items are plastic containers, such as cups, bowls, bags, and disposable gloves. Some patients prefer to enclose ice cubes in a small handcloth and then wrap the cloth with plastic wrap. A bag of frozen vegetables works well, too. Any container holding ice must be closed securely after the ice is inserted.

If the patient has ice pops in his freezer, he can make an ice pack by filling a paper cup with water, standing an ice pop stick in the cup, and placing it in the freezer. After the water freezes, he peels the paper cup off the ice and holds it with the protruding handle. Before applying the ice, however, he must cover the affected area with a cloth.

To make a moldable ice pack, recommend that the patient fill the finger of a nonsterile disposable glove with 70% isopropyl alcohol and fill the rest of the glove with water. Then he must shake the glove gently to mix, tie a knot at its wrist, and place it in the freezer. Within a short time, the liquid will become slushy and mold easily to almost any shape desired.

Whatever items the patient uses for cold therapy, warn him never to place the ice pack directly on his skin because this can cause frostbite. Also warn him not to apply ice for more than 20 minutes at a time. (See *Safety tips for cold therapy*.)

Personal items

To stay warm, your patient can use a bath towel instead of a shawl if he doesn't have one. Tell him to fold the towel into a large triangle and drape it around his shoulders; he should fasten it at the base of his neck with a large safety pin or adhesive tape.

To make a robe from a blanket, instruct the patient to fold over one edge of the blanket to create a collar, place the collar edge over his shoulders and arms, bring the blanket edges around to his front, and secure the open edges. To make sleeves, he can turn back the long ends covering his arms, rolling them until his hands are exposed. Then he can fasten the edges of the blanket around the arms and secure the sides. Tell him to keep securing the sides until all openings along the length of the blanket are closed.

Communication aids

If your patient has a speech impairment, help him find other ways to communicate, such as lipreading or using a communication board. If his manual dexterity is good, he may be able to communicate adequately with paper and pencil or an Etch-a-Sketch.

A communication board lets the patient express himself by pointing to words, letters, pictures, or phrases on the board. Boards come in manual versions and those that operate on a home computer. If the patient uses a board, make sure he can see it clearly. Help him decide how he'll identify the figure or character on the board. If he can't lift an arm to point, he can get a special pointer that requires only slight hand or arm movement. A speech pathologist can help determine which board best suits your patient's needs and can teach him how to use it.

If your patient can't afford a commercially available communication board, you or a caregiver can create one by cutting out pictures from magazines, books, or newspapers that express various needs and taping or pasting them onto a piece of cardboard or the pages of a writing tablet. For example, a picture of a toilet indicates the need to go to the bathroom, a picture of a glass of water signals thirst, a picture of food shows hunger, and a picture of a television set indicates the desire to watch TV. Advise the patient to keep the board near him at all times.

Special considerations

- ◆ To identify the assistive devices that will best promote your patient's independence, assess his functioning level. Consult an occupational therapist, if necessary, for advice on appropriate substitutes for medical equipment and supplies.
- ◆ Enlist the patient's help to improvise medical supplies. Suggest items that other patients have used, and ask if the patient has similar items in the home. Explain how the improvised item will help him, and ask him to help you make it, if possible.
- ◆ Give the patient a written instruction sheet explaining how to use the improvised equipment, and observe him use it.
- ◆ Make sure all improvised equipment is safe.
- ◆ Tell the patient how to care for any improvised medical supplies and equipment and how to make replacements in case of damage. If he's using an item made from cardboard, instruct him to replace it if it becomes damp and soft.
- ◆ If your patient refuses to use improvised equipment, find out what his objection is and provide more teaching as appropriate. For instance, if he doesn't see the need for the item, explain how it can help prevent injury or promote independence. If he continues to refuse the improvised item, ask a social worker for the names of organizations that might be able to provide the item without charge.
- ◆ Document in the patient's record the type of improvised item he's using and how the item was made. Also document all efforts made to help the patient become more independent.

◆ SPECIAL CALLING DEVICES

Getting others' attention and obtaining help in an emergency are crucial

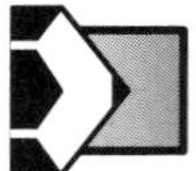

TEACHING POINTS

Using a personal emergency response system

To help your patient use his special calling device effectively, provide the following instructions:

◆ Place the calling device in a central location so you can reach it quickly in case of an emergency.

◆ Wear the neck pendant inside your clothing so the cord won't get tangled or caught if you fall, which could cause you to choke.

◆ If the device must be plugged in, be sure to use a grounded electrical source.

◆ Keep cords and wires away from high-traffic areas to help prevent falls.

◆ Protect the device from liquids and accidental damage.

to the home care patient. Advise a bedbound or chairbound patient to use a bell or another call device rather than calling a caregiver when he needs something. If the patient can't afford a bell, tell him to make one by inserting small stones, marbles, or other small, hard items through the pop-top opening of an empty soda can. Instruct him to tape the can shut to keep the items from falling out and to cover sharp edges. To keep the improvised bell within easy reach, tell him to attach it to a string.

Personal emergency response system

To ensure that your patient — especially a frail, older patient — can get help in an emergency, urge him to enroll in a personal emergency response system or a telephone alert system. Marketed under such brand names as Vitalink, Lifeline, and Communicall, these systems link the patient's home to a central monitoring station. When an emergency occurs, the patient presses a button on a home console, which signals the central monitoring station. The station then notifies a designated contact person to check on the patient. If the contact person isn't available, the station contacts the appropriate emergency response team. (See *Using a personal emergency response system*.)

Some personal emergency response systems eliminate the need for a contact person by immediately activating a medical alert when signaled by the patient. Still others are voice-activated; the patient presses an emergency activation button on a neck pendant to speak directly to someone at the monitoring station.

To use one of these systems, the patient usually pays an initial activation fee of about $25 to $75, plus a monthly fee of about $25 to $45 for ongoing use. Although Medicare doesn't reimburse this cost, some private insurers may — especially if the patient is susceptible to falls. If necessary, the social worker may be able to help your patient obtain a personal emergency response system. Various organizations provide these systems free of charge or at a reduced cost if the patient meets certain requirements.

Telephone alert system

A telephone alert system is available from the local telephone company for certain patients with limited resources. The social worker can help your patient complete the necessary forms to apply for the system. If possible, also suggest that your patient use a telephone equipped with automatic-dialing or speed-dialing options for use in an emergency; the patient or family member need only press a single preprogrammed key on the telephone keypad to reach the doctor or get emergency help.

Telecommunications relay services

If your patient has a hearing or speech impairment, tell him about the telecommunications relay services available from some local telephone companies. Using a typewriter-like device called a text telephone, the patient can type a message to communicate with someone who has intact speech and hearing. Messages are relayed by specially trained communication assistants who are available 24 hours a day.

Special considerations

◆ If your patient has a personal emergency response system or another special calling device, make sure he knows how to use it properly.

◆ If the patient's telephone has memory features or programmable numbers, help him program the numbers of the emergency medical service, his doctor, and other crucial persons, Make sure he knows which preset number to press for each.

◆ If the patient has impaired vision, advise him to get a telephone with oversized numbers if possible.

◆ If your patient lacks a telephone or emergency calling device and refuses assistance to obtain one, write down the telephone numbers of his family members or neighbors and ask these people if your agency can call them regarding the patient's status in an emergency.

◆ ADAPTING YOUR PATIENT TEACHING

Teaching is perhaps the most important role of a home nurse. Home visits to teach a patient or caregiver how to manage ordered treatments are reimbursable. (See *Reimbursable teaching activities,* page 326.)

As with any patient, you'll need to prepare a specific teaching plan and modify it according to your home patient's needs. In your plan, be sure to indicate whether your teaching on a particular topic represents the patient's initial instructions or a review of teaching previously given in a health care facility. Also note whether you must provide any repeat teaching or training because the patient or caregiver is performing a task improperly.

To prepare your teaching plan, you'll need to assess your patient's learning needs, learning style, and educational level, and then gear your teaching technique and tools accordingly. Teaching techniques include demonstration, practice, and return demonstration (most appropriate for care procedures); role playing; and lectures. Teaching tools include printed materials, audiotapes, and videotapes.

Using printed materials

You can present background information and explain procedures with books, pamphlets, and other printed materials. These allow the patient to read and reread information at his convenience. Printed materials can be prepared and adapted to meet almost any patient learning need.

When recommending printed materials, be sensitive to the patient's ability or inability to read and absorb information. He may be too embarrassed to admit he's not a skilled reader; if the material proves too complex

Reimbursable teaching activities

Federal guidelines allow reimbursement for home visits by a registered nurse when the visits are made to provide patient teaching on the following topics:
◆ bowel or bladder training
◆ care and application of special dressings or treatments (such as those used to treat widespread fungal infections or skin deterioration after radiation therapy)
◆ care and maintenance of peripheral and central venous lines
◆ care of the bedbound patient
◆ complete diabetes management for a newly diagnosed diabetic (including home glucose monitoring, signs and symptoms of hypoglycemia and hyperglycemia, skin and foot care, insulin administration, and dietary modifications)
◆ home safety
◆ new or exacerbated disease processes (including precautions and complications)
◆ ostomy care
◆ pain management
◆ preparation and maintenance of a therapeutic diet
◆ procedure for accessing emergency services
◆ urinary self-catheterization
◆ self-administration of gastrostomy or enteral feedings
◆ self-administration of injectable medications
◆ self-administration of medical gases
◆ self-administration of oral medications (including adverse effects and interactions with food and other medications)
◆ wound care.

or difficult, he may quickly lose the motivation to learn.

Some home health agencies prepare their own patient-education materials to fit patients' needs. Such materials may come in two versions — one for the patient and one for the nurse. The patient's version, written in lay terms, addresses him directly; the nurse's version tells you exactly how to instruct the patient.

However, developing patient-education materials can be time-consuming and expensive, so your home health agency may encourage you to use existing printed materials. To obtain them, you may need to consult a hospital librarian or inservice instructor. Other reliable sources include pharmaceutical and medical supply companies and national associations and foundations (such as the American Heart Association). These sources usually have large supplies of patient-teaching materials written with the layperson in mind. Many are provided free of charge; some are offered at a nominal cost.

If your agency wants to adapt some of these materials, be aware that it must obtain permission from the publisher to reprint or photocopy the pages for patient use, unless there's a general permission statement at the front of the book or on each page stating that the material can be reproduced for individual patient use.

Although prepackaged references can save you time, they're no substitute for your personal teaching; they only supplement it. Be sure to mark significant passages for your patient and review the information with him.

Teaching about medications

Written materials are usually preferred for teaching a patient about medications. If possible, provide a separate instruction sheet for each medication the patient takes, and review only one sheet per visit. On your next visit, test your patient's knowledge of the medication covered during the previous visit. If necessary, review your instructions on that drug; otherwise, go on to the second medication. Follow this approach on subsequent visits until the patient shows sufficient knowledge of all prescribed medications.

If your patient must self-administer injections, provide thorough instruction and plenty of time for him to master this skill. Begin such teaching early on in your visits. As a learning aid, provide an illustration with recommended injection areas highlighted.

If your patient is taking insulin, stress the importance of rotating injection sites. Offer tips and techniques for injecting hard-to-reach areas, such as leaning against a door frame to reach the back of the upper arm.

Reviewing printed materials

Be sure to read printed teaching materials — especially medication instructions — before giving them to your patient. Review them closely for accuracy and suitability. Most patient-education materials should be written for a sixth-grade reading level; a more advanced reading level will only confuse the average patient, as will medical terminology.

Does the material contain photos, illustrations, or diagrams? Generally, the more pictures the printed materials contain, the better the patient will retain what he's learning. Also check whether the print is large enough for him to read; if it's too small, consider enlarging individual pages by using a photocopy machine that can make enlargements.

Helping foreign-language patients

If your patient speaks and understands only a foreign language, perhaps a family member can translate printed materials. Or find out if the state Health and Human Services Department or a pharmaceutical company can provide printed teaching material in the patient's native language. For instance, the manufacturer of Coumadin (warfarin) offers home care instructions on this medication in more than 15 languages.

Using audiotapes

You may want to use audiotapes to teach auditory and performance skills or if your patient can't read or is visually impaired. Possible sources of patient-teaching cassettes include consumer health publishers and pharmaceutical companies.

If these resources aren't available, you can prepare your own audiotapes simply by recording yourself during a teaching session. Bring a tape recorder and plenty of audiotape to the session. If your patient speaks a foreign language, ask an interpreter to record your instructions in his native language. Leave the finished tape in the home so the patient or home caregiver can review it between visits.

Using videotapes

If your patient has a television and videocassette recorder, you can provide educational videotapes for him to watch. Be sure to leave written instructions to reinforce the videotaped instructions. For a list of relevant videotapes available for purchase, contact consumer health publishers and pharmaceutical companies. Some home health agencies may produce their own patient-teaching videos.

If you own a camcorder, consider preparing your own videos. A customized videotape is especially useful if you're teaching a complex procedure. Your home health agency may be able to provide an appropriate setting to use as a studio. To make the videotape, gather the required equipment, and then ask a friend or colleague to videotape you as you provide instructions or demonstrate a care procedure. If you're making a tape for a foreign-language patient, ask an interpreter to translate your words into the patient's native language as you provide instructions or perform the procedure on camera.

If you can't leave a purchased videotape with the patient for ongoing use, you may be able to make a copy of it. First, though, examine the label for a written permission statement.

Special considerations

◆ Be aware that a patient under physical or emotional stress, such as from poor health or an adverse effect of treatment, won't respond well to teaching. Don't force your teaching on him; instead, wait until he starts to show interest in learning. If a caregiver is available and willing to learn, start instructing this person during your early visits.

◆ Adjust your teaching pace to the topic and your patient. Be sure to use a slower pace for an elderly, debilitated patient.

◆ Break complex procedures into small sections to avoid overwhelming your patient. For example, when teaching about wound care, first describe which supplies to gather; next, how to remove and discard the old dressing; and then, how to examine the wound. Ideally, you should teach simple wound care over at least five sessions. If your time is too limited for this, cover more than one step during each visit.

◆ If your patient has an I.V. line or a feeding tube, teach a caregiver how to care for the line or tube in case of an emergency. If the patient lives alone, get the phone numbers of persons who may be available to help him in an emergency.

◆ Before concluding that your patient can perform self-care independently, review his technique during each step of the procedure you've taught him.

◆ If your patient received instructions in an acute care facility, reinforce those instructions because he may have forgotten them or may be using different equipment and supplies at home.

◆ Never force your teaching on a patient or home caregiver. Remember, the patient has the right to refuse care. If the patient or caregiver is unwilling or unable to learn crucial information and skills, you'll need to make other care arrangements. If the patient is elderly, contact a local center for the aging; it may be able to help him with his daily injections or ongoing personal hygiene needs.

◆ Document your teaching and the patient's response during every home visit.

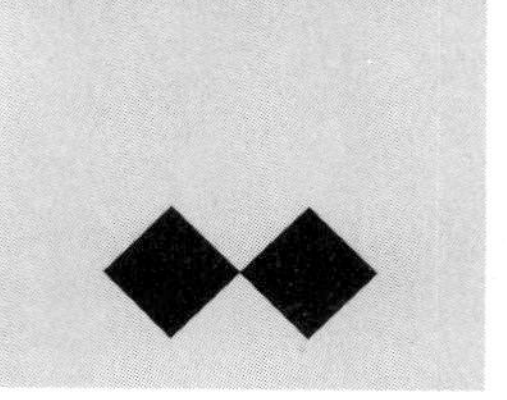

CHAPTER 11

Providing wound care

The principles of wound care — and many of the techniques for performing it — have remained essentially unchanged over the years. But that doesn't make wound care any less important than high-tech or specialized procedures created by new medical treatments and machines. In fact, effective wound care goes a long way toward maintaining patient comfort, decreasing anxiety, and reducing the risk of infection.

When caring for a patient who has a wound, you'll carry out procedures that help prevent infection by stopping pathogens from entering the wound or growing in it. Besides promoting patient comfort, such procedures protect the skin surface from maceration and excoriation caused by contact with irritating drainage. They also allow you to measure wound drainage and thus to monitor your patient's fluid and electrolyte balance.

As a home health nurse, you're in an excellent position to evaluate how well your patient's wound is healing. Ongoing assessment and early identification of poor healing are essential in guiding treatment and in preventing infection and other complications.

This chapter provides step-by-step instructions in essential wound care procedures. It explains how to clean a closed surgical wound, apply a topical dressing or pouching system, and deal with such emergencies as wound dehiscence and evisceration. It describes how to assess wound healing, remove sutures and skin staples, manage a closed-wound drain, and measure and evaluate wound drainage.

The chapter also details the techniques you'll use to irrigate, measure, and pack a wound; it also describes mechanical debridement. It concludes with a detailed discussion of pressure ulcers. For each wound care procedure, you'll find teaching tips that will help the patient or a home caregiver learn how to care for the wound.

Checking the doctor's orders

Orders for wound care must include the frequency of visits to perform such care, the expected end-point for daily visits (if ordered), supplies to be used, and specific wound care techniques to be used. Before going on a wound care visit, make sure your orders are complete.

Finding a willing caregiver

Many third-party payers have reduced the number of visits permitted for wound care. For this reason, make every effort to find a family member or friend of the patient who's willing to learn wound care and perform it regularly for him. Otherwise, you'll need to thoroughly document the reason for making ongoing nursing visits to provide wound care.

◆ CARING FOR A CLOSED SURGICAL WOUND

The care you provide for a closed surgical wound focuses on preventing infection while promoting healing. The most common methods of caring for a closed surgical wound include a topical dressing and a pouching system.

A topical dressing is preferred unless the wound is producing large amounts of drainage that is caustic to the skin. If wound drainage is excessive and may excoriate the skin, a pouching system is a better choice.

Equipment and preparation

Unless the doctor orders otherwise, use clean technique when caring for a closed surgical wound in the patient's home. Before you leave for the patient's home, review the procedure you'll use for the ordered wound care and select appropriate patient-teaching materials. Also assemble the following items:

◆ doctor's order identifying the type of dressing to use
◆ prescribed dressing treatment
◆ antiseptic solution, as ordered
◆ sterile 4″ × 4″ gauze sponges
◆ large sterile pads, if indicated
◆ sterile cotton-tipped applicators
◆ collection pouch with drainage port (if the patient has a pouch for drainage)
◆ hypoallergenic tape
◆ sterile and clean disposable gloves
◆ gown, face shield, or goggles, as indicated, for standard precautions
◆ waterproof trash bag
◆ soap, paper towels.

Implementation

When you arrive at the patient's home, explain what you'll be doing before you get started. Then assist him to a comfortable position that provides privacy. Spread a clean towel or pad near the patient and assemble your dressing supplies on it to prevent contamination. Wash your hands and put on clean gloves.

Removing the old dressing

Remove the old dressing gently to avoid causing or worsening skin excoriation from the tape. Inspect the old dressing to assess the type, color, amount, and odor of any drainage. Then discard the dressing in the waterproof trash bag. Remove your gloves and wash your hands.

Cleaning the wound

Now put on another pair of clean gloves. Open the package of gauze pads, and saturate them with the prescribed antiseptic solution. Squeeze any excess solution from the pads, and begin cleaning the wound. Always wipe from the clean area toward the less clean area — usually from the top of the incision line to the bottom (as shown below).

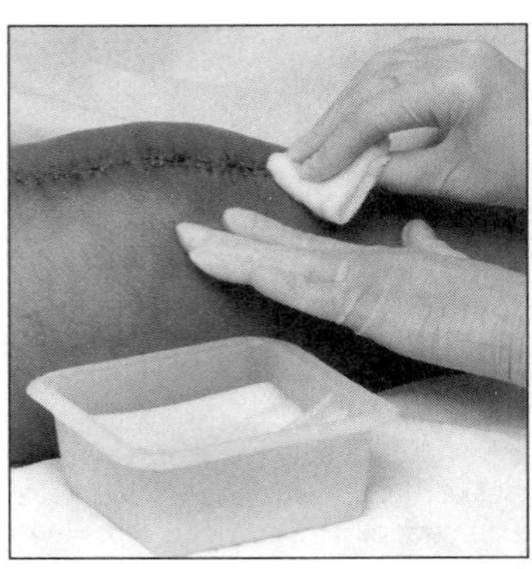

Clean as close to the incision line as possible, moving outward with each subsequent stroke. Use one gauze pad to clean one side of the wound, and discard it after use. Then, with a new saturated gauze pad, clean the other side of the incision line and discard that pad after use.

For crusted exudate or drainage, saturate a cotton-tipped applicator with antiseptic solution and apply it gently to the crusted areas to loosen them. Then, using a clean applicator, remove crusts from the incision area. Continue to clean the wound and incision line until you've covered the entire area.

Apply the prescribed topical antimicrobial ointment or solution with a saturated gauze pad or a clean cotton-tipped applicator. Take care not to disrupt any sutures, staples, or Steri-Strips while applying the medication.

If necessary, clean the skin surrounding the wound with soap and warm water. Thoroughly dry the skin before applying a new gauze dressing. Cover the incision line with gauze pads and apply enough tape to secure the gauze.

Discard all used items in the waterproof trash bag. Remove your gloves and wash your hands. Provide for patient comfort.

Pouching a wound

If the patient has a significant amount of wound drainage, or if drainage has damaged the surrounding skin, you may use a pouching system. If the doctor orders one, explain the procedure to the patient, and assist him to a comfortable position that provides privacy.

Assemble all supplies near the patient, placing a clean towel or pad under them to prevent contamination. Then wash your hands and put on nonsterile gloves.

If an old pouch is in place, remove it and inspect for drainage type, color, amount, and odor. Then discard it in the waterproof trash bag and close the bag securely.

Measure the wound, tracing its size onto the backing of the wound pouch. Cut the pouch backing about ⅛″ (0.3 cm) larger than the size of the wound (as shown below).

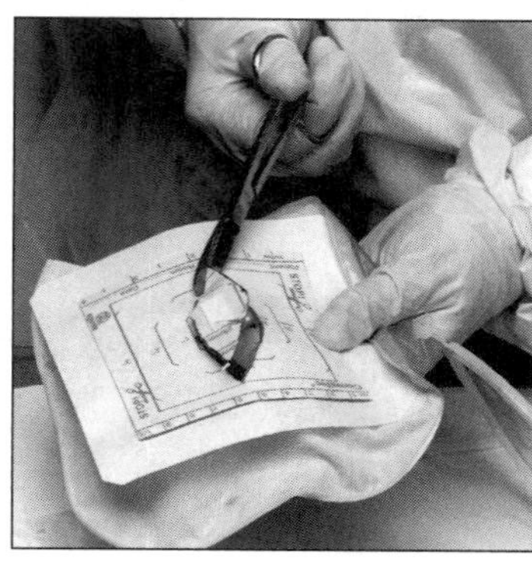

Remove your gloves and wash your hands. Then put on another pair of clean disposable gloves. Wash the skin with soap and warm water, and dry it thoroughly. Provide wound care as prescribed.

If necessary, paint the skin around the wound with a pad saturated with skin preparation solution. Allow the solution to dry before applying the pouch.

Remove the backing from the pouch adhesive and apply the pouch to the skin over the drainage portion of the wound. The drainage port on the pouch should be at the bottom of the wound and in the closed position. Make sure the pouch is affixed firmly to the patient's skin.

Remove all used disposable items and discard them in the waterproof trash bag. Remove your gloves and wash your hands. Make the patient comfortable.

Dealing with wound dehiscence and evisceration

When inspecting your patient's wound, stay alert for dehiscence and evisceration. *Dehiscence* occurs when the layers of a surgical wound separate. It may be partial and superficial

Responding to wound dehiscence

If wound dehiscence occurs, contact the doctor immediately. Help the patient into a reclining position and reassure him to help him stay calm. Cover the wound with gauze pads or sponges soaked in sterile normal saline solution. Then cover the wound with dry sterile gauze sponges and tape them in place. Stay with the patient until the doctor provides further instructions.

If the wound eviscerates, contact emergency medical services and prepare the patient for transport to an acute care facility. Cover the entire eviscerated area with sterile gauze pads or sponges saturated with sterile normal saline solution. Calm the patient, monitor his vital signs, and continue to assess the condition of the evisceration until emergency help arrives. Call the acute care facility where the patient will be taken to inform them of the patient's arrival and condition.

or complete, with disruption of all layers.

Dehiscence commonly occurs 3 to 11 days after wound formation. Depending on the degree of dehiscence, the patient might need additional sutures or topical skin closures, such as Steri-Strips or butterfly adhesive strips, to keep the wound closed. (See *Responding to wound dehiscence*.)

Dehiscence occurs primarily in abdominal wounds after a sudden strain, such as coughing, vomiting, or sitting up in bed. Obese patients are at high risk because of the constant strain placed on the wound and poor healing of fatty tissue.

Suspect *evisceration* if you can see body organs through the wound edges. In this medical emergency, all wound layers separate; you must act quickly to protect exposed tissues from infection and exposure.

Special considerations

◆ A closed surgical wound with insignificant drainage rarely requires numerous nursing visits if a home caregiver learns to care for the wound or if the patient can care for it himself. However, the patient who has a wound in a hard-to-reach area — or no in-home caregiver — will need nursing care until the wound no longer requires a dressing.
◆ If sterile technique is required, teach the patient or caregiver how to perform it.
◆ Instruct the patient to inspect the wound often and to report symptoms of infection — a low-grade fever; localized redness, pain, swelling, and warmth; or a change in drainage amount, color, or odor. Leave appropriate printed materials with him so he or a caregiver can review wound care techniques and eventually perform them independently.
◆ When documenting your care for a patient with a closed surgical wound, include the presence or absence of sutures, staples, or Steri-Strips; the wound's condition; evidence of healing; the presence or absence of infection; the date the patient will return to the doctor for suture or staple removal; and any teaching you provided.

◆ REMOVING SUTURES

When removing sutures from a healed wound, your goal is to avoid damaging newly formed tissue. The timing of suture removal depends on the shape, size, and location of the sutured incision; the presence or absence of inflammation, drainage, and infection; and the patient's general condition.

Techniques for removal depend on the method of suturing, but all require sterile technique to prevent contamination.

Equipment and preparation

Gather the following supplies:

◆ doctor's order to remove sutures at home
◆ suture removal kit (including sterile forceps and sterile suture scissors)
◆ antimicrobial solution
◆ Steri-Strips or butterfly adhesive strips (optional)
◆ waterproof trash bag
◆ prescribed topical dressing supplies
◆ sterile and clean disposable gloves
◆ gown, mask, and goggles, as indicated, for standard precautions
◆ soap, paper towels.

Place the supplies near the patient. Open the waterproof trash bag and place it near the bed. Position the bag properly to avoid reaching across the sterile field or the suture line when disposing of soiled articles. Form a cuff by turning down the top of the trash bag to provide a wide opening and prevent contamination of instruments or gloves that might touch the bag's edge.

Implementation

Explain the procedure to the patient. Assure him that it's usually painless, but that he may feel a tickling sensation as the stitches come out. Explain to him that because his wound is healing properly, removing the stitches won't weaken the incision.

Provide privacy, and position the patient so he's comfortable without placing undue tension on the suture line. Have him recline if possible, because some patients become dizzy or nauseated during the procedure. Adjust the light so it shines directly on the suture line.

Wash your hands. If the wound has a dressing in place, put on clean gloves and carefully remove it. Then discard the dressing and the gloves in the waterproof trash bag.

Observe the wound for possible gaping, drainage, inflammation, signs of infection, or embedded sutures. Contact the doctor if the wound isn't healing properly. The absence of a healing ridge under the suture line after 5 to 7 days suggests that the line needs continued support and protection during healing.

If the wound looks ready to have its sutures removed, establish a sterile work area. Put on sterile gloves and open the suture removal kit. Using sterile technique, clean the suture line. The cleaning process should moisten the sutures sufficiently to promote their removal. Then proceed according to the type of sutures you're removing. (See *Removing sutures,* pages 334 and 335.)

After you've removed the sutures, clean the incision line with sterile gauze pads soaked in an antimicrobial solution. If necessary, apply Steri-Strips or butterfly adhesive strips to support the incision line. Cover the incision line with sterile or clean gauze pads, and secure the pads with adhesive tape.

Discard your gloves and wash your hands. Properly clean or dispose of soiled supplies and equipment. Make the patient comfortable.

Removing sutures

The method used to remove sutures depends largely on the type of sutures in the wound. The illustrations below show removal steps for four common suture types. Regardless of the type, be sure to grasp and cut the sutures in the correct place to avoid pulling the exposed (thus contaminated) suture material through subcutaneous tissue.

Plain interrupted sutures

Using sterile forceps, grasp the knot of the first suture and raise it off the skin. This will expose a small portion of the suture that was below skin level.

Place the rounded tip of sterile curved-tip suture scissors against the skin and cut through the exposed portion of the suture. Still holding the knot with the forceps, pull the cut suture up and out of the skin in a smooth continuous motion to avoid causing the client pain. Discard the suture.

Repeat the process for every other suture, initially. If the wound doesn't gape, you can then remove the remaining sutures as ordered.

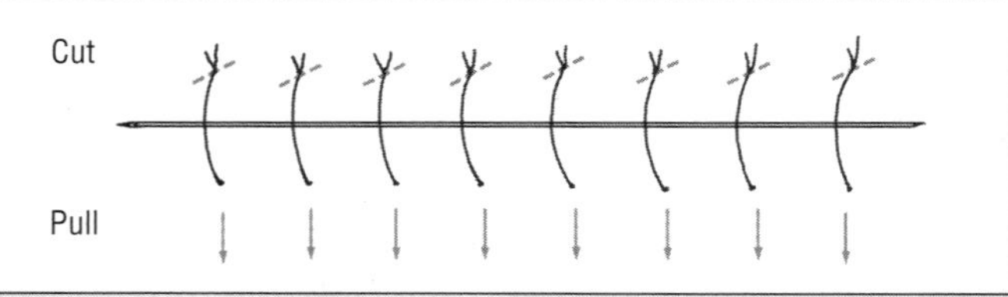

Mattress interrupted sutures

If possible, remove the small visible portion of the suture opposite the knot by cutting it at each visible end and lifting the small piece away from the skin to prevent pulling it through and contaminating subcutaneous tissue. Then remove the rest of the suture by pulling it out in the direction of the knot (as shown below). If the visible portion is too small to cut twice, cut it once and pull the entire suture out in the opposite direction.

Repeat for the remaining sutures and monitor the incision carefully for infection.

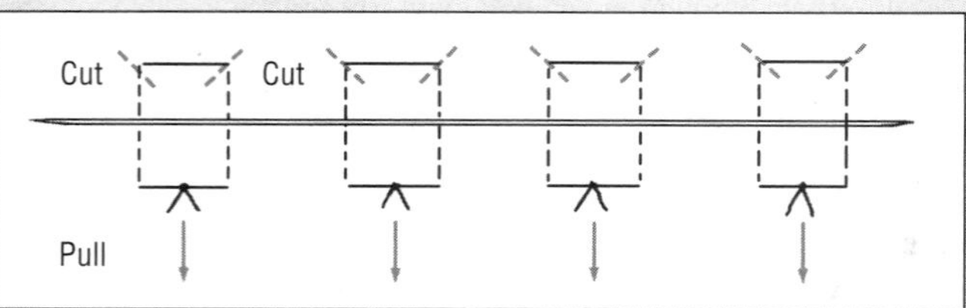

Removing sutures *(continued)*

Plain continuous sutures

Cut the first suture on the side opposite the knot. Next, cut the same side of the next suture in line. Then lift the first suture out in the direction of the knot. Proceed along the suture line, grasping each suture where you grasped the knot on the first one.

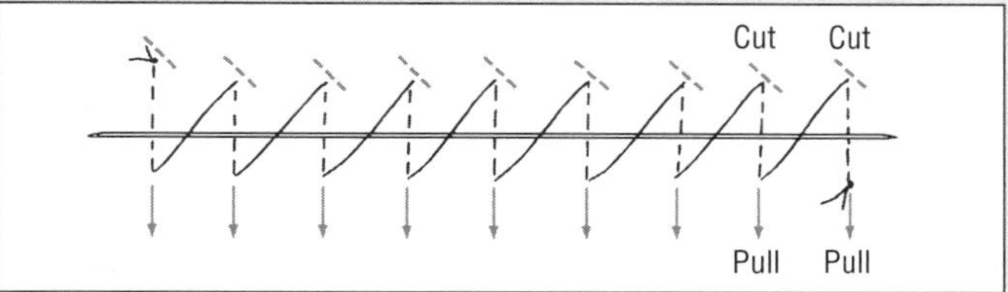

Mattress continuous sutures

Follow the procedure for removing mattress interrupted sutures, first removing the small visible portion of the suture, if possible, to prevent pulling it through and contaminating subcutaneous tissue. Then extract the rest of the suture in the direction of the knot.

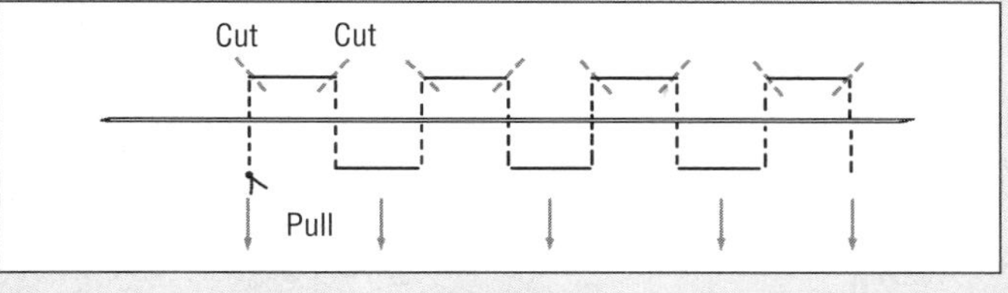

Special considerations

◆ If wound dehiscence occurs during suture removal, apply butterfly adhesive strips or Steri-Strips to support and approximate the edges. Call the doctor immediately so the wound can be repaired.

◆ Instruct the patient to call his doctor at once if he observes wound discharge or other abnormal changes. Point out that the redness surrounding the incision should gradually disappear and that, after a few weeks, only a thin line should show.

◆ Document the date and time of suture removal, type and number of sutures removed, appearance of the suture line, any signs of complication, any dressings or butterfly adhesive strips applied, and the patient's tolerance of the procedure.

◆ REMOVING STAPLES

Occasionally, you may be ordered to remove skin staples for a patient in the home. Used instead of standard sutures to close surgical wounds, staples can secure a wound more quickly than sutures. They may substitute for surface sutures where cosmetic results aren't a prime consideration, as in abdominal closure. When prop-

Removing staples

Position the extractor's lower jaws beneath the span of the first staple (as shown in the first illustration). Squeeze the handles until they're completely closed; then lift the staple away from the skin (as shown in the bottom illustration). The extractor changes the shape of the staple and pulls the prongs out of the intradermal tissue.

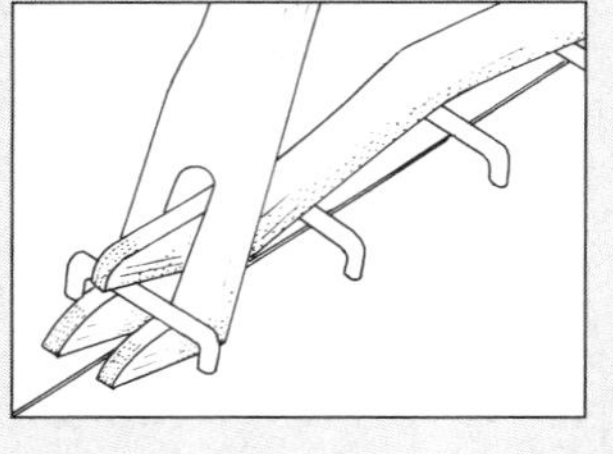

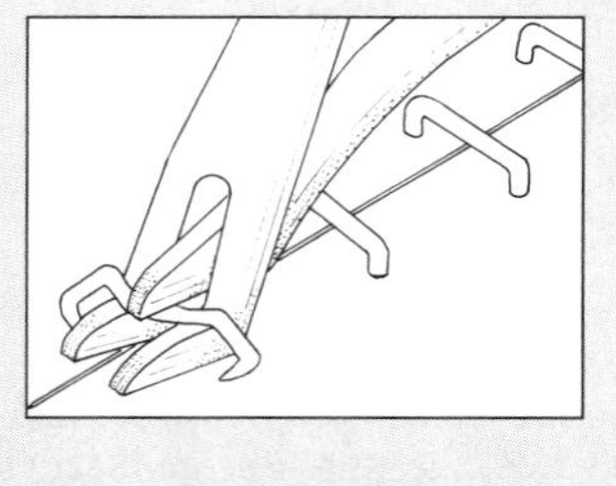

erly placed, staples distribute tension evenly along the suture line with minimal tissue trauma and compression, promoting healing and minimizing scarring.

Equipment and preparation

Gather the following supplies:

- ◆ doctor's order to remove staples at home
- ◆ sterile staple extractor
- ◆ sterile and clean disposable gloves
- ◆ gown, mask, and goggles, as indicated, for standard precautions
- ◆ prescribed topical dressing supplies
- ◆ Steri-Strips or butterfly adhesive strips (optional)
- ◆ waterproof trash bag
- ◆ soap, paper towels.

Assemble all supplies near the bedside. Open the waterproof trash bag and place it near the bed, positioning it so you won't have to reach across the sterile field or the wound to dispose of soiled items. Turn down the edge of the bag to form a cuff.

Implementation

Explain the procedure to the patient. Tell him that he may feel a slight pulling or tickling sensation. Reassure him that removing the supporting staples or clips won't weaken the incision line. Provide privacy, and help the patient to a comfortable position that doesn't place undue tension on the incision.

Wash your hands. If the wound has a dressing, put on clean gloves and carefully remove it. Discard the dressing and gloves in the waterproof trash bag. Assess the wound, and note any gaping, drainage, inflammation, or other signs of infection (which must be reported to the doctor).

Establish a sterile work area. Open the package containing the staple extractor, then put on sterile gloves.

Wipe the incision site gently with gauze sponges soaked in antimicrobial solution. Pick up the staple extractor. Starting at one end of the incision, remove the first staple. Hold the extractor over the trash bag, and release the handle to discard the staple. Repeat the procedure for each staple until all staples are removed. (See *Removing staples*.)

Then clean the incision line. Apply Steri-Strips or butterfly adhesive strips, if needed, for support. Cover the incision with sterile or clean gauze pads, and secure the pads with adhesive tape. Remove your gloves and wash your hands. Properly dispose of soiled supplies and equipment. Make the patient comfortable.

Special considerations

◆ Before beginning the procedure, carefully check the doctor's order for the time and extent of staple removal. You may need to remove only alternating staples or clips initially, leaving the others in place for another day or two to support the incision.
◆ When removing a staple, place the extractor's jaws carefully between the patient's skin and the staple to avoid patient discomfort.
◆ If wound dehiscence develops after staples are removed, apply butterfly adhesive strips or Steri-Strips to approximate and support the wound's edges. Call the doctor immediately so the wound can be repaired.
◆ Teach the patient or a caregiver how to remove the dressing and care for the wound. Instruct him to call the patient's doctor immediately if he observes wound discharge or any other abnormal change. Tell him that the redness surrounding the incision should gradually disappear and that, after a few weeks, only a thin line should show.
◆ Document the date and time of staple removal, the number of staples removed, the appearance of the incision, any dressings or butterfly adhesive strips applied, any signs of complication, and the patient's tolerance of the procedure.

◆ MANAGING A CLOSED-WOUND DRAIN

Typically inserted during surgery in anticipation of substantial postoperative drainage, a closed-wound drain consists of a perforated tube connected to a mechanical vacuum unit. The perforated end of the tubing lies within the wound (although usually not within the suture line) to preserve wound integrity.

Closed-wound drains promote healing and prevent fluid accumulation at the wound site. Fluid removal decreases the need for frequent dressing changes and reduces the risk of wound infection and skin breakdown. The most commonly used closed-wound drains are the Hemovac and Jackson-Pratt drains.

With more patients now returning home with closed-wound drains, you must know how to care for these drains expertly, troubleshoot problems, and teach the patient or caregiver how to manage a drain.

Equipment and preparation

Before you leave for the patient's home, select appropriate teaching materials. Find out what type of drainage system the patient has by contacting the doctor or the acute care facility where the drain was placed.

Also obtain the following information:
◆ drain location
◆ amount of drainage collecting, on average, over a set period of time
◆ drainage color, consistency, and odor
◆ presence of any sutures
◆ type of dressing to apply over the drainage site.

Then assemble the following items:
◆ doctor's order for drain removal
◆ irrigation tray or other receptacle for drainage collection
◆ graduated biohazard cylinder
◆ povidone-iodine sponges
◆ topical antimicrobial ointment as prescribed
◆ sterile and nonsterile 4″ × 4″ gauze pads
◆ disposable measuring tape

◆ several pairs of sterile disposable gloves
◆ gown, mask, and goggles, as indicated, for standard precautions
◆ waterproof trash bag
◆ soap, paper towels.

Implementation

When you arrive at the patient's home, explain the procedure, provide privacy, and help the patient to a comfortable position. Wash your hands and put on gloves.

If the site is covered by a dressing, remove it to expose the drain insertion site, wound, drain tubing, and drain. Remove any tape from around the drain and straighten the tubing. Examine the tubing for kinks and tears. If the drain is sutured in place, assess suture integrity. Measure the entire length of the tubing and document your findings.

Analyze the skin around the insertion site. Check for signs of pulling or tearing as well as swelling and infection of the wound and surrounding skin (as shown below).

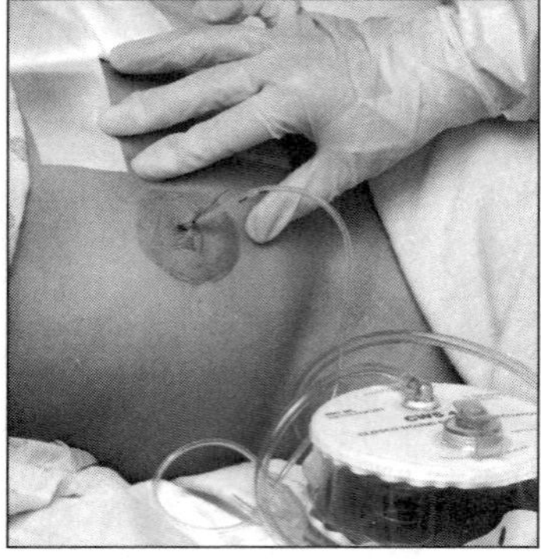

Remove your gloves and wash your hands. Put on another pair of gloves.

Provide wound care at the drain insertion site. Clean the entire area with povidone-iodine sponges, starting at the insertion site and moving outward. Continue to clean the perimeter around the insertion site until the entire wound area has been cleaned. If necessary, repeat the procedure.

If ordered, apply a topical antimicrobial ointment at the drain insertion site, and cover the site with a sterile gauze dressing. Tape drainage tubing in place as appropriate to prevent it from catching on items and being pulled out of place (as shown below). Provide wound care to the drain site as prescribed.

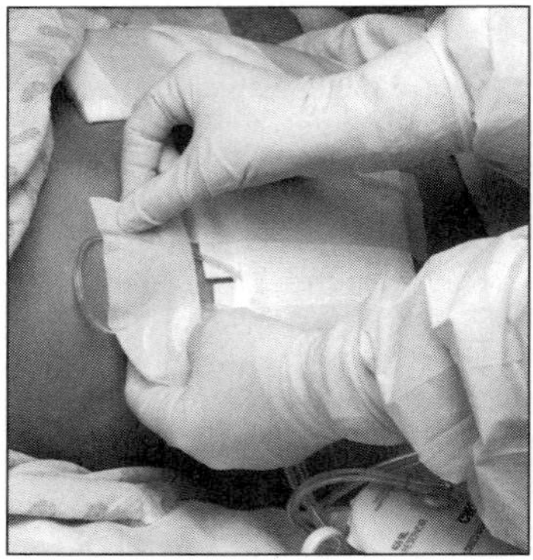

Remember that the drain wound and surgical wound are two separate wounds and should be cared for separately. When you've finished caring for the drain wound, provide care for the surgical wound, as ordered. Don't tape both dressings together.

Once you've completed wound care, remove your gloves and wash your hands. Then put on a clean pair of gloves. Position the irrigation tray or other drainage receptacle so that the drain can empty. Holding the drain in your nondominant hand, open the drain spout with your dominant hand. Carefully pour the drain contents into a graduated biohazard receptacle.

Then apply pressure to the drain unit and close the drainage spout snugly (as shown at the top of the next page).

Inspect the drain unit to make sure there's no air leak. Secure the drain tubing to the patient by looping the

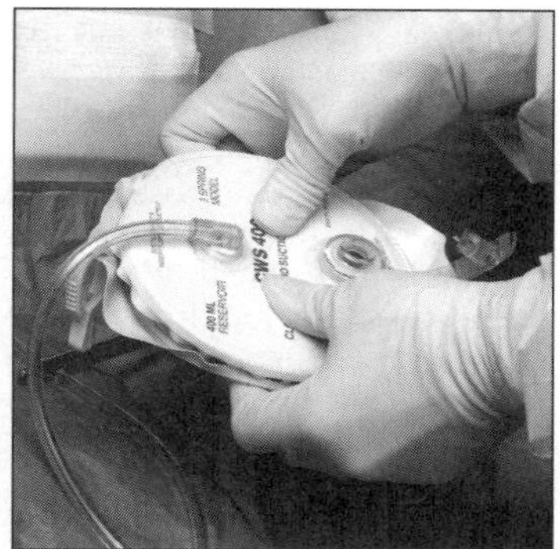

tubing and then taping it. Fasten the drain collection unit to the patient's clothing if he's ambulatory or to the bed if he's bedbound. To promote drainage, make sure the drain unit is below wound level.

Before discarding the drainage, assess and document its amount, color, consistency, and odor. Rinse and clean all reusable items and store them for later use. Discard used disposable items in the waterproof trash bag. Remove your gloves, wash your hands, and make the patient comfortable.

Caring for a Penrose drain

If the patient has a Penrose drain, it may lie directly under the gauze dressing, extend through the dressing, and connect to a drainage bag or suction apparatus. To prevent the drain from slipping into the wound, it may be attached by a clip or safety pin.

Expect the dressings around a Penrose drain to be highly saturated, especially if the drain isn't connected to a collection device. To collect the additional drainage, place additional layers of gauze or heavy pads on top of the dressing.

When caring for a Penrose drain, remove the old dressing, assess the drainage, and care for the drain site and surrounding skin. Then cover the site with a reinforced gauze dressing (as shown below) and tape the dressing securely.

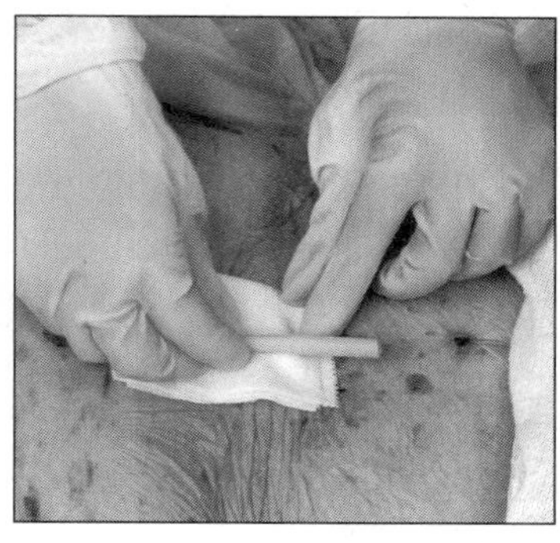

Regularly measure the length of drain that's exposed through the skin; notify the patient's doctor if it increases or decreases.

Special considerations

◆ Depending on the type of surgery the patient had, there may be more than one drainage tubing site. If so, perform care for each wound.
◆ Ensure the integrity of the drain until its removal. After removal, perform wound care similar to that for a closed surgical wound (with or without packing or wound pouching).
◆ Teach the patient or a caregiver how to care for the wound and drain. Explain how often to empty the drainage container, how to measure and document the amount of drainage, how to assess drainage characteristics, and how to detect signs and symptoms of infection.

Instruct the patient or caregiver to contact the home care agency right away if he detects a sudden change in drainage (especially if a profusely draining wound suddenly stops draining), if the drain becomes accidentally dislodged from the wound bed, or if he suddenly sees bright red drainage, clots, or other material in the tubing or collection chamber.

Also instruct him to report signs and symptoms of wound infection, including fever, chills, increased tenderness around the wound or drain site, pain, and yellow, green, or purulent drainage.

◆ IRRIGATING A WOUND

Wound irrigation removes cell debris and drainage from an open wound. Flushing these products from the wound bed promotes healing from the inside tissue layers to the outer skin surface. For most patients, you'll perform wound irrigation using sterile technique, then apply a sterile dressing.

Equipment and preparation

If an irrigation kit isn't available, gather the following items:

◆ doctor's order for wound irrigation, specifying the irrigating solution, frequency of irrigation, and any use of mechanical devices (such as an oral irrigation device [WaterPik] or a home whirlpool)
◆ prescribed irrigating solution
◆ emesis basin or clean bowl
◆ plastic sheets or towels
◆ sterile soft catheter
◆ sterile 35-ml syringe
◆ dressing supplies, as ordered
◆ mechanical irrigation device, if ordered
◆ sterile and clean gloves
◆ goggles, mask, and gown, as indicated, for standard precautions
◆ disposable wound measurement guide or paper measuring tape
◆ waterproof trash bag
◆ soap, paper towels.

Before you arrive at the patient's home, review the ordered procedure for wound irrigation. Make sure you have enough irrigating solution and dressing supplies. If you plan to instruct the patient on independent wound care during this visit, select appropriate teaching materials.

Implementation

At the patient's home, assemble all supplies on a sterile drape or clean towel near the patient. Wash your hands. Check the sterilization date and the date that each bottle of irrigating solution was opened; don't use any solution that's been open longer than 24 hours.

Explain the procedure to the patient and help him to a comfortable position that provides privacy. Place a plastic sheet, drape, or towel under him to protect the clothing or bedding.

Put on clean gloves, remove the old dressing from the wound (if present), and discard it in the waterproof trash bag. Analyze the wound for size, depth, width, drainage, color, and presence or absence of granulation tissue. After measuring the wound, discard the wound measurement guide or paper tape. Remove your gloves and wash your hands.

Warm the prescribed irrigating solution (usually normal saline solution) to at least room temperature. *Important:* Don't use a microwave to warm the solution.

Pour the warm solution into a sterile container. Place the clean bowl or emesis basin at the lower end of the wound to catch the solution.

Put on sterile gloves and attach the soft catheter to a 35-ml sterile syringe. Fill the syringe with irrigating solution. Take care not to contaminate the tip of the catheter.

Irrigate the entire wound, starting at the center of the wound and working outward. Gently instill a slow, steady stream of irrigating solution into the wound until the syringe empties. (See *Irrigating a deep wound.*) Make sure the solution flows from

Irrigating a deep wound

Position the patient so that an emesis basin can be placed under the wound. Hold the syringe so that the tip of the irrigating catheter is 1″ to 2″ (2.5 to 5 cm) from the wound. Push down on the plunger to flush the surface of the wound with the irrigant (as shown below). Point the tip of the catheter into all areas of the wound bed. Use the full force of the solution to debride loose tissue. To avoid damaging new granulation tissue, change to a gentle stream in these areas.

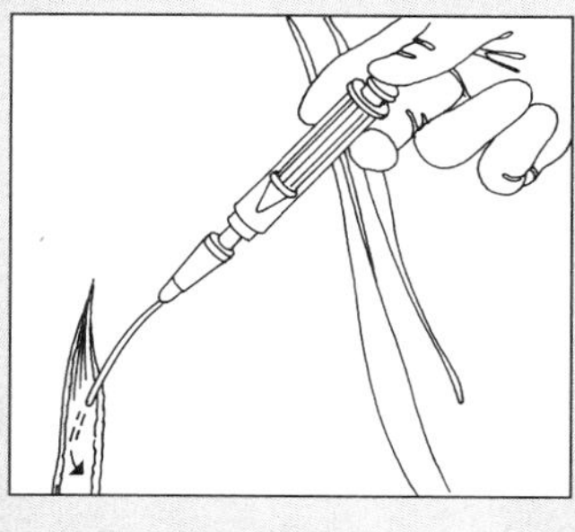

Refill the syringe, and repeat the procedure until you've irrigated all areas of the wound. Leave the emesis basin under the wound to collect excess drainage (as shown below).

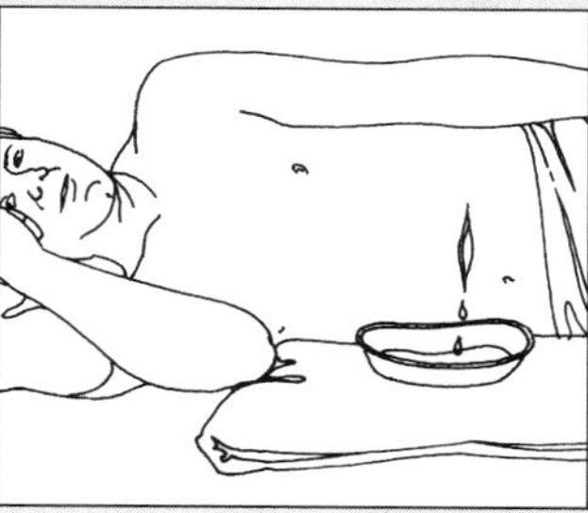

Then place the syringe and catheter in the irrigant container. Use the dry sterile gauze to gently blot — not rub — the skin surrounding the wound.

If the patient reports pain during the procedure, consider adjusting the irrigation schedule to coincide with his pain medication's peak effect.

the clean to the dirty area of the wound and reaches all areas of the wound. Also be sure to irrigate all pockets or sinus tracts. The irrigating solution should drain out from the wound into the emesis basin or bowl.

Continue irrigating until you've administered the prescribed amount of solution and all the solution has drained from the wound. (Alternatively, you can use 4″× 4″ gauze pads to absorb the irrigating solution.) Then remove the basin or bowl.

Make sure all surrounding skin is dry. Then pack and dress the wound as prescribed. Discard used disposable items in the waterproof trash bag. Remove and discard your gloves, wash your hands, and provide for patient comfort.

Tailoring wound care to wound color

If your patient has an open wound, assess how well it's healing by inspecting its color. Also use the wound's color to guide your management approach.

Red wounds. Red, the color of healthy granulation tissue, indicates normal healing. When a wound begins to heal, a layer of pale pink granulation tissue covers the wound bed. As this layer thickens, it becomes beefy red.

Cover a red wound, keep it moist and clean, and protect it from trauma. As ordered, use a transparent dressing (such as Tegaderm or Op-Site), a hydrocolloid dressing (such as DuoDerm), or a gauze dressing moistened with sterile normal saline solution or impregnated with petroleum jelly or an antibiotic.

Yellow wounds. Yellow is the color of exudate produced by microorganisms in an open wound. When a wound heals without complications, the immune system removes microorganisms. But if there are too many microorganisms to remove, exudate accumulates and becomes visible. Exudate usually appears whitish yellow, creamy yellow, yellowish green, or beige. Water content influences the shade: Dry exudate appears darker.

If your patient has a yellow wound, clean it and remove exudate using high-pressure irrigation as ordered. Then cover it with a moist dressing. As ordered, use absorptive products (for example, Debrisan beads and paste) or a moist gauze dressing with or without an antibiotic. The patient's doctor also may order hydrotherapy with a whirlpool or high-pressure irrigation. Help the patient make arrangements to receive these treatments as an outpatient in a rehabilitation center of a local hospital, if appropriate.

Black wounds. Black, the least healthy color, signals necrosis. Dead, avascular tissue slows healing and provides a site for microorganisms to proliferate.

Usually, the doctor orders debridement of a black wound. After removing dead tissue, apply a dressing as ordered to keep the wound moist and guard against external contamination. As ordered, use enzyme products (such as Elase or Travase), surgical debridement, hydrotherapy with a whirlpool or high-pressure irrigation, or a moist gauze dressing.

Multicolored wounds. You may note two or even all three colors in a wound. In this case, you'd classify the wound according to the least healthy color present. For example, if your patient's wound is both red and yellow, classify it as a yellow wound.

Using a mechanical irrigating device

When using a mechanical device — such as a high-pressure oral irrigating system or a whirlpool — to remove debris from the wound, make sure you don't cause further injury to the wound bed during the procedure. Always use a steady stream of irrigant (syringe) instead of a sporadic stream (bulb syringe).

The best pressure for wound irrigation is 8 lb/square inch. However, oral irrigating devices typically deliver pressure at 50 to 70 lb/square inch, which can damage the wound bed and hinder healing. To lower the pressure, use a 35-ml syringe with a soft catheter.

A whirlpool is usually indicated to promote removal of thick exudate, slough, or necrotic tissue. Although it's effective for wound irrigation, a pressurized rinse may be a better choice for removing bacteria. A whirlpool is rarely indicated to irrigate a clean wound because it can damage granulation tissue.

Before using a mechanical irrigating device, clean the surrounding skin with a topical antiseptic solution or with soap and water, as prescribed. After you've removed all debris and drainage, inspect the wound bed for signs of healing or infection.

Special considerations

◆ Use sterile technique when irrigating a wound, unless ordered otherwise.

◆ Instruct a caregiver, if available, on the appropriate technique for irrigating and caring for the patient's wound.

◆ PACKING A WOUND

Packing a wound promotes healing from the inner tissue layers of the wound to the outer skin surface. It's commonly ordered for a patient who's recovering from abdominal surgery or who has experienced a wound complication, such as infection, necrosis, hematoma, or sinus tract formation. Wound packing usually calls for sterile technique. (See *Packing a wound.*)

Equipment and preparation

Gather the following supplies:

◆ doctor's order specifying the type of packing material, packing solution, and frequency of packing
◆ sterile normal saline solution or other packing solution
◆ sterile disposable gloves and several pairs of clean disposable gloves
◆ gown, mask, and goggles, as indicated, for standard precautions
◆ sterile cotton-tipped applicators
◆ sterile gauze packing (¼″, ½″)
◆ sterile and nonsterile 4″ × 4″ gauze pads
◆ two sterile suture removal kits (including sterile forceps and sterile scissors)
◆ heavy gauze pads (such as ABD pads)
◆ adhesive tape, Montgomery straps, or abdominal binder
◆ sterile drape or towel
◆ waterproof trash bag
◆ soap, paper towels.

Also gather appropriate teaching materials so you can begin instruction on wound packing.

Packing a wound

Using sterile forceps, pack the wound with sterile moist gauze pads (as shown here).

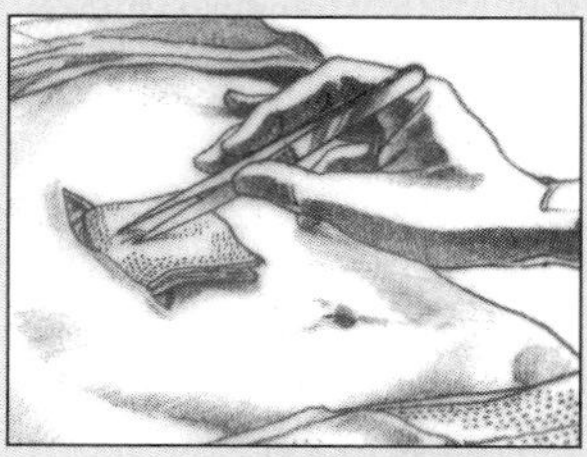

Loosely pack the wound cavity carefully with fluffed, moist sterile gauze pads. Make sure that all wound surfaces are covered and kept moist so that complete debridement can take place and granulation tissue can maintain hydration.

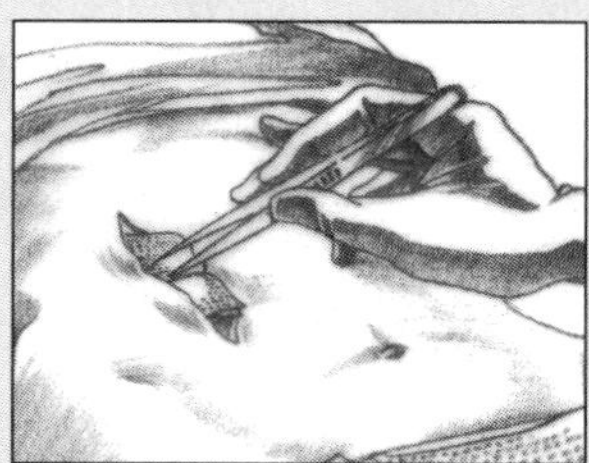

Remember to pack the wound only until the wound surfaces and edges are covered. Packing that overlaps the edge can cause maceration of surrounding tissues.

Implementation

Explain the purpose of wound packing to the patient. Provide privacy and help him to a comfortable position. Then arrange all supplies near the patient. Place a disposable drape or

How to make Montgomery straps

An abdominal dressing requiring frequent changes can be secured with Montgomery straps to promote the patient's comfort. If ready-made straps aren't available, follow these steps to make your own.

Cutting and folding the tape strips

Cut four to six strips of 2″ to 3″ (5 to 7.6 cm) nonallergenic tape of sufficient length to allow the tape to extend about 6″ (15 cm) beyond the wound on each side. (The length of the tape varies, depending on the patient's size and the type and amount of dressing.)

Fold one end of each strip 2″ or 3″ back on itself (sticky sides together) to form a nonadhesive tab. Then cut a small hole in the folded tab's center, close to its top edge. Make as many pairs of straps as you'll need to snugly secure the dressing.

Applying the straps

Clean the patient's skin to prevent irritation. After the skin dries, apply a skin protectant.

Then apply the sticky side of each tape to a skin barrier sheet composed of opaque hydrocolloidal or nonhydrocolloidal materials, and apply the sheet directly to the skin near the dressing.

Next, thread a separate piece of gauze tie, umbilical tape, or twill tape (about 12″ [30.5 cm] long) through each pair of holes in the straps and fasten each tie as you would a shoelace. Don't stress the surrounding skin by securing the ties too tightly. Repeat this procedure according to the number of Montgomery straps needed.

Replace Montgomery straps whenever they become soiled (every 2 or 3 days). If skin maceration occurs, place new tapes about 1″ (2.5 cm) away from any irritation.

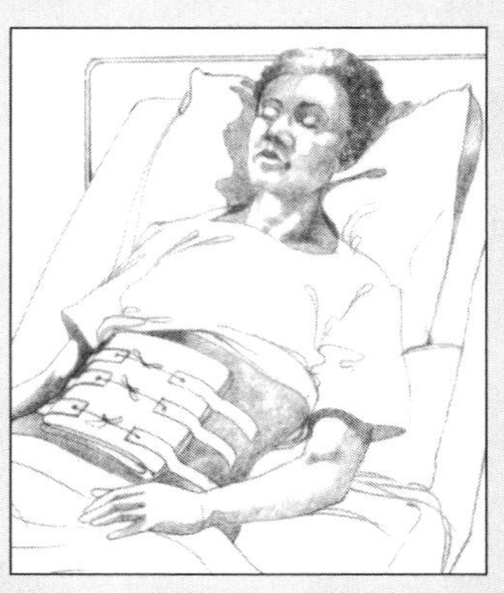

clean towel under him to protect his clothing or bedding.

Wash your hands and put on clean gloves. Remove the tape from the old dressing. Then remove the top layer of gauze and assess the wound for drainage and other characteristics. Discard the old dressing in the waterproof trash bag.

Remove the used gloves and wash your hands. Then put on new clean gloves. With the sterile forceps from a suture removal kit, remove the packing from the wound. Analyze the packing for the amount and color of drainage, and measure the length of packing used in the previous packing session.

Provide wound care according to the doctor's order. Clean the surrounding skin with warm water and dry it thoroughly. Inspect the entire area for signs of healing or infection. Measure the depth and width of the wound and assess the color of the wound bed.

Remove the used gloves and wash your hands. Then prepare to apply a sterile dressing. Open all sterile packages without contaminating them. Place a sterile drape over the wound site.

Put on the mask, gown, and sterile gloves. Using sterile technique, saturate the sterile packing in the prescribed solution, if ordered. If dry packing is ordered, begin placing sterile packing in the wound using the sterile forceps. To make sure all areas in the wound are packed, use a sterile cotton-tipped applicator to help place the packing.

After the wound has been packed, place dry gauze over the entire wound area. If the packing is moist, place heavy gauze pads over the wound site. Secure the entire dressing with adhesive tape, Montgomery straps, or an abdominal binder. (See *How to make Montgomery straps*.)

Discard all used disposable items in the waterproof trash bag. Label the opened bottle of packing material with the date, time, and your name. Remove your gloves and wash your hands. Make the patient comfortable.

Special considerations

◆ Thoroughly document all wound care to indicate the need for ongoing home care visits and thus ensure reimbursement. Be aware that the frequency of reimbursed nursing visits may decrease if a willing caregiver is available to pack the patient's wound. However, weekly nursing visits will still be required to assess wound healing and evaluate this caregiver's technique.

◆ CARING FOR PRESSURE ULCERS

A pressure ulcer is a localized area of tissue necrosis that results when pressure — applied with great force over a short period or with less force over a longer period — impairs circulation, thus depriving tissue of oxygen and other nutrients. This process damages skin and underlying structures. Untreated, the ischemic lesion can lead to necrosis and serious infection.

Successful treatment of pressure ulcers involves relieving pressure, restoring circulation and, if possible, resolving or managing related disorders. Typically, you'll apply a topical agent directly to the wound and cover it with a dressing. However, specific treatment varies with the ulcer's characteristics. (See *Stages of pressure ulcers,* page 346.)

Predisposing factors

Pressure, shear, friction, and moisture combine to produce pressure ulcers. *Pressure* — the force exerted on an area — is the most essential factor in ulcer development. Applying pressure to the skin in excess of venous capillary pressure (higher than 30 to 40 mm Hg) leads to localized tissue ischemia. The degree of tissue necrosis varies when pressure is applied over a bony prominence; pressure is greatest over the bone and diminishes outward. The result is a cone-shaped area of necrosis beneath the skin surface, commonly presenting as a closed ulcer.

Shear occurs when layers of tissue slide over each other, causing kinking or tearing of tissue and blood vessels. Shear commonly results when

Stages of pressure ulcers

To select the most effective treatment for a pressure ulcer, you first need to assess its characteristics. The pressure ulcer stages described below, used by the National Pressure Ulcer Advisory Panel and the Agency for Health Care Policy and Research, reflect the anatomic depth of exposed tissue. Keep in mind that if the wound contains necrotic tissue, you won't be able to determine the stage until you can see the wound base.

Stage 1
A reddened area of intact skin that doesn't blanch

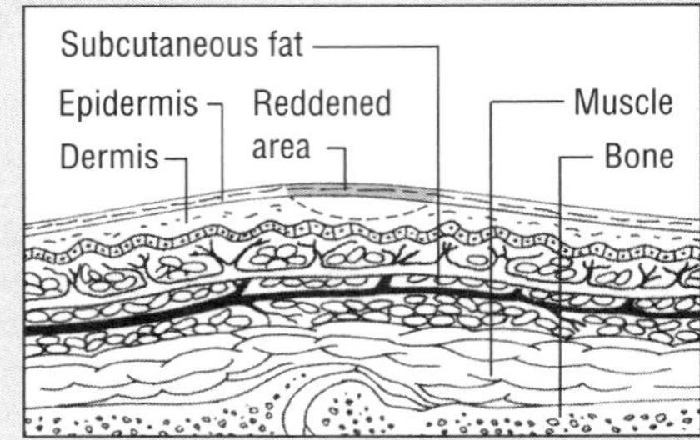

Stage 2
Partial-thickness skin loss involving the epidermis, dermis, or both; ulcer appears as an abrasion, a blister, or a shallow crater

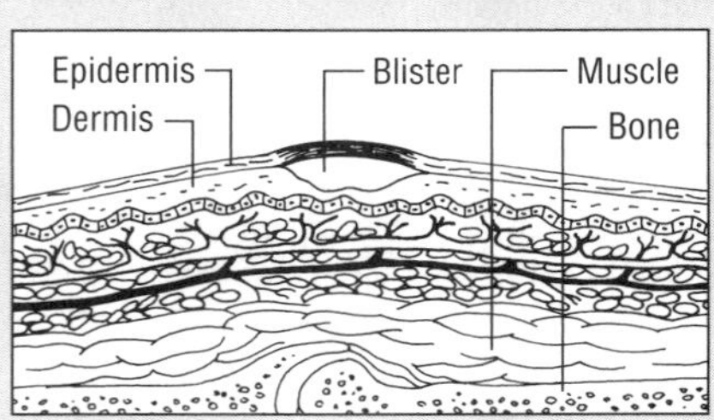

Stage 3
Full-thickness wound that penetrates subcutaneous tissue and may extend to but not through underlying fascia; a deep crater that may undermine adjacent tissue

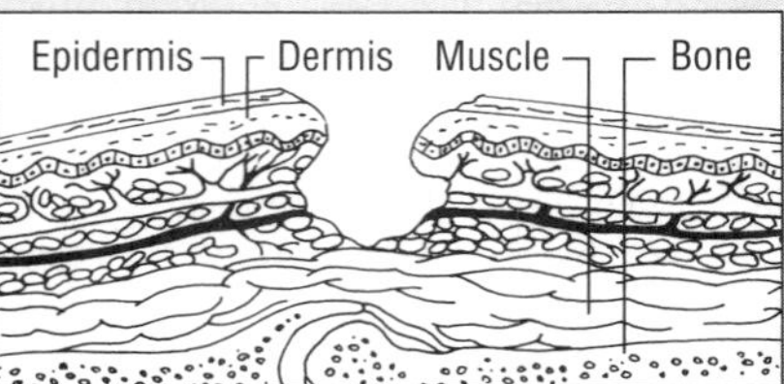

Stage 4
Extensive destruction, tissue necrosis, or damage to muscle, bone, or supporting structures (such as tendons and joint capsules)

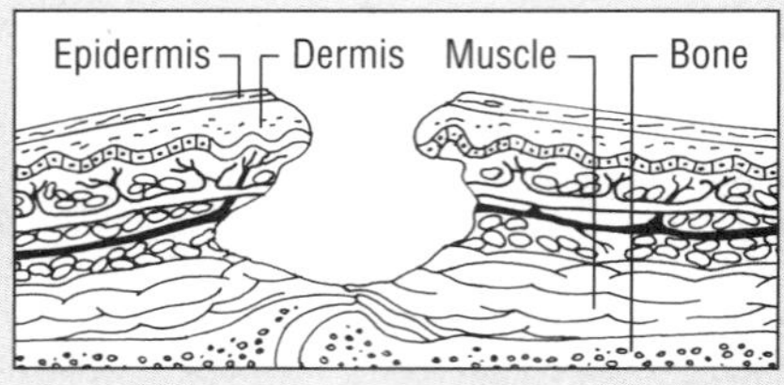

a patient slides down from a semi-sitting position in bed.

Friction is the force created when two surfaces come in contact with and move across each other. It can occur when a patient is pulled across a surface, such as a bed. Friction that breaks the outer skin surface can create a future ulcer site.

Moisture may result from contact with such substances as urine, feces, wound drainage, or perspiration. Such contact leads to skin maceration, increasing the risk of ulceration.

High-risk patients

Many home care patients are prone to developing pressure ulcers because of their underlying health condition and physical debilitation. Specific patients at high risk for pressure ulcers include:

- ◆ elderly, immobilized, or debilitated patients with chronic illness
- ◆ patients with altered mental status
- ◆ patients with decreased sensory or motor sensation, as from a cerebrovascular accident, peripheral vascular disease, or diabetes.

Most pressure ulcers develop over bony prominences, where friction and shearing force combine with pressure to break down skin and underlying tissues. (See *Common pressure ulcer sites,* pages 348 and 349.) Other conditions that increase the risk of pressure ulcer development include anemia, diaphoresis, edema, fever, incontinence, jaundice, malnutrition, obesity, pruritus, and xerosis.

Assessment guidelines

Be sure to assess all home care patients for the risk for pressure ulcers. Factors to evaluate include:

- ◆ general physical condition
- ◆ weight
- ◆ daily nutritional intake (also socioeconomic status if nutritional intake is an issue)
- ◆ fluid or hydration status
- ◆ bladder and bowel continence
- ◆ level of responsiveness
- ◆ mobility
- ◆ presence or absence of chronic debilitating disease.

Equipment and preparation

Gather the following supplies:

- ◆ doctor's order for the topical agent or dressing
- ◆ prescribed topical agent (See *Guide to topical agents for pressure ulcers*, page 350.)
- ◆ irrigating tray (including a large piston syringe)
- ◆ sterile normal saline solution
- ◆ sterile 4″ × 4″ gauze pads
- ◆ clean towels or disposable pads
- ◆ wound measuring guide or tape
- ◆ several pairs of disposable gloves (sterile or clean, as ordered)
- ◆ gown, mask, goggles, as indicated, for standard precautions
- ◆ waterproof trash bag
- ◆ soap, paper towels.

Explain the procedure to the patient and assist him to a comfortable position that provides privacy. Place a disposable drape or clean towel under him to protect clothing or bedding.

Assemble your supplies at the patient's bedside. Loosen the lids on cleaning solutions and medications so you can remove them easily. Loosen existing dressing edges and tapes before putting on gloves. Place a waterproof trash bag near the bed to hold used dressings and refuse. Then wash your hands and put on clean disposable gloves.

Cleaning the pressure ulcer

If you plan to irrigate the ulcer, prepare the irrigating solution and fill the piston syringe. Remove the old dressing and any layers of medication-soaked gauze. Assess the characteristics of the drainage and

Common pressure ulcer sites

Common sites where pressure ulcers develop include the sacrum, coccyx, ischial tuberosities, and greater trochanters. Patient positioning plays a role in the site of ulcer development, as these illustrations show.

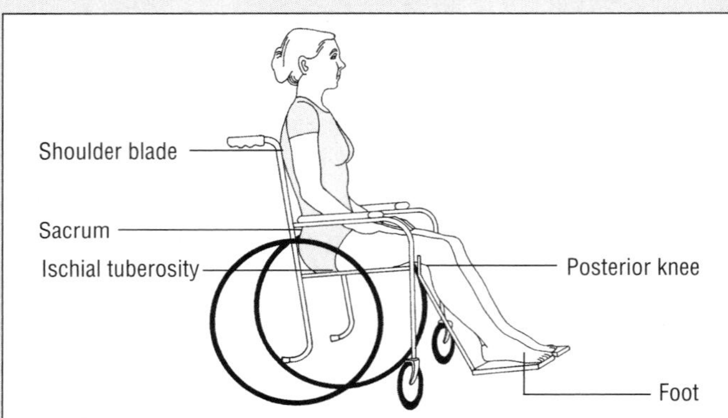

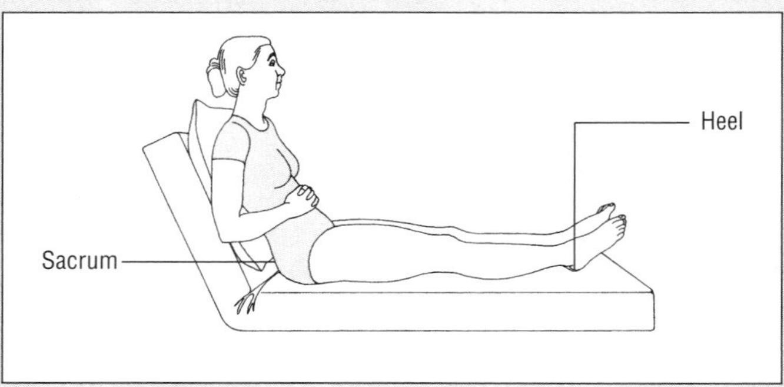

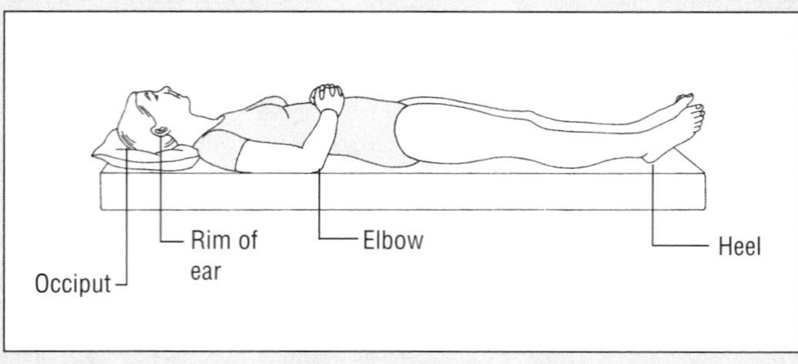

Common pressure ulcer sites *(continued)*

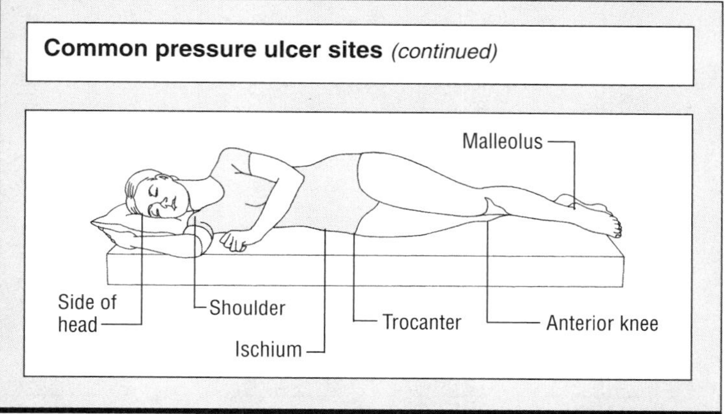

other material. Then discard the old dressing in the trash bag.

Inspect the wound, noting any new areas of necrosis. Using a wound measuring guide or tape, measure the depth and perimeter of the wound; document any change from your last visit.

Remove your gloves, wash your hands, and put on sterile or clean disposable gloves, as ordered. Irrigate the wound and provide wound care, as ordered. Clean the surrounding skin with warm water and dry it thoroughly. Remove your gloves and wash your hands. Then prepare to apply the ordered topical dressing.

Applying a saline gauze dressing

Irrigate the pressure ulcer with normal saline solution. Blot the surrounding skin dry. Then moisten a gauze dressing with saline solution. Gently place it over the surface of the ulcer. If the wound has opposing surfaces, gently place a saline-saturated gauze dressing between them. Don't pack the gauze tightly because you could damage the tissues. Finish dressing the wound with dry sterile gauze and tape it securely.

Applying a hydrocolloid dressing

Irrigate the pressure ulcer with normal saline solution. Blot the surrounding skin dry. Then choose a clean, dry, presized hydrocolloid dressing, or cut one to extend about 1″ (2.5 cm) beyond the ulcer's edges. Remove the dressing from its backing, pull the release paper from the adherent side of the dressing, and apply the dressing to the wound. Carefully smooth out wrinkles as you apply the dressing.

If you need to secure the dressing's edges with tape, apply a skin sealant to the intact skin around the ulcer. After the area dries, tape the dressing to the skin to protect the skin and help the tape adhere. Don't use tension when applying the tape.

Remove your gloves and discard them in the trash bag. Dispose of refuse and wash your hands.

Applying a transparent dressing

Irrigate the pressure ulcer with normal saline solution. Blot the surrounding skin dry. Then clean and dry the wound as described above. Select a dressing to extend about 2″ (5 cm) beyond the ulcer's edges. Gently lay the dressing over the ulcer without stretching it. Press firmly on

Guide to topical agents for pressure ulcers

Topical agents	Nursing considerations
Antibiotics bacitracin, Neosporin Ointment, Polysporin Ointment	◆ Use only for early ulcers because these agents may not penetrate sufficiently to kill deeper bacterial colonies.
Circulatory stimulants Granulex, Proderm	◆ Use to promote blood flow. Both contain balsam of Peru and castor oil; Granulex also contains trypsin, an enzyme that promotes debridement.
Enzymes collagenase (Santyl), fibrinolysin and desoxyribonuclease (Elase), sutilains (Travase)	◆ Apply collagenase in thin layers after cleaning the wound with normal saline solution. ◆ Promote effectiveness by avoiding concurrent use of collagenase with agents that decrease enzymatic activity, including detergents, hexachlorophene, antiseptics with heavy-metal ions, iodine, or such acid solutions as Burow's solution. ◆ Use collagenase and sutilains cautiously near the patient's eyes. If contact occurs, flush the eyes repeatedly with normal saline solution or sterile water. ◆ Use fibrinolysin and desoxyribonuclease only after surgical removal of dry eschar. ◆ If using sutilains and topical antibacterials, apply sutilains ointment first. ◆ Store sutilains at 35.6° to 50° F (2° to 10° C). ◆ Avoid applying sutilains to ulcers in major body cavities, to areas with exposed nerve tissue, or to fungating neoplastic lesions. Do not use sutilains in women of childbearing age or in patients with limited cardiopulmonary reserve.
Exudate absorbers dextranomer beads (Debrisan)	◆ Use dextranomer beads on secreting ulcers. Discontinue use when secretions stop. ◆ Clean, but don't dry, the ulcer before applying dextranomer beads. Don't use in tunneling ulcers. ◆ Remove gray-yellow beads (indicating saturation) by irrigating with sterile water or normal saline solution. ◆ Use cautiously near the eyes. If contact occurs, flush the eyes repeatedly with normal saline solution or sterile water.
Isotonic solutions normal saline solution	◆ Moisturize tissue without injuring cells.

its edges to promote adherence. Although these dressings are self-adhesive, you may have to tape the edges to prevent curling.

If necessary, aspirate accumulated fluid with a 21G needle and syringe. Then clean the aspiration site with an alcohol sponge, and cover it with another strip of transparent dressing.

Applying an alginate dressing

Irrigate the pressure ulcer with normal saline solution. Blot the surrounding skin dry. Then apply the alginate directly to the ulcer surface. Cover the area with sterile 4″ × 4″ gauze pads, and tape the dressing in place. Depending on the amount of exudate, you may need to use additional gauze pads or an abdominal dressing. Stop using the alginate dressing once drainage stops or the wound bed looks dry.

Applying a foam dressing

Irrigate the pressure ulcer with normal saline solution, and blot the surrounding skin dry. Then gently lay the foam dressing over the pressure ulcer. Cover it with sterile 4″ × 4″ gauze pads, and tape the dressing in place.

Applying a hydrogel dressing

Irrigate the pressure ulcer with normal saline solution. Blot the surrounding skin dry. Then apply gel to the wound bed. Cover with sterile 4″ × 4″ gauze pads, and tape in place.

Completing the procedure

Remove all used items from the area. Discard disposable items in the trash bag. Label any opened bottles of irrigating solution with the date, time, and initials of the person who opened them. Remove your gloves and wash your hands. Make the patient comfortable.

When to change dressings

The frequency of dressing changes depends on the type and amount of drainage that's coming from the wound.

- ◆ A moist saline gauze dressing usually should be changed as often as needed to keep the wound moist — typically two to four times a day.
- ◆ A hydrocolloid dressing should be changed every 2 to 7 days, if the patient complains of pain, or if the dressing is coming off or leaking.
- ◆ A transparent dressing should be changed every 3 to 7 days according to the amount of drainage, or if the dressing leaks.
- ◆ An alginate dressing with heavy drainage should be changed once or twice a day for the first 3 to 5 days, or every 2 to 4 days for less profuse drainage.
- ◆ A foam dressing should be changed when the foam becomes saturated with drainage.
- ◆ A hydrogel dressing should be changed every day or as needed to keep the wound bed moist.

Special considerations

- ◆ The best treatment for pressure ulcers is prevention. Instruct all patients and caregivers in the importance of frequent position changes. Teach them how to use pillows to support bony prominences and thus help prevent pressure ulcer formation. Also teach them proper skin care, describe ways to relieve pressure and friction, and emphasize the importance of maintaining adequate nutrition and hydration.
- ◆ If the patient is bedbound, he may need a special mattress. As appropriate, suggest such a mattress, and coordinate the ordering and installation by contacting the durable medical equipment company that's affiliated with your home care agency.

◆ Frequently update the patient's doctor on the status of the pressure ulcer, including its appearance and signs of healing or worsening necrosis. The doctor may choose to modify the treatment plan according to healing progress. A poorly healing pressure ulcer may require further medical intervention, such as surgical debridement.

◆ DOCUMENTING WOUND CARE

Wound care is closely scrutinized by health insurance providers and other regulatory agencies. For each visit you make to provide wound care, your documentation must include:

◆ actual wound care and dressing provided
◆ observation and assessment of the wound, including the degree of healing
◆ instructions given to the patient or home caregiver on performing independent wound care.

Also make sure your documentation specifies wound size and location, the type and amount of drainage present, and the wound's potential for healing.

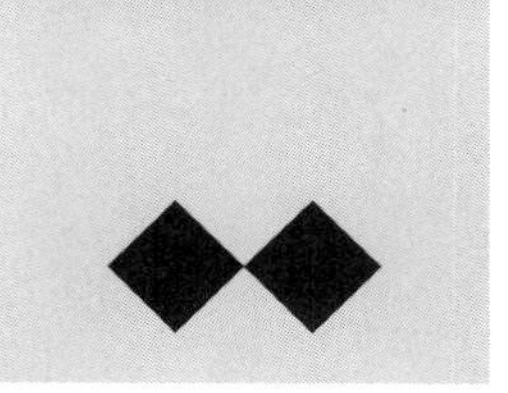

CHAPTER 12

Providing high-tech home care

As patients leave acute care facilities sooner than ever, home care grows more and more complex. These days, you may be expected to deliver high-tech care that even a few years ago wouldn't have taken place at home. It's important for you to understand these sophisticated procedures and to learn how to deliver them with efficiency and expertise.

◆ I.V. PROCEDURES

According to Medicare reimbursement guidelines, the administration of I.V. therapy in a patient's home is considered a reasonable and necessary procedure if the medication (or fluid) being delivered has been deemed safe and effective for the patient's condition. Intermittent home nursing care for I.V. therapy is permitted as long as the medication can't be taken orally.

Federal reimbursement also applies to teaching, care, and maintenance of peripheral and central venous lines and the administration of I.V. medications through such lines. Likewise, the use of infusion pumps is reimbursable if ordered by a doctor in conjunction with a course of treatment that's appropriate for the patient's diagnosis.

Administering peripheral I.V. therapy

Administration of peripheral I.V. therapy is becoming more common in the home setting. If your agency provides home I.V. therapy, be sure to study the appropriate policies. And make sure you're competent in all aspects of I.V. therapy procedures. Before receiving I.V. therapy, the patient may have to sign a special consent form just for that procedure. Be sure to check your agency's policy.

Make sure the doctor's order for I.V. therapy includes the type of solution, any medication additives and specific doses, the total volume to be infused, and the hourly rate. Types of I.V. fluids most commonly infused in the home setting include normal saline solution, lactated Ringer's solution (with or without dextrose), dextrose, and sterile water combinations. You may also give I.V. pain medications and antibiotics.

Once you receive an order for I.V. therapy, ask the home care pharmacist to prepare the solution and infusion supplies.

Equipment and preparation

To administer peripheral I.V. therapy, gather the following equipment: ◆ alcohol swabs ◆ gloves (gown and goggles are optional) ◆ topical antimicrobial ointment ◆ tourniquet ◆

two I.V. catheters (20G or 22G for peripheral fluids and medications) ◆ 2″ × 2″ gauze pads ◆ transparent semipermeable dressing ◆ hypoallergenic tape ◆ sharps container ◆ infusion items (I.V. fluids, tubing, pole) ◆ optional: arm board, warm packs.

To prepare for the infusion, remember to compare the I.V. fluid or medication label to the doctor's order. Also check the expiration date on the infusion and on all infusion supplies.

Implementation

Explain the procedure to the patient and answer any questions he may have. Help him to a comfortable position that exposes his forearm or hand. Wash your hands and arrange all equipment within easy reach.

Put on a pair of clean gloves and use other standard precaution equipment as necessary. Using aseptic technique, set up the I.V. infusion or medication infusion. Remove the tubing from the package, roll the flow regulator to the top of the tubing (just below the drip chamber), and clamp it closed.

Holding the infusion solution, remove the protective covering on the tubing and on the infusion bag. Spike the tubing into the infusion bag, and hang the bag on a pole or another available hook (such as a door or a bedpost).

Gently squeeze the drip chamber until it's about half full. Open the flow regulator on the tubing, prime the tubing, and then reclamp the flow regulator. Hang the primed tubing over the bag or other convenient location until needed. Time the infusion bag with an I.V. time tape if you won't be using an infusion pump.

Look over the patient's blood vessels to find a likely access site. Also think about the reasons for the infusion and the type and length of the infusion. Bearing that in mind, use the smallest possible catheter, and place it in the patient's nondominant hand or arm. Try to use his forearm rather than his hand, if possible.

Apply the tourniquet about 2″ to 6″ (5 to 15 cm) above the intended puncture site. Lightly palpate the vein and stretch the skin around the vein to see if the vein will roll. If it feels hard or ropelike, you might have trouble accessing it. Instead, look for a spongy, firm vein.

Open one of the packets containing alcohol swabs and clean the intended puncture site. Work from the intended site outward in a circular motion. Clean about 1″ to 1½″ (3 to 4 cm) around the intended infusion site.

Select a catheter and pick it up in your dominant hand. With your nondominant hand, secure the skin around the intended site. Hold the catheter parallel to the skin. While tightly stretching the skin, insert the catheter, bevel up, at a 30-degree angle. Once you've punctured the skin, slowly drop the angle of the catheter and move the needle forward until the entire needle enters the vein. Watch for the catheter to fill with blood (blood return).

Stabilize the needle while advancing the catheter. Release the tourniquet. Remove the needle and attach the I.V. tubing to the catheter. Discard the needle in the sharps container.

Turn on the flow regulator on the tubing and adjust the rate. Watch the puncture site and surrounding skin for signs of infiltration, including redness, swelling, coolness, and patient complaints of pain or discomfort. If you suspect infiltration, turn off the infusion, remove the tubing, and pull the catheter out of the vein. Apply warm compresses to the infiltrated site. Prepare to place another catheter in a spot removed from the area you just accessed.

If the venipuncture site shows no evidence of infiltration, apply a dressing over the puncture site. Either make an occlusive dressing with topical antiseptic, a sterile 2″ × 2″ gauze pad, and adhesive tape, or apply a transparent semipermeable adhesive dressing.

To do so, first make sure the insertion site is clean and dry. Then remove the dressing from the package and, using aseptic technique, remove the protective seal. Avoid touching the sterile surface. Place the dressing directly over the insertion site and the hub (as shown below). Don't cover the tubing. Also, don't stretch the dressing; doing so may cause itching. Tuck the dressing around and under the catheter hub to make the site impervious to infectious microorganisms.

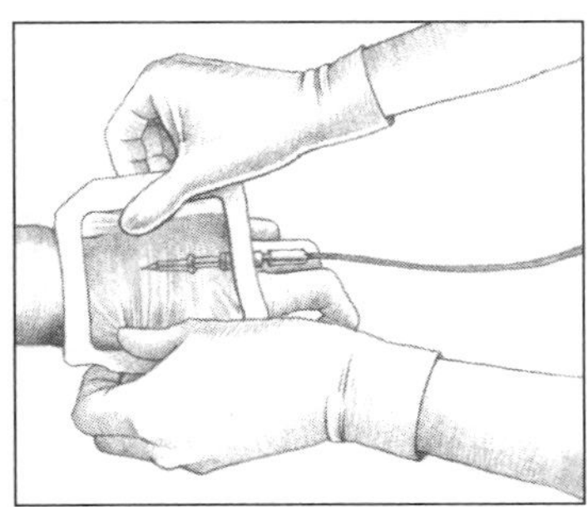

If you use a transparent dressing, secure it with tape. On one piece of tape, label the catheter insertion site with the catheter gauge, the date and time of insertion, and your initials.

Using one of several acceptable methods, tape the tubing near and around the venipuncture site and along the patient's arm, avoiding direct taping over the site. (See *How to tape a venipuncture site*, pages 356 and 357.) If the site is near a joint, use an arm board to temporarily immobilize the joint and keep from accidentally dislodging the catheter.

Place blood-contaminated items in a biohazard container and used sharps in the sharps container. Help the patient to a comfortable position that facilitates the flow of infusion. Place other used items in the plastic trash bag. Then remove your protective gear and wash your hands. Don't discard your goggles unless they're disposable.

When the infusion is finished, wash your hands and put on clean gloves and other protective items, as needed. Clamp the flow regulator on the tubing. If the patient will receive no more infusions, prepare to remove the entire catheter. Take at least two sterile 2″ × 2″ gauze pads and place them over the venipuncture site. Applying gentle pressure, slowly withdraw the catheter from the skin and place the gauze over the site. Apply pressure to the site to ensure blood clotting. Once the bleeding has stopped, apply an occlusive taped dressing over the puncture site.

If the patient will receive more infusions, see "Using an intermittent infusion device" later in the chapter.

Teaching points

Patients who need long-term peripheral I.V. therapy will either have to learn how to provide the therapy themselves or have another home caregiver learn how to do it. Cover these topics when teaching I.V. therapy procedures:

◆ *hand washing before working with the I.V. supplies, before starting an infusion, and after completing an infusion*

◆ *proper storage of solutions and supplies in the home, including which solutions should be refrigerated and then brought to room temperature before infusing*

How to tape a venipuncture site

If you'll be using tape to secure the venipuncture device to the insertion site, use one of these common methods described below.

Chevron method

If you're using the chevron method to secure a venipuncture device, cover the site with an adhesive bandage or a sterile 2″ x 2″ gauze pad. Then cut a long strip of 1/2″ tape and place it, sticky side up, under the needle and parallel to the short strip of tape (as shown below).

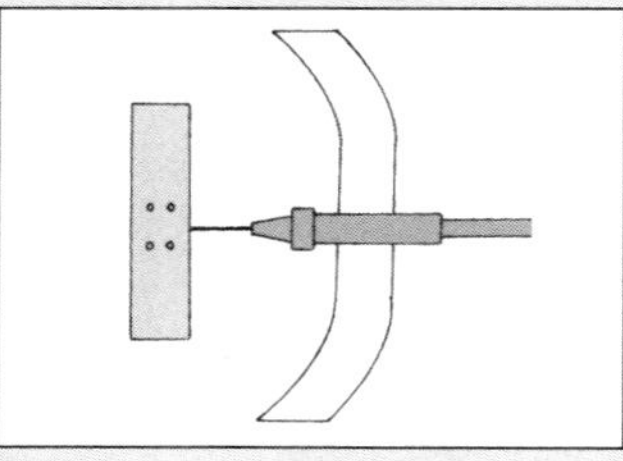

Cross the ends of the tape over the needle so the tape sticks to the patient's skin, forming a chevron (as shown below).

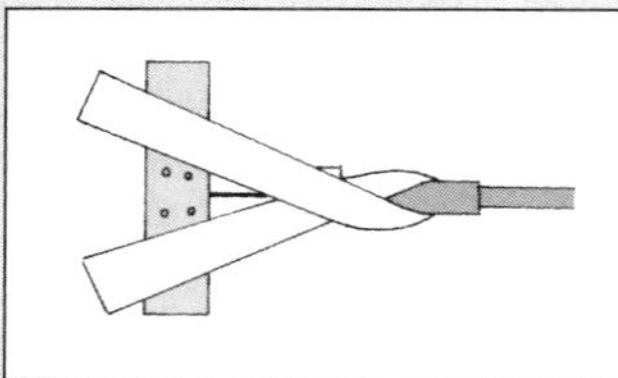

Then apply 1″ tape across the two wings of the chevron. Loop the I.V. tubing and secure it with more tape. Label the tape with the date and time of insertion, the type and gauge of the venipuncture device, and your initials (as shown below).

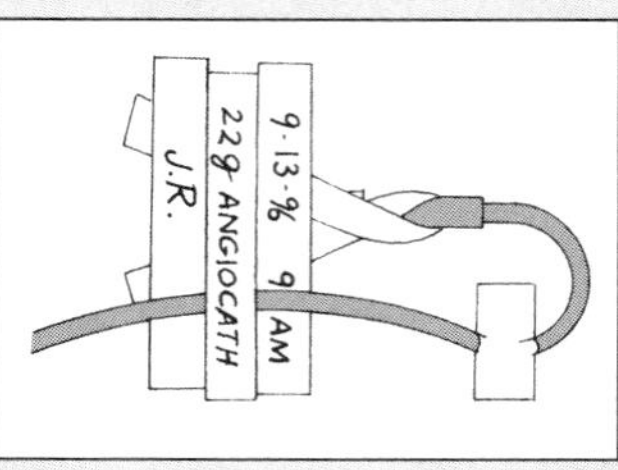

U method

To secure a winged venipuncture device using the U method, cover the site with an adhesive bandage or a sterile 2″ x 2″ gauze pad. Then place a 2" (5-cm) strip of 1/2″ tape, sticky side up, under the tubing (as shown below).

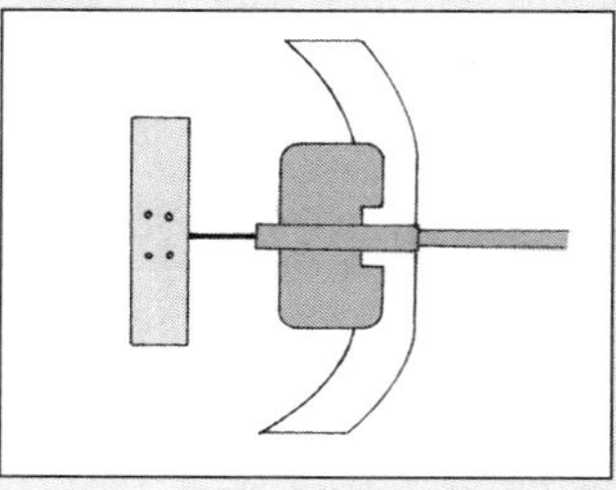

Bring up each side of the tape and fold it over the wings of the needle. Affix each side of the tape parallel to the tubing (as shown below).

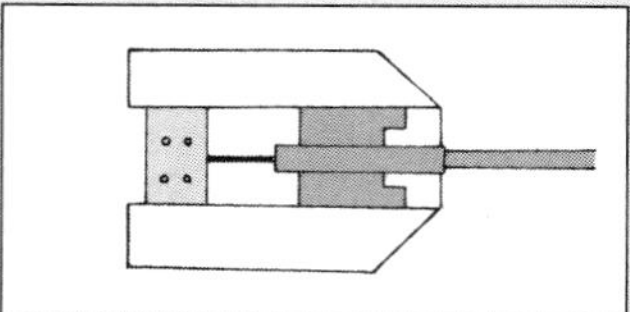

How to tape a venipuncture site *(continued)*

Next, apply tape as you would with the chevron method. Label the tape with the date and time of insertion, the type and gauge of the venipuncture device, and your initials (as shown below).

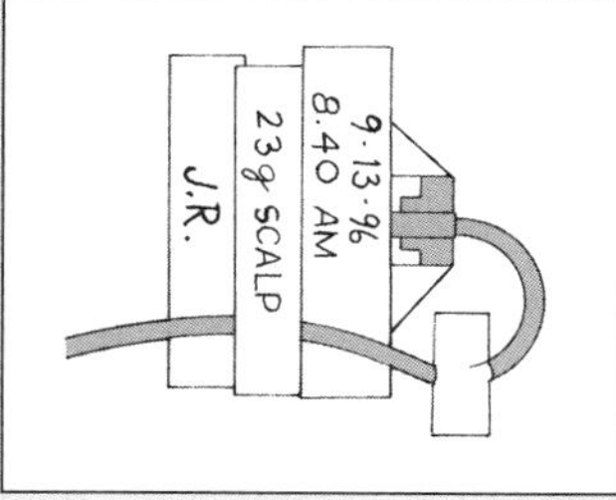

H method

To secure a winged venipuncture device using the H method, cover the venipuncture site with an adhesive bandage or a 2″ x 2″ gauze pad and cut two strips of ½″ tape. Then place one strip of tape over each wing, keeping the tape parallel to the needle (as shown above right).

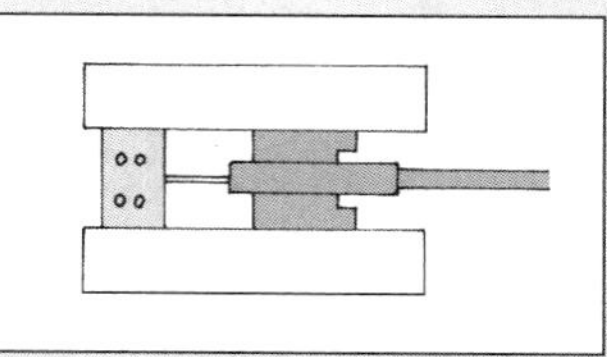

Next, place one or more strips of 1″ tape perpendicular to the first two strips. Put them either directly on top of the wings or just below the wings, directly on top of the tubing.

On the last piece of tape, write the date and time of insertion, the type and gauge of the venipuncture device, and your initials (as shown below).

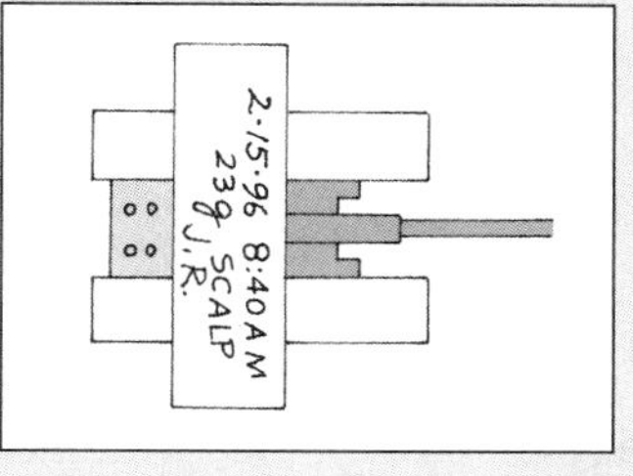

◆ *how to check the I.V. site for signs of infiltration, phlebitis, and infection (If the site is red or painful, tell the patient not to use the catheter. Instead, he should call you to have another catheter placed.)*

◆ *how to flush the catheter with normal saline solution and heparin (If the home infusion set doesn't come with prefilled syringes, teach the patient or caregiver how to draw up the normal saline solution and heparin.)*

◆ *correct procedure for opening I.V. tubing, rolling the clamp to the top of the drip chamber, spiking the infusion bag, squeezing the drip chamber, and priming the tubing; stress the importance of removing all air from the tubing before attaching it to the catheter*

◆ *how to attach the tubing to the catheter, using aseptic technique*

◆ *how to count drops in the drip chamber to ensure a correct flow rate*

◆ *the correct way to discontinue an infusion and flush the catheter after the infusion*

◆ *standard precautions and proper disposal of contaminated items (Tell the patient or caregiver to call you when the sharps container gets full.)*

◆ *how to change the I.V. dressing if it becomes loose or damp*

◆ how to apply a gauze dressing to stop the bleeding if the catheter becomes loose or begins to fall out (Instruct the patient or caregiver to hold pressure over the puncture site for a full minute or until bleeding has stopped before applying an occlusive dressing. Then he should let you know that the catheter became dislodged or fell out.)

◆ the proper way to time an I.V. infusion. (Demonstrate how to write down the date and time the infusion was started and discontinued.)

Provide the patient with additional information to help him detect and respond to catheter problems. Address the topics that follow.

Slowed or stopped infusion. If the infusion slows or stops, teach the patient to look for swelling, pain, or hardness around the needle or catheter site. If any of these signs is present, tell him to shut off the infusion and call you right away.

If the infusion slows or stops but the patient sees no signs of infiltration, tell him to make sure that the tubing isn't twisted or kinked and that his arm is still in the proper position. If he finds no apparent problems, he'll need to call you for an evaluation.

Fluid overload. Tell the patient that symptoms of fluid overload include coughing, shortness of breath, facial flushing, a rapid pulse rate, and dizziness. If these symptoms arise, instruct the patient to turn off the infusion and call you.

Air embolus. If the patient develops extreme shortness of breath, blue lips and nailbeds, anxiety, rapid pulse, and feelings of faintness, this could mean that air has entered his bloodstream. This is a medical emergency; tell the patient or caregiver to call the emergency medical service at once. Tell the patient to lie down on his left side with his head down until the emergency service arrives.

Contamination. If the patient develops a fever, chills, backache, headache, nausea, vomiting, flushing, or dizziness, the I.V. equipment or solution could be contaminated. If this rare situation arises, instruct him to stop the infusion, to call you, and not to discard the used equipment. Tell the patient or a caregiver to call the emergency medical service or go to the nearest emergency department if the patient's symptoms worsen before you arrive.

Ask the patient or caregiver to call your agency if they need more supplies, if complications develop, or the patient is hospitalized.

Special considerations

During each visit, examine the catheter site for signs and symptoms of phlebitis, infiltration, and infection. (See *Gauging phlebitis*.) Also inspect the site before, during, and after the infusion.

Change the gauze dressing at the puncture site when it is damp, loosened, or soiled or according to agency protocol. Change occlusive transparent dressings at least once weekly. Change the primary tubing on a continuous infusion every 3 days and on an intermittent infusion (secondary or piggyback tubing) every day. Luer-lock caps used for intermittent therapy should be changed at least weekly.

Evaluate the catheter site daily, and change it at least every 72 hours — more often if complications develop. If venous access is limited, the catheter may remain in place for up to 7 days if the patient has no signs or symptoms of infection. Obtain a doctor's order for the extended dwell time.

Check all I.V. solutions for expiration date, cracks, discoloration, or particulate matter before giving them to the patient. Check all I.V. labels for the correct patient name, medication, dosage, and expiration date.

If an infusion has been hanging for more than 24 hours, discard it and hang a new bag. If you add a medication, place a label on the infusion that includes the name of the medication, dose, time, date, and your initials.

Typically, first doses of I.V. medications aren't given at home. Instead a nurse at an acute care setting or outpatient facility may need to give the first dose. Once the first dose has been administered and if the patient suffered no acute reactions, subsequent doses may be administered in the home. Check your agency's policy for any additional instructions.

Make sure your documentation describes the procedure, patient's response, adverse reactions, size and length of I.V. catheter, location of the catheter, appearance of the venipuncture site, type of dressing and condition, instructions provided to the patient and other home caregivers, and their response to instruction. If the patient will be on long-term home I.V. therapy, continue instructing the patient or caregiver, and continue supervising the infusion process when administered by someone other than a nurse.

Gauging phlebitis

The Intravenous Nurses Society recommends that you use this scale to rate and document your patient's phlebitis.

1+ phlebitis
- ◆ Pain at the site
- ◆ Erythema, edema, or both
- ◆ No streak
- ◆ No palpable cord

2+ phlebitis
- ◆ Pain at the site
- ◆ Erythema, edema, or both
- ◆ Streak visible
- ◆ No palpable cord

3+ phlebitis
- ◆ Pain at the site
- ◆ Erythema, edema, or both
- ◆ Streak visible
- ◆ Palpable cord

Using an intermittent infusion device

Also called a heparin lock, an intermittent infusion device allows an I.V. catheter to be accessed intermittently. It's ideal for patients who need venous access for I.V. medications and periodic fluids. A heparin lock is better than a keep-vein-open infusion for home care patients because it reduces the risk of accidental fluid overload, is less expensive to maintain, has a lower risk of contamination and infection, and increases patient comfort and mobility. The intermittent infusion device requires flushing before and after use.

Equipment and preparation

Obtain the following equipment for an intermittent infusion device: ◆ heparin lock (luer-lock injection cap or needleless connector) ◆ 25G needle ◆ 3-ml syringe ◆ heparin solution 1:10 multi-use vial ◆ normal saline solution multi-use vial (Some agencies are reimbursed for prefilled heparin and saline flush solution syringes.) ◆ tourniquet ◆ alcohol swabs ◆ venipuncture equipment (if placing a catheter for intermittent use) ◆ gauze pads for a sterile dressing ◆ hypoallergenic tape ◆ transparent

Drugs not compatible with heparin

The following drugs are not compatible when used in the same syringe with heparin:

- ◆ atropine
- ◆ chlorpromazine
- ◆ diazepam
- ◆ droperidol
- ◆ erythromycin
- ◆ gentamycin
- ◆ hydrocortisone
- ◆ hydroxyzine
- ◆ meperidine
- ◆ morphine
- ◆ pentazocine
- ◆ promethazine
- ◆ quinidine
- ◆ tetracycline
- ◆ tobramycin
- ◆ vancomycin.

When using these drugs, you'll have to flush the access device with normal saline solution before and after administration.

semipermeable dressing (optional) ◆ sharps container ◆ hand-washing supplies.

Check the flush solution for expiration date. Prepare patient-education materials before your visit. If you're using heparin, determine whether the prescribed I.V. medications are compatible with heparin. (See *Drugs not compatible with heparin*.) For incompatible drugs, flush the device with normal saline solution before administering medications.

Implementation

Explain the procedure to the patient. Wash your hands, and assemble the equipment on a clean, convenient work area. Help the patient to a comfortable position with easy access to his forearm or hand.

Gently remove the tape around the connection site and remove the tubing. Protect the end of the tubing with either a cap or a sterile needle. Place the tubing near the empty infusion solution for later use.

Prepare to flush the catheter by drawing up 2 ml of sterile normal saline solution into a syringe.

Clean the outer cover of the connector or cap with an antiseptic swab, and let it air-dry. Attach the syringe and flush the catheter. Withdraw the used syringe and place it in the sharps container.

If your agency's protocol requires the use of a heparin flush, draw the heparin solution into a syringe and inject it slowly through the lock into the catheter. Observe the venipuncture site for signs of infiltration. After injecting the heparin, maintain positive pressure on the plunger to prevent blood from backing up into the catheter tip. Withdraw the used syringe and place it in the sharps container. Discard used disposable items, remove your gloves, and wash your hands.

If you're using the intermittent device for antibiotic administration, explain the procedure to the patient. Assemble equipment at a convenient work area. Help the patient to a comfortable position, exposing the intermittent device.

Wash your hands and put on a pair of clean gloves. Taking the infusion set tubing, roll the clamp closed and spike the bag of medication. Hang the medication bag on an I.V. pole or other device, gently squeeze the drip chamber until it's half full, and prime the tubing.

Following aseptic technique, clean the rubber resealable port on the intermittent cap with an alcohol swab. Gently insert the needle or needleless device into the cap. Tape the I.V. tubing to the patient's arm to prevent pulling on the catheter.

Turn on the infusion and regulate the flow. Observe the site for a few minutes for signs of infiltration. Provide for patient comfort, and remove used items from the environment. Remove your gloves and wash your hands. Monitor the I.V. site and flow rate periodically during the infusion.

When the medication has finished infusing, wash your hands and put on a pair of gloves. Clamp the tubing, remove the tape from around the tubing on the patient's arm, and disconnect the needle or needleless connector from the intermittent infusion device. Flush the catheter with normal saline solution (or heparin solution if protocol requires; if the medication isn't compatible with heparin, flush the catheter first with normal saline solution, then with heparin).

Teaching points

If your patient has an intermittent infusion device, give him these instructions:

◆ *Always wash your hands before touching the device or its dressing.*

◆ *Cover the device and the dressing with plastic wrap before bathing.*

◆ *Check the insertion site every 2 hours. If you don't have a fever and the site doesn't hurt when you press on it, you don't have to remove the dressing to inspect the skin. If you have a fever or the site hurts when you press on it, remove the dressing, inspect the skin, and call the home care nurse. Call immediately if the site is swollen or red.*

◆ *To change the dressing, get two 4" × 4" or 2" × 2" gauze pads and tape. Wash your hands, remove the old dressing, and throw it away. Wash your hands again and inspect the insertion site for redness, swelling, or tenderness. Place the two gauze pads (either 2" or 4") over the device and insertion site. Avoid touching the site or keeping the device exposed. Apply tape to the gauze to secure the dressing and make the dressing occlusive.*

◆ *If the catheter becomes dislodged from the vein, remove the dressing, remove the tape from the intermittent device in your arm, and remove the catheter. Then apply pressure over the puncture site for at least 1 minute or until the bleeding stops. Cover the insertion site with a 2" × 2" gauze pad and tape or with an over-the-counter bandage. Call the home care nurse immediately to place another catheter.*

If the patient will be flushing his intermittent device, give him these instructions:

◆ *Gather all of the necessary equipment: normal saline solution, sterile 3-ml syringes with 25G ⅝" needles or needleless connectors, alcohol swabs.*

◆ *Wash your hands and open one antimicrobial pad to wipe off the top of the saline solution vial.*

◆ *Open the packet of alcohol swabs and gently wipe off the resealable rubber cap on the intermittent device. Let the cap air-dry.*

◆ *Uncap one of the 3-ml syringes and inject 1 to 2 cc of air into the vial. Don't remove the needle and syringe from the vial.*

◆ *Turn the bottle upside down so the syringe plunger is facing the floor. Slowly withdraw 1 to 2 ml of saline into the syringe.*

◆ *Gently pull the needle and syringe out of the vial.*

◆ *Inspect the syringe and saline for air bubbles. Tap the barrel of the syringe gently to force the air bubbles to rise to the top of the syringe. Once all of the air is in the top of the syringe, gently expel it.*

◆ *Insert the needle of the syringe through the center of the cap on the intermittent device or attach it to a needleless connector.*

◆ *Inject all of the saline through the cap, but don't force the injection. If you feel resistance, stop injecting, pull the needle out, and call the home care nurse.*

◆ *After injecting all of the saline, remove the needle and syringe and place them in the sharps container.*

◆ *Discard all used supplies and wash your hands.*

Special considerations

Consider teaching the patient how to maintain an intermittent device flushing log that includes the date and time of each flush and the date of each dressing change. Peripheral I.V. lines used intermittently must be flushed with heparin at least once daily to maintain patency.

Using an infusion pump

Depending on the solution or medication ordered, I.V. therapy may need to be administered with a pump. Pumps measure the flow rate of I.V. infusions by milliliters per hour. Many pumps used in the home are compact and attach to the patient's belt or waist band to permit ambulation. Check with your agency to determine the types of pumps and medications that are reimbursable through home care.

Controllers regulate gravity flow by compressing the I.V. tubing. They count drops rather than measuring flow rates and are considered less accurate than volumetric pumps. Controllers are either electronic (which means they have an "eye" that counts the number of drops going through the drip chamber) or in-line (which means they deliver the prescribed flow when you set the dial).

Pumps, used for highly accurate delivery of fluids or drugs, have internal mechanisms to infuse the solution at the set rate under pressure. The pump applies pressure to the I.V. tubing to force the solution through it. Pressures on infusion pumps can range from 10 to 45 psi.

Pumps and controllers have detectors and alarms that automatically signal the end of an infusion, air in the line, low battery power, or an occlusion or inability to deliver the fluid at the set rate. Depending on the pump and problem, the pump might sound or flash an alarm, shut off, or switch the flow to a keep-vein-open rate.

Home care agencies will either contract with a home infusion company to have the infusion pump delivered directly to the home or will have an infusion division with the home care agency.

Equipment and preparation

The equipment needed to set up an infusion pump includes: ◆ the ordered pump ◆ I.V. pole (unless the pump is ambulatory) ◆ two sets of pump-specific tubing ◆ alcohol swabs ◆ clean gloves ◆ hand-washing supplies ◆ I.V. solution for infusion or medication.

Review the operation of the pump with the home infusion representative before using it in the patient's home. Read the entire operating manual, and study the correct way to load the pump and place the tubing. Find out if the pump needs to be plugged into a power source during or after use, how long the pump will work on battery, and whether the patient will need to charge the battery at home between uses. Some models operate on disposable batteries. (Make sure you have spare batteries on hand.)

Prepare the pump for use by first attaching it to an I.V. pole. Open one set of the infusion tubing, spike the I.V. solution or medication bag, and prime the tubing. Insert the tubing through the pump according to the manufacturer's instructions.

Additional equipment needed to set up a controller includes: ◆ in-line I.V. controller ◆ two sets of I.V. tubing compatible with the ordered controller.

Review the operation of the controller before administering the infusion. Make sure that the I.V. infusion set is compatible with the controller.

Implementation

Contact the patient before your visit if the pump and I.V. supplies will be delivered directly to the patient's home. Also call just before the scheduled time to verify that all equipment has arrived.

Explain the procedure to the patient, emphasizing the reason why the ordered infusion must be delivered through a pump. Wash your hands and arrange all equipment within easy reach. Put on a pair of clean gloves and help the patient to a comfortable position, exposing the I.V. venipuncture site. Insert an I.V. catheter if one isn't already present.

Assess the ordered infusion for accuracy, expiration date, patient name, and any medications or additives. Compare the solution with the doctor's order.

Set the pump to infuse at the ordered rate. Make sure all alarms are turned on and the pump is plugged into an electrical source, if necessary.

Prepare the I.V. infusion and prime the tubing. Attach the tubing to the patient's catheter. Turn the pump on, and observe the infusion for at least 5 minutes.

Once you determine that the infusion is being delivered successfully, secure the I.V. tubing near and around the catheter site. Don't put tape over any transparent semipermeable dressings. Note the date and time the infusion was started. Discard used disposable items, provide for patient comfort, remove your gloves, and wash your hands.

If you'll be using an electronic controller for your patient's infusion, make sure the controller is either delivered directly to the patient's home or available for delivery at the time of your visit. Review its operation with the patient.

Explain the procedure to the patient, and help him to a comfortable position. Place all needed equipment within easy reach. Wash your hands, put on gloves, and place the controller on the I.V. pole. Spike the infusion solution with controller-compatible tubing, and fill the drip chamber half full. Rotate the solution in the drip chamber to ensure adequate sensing by the controller.

Prime the entire length of the tubing. Position the drop sensor of the controller above the fluid level in the chamber and below the drop port to ensure correct drop counting.

Place the designated section of the tubing within the controller and close the door, securing the tubing. Open the drip chamber wide and prepare to attach the tubing to the patient's catheter.

Ensure the correct rate by making sure the controller is positioned at least 30″ (76 cm) above the infusion site. Monitor the accuracy of the infusion rate for at least 2 minutes. Observe the infusion site for signs of infiltration. Recheck the accuracy of the controller.

The tubing in a controller should be moved every few hours to prevent permanent compression or damage to the tubing (as shown below).

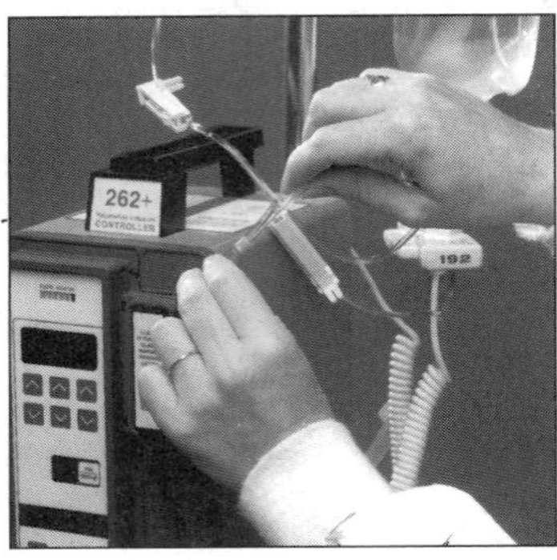

If you'll be using an in-line controller, prepare the infusion tubing and place the flow dial mechanism at the end closest to the infusion site. Attach an extension tubing set to one end of the controller for attachment to the patient's catheter. Prime the tubing and attach to the patient. Set the infusion rate on the control dial, open the clamp on the tubing, and observe the drip rate. Adjust the control dial to deliver the prescribed drops per minute.

Teaching points

◆ *Make sure the patient and other home caregivers thoroughly understand the function and operation of the infusion pump or controller apparatus.*

◆ *Instruct the patient and the caregiver on the proper functioning of the pump, the alarms, and pump care. Have on hand a back-up solution and infusion set in case the pump fails or a power failure lasts long enough to exhaust the battery.*

◆ *Instruct the patient and other home caregivers about the signs and symptoms of infiltration. Also tell them that pumps will continue to deliver fluids at the set amount, even if the catheter becomes dislodged. Explain that fluids will be administered into the subcutaneous tissue until a sufficient obstruction is met.*

◆ *Instruct the patient and other home caregivers on the way to count drops per minute with a controller.* *(See* Counting drops per minute.*)*

◆ *Ongoing evaluation of the effectiveness of the controller to deliver ordered fluid amounts is necessary for effective I.V. therapy and treatment.*

Special considerations

If a pump is used for infusing fluids over several hours, set the pump volume for at least 50 ml less than the bag holds. This will provide additional time for the patient or other home caregiver to change the bag before the fluid runs out, preventing air from entering the tubing and possibly causing an air embolism.

Maintaining a long-term CV catheter

Central venous (CV) catheters are inserted — usually in an acute care or outpatient facility — in patients who need long-term fluid replacement or medications but have no other venous access sites. The traditional catheter site is the subclavian vein, but the jugular vein can also be used. Working with CV catheters in the home setting requires special training.

Home care nurses typically use CV catheters for serum studies and giving medications, total parenteral nutrition (TPN), fluids, or chemotherapy. The care of a central venous catheter includes irrigation (routine catheter maintenance), laboratory specimen collection, dressing changes, cap changes, and site assessment.

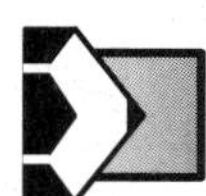

TEACHING POINTS

Counting drops per minute

If your patient will be using a controller to deliver I.V. infusions, you'll need to teach him how to count the drip rate. Here's what to tell him:

◆ Because different types of I.V. tubing deliver different amounts of fluid or medication per minute, you'll need to learn how to count drops per minute to make sure you're receiving the proper amount.

◆ Start by looking at the table below. You should see the name of the tubing you're using and the number of drops per minute needed to deliver certain amounts of fluid or medication. Find your ordered infusion rate.

◆ Once the medication or fluid is attached to your arm through the tubing, you'll need to set the control clamp. This regulates how much fluid goes through the tubing and into your body.

◆ To set the control flow, stand next to the I.V. pole. Keep the arm with the I.V. line in it next to your side. Taking the clamp in your other hand, gently unroll it with your thumb. Watch for fluid to begin dripping in the chamber. Make the drops go very slowly until you're ready to start timing them.

◆ Count the drops for 1 minute.

◆ Adjust the clamp until the number of drops per minute equals the number you're supposed to receive.

◆ When the infusion is finished, clamp the tubing and disconnect it from your arm.

Ordered volume

		Drops/minute to infuse							
Administration set	**Drip factor drops = 1 ml**	100 ml/hr	250 ml/1hr	500 ml/24hr	1000 ml/24hr	1000 ml/20hr	1000 ml/10hr	1000 ml/8hr	1000 ml/6hr
Macrodrip									
Abbott	15	25	62	5	10	12	25	31	42
Baxter Healthcare	10	17	42	3	7	8	17	21	28
Cutter	20	34	83	7	14	17	34	42	56
IVAC	20	34	83	7	14	17	34	42	56
McGaw	15	25	62	5	10	12	25	31	42

Several different catheters are available for central venous access. Common ones include the Groshong, Hickman, and Broviac.

The *Groshong catheter* is a long tunneled catheter ideal for long-term therapy. It has one, two, or three lumens and ports and a pressure-sensitive two-way valve that reduces the need for frequent flushing. It must be surgically inserted and tears and kinks easily. It must be flushed with enough saline solution to clear the entire length of the catheter, especially after being used for serum blood samples.

The *Hickman catheter* is another long tunneled catheter that's ideal for long-term therapy. It has single and double lumens and ports. Because it has an open end with a clamp, the catheter must be clamped with a nonserrated clamp any time it becomes disconnected or opens. It must be surgically inserted and tears and kinks easily.

The *Broviac catheter* is identical to the Hickman except it has a smaller inner lumen. Consequently, it may make a good choice for pediatric and geriatric patients. It has only one port.

For more information on peripherally inserted central catheters, see "Using a PICC line" later in the chapter.

Equipment and preparation

The equipment and preparation needed before working with a CV catheter will depend on the type of catheter to be used and the procedure to be performed.

Flushing. If you need to flush the catheter as part of routine care, you'll need the following equipment and preparation: ◆ 10-100 U/ml heparin solution ◆ sterile normal saline solution for infusion ◆ needleless system or 10-ml syringes with 23G 1″ needles (note that CV catheters should be flushed with a 10-ml or larger syringe so infusion pressure doesn't exceed 25 to 40 psi) ◆ alcohol swabs ◆ clean gloves ◆ sharps container ◆ hand-washing supplies.

If prefilled heparin and saline syringes are not available through home infusion companies, prepare to fill them just before the irrigation. If prefilled syringes will be kept in the agency's medication refrigerator or the patient's home, identify on the syringe the name of the solution, date filled, intended use, and expiration date on the solution bottle. The optimum practice is to prepare syringes at the time of intended use rather than prefilling them.

Serum studies. If the catheter will be used for serum laboratory studies, the following equipment is needed: ◆ blood sample tubes ◆ 20-ml and 10-ml syringes with 20G 1″ needles or a needleless connector ◆ laboratory requisitions ◆ alcohol swabs ◆ clean gloves ◆ sharps container ◆ hand-washing supplies ◆ 10-100 U/ml heparin solution ◆ sterile normal saline solution for infusion ◆ 10-ml syringes with 23G 1″ needles.

To prepare for accessing the central venous line for serum laboratory studies, you'll need to ensure that there are enough test tubes for blood samples and that the required catheter irrigation equipment is available.

Changing the dressing. If you're planning to change the dressing on the catheter, the following equipment and preparation is needed: ◆ disposable CV catheter dressing change kit (includes three alcohol swabs, three povidone-iodine swabs, one benzoin swab, tape, face mask, sterile gloves, sterile drape) ◆ transparent semipermeable adhesive dressing ◆ clean gloves ◆ sharps container ◆ hand-washing supplies.

Your agency's policy may dictate whether the dressing change is to be done with sterile or clean technique. Coordinate the frequency of dressing changes with other scheduled skilled activities, such as cap changes, blood draws, or routine irrigations.

Changing the catheter cap. If you're planning to change the catheter cap, the following equipment and preparation is needed: ◆ injection cap for the catheter ◆ tape ◆ hemostats or other clamps ◆ clean 4″ × 4″ gauze pad ◆ sterile normal saline solution for infusion ◆ 10-ml syringe with 23G 1″ needle ◆ alcohol swabs ◆ clean gloves ◆ sharps container ◆ hand-washing supplies.

Coordinate changing the cap on the catheter with other scheduled skilled activities.

Implementation

The implementation needed when working with a CV catheter will depend on the type of catheter and procedure to be performed.

Flushing. Explain the procedure to the patient, and help him to a comfortable position that exposes the catheter and the site. Wash your hands and assemble all equipment within easy reach. Put on gloves and prepare the syringes—one of normal saline solution and one of heparin—for each port. With an alcohol swab, clean the first port to be flushed. Allow to air-dry.

Depending on the catheter being flushed, a clamp may need to be released. Be sure to release any clamps before irrigating.

Take one of the normal saline–filled syringes, inject the needle into the port cap (or insert the needleless connector into the port), and inject 2.5 ml of normal saline solution. Remove the needle and syringe or the needleless connector, and place it in the sharps container. With one heparin syringe, place the needle into the port and begin injecting the heparin at a rate of 0.5 ml/second.

While withdrawing the heparin syringe, maintain pressure on the plunger to avoid a backflow of blood into the lumen. Reclamp the catheter, if necessary, and withdraw the heparin needle and syringe and place them in the sharps container.

Discard any used disposable supplies, and provide for patient comfort. Remove your gloves and wash your hands.

Serum studies. Explain the procedure to the patient, and help him to a comfortable position that exposes the catheter. Wash your hands and put on clean gloves. Assemble all equipment within easy reach. Prepare irrigation syringes for flushing the catheter after drawing blood. Review all orders for laboratory specimens, and have the appropriate color-coded tubes available.

With an alcohol swab, clean the port that will be used for drawing blood. Allow the port to air-dry.

Depending on the catheter being used, a clamp may need to be released. Be sure to release any clamps before drawing blood.

Taking one of the 10-ml syringes, insert the needle or needleless connector into the cleaned port. Gently aspirate about 7 ml of blood through the catheter. Remove the needle and syringe or the needleless connector from the port and discard it, with the blood intact, in the sharps container.

Now take one of the 20-ml syringes and gently insert the needle or needleless connector into the port. Gently withdraw the amount of blood needed for the samples. When filled, remove the needle from the port and inject the blood into the test tubes for analysis. If more than 20 ml of blood is required for all tests ordered, use another 20-ml syringe and insert the needle or needleless connector into the port. Continue to withdraw blood until all of the test tubes are filled.

When you've finished collecting the blood samples, dispose of all sharps used to draw blood in the appropriate sharps container. Taking one syringe filled with normal saline solution, flush the port just used with a "pulsing" motion. This will help prevent fibrin formation and buildup in the catheter. Remove the saline syringe and discard it in the sharps container. With the heparin-filled syringe, flush the port, being sure to keep positive pressure on the plunger as you withdraw the needle on the syringe.

Discard this used syringe in the sharps container. Discard other used items and provide for patient comfort. Remove your gloves and wash your hands.

Changing the dressing. Explain the procedure to the patient, and help him to a comfortable position that exposes the catheter. Wash your hands and place the dressing tray on a clean, dry surface. Carefully unwrap the tray, including the sterile gloves. Try to avoid accidentally contaminating the contents.

Put on a pair of clean gloves and the face mask. Remove and discard the old dressing, being careful not to dislodge the catheter.

Examine the catheter site for any signs of infection, including redness, swelling, drainage, or patient complaints of pain.

Remove your gloves and wash your hands. Put on the sterile gloves, using aseptic technique. Continue with aseptic technique to clean the catheter insertion site. Take one alcohol swab and begin cleaning the insertion site. Start at the site and move outward in a circular motion to clean an area about 1½" to 2" (4 to 6 cm) in diameter. Discard the used swab and pick up a new one. Repeat this cleaning procedure with two more alcohol swabs. Never go back to the catheter site with a swab that has been used to touch skin removed from the site.

After three alcohol swabs have been used to clean the site, allow the skin to air-dry.

Repeat the entire cleaning process with the three povidone-iodine swabs (as shown below). Be careful not to dislodge the catheter during cleaning and not to touch a used swab on the catheter site.

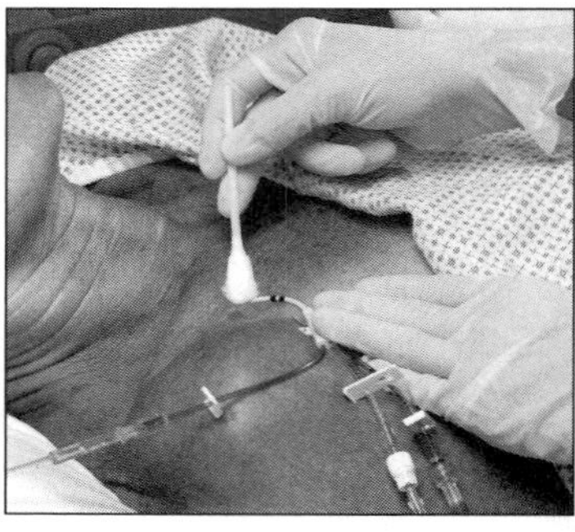

Allow the povidone-iodine to air-dry. Then take the benzoin swab and either paint an area on the skin where the new dressing will go or paint the dressing itself.

Take the adhesive dressing and apply it over the catheter site. If the dressing has been known to become loose, at this time apply adhesive tape over the periphery of the dressing (in the form of a picture frame) to secure it in place. Then take the ports of the catheter and loop them, cap pointing up, on the dressing.

With adhesive tape, secure the loop to the dressing to prevent accidental tugging or dislodgment of the catheter.

On a small piece of tape, write the date, time, and initials of the person who performed the dressing change, and place it on the completed dressing.

Discard all used items and provide for patient comfort. Remove the sterile gloves and face mask, and wash your hands.

Changing the catheter cap. Explain the procedure to the patient, and help him to a comfortable position that exposes the catheter. Wash your hands and put on a pair of gloves. Close the clamp on the catheter if it has one (as shown below). If it doesn't have one, check with the manufacturer before using a hemostat to clamp the catheter. Some catheters, like the Groshong, can be damaged by using a hemostat.

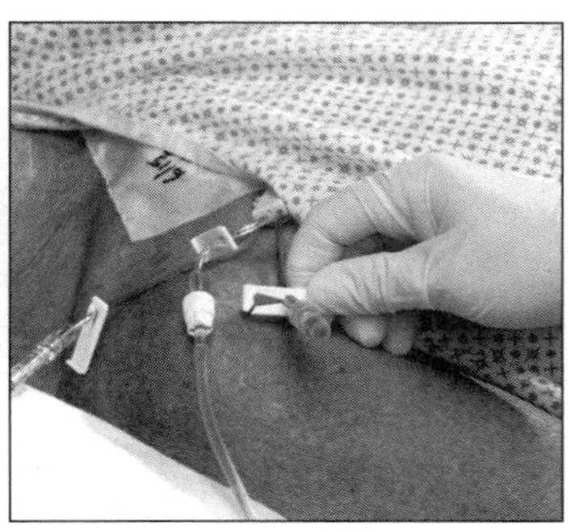

Remove any tape around the connection between the injection cap and the catheter. Taping the connection helps prevent the cap from accidentally becoming dislodged. Don't cut the tape with scissors because the catheter can be damaged.

Hold the end of the catheter between your index finger and thumb. Clean the connection with an alcohol swab. Allow the connection to air-dry.

Slowly unscrew the old injection cap and discard it. Touch only the outside rubber port when you pick up the new cap. Gently remove the protective covering from the end of the new cap and discard it. Screw the new injection cap onto the catheter (as shown below). Take care not to touch the tip of the catheter or the injection cap.

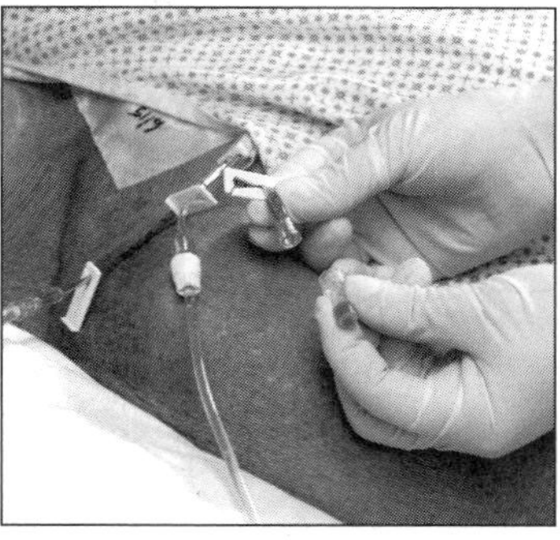

Release the clamp on the catheter for a minute only to make sure that the cap is applied correctly and the connection is not leaking. Then reclamp the catheter.

Tape the connection. Make tabs on the ends of the tape by folding back about ½" (1.3 cm). The tabs on the tape will be helpful when the cap needs changing again. Write the date and time of the cap change on the tape.

Discard all disposable items used, and provide for patient comfort. Remove your gloves and wash your hands.

Teaching points

◆ *Demonstrate the correct way to irrigate the catheter's ports. Observe the patient or other home caregivers perform the skill. Document the pa-*

tient's or caregiver's ability to perform irrigations. Offer additional instruction as needed.

◆ *A patient probably won't be asked or expected to draw his own blood for laboratory analysis. If he is, instruct him on the importance of adequate catheter irrigation after drawing blood.*

◆ *Teach the patient or home caregiver how to change the dressing. Demonstrate the correct procedure and then observe the return demonstration. Stress the importance of not moving the catheter around haphazardly. Teach him how to correctly loop the catheter, ensuring easy access while protecting the integrity of the dressing.*

◆ *Remind any patient with a long-term catheter to secure the catheter to prevent dangling. Keep a clamp or hemostat with 4" × 4" gauze in the home in case the catheter is damaged or cut. Instruct the patient to call the home health agency or go immediately to the emergency department if the catheter is accidentally severed.*

◆ *Teach the patient to clamp the catheter between his body and the damaged area to keep air from entering the vein and blood from leaking out of the catheter.*

◆ *Remind the patient and caregiver to contact the home infusion company when they need supplies. Depending on your agency's policy, the patient and home caregivers may be allowed to use clean technique.*

◆ *Teach the patient or home caregiver how to change the injection cap or needleless connector on the catheter. Provide instructions verbally while performing the skill.*

Special considerations

If you can't irrigate the catheter, don't force the solution into the catheter. Help the patient change positions, cough, deep-breathe, or raise his arms over his head. If you still can't irrigate the catheter, contact the doctor and prepare the patient for possible transport to unblock or replace the catheter. With special training, you may be able to use a declotting agent to declot the catheter. (See *Clearing an occluded catheter*.)

Thorough irrigation is required after you use a catheter to draw blood. If you're using a Groshong catheter, be sure to use enough normal saline solution to ensure complete catheter irrigation. Heparin might not be ordered as part of the irrigation procedure.

Instruct the patient and home caregivers in the signs and symptoms of infection, including redness, swelling, drainage, and complaints of pain. Signs of a systemic infection include fever, lethargy, change in appetite, and general malaise.

The cap should be changed at least weekly. In some situations — such as frequent access of the device through the cap, administration of 3-in-1 TPN solutions, or an immunocompromised patient — more frequent changes are required.

Each time blood is drawn through the device, the cap should be changed. When changing the cap, clamp the catheter or coach the patient to perform Valsalva's maneuver to increase intrathoracic pressure and reduce the risk of air embolism. Don't use Valsalva's maneuver with patients who have increased intracranial pressure or who aren't alert or cooperative.

Teach the patient ways to prevent air embolism, such as:

◆ removing all air from syringes and tubing before injecting or infusing into the catheter

◆ using tubing and injection caps with locking connections (luer-lock); if these aren't available, teach the patient how to secure the connections with tape

CRITICAL DECISIONS

Clearing an occluded catheter

If your patient's catheter is occluded, follow the steps described below to help clear the obstruction.

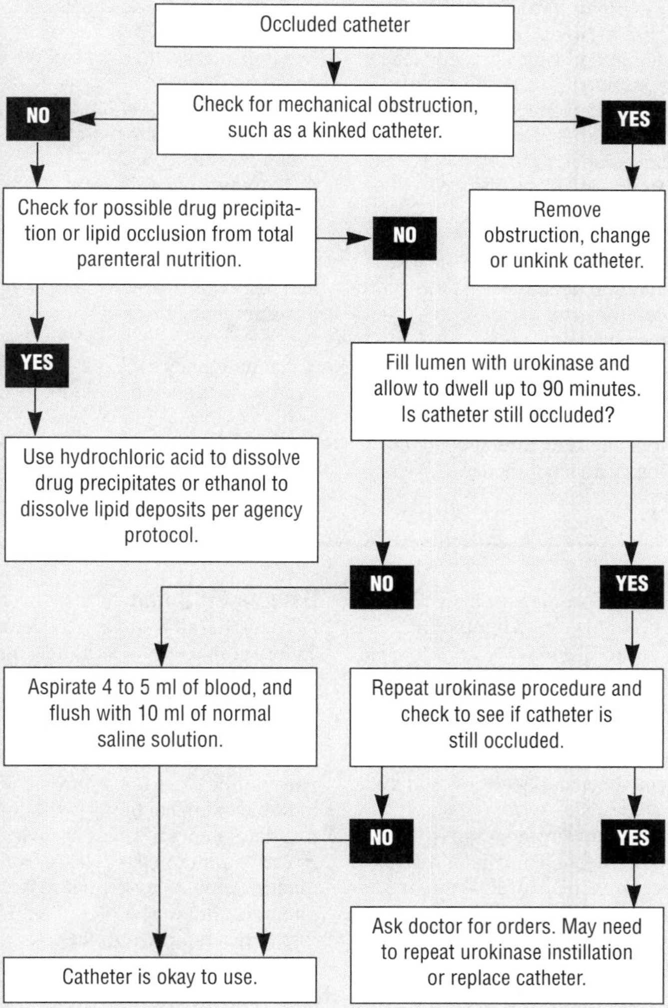

Occluded catheter

↓

Check for mechanical obstruction, such as a kinked catheter.

- **YES** → Remove obstruction, change or unkink catheter.
- **NO** → Check for possible drug precipitation or lipid occlusion from total parenteral nutrition.
  - **YES** → Use hydrochloric acid to dissolve drug precipitates or ethanol to dissolve lipid deposits per agency protocol.
  - **NO** → Fill lumen with urokinase and allow to dwell up to 90 minutes. Is catheter still occluded?
    - **NO** → Aspirate 4 to 5 ml of blood, and flush with 10 ml of normal saline solution. → Catheter is okay to use.
    - **YES** → Repeat urokinase procedure and check to see if catheter is still occluded.
      - **NO** → Catheter is okay to use.
      - **YES** → Ask doctor for orders. May need to repeat urokinase instillation or replace catheter.

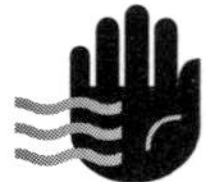

EMERGENCY INTERVENTIONS

Responding to an air embolism

An air embolism is a life-threatening complication of central venous catheters. Signs and symptoms include extreme shortness of breath, anxiety, cyanosis, coughing, chest pain, and loss of consciousness. Without immediate interventions, the patient could die. If you suspect an air embolism do the following:

◆ Stop infusions and clamp the catheter.

◆ Turn the patient onto his left side, with his head down, to encourage air to flow into the right ventricle and allow blood to perfuse the lungs.

◆ Assess the patient's cardiopulmonary status, and immediately measure his vital signs. Prepare to administer cardiopulmonary resuscitation if required.

◆ Activate the emergency medical service (EMS) if the patient's cardiopulmonary status is unstable or if he's unconscious. Stay with him until the EMS arrives and transports him to an emergency care facility.

◆ Notify the doctor and home health agency of the patient's status and location.

◆ Document the date, time, symptoms, emergency actions taken, patient's response to treatment, time the EMS was called and responded, actions taken by the emergency team, and patient's location.

◆ If your agency requires it, fill out an occurrence or incident report.

◆ always clamping the catheter when changing or removing the injection cap. (See *Responding to an air embolism.*)

The procedure used to repair a damaged Hickman catheter is similar to that used for a Groshong catheter. Check the manufacturer's guidelines to repair catheters.

Document any situation in which a catheter becomes damaged and the steps taken to repair it. Notify the patient's doctor of repairs made, and implement orders for follow-up care. Depending on your agency's policies, you may need to complete an occurrence or incident report.

Using a PICC line

A peripherally inserted central catheter (also known as a PICC line) is used for patients who need CV therapy for a few days to several months or for those who require repeated venous access. A PICC line is commonly used for a patient with multiple trauma or burns to the chest, respiratory compromise, chronic obstructive pulmonary disease, a mediastinal mass, cystic fibrosis, or pneumothorax. The use of a PICC line helps avoid complications that might result if a central venous catheter were used.

PICC lines are becoming more common in home care patients. The line is easier to insert and provides a safe, reliable access site for medications and fluids. Home care patients with PICC lines can receive TPN, chemotherapy, antibiotics, narcotics, analgesics, and blood products. Ideally, a PICC line should be used early in therapy and not as a last resort for patients with sclerosed or damaged veins from repeated punctures.

PICC lines are soft and flexible and range in diameter from 16G to 23G and in length from 16″ to 24″. PICCs are available with either single or double lumens and with or without a guide wire. The use of a guide wire during insertion stiffens the catheter, easing its advancement. However, it can damage the vessel if used improperly.

Patients who are candidates for a PICC line must have a peripheral vein large enough for a 14G or 16G introducer needle and a 3.0G to 4.0G catheter. The line is inserted through the basilic, median cubital, or cephalic vein. The catheter is then threaded centrally to the superior vena cava. A catheter placed in the subclavian vein is called a midclavicular catheter.

Equipment and preparation

The equipment needed to insert a PICC line is as follows: ◆ PICC line insertion tray (single-lumen #3 French or double-lumen #4 French) ◆ two sterile 10-ml syringes with needles ◆ sterile luer-lock injection cap or reflux valve ◆ sterile 3″ luer-lock extension set ◆ 10-ml vial of heparin 10-100 U/ml ◆ 10-ml vial of bacteriostatic normal saline solution ◆ 3″ × 4″ transparent occlusive dressing ◆ tourniquet ◆ 2″ × 2″ gauze pads ◆ 4″ × 4″ gauze pads ◆ povidone-iodine and alcohol swabs ◆ povidone-iodine ointment ◆ sterile and nonsterile measuring tape ◆ adhesive tape ◆ sterile drape or towels ◆ sterile gloves ◆ clean gloves ◆ gown, mask, goggles ◆ sharps container ◆ handwashing supplies.

Before arriving at the patient's home, gather all required and spare supplies. If the line is being placed for infusion, prepare the required infusion for transport to the patient's home. If working with a home infusion company, contact them before the line is placed to ensure that fluid and other supplies are delivered to the home beforehand.

If the line will be placed in the superior vena cava, contact the mobile X-ray company and tell them you need a post–PICC line insertion X-ray. (Make sure they can read the X-ray on the premises.) Check with your home care agency for guidelines regarding the need for an X-ray to confirm placement.

Implementation

To manage a PICC line, you'll need to be prepared to perform several procedures.

Inserting the line. Explain the procedure to the patient. Then help the patient to a comfortable, reclining position. Expose the arm in which the line will be placed. Wash your hands and assemble all equipment in a convenient and clean work area.

Begin by evaluating the antecubital veins for possible insertion. With the nonsterile measuring tape, measure the patient for the desired final tip location. Place the patient's arm at a 45-degree angle from his body.

If the catheter will be placed in the subclavian vein, measure and record the distance from the insertion site to the sternal notch (as shown below). If none of the catheter will be left out at the site, cut the catheter 1″ (2.5 cm) shorter than the distance measured. If 1″ of catheter will be left out at the insertion site, cut the full length from the insertion site to the sternal notch.

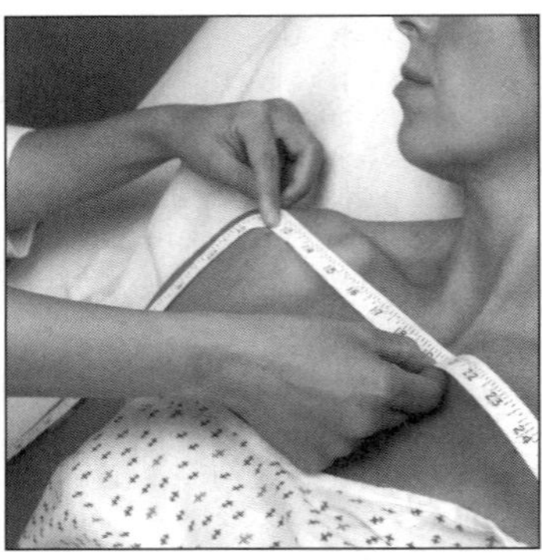

If the catheter will be placed in the superior vena cava and 1″ will be exposed at the insertion site, measure from 1″ below the insertion site to the third intercostal space. If the intercostal spaces aren't palpable, estimate the length by measuring one-third of the distance from the sternal notch to the xiphoid process. Catheters being placed through the left antecubital region will be slightly longer because the catheter will cross over the chest to reach the superior vena cava.

Now wash your hands and put on a mask and goggles. Open the sterile PICC line tray. Make sure the patient is in the proper position: head down and body as flat as comfortably possible, with a clothing protector under the arm you'll be using. Make sure you have adequate work space and lighting. Put the tourniquet around the patient's arm, but don't tie it.

Put on the sterile gloves and gown. Taking a sterile drape or towel, place it under the patient's arm.

With the alcohol swabs, begin to clean the puncture site. Clean for a full 3 minutes with the alcohol swabs. Then clean for a full 3 minutes with the povidone-iodine swabs. Clean in a circular motion, beginning at the intended site and working outward.

While the antimicrobial antiseptic is drying on the skin, measure the desired length of the catheter with the sterile measuring tape. Do not touch the catheter with gloved hands. Use forceps or hemostats to manipulate the catheter.

Pull the guide wire out of the catheter, ¼″ to ½″ (0.7 to 1.25 cm) shorter than the desired length. Bend the guide wire at the hub to prevent movement. With the sterile scissors, cut the catheter to the desired length.

Draw up 5 ml of normal saline solution and 5 ml of heparin solution in separate syringes. Prime the extension tubing (as shown below).

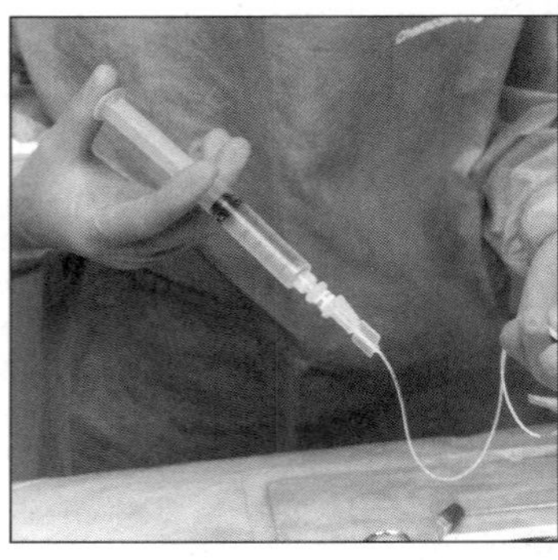

Position a fenestrated drape over the prepared puncture area. Place sterile 4″ × 4″ gauze pads around the puncture area to absorb blood flow. Tighten the tourniquet around the patient's arm. Remove the used sterile gloves, and use a waterless antiseptic hand cleaner. Put on another pair of sterile gloves.

Prepare to puncture the skin by taking the catheter and needle in your dominant hand. With your nondominant hand, stabilize the vein and skin. Puncture the vein at a 10-degree angle. A successful puncture will show a blood return in the flashback chamber. Without changing the needle position, gently advance the plastic introducer sheath into the vein (as shown below) about ¼″ (0.7 cm). Carefully remove the needle while stabilizing the plastic sheath within the vein.

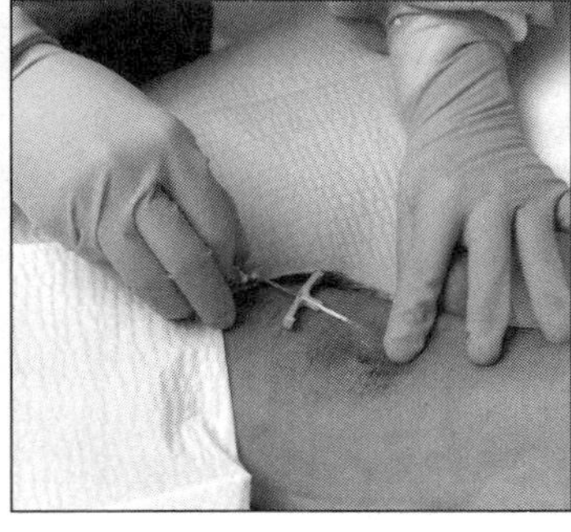

To reduce blood flow, gently apply pressure above the introducer with your finger or by using sterile 2″ × 2″ gauze pads to occlude the end of the introducer.

Taking a pair of sterile forceps, insert the catheter into the introducer sheath, and advance it a few inches into the vein. With a sterile gauze pad, release the tourniquet on the patient's arm. Advance the catheter in short amounts until about 5″ to 7″ (13 to 18 cm) of it is placed.

Ask the patient to turn his head toward his arm and place his chin on his chest. This movement will occlude the jugular vein and aid the catheter's placement into the subclavian vein.

Continue advancing the catheter until 3″ to 4″ (7.5 to 10 cm) remain. Remove the introducer and peel it away. The extra catheter length aids in removing the introducer.

Continue to advance the catheter until all but 2″ (5 cm) remain. Remove the guide wire by stabilizing the catheter with one hand and gently pulling out the guide wire with the other. Do not pull vigorously or suddenly. Once the guide wire is removed, place a thumb over the hub of the catheter to prevent an inflow of air.

Flush the catheter with a syringe filled with 3 ml of normal saline solution. Withdraw blood to confirm that the catheter tip is within the vascular system. Flush the catheter with 3 to 5 ml of heparin solution. Connect the capped extension set to the hub of the catheter.

Apply a sterile occlusive dressing over the site by first cleaning the site with antimicrobial pads. Pull the catheter out 1″ (2.5 cm) and in an L shape to prevent kinking and occlusion at the bend of the arm. Apply Steri-Strips over the catheter to secure it.

Place folded 2″ × 2″ sterile gauze pads under the length of the hub and extension tubing. Cover the entire site with occlusive transparent dressings so that the site is covered from 1½″ (3.8 cm) above the exit site. This dressing will need to remain intact until your next scheduled visit.

Discard all used sharps in the sharps container. Provide for patient comfort and catheter safety. Remove your sterile gown and gloves and discard them. Disinfect reusable goggles and store them for later use. Document the procedure and the patient's response.

Once inserted, the PICC line may be used for fluid infusions and medication administration. Before using the line, the tip placement should be checked by X-ray. Check your agency policy for specific guidelines.

Another way to check line placement is to first clamp the extension tubing and then attach a syringe to the hub and aspirate for blood return. Discard any blood-filled syringes in the sharps container. Flush the catheter with normal saline solution after checking for blood return. This method should be used in place of X-ray verification only when X-rays aren't available.

Changing the dressing. The original dressing will need to be changed, using aseptic technique, within 1 or 2 days after placing the PICC line. To change it, help the patient to a comfortable position and expose the insertion site. Wash your hands and put on a pair of clean gloves.

Slowly peel away the transparent occlusive dressing, taking care not to dislodge the catheter or move it around inside the vein. Start removing the occlusive dressing at the farthest point away from the insertion site, and finish at the site.

Remove the 2″ × 2″ gauze pads placed during insertion. Also change the Steri-Strips each time you change the dressing. Inspect the insertion site for signs of complications.

After removing your gloves, wash your hands and put on a mask and sterile gloves. Use sterile technique when performing the dressing change.

Clean the insertion site with alcohol swabs followed by povidone-iodine swabs. Allow the skin to air-dry.

Apply new Steri-Strips to anchor the wing tips of the catheter hub to the skin. Replace the 2″ × 2″ gauze pads if necessary.

Apply a new sterile transparent dressing over the entire catheter site and at least 1½″ (3.8 cm) above the exit site. Secure any tubing to the outer periphery of the transparent dressing with adhesive tape.

Remove and discard used disposable items. Provide for patient comfort. Remove your sterile gloves and mask, and wash your hands.

Removing the line. If the catheter is no longer needed for infusion therapy or if it becomes damaged, broken, or occluded, it will need to be removed.

Start by explaining the procedure to the patient; then help him into a comfortable position that exposes the catheter insertion site. Wash your hands and put on clean gloves.

Remove the transparent dressing and loosen any taped connections around the extension tubing. Then remove your gloves, wash your hands, and put on sterile gloves.

Stabilize the catheter at the hub with your nondominant hand. With the other hand, gently tug on the PICC line, removing a few centimeters at a time. It should come out easily. If you feel resistance, apply tension to the line by taping it down. Then attempt to remove it again in a few minutes.

Once you've successfully removed the catheter, apply manual pressure to the site with folded sterile gauze pads for at least 1 minute. Then cover the site with povidone-iodine ointment, and tape a new folded gauze pad into place. Inspect the PICC to ensure that the entire line was removed intact. You can verify that the line was completely removed by measuring the removed line and comparing this length with the length of the line when it was inserted.

Discard the used PICC line in a sharps container. Discard used disposable items and provide for patient comfort. Remove your gloves and wash your hands.

Teaching points

◆ *Teach your patient with a PICC line how to administer his own fluids or medications. Instruct other home caregivers on how to care for the line and administer medications and fluids.*

◆ *Teach the patient and home caregivers how to flush the line, but only establish a routine flushing schedule if the catheter isn't routinely used for fluids or medications. A flush of 2 ml of 10-100 U/ml heparin solution every 12 hours is sufficient to flush the PICC line if the catheter is not used daily.*

◆ *Teach the patient and home caregivers to inspect the insertion site daily. They should inspect the catheter and check for any bleeding, redness, drainage, or swelling. Instruct the patient to contact you if he observes any of those signs.*

Special considerations

You'll need special training, as defined by your agency and state authorities, before you'll be able to insert PICC lines.

In the home setting, the dressing on a PICC line should be changed every 5 to 7 days. However, because of the location of the catheter, the patient may not be able to change the dressing himself. So you may need to teach another caregiver in the home how to do it. Be careful, however, to choose a person who you believe capable of learning and performing the procedure correctly and carefully. Remember that the catheter may not be sutured in place, and the procedure requires sterile technique. If you suspect that the integrity of the dressing or the catheter is being compromised, perform the dressing changes yourself.

Be sure to have an adequate length of extension tubing attached to the catheter hub, especially if the patient will be administering his own fluids or medications through the line. Change the extension tubing weekly, along with the dressing change.

PICC lines traditionally cause fewer and less severe complications than CV access lines, but they may cause some. (See *Correcting PICC problems,* pages 378 and 379.) The most common complication, phlebitis, can occur within the first 48 to 72 hours after placement. Phlebitis is more common in left-sided insertions and when a large-gauge catheter is used. Application of moist heat during the first 24 hours after insertion may prevent phlebitis. Also, wearing powder-free gloves during insertion eliminates particulate contact with the catheter, which can be a source of phlebitis.

Air embolism is a smaller risk with PICC lines than it is with CV lines because PICC lines are inserted below the level of the heart.

Patients may complain of pain during insertion and throughout therapy, mainly because of the fluid or medication being infused. Sudden onset of pain should be investigated.

Vigorous flushing can cause the catheter tip to migrate. Teach the patient and other home caregivers to flush gently to avoid this complication.

If not adequately flushed or heparinized, the line can clot as well. Catheter occlusion is a common complication that will necessitate either instillation of declotting medication (such as urokinase) or replacement of the catheter. Avoid this complication by thorough flushing with each use and thorough education if the patient will be caring for his own line.

Correcting PICC problems

Problem	Causes	Interventions
Damaged or broken catheter	◆ Pinholes, leaks, or tears in catheter	◆ Examine the catheter for drainage after flushing. ◆ Follow the recommended clamping procedure. ◆ Remove the catheter, if ordered. ◆ To prevent catheter damage, avoid using sharp objects near the catheter and avoid inserting needles longer than 1″ through the injection cap.
Disconnected catheter or loose connections	◆ Patient movement ◆ Catheter not securely connected to extension tubing	◆ Tighten all loose connections. ◆ If extension tubing or cap disconnects, clamp the catheter. ◆ Clean the catheter hub or extension tubing with alcohol or povidone-iodine solution to ensure a tight connection. ◆ Change the extension tubing. Don't reconnect contaminated tubing. ◆ Connect clean I.V. tubing or a heparin lock to the site, and restart the infusion.
Fluid won't infuse	◆ Closed clamp ◆ Displaced or kinked catheter ◆ Thrombus	◆ Check the infusion system and clamps. ◆ Change the patient's position. ◆ Remove the dressing and examine the external portion of the catheter. If a kink isn't apparent, consider assessing the catheter's position by X-ray. ◆ Have the patient cough, breathe deeply, or perform Valsalva's maneuver. ◆ Try to withdraw blood.

Correcting PICC problems *(continued)*

Problem	Causes	Interventions
Occlusion	◆ Thrombus ◆ Improper flushing ◆ Decreased flow rate ◆ Precipitate formation from infusion of incompatible substances ◆ Catheter improperly positioned in vein; catheter tip against vessel wall	◆ Reposition the patient and check for flow. ◆ Attempt to aspirate the clot, but don't force it. ◆ Notify the doctor. ◆ If ordered, infuse a thrombolytic agent, such as streptokinase or urokinase, to dissolve the occlusion. ◆ If necessary, remove the catheter (may be repositioned in the vein with confirmation by X-ray).
Inability to draw blood	◆ Closed clamp ◆ Displaced or kinked catheter ◆ Thrombus ◆ Catheter movement against vessel wall with negative pressure	◆ Change the infusion system and clamps. ◆ Change the patient's position. ◆ Remove the dressing and examine the external portion of the catheter. ◆ Have the patient cough, breathe deeply, or perform Valsalva's maneuver. ◆ Obtain an X-ray order to verify placement of the catheter.

Maintaining a vascular access port

An implanted vascular access device is inserted surgically, by a doctor, with local anesthesia. Access devices are considered for patients when an external CV access line is not desirable or cannot be inserted.

The device consists of a catheter attached to a reservoir that's covered by a self-sealing rubber septum. The most popular access device is the vascular access port (VAP). Implanted in a pocket under the skin, a VAP functions like a long-term CV access line, minus the external parts. The attached indwelling catheter tunnels through subcutaneous tissue, and its tip lies in a central vein, such as the subclavian. VAPs can also be used for arterial access. They also can be implanted in the epidural space, peritoneum, and pericardial and pleural cavities.

VAPs come in two types: top entry and side entry. The reservoir on the port can be made of titanium, stainless steel, or molded plastic. In a top-entry device, the needle enters the port perpendicular to the reservoir (as shown in the top illustration below). In a side-entry device, the needle enters the port through the septum that lies parallel to the reservoir (as shown in the bottom illustration below). A needle stop prevents the needle from coming out the other side.

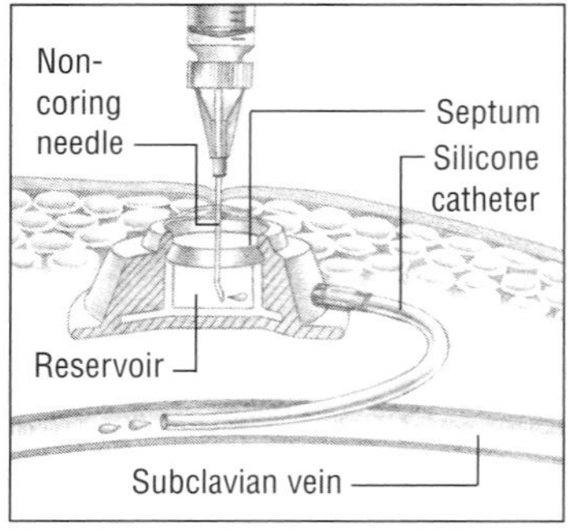

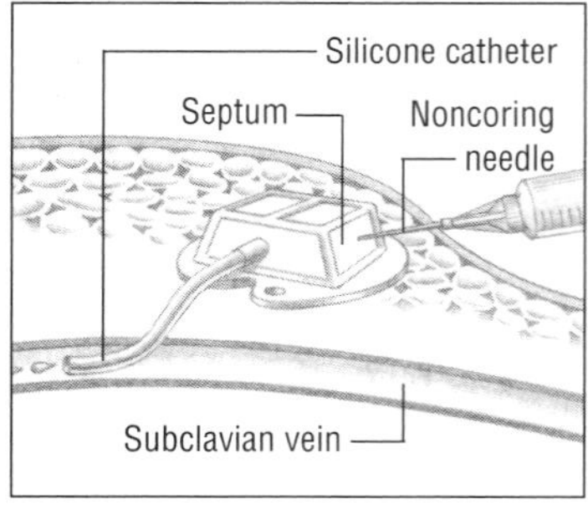

VAPs are used to deliver continuous or intermittent infusions of medication, chemotherapy, TPN, fluids, or blood products.

Implanted devices are easier to maintain than external devices. VAPs require heparinization only once after each use or monthly if not in use. The risk for infection is reduced because no exit site exists to allow entry of microorganisms. Dressings are required only while the port is accessed. In addition, patients with VAPs have fewer activity restrictions because the device has no external parts.

Many patients find the VAP easier to accept than an external device because the device is completely covered with skin and creates only a slight protrusion. However, because the device is implanted, some patients might find it more difficult to manage, particularly if they need to administer fluids or medications frequently.

Patients who fear or dislike needle punctures might be uncomfortable with a VAP as well, because accessing the device requires inserting a needle through the subcutaneous tissue. Also, the implantation and removal of the device requires a surgical procedure and associated hospitalization.

Because of the high cost of a VAP, it is usually viewed as worthwhile only for patients who require infusion therapy for at least 6 months. A VAP is usually contraindicated in patients who haven't been able to tolerate other implantable devices and in patients who might develop an allergic reaction to the VAP material.

Equipment and preparation

The VAP will be implanted in the hospital by a doctor. You can then use the port at the patient's home to administer medications, draw blood, or provide continuous or intermittent infusions of fluids, TPN, medications, chemotherapy, and pain management. To care for a VAP, you'll need specific I.V. therapy certification. Before arriving at the patient's home, find out whether the access port is on the top or the side.

Bolus doses. If you're using the VAP to infuse bolus medications or fluids, you'll need the following equipment: ◆ one right-angle noncoring Huber needle with integrated 6″ extension tubing with clamp ◆ vial of 10-100 U/ml heparin solution for infusion ◆ vial of sterile normal saline solution ◆ 5- and 10-ml syringes ◆ medication for infusion or I.V. fluids with tubing ◆ topical antimicrobial pads (povidone-iodine and alcohol) ◆ disposable sterile gloves ◆ sharps container ◆ hand-washing supplies.

Continuous doses. If using the VAP to administer continuous medications, the following equipment is needed: ◆ one right-angle noncoring Huber needle with integrated 6″ extension tubing with clamp ◆ vial of 10-100 U/ml heparin solution ◆ vial of sterile normal saline solution ◆ 5- and 10-ml syringes ◆ medication for bolus ◆ topical antimicrobial pads (povidone-iodine and alcohol) ◆ disposable sterile gloves ◆ sharps container ◆ hand-washing supplies.

Drawing blood. If you're using the VAP to draw blood, the following equipment is needed: ◆ one right-angle noncoring needle with integrated 6″ extension tubing with clamp ◆ 10-100 U/ml heparin solution for infusion ◆ sterile normal saline solution ◆ 5- and 10-ml syringes ◆ one or two 20-ml syringes for blood sampling ◆ laboratory specimen tubes ◆ laboratory requisitions ◆ topical antimicrobial pads (povidone-iodine and alcohol) ◆ disposable sterile gloves ◆ sharps container ◆ hand-washing supplies.

Handling a clot. If a clot forms in the port, you may have to instill a declotting agent. Equipment needed to declot a port includes: ◆ doctor-prescribed thrombolytic agent (such as urokinase) ◆ sterile normal saline solution for infusion ◆ 3-ml syringes with 1″ needles ◆ one straight, noncoring needle with integrated extension tubing and clamp ◆ topical antimicrobial pads (povidone-iodine and alcohol) ◆ disposable clean gloves ◆ sharps container ◆ hand-washing supplies.

Implementation

Your implementation will depend largely on what you're administering.

Bolus doses. Explain the procedure to the patient, and help her into a comfortable position that allows easy access to the port. Assemble all your equipment within easy reach. Wash your hands and set up supplies on a sterile field. Then put on a pair of sterile gloves.

Palpate the area over the device, and assess it for signs of infection and skin breakdown (as shown below). You can place an ice pack over the site for several minutes to ease discomfort from the needle puncture.

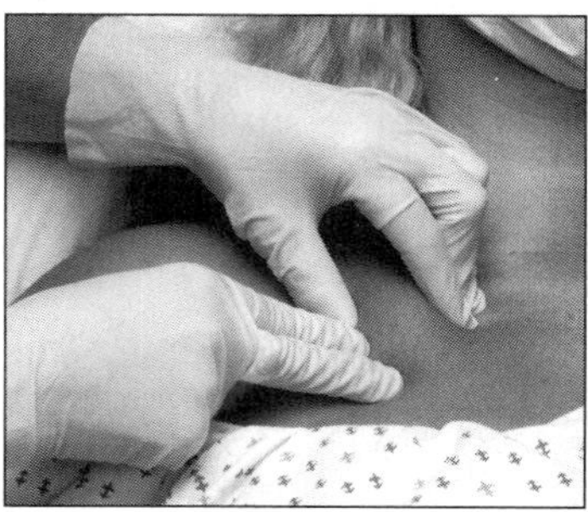

Clean the skin over the implanted device with an alcohol pad. Start cleaning at the center of the port, and work in a circular motion, 1½″ to 2½″ (4 to 6 cm) outward. Discard the used pad. Then repeat the cleaning procedure two more times with two more alcohol pads.

Using the povidone-iodine pads, continue cleaning until the site has been cleaned three times with the povidone-iodine. Allow the skin to air-dry.

Attach a syringe filled with 10 ml of normal saline solution to the extension tubing on the noncoring needle. Flush the tubing and the needle.

Palpate the location of the device's septum to access the portal septum. To use a top-entry port, anchor the port between the thumb and forefinger of one hand to stabilize it. Firmly push the needle through the skin and portal septum at a 90-degree angle until it hits the bottom of the portal chamber (as shown below). You may hear a click as the needle touches the bottom of the portal chamber.

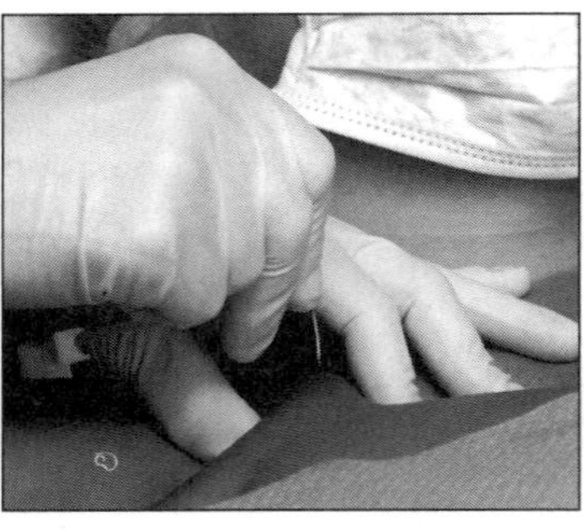

To use a side-entry port, insert the needle parallel rather than perpendicular to the reservoir (as shown below).

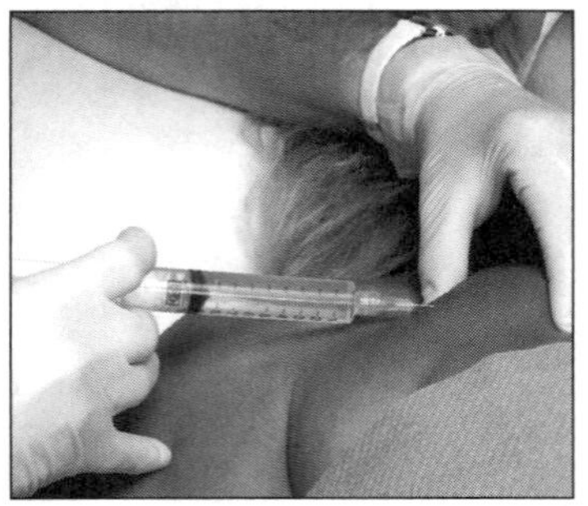

Check for blood return and flush the system with 10 ml of normal saline solution to ensure patency. Secure the noncoring needle to the skin with a small piece of tape.

Clamp the extension tubing on the needle and remove the syringe. Discard the used syringe in the sharps container.

Take up the medication for bolus delivery (in a syringe), and attach the syringe to the extension tubing. Release the clamp and inject the medication bolus through the tubing into the port (as shown below).

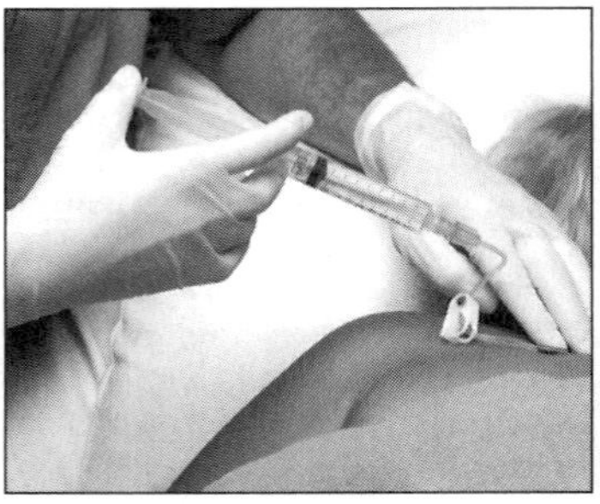

After injecting the medication, reclamp the tubing, remove the syringe, and discard it in the sharps container.

Taking another syringe filled with 10 ml of normal saline solution, attach it to the extension tubing, release the clamp, and flush the port. Remove the normal saline flush syringe, and attach a syringe filled with 5 ml of heparin solution. Flush the port with the heparin solution. Continue to maintain positive pressure on the plunger of the heparin syringe with one hand as the other hand closes the clamp on the extension tubing. Do not remove the syringe from the tubing. While stabilizing the port, remove the needle.

Remove and discard all used items, and provide for patient comfort. Remove your gloves and wash your hands.

Continuous doses. Explain the procedure and help the patient to a comfortable position that allows easy access to the port. Assemble all necessary equipment within easy reach. Prepare the medication or fluid for infusion by opening the tubing, closing the clamp, spiking the solution bag, and priming the tubing. If using an infusion pump, make sure you have appropriate, compatible tubing. Wash your hands and set up a sterile field. Then put on a pair of sterile gloves.

Clean the skin over the implanted device with an alcohol pad. Start cleaning at the center of the port, and work in a circular motion, 1½″ to 2½″ (4 to 6 cm) outward. Discard the used pad. Repeat the cleaning procedure with two more alcohol pads.

Using povidone-iodine pads, continue cleaning until the site has been cleaned three times with povidone-iodine. Allow the skin to air-dry.

Attach a syringe filled with 10 ml of normal saline solution to the extension tubing on the noncoring needle. Flush the tubing and the needle.

Palpate the location of the device's septum to access the portal septum. While stabilizing the port with one hand, firmly push the needle through the skin and portal septum at a 90-degree angle (or parallel to the port if using a side-entry model) until it hits the bottom of the portal chamber. You may hear a click as the needle touches the bottom of the portal chamber.

Check for blood return, and flush the system with 10 ml of normal saline solution to ensure patency.

Secure the noncoring needle with Steri-Strips or ½″ tape. Roll a 2″ × 2″ piece of gauze under the needle for stabilization, if necessary, and apply a transparent adhesive dressing over the noncoring needle. (See *Continuous infusion: Securing the needle*.)

Continuous infusion: Securing the needle

When starting a continuous infusion, you need to secure the right-angle, noncoring needle to the skin. If the needle hub isn't flush with the skin, place a folded sterile dressing under the hub (as shown below). Then apply adhesive skin closures across it.

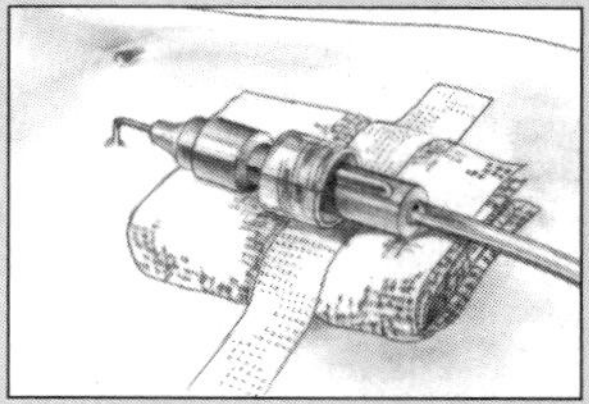

Secure the needle and tubing using the chevron taping technique (as shown below).

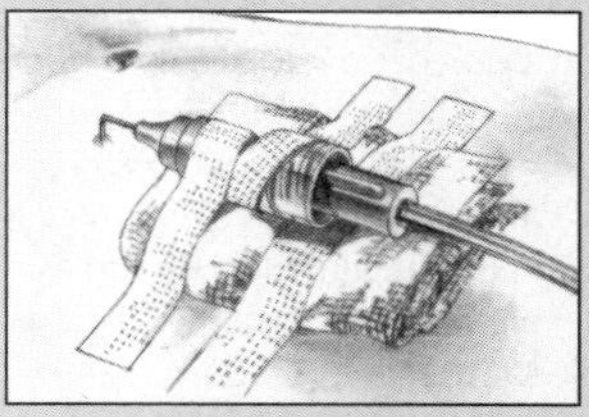

Apply a transparent semipermeable dressing over the entire site (as shown below).

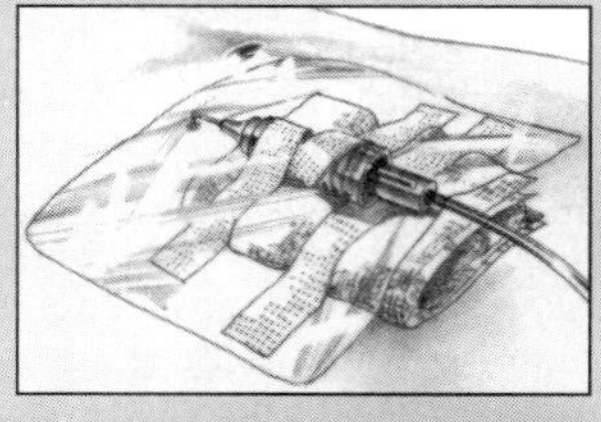

Clamp the extension tubing on the needle, and remove the syringe. Discard the used syringe in the sharps container.

Connect the I.V. infusion tubing to the extension tubing. Release the clamp on the extension tubing, and begin the infusion. Secure all connections with tape. Loop the extension tubing and secure with tape.

After the infusion is finished, reclamp the extension tubing, remove the infusion tubing, and discard it in the appropriate trash container.

Flush the extension tubing and port first with a syringe filled with 10 ml of normal saline solution. Then flush with a syringe filled with 5 ml of heparin solution for infusion. Continue to maintain positive pressure on the plunger of the heparin syringe with one hand while closing the clamp on the extension tubing. Do not remove this syringe from the tubing. While stabilizing the port, remove the needle.

Remove all used items. Discard the disposable ones and provide for patient comfort. Remove your gloves and wash your hands.

Drawing blood. Explain the procedure to the patient, and help him to a comfortable position that allows easy access to the port. Assemble all of the necessary equipment on a sterile field and within easy reach. Wash your hands and put on sterile gloves.

Clean the skin over the implanted device with an alcohol pad. Start cleaning at the center of the port, and work in a circular motion, 1½″ to 2½″ (4 to 6 cm) outward. Discard the used pad. Repeat the cleaning with two more alcohol pads. Then, using the povidone-iodine pads, continue cleaning until the site has been cleaned three times with the povidone-iodine. Allow the skin to air-dry.

Attach a syringe filled with 10 ml of normal saline solution to the extension tubing on the noncoring needle. Flush the tubing and the needle.

Palpate the device to find the portal septum. While stabilizing the port with one hand, firmly push the needle through the skin and portal septum at a 90-degree angle (with a side-entry port, enter the skin parallel to the port) until it hits the bottom of the portal chamber. You may hear a click as the needle touches the bottom of the portal chamber.

Check for blood return to verify correct needle placement and to prevent inadvertently injecting the normal saline solution into subcutaneous tissue. Flush the system with 10 ml of normal saline solution to ensure patency. Using the same syringe, aspirate about 5 to 10 ml of blood. Clamp the extension tubing and disconnect the blood-filled syringe. Discard it in the sharps container. This is done to ensure that the blood sample is as free as possible from medications, normal saline solution, or heparin.

Attach a 20-ml syringe to the extension tubing, and release the clamp. Slowly withdraw the amount of blood needed for laboratory studies into the syringe. Clamp the extension tubing, remove the syringe, and inject the blood into the laboratory tubes. Continue to aspirate for blood until all required tubes are filled.

Clamp the extension tubing on the needle and remove the syringe. Discard the used syringe in the sharps container.

Taking another syringe filled with 10 ml of normal saline solution, attach it to the extension tubing, release the clamp, and flush the port. Remove the normal saline flush syringe, and attach a syringe filled with 5 ml of heparin solution for infusion. Flush the port with the heparin solution. Continue to maintain positive pressure on the plunger of the heparin syringe with one hand while closing the clamp on the extension tubing. Do not remove the syringe from the tubing. While stabilizing the port, remove the needle.

Remove and discard all used items and provide for patient comfort. Remove your gloves and wash your hands.

Handling a clot. Explain the procedure to the patient, and help him to a comfortable position that allows easy access to the port. Assemble all necessary equipment within easy reach. Wash your hands and put on a pair of sterile gloves.

Clean the skin over the implanted device with an alcohol pad. Start cleaning at the center of the port, and work in a circular motion, 1½″ to 2½″ (4 to 6 cm) outward. Discard the used pad. Repeat the cleaning with two more alcohol pads.

Using the povidone-iodine pads, continue cleaning until the site has been cleaned three times with the povidone-iodine. Allow the skin to air-dry.

Attach a syringe filled with 10 ml of normal saline solution to the extension tubing on the noncoring needle. Flush the tubing and the needle.

Palpate the location of the device's septum, and stabilize and access the port as described previously.

Draw up 1 ml of urokinase and 1 ml of normal saline solution into a 3-ml syringe. Connect the syringe to the integrated extension tubing on the noncoring needle. Unclamp the tubing. Slowly inject the urokinase into the occluded lumen and port. Wait 10 minutes.

Using the same syringe, attempt to aspirate the residual clot. If unsuccessful, refill a syringe with 1 ml of normal saline solution and 1 ml of urokinase, and reflush the port. Wait 20 minutes. Attempt to aspirate the residual clot.

If successful, take another syringe filled with 10 ml of normal saline solution, attach it to the extension tubing, release the clamp, and flush the port. Remove the normal saline flush syringe, and attach a syringe filled with 5 ml of heparin solution for infusion. Flush the port with the heparin solution.

Continue to maintain positive pressure on the plunger of the heparin syringe with one hand while closing the clamp on the tubing. Stabilize the port while removing the needle.

If you're unable to aspirate the residual clot, contact the doctor for further instuctions. The VAP might need to be surgically removed and replaced.

Remove and discard all used items and provide for patient comfort. Remove your gloves and wash your hands.

Teaching points

- *Instruct the patient with a VAP thoroughly about nursing procedures and follow-up visits to ensure safety and successful treatment. If the patient or a home caregiver will be accessing the port, explain that the most uncomfortable part of the procedure is the actual insertion of the needle through the skin into the port. Once the needle is in the port, the patient will likely only feel pressure. Over time and with many accesses, the skin over the port will become desensitized. Until that occurs, the patient can use ice or a topical anesthetic to reduce the discomfort associated with the needle puncture.*
- *Teach the patient the proper way to insert the needle. Make sure the patient and other home caregivers learn to push the needle until they can feel the back of the port. Patients tend to*

Risks of VAP therapy

Use this chart to help determine interventions appropriate for complications associated with venous access ports (VAPs).

Complications and possible causes	Signs and symptoms	Nursing actions
EXTRAVASATION		
◆ Needle incorrectly inserted into the port ◆ Needle position not confirmed ◆ Needle pulled out of the septum ◆ Infusion of vesicant drugs	◆ Patient complaints of burning sensation ◆ Swelling in and around subcutaneous (S.C.) tissue ◆ Needle dislodged in S.C. tissue	*Interventions:* ◆ Stop the infusion. ◆ Notify the doctor. ◆ Prepare to administer an antidote, if ordered. ◆ Remove the needle if possible. *Prevention:* ◆ Teach the patient how to access the port, verify needle placement, and secure the needle before starting an infusion.
FIBRIN SHEATH FORMATION		
◆ Platelets adhered to catheter	◆ Blocked port and catheter lumen ◆ Inability to flush the port or administer infusion ◆ Swelling, tenderness, and erythema in the neck, chest, and shoulder area	*Interventions:* ◆ Notify the doctor. ◆ Prepare to perform declotting procedure, if trained to do so. *Prevention:* ◆ Administer only compatible medications and fluids through the port. ◆ Don't use the port to draw blood for laboratory specimens. ◆ Use the port only to infuse fluids and medications.
INFECTION OR SKIN BREAKDOWN		
◆ Infected incision or port pocket ◆ Poor postoperative healing	◆ Redness and warmth at the port site ◆ Oozing or purulent drainage at the port site or in the pocket ◆ Fever	*Interventions:* ◆ Notify the doctor. ◆ Give antibiotics as prescribed. ◆ Apply warm soaks for 20 minutes four times daily. ◆ Assess the site daily for redness; document drainage.

Risks of VAP therapy *(continued)*

Complications and possible causes	Signs and symptoms	Nursing actions
INFECTION OR SKIN BREAKDOWN *(continued)*		
		Prevention: ◆ Teach the patient how to inspect the site for signs of infection, including redness, swelling, drainage, or skin breakdown.
THROMBOSIS		
◆ Frequent use of the port for blood sampling ◆ Use of the port to infuse packed red blood cells (RBCs) or other blood products	◆ Inability to flush the port ◆ Inability to administer medications or fluids through the port	*Interventions:* ◆ Notify the doctor. ◆ Prepare to perform declotting procedure, if trained to do so. *Prevention:* ◆ Give packed RBCs piggybacked with a normal saline infusion. ◆ Give blood products with an infusion pump, ◆ Flush the port between units of blood for multiple infusions. ◆ Flush the port thoroughly if using for blood sampling.

stop short of the back of the port, leaving the bevel of the needle in the rubber septum. Also, teach the patient not to twist the needle while inserting because it could damage the septum.

◆ *If the device isn't used often, teach the patient and home caregivers to flush it monthly with normal saline solution and heparin to keep the port viable.*

◆ *If the VAP has a double port, remind the patient that it's even more important to flush the device regularly and to use a new needle for each port.*

Special considerations

If the VAP is being used for a continuous fluid infusion, the needle will need to be changed every 7 days. Secure the needle with a sterile dressing to keep it secure in the port.

VAPs are not problem-free. (See *Risks of VAP therapy*.) Common problems with this device include an inability to flush the device, draw blood, or palpate the device. *If you can't flush the device or draw blood,* do the following:

◆ Check the tubing to make sure it's not kinked or clamped.

◆ Reposition the patient by raising the arm on the same side of the port, rolling the patient to his other side, or having the patient cough, sit up, or take a deep breath. You can also try infusing 10 ml of normal saline solution through the catheter or changing the noncoring needle.

◆ Make sure the needle has been correctly placed, and aspirate for blood return.

◆ Suspect clot formation in the port, and obtain an order from the doctor for a declotting agent.

◆ Notify the doctor if the catheter has moved or the port has rotated from its usual position.

If you can't palpate the device, do the following:

◆ Locate the portal chamber scar.

◆ Use deep palpation to try to locate the device.

◆ Use a longer noncoring needle (1½″ or 2″) to gain access to the port.

Other complications associated with VAP therapy include site infection or skin breakdown, extravasation, thrombosis, and fibrin sheath formation.

Maintaining an implantable pump

The use of implantable pumps is slowly increasing. Currently, pumps are being implanted primarily in independent patients capable of a high degree of self-management. Implantable pumps are of great advantage to patients requiring long-term infusions because they help to minimize negative effects on body image.

First developed to simplify long-term insulin administration in diabetic patients, they now are also used to deliver chemotherapeutic agents, intraspinal narcotics, intra-articular antibiotics, and intrathecal muscle relaxants.

The pump typically is surgically implanted in a subcutaneous pocket of the lower abdomen or subclavian fossa, where it can remain for years, if necessary.

The pump has a reservoir that needs periodic refilling through a small septum (as shown below). If you've been authorized by your home care agency to refill your patient's reservoir, you'll do so at scheduled intervals to make sure he receives a consistent dosage. For some medications, the patient may need to have the pump refilled at an acute care or outpatient facility.

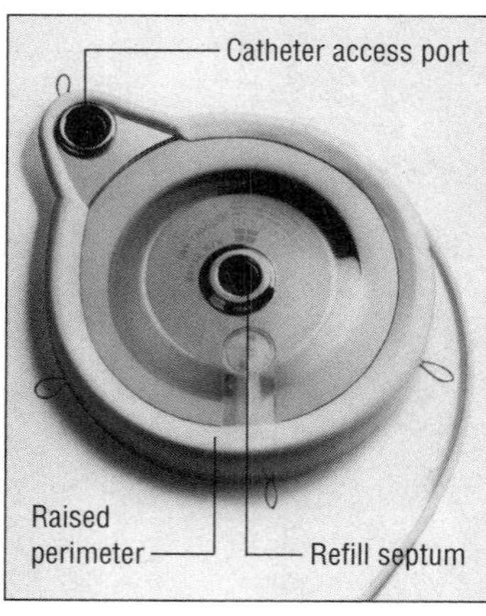

Your role in caring for a home-based patient with an implanted pump includes:

◆ monitoring the effectiveness of the medication being administered

◆ examining the site for signs and symptoms of infection

◆ communicating about the patient's care and refilling schedule with staff at the acute care or outpatient facility, as needed

◆ instructing the patient on self-care techniques to ensure pump integrity

◆ instructing the patient on signs and symptoms associated with pump failure.

Equipment and preparation

If you're trained to refill implanted pumps and assigned to do so by your agency, you'll probably need the following equipment: ◆ information about the pump ◆ dressing change supplies if needed ◆ sterile and nonsterile gloves ◆ standard precaution supplies ◆ sharps container ◆ plastic disposable trash bags ◆ handwashing supplies.

Some implantable pump manufacturers supply a pump-specific refill kit, which may or may not be reimbursable. Check with your home care agency about the use of these kits.

Implementation

Contact the patient before making the home visit to see if he needs any specific supplies. When you arrive, wash your hands and arrange needed supplies within easy reach.

Begin the visit by assessing the patient's vital signs. Analyze the site of the implanted pump. Inspect the skin and surrounding area for any signs of infiltration, breakdown, redness, swelling, or drainage. Document the condition of the skin.

Evaluate the pump by noting if the settings are correct and if the infusion has a sufficient quantity of medication. Check all connections and any battery back-up packs for maximum functioning.

Perform diagnostic tests to help evaluate whether the infusing medication is sufficient. For example, use a glucometer to check blood glucose level, perform urine tests for glucose and ketone levels, and draw blood for such tests as fasting blood glucose, hematocrit, hemoglobin, or complete blood count (CBC) and differential for chemotherapy infusion.

Depending on the location of the pump, you may need to change a dressing. If you do, wash your hands and assemble all needed supplies. Help the patient to a comfortable position, and expose the pump site and dressing area. Remove the old dressing and discard it. Then remove your soiled gloves and discard them.

Wash your hands and put on a fresh pair of sterile gloves to assess the site. Clean it with a prescribed antimicrobial solution or pads. Allow the site to air-dry. Apply an antimicrobial ointment or other treatment to the affected area.

Cover with sterile gauze pads and tape securely. Label with the date, time, and your initials on top of the dressing.

To refill an implantable pump, first explain the procedure to the patient. Then help him into a comfortable position, and expose his abdomen. Open the refill kit (or gather your supplies on a sterile field). Wash your hands and put on gloves.

Palpate the pump by feeling the raised outer perimeter (as shown below). Near the center is the refill septum where you'll infuse the medication. The catheter access port is located near the pump's perimeter and is used only for bolus doses.

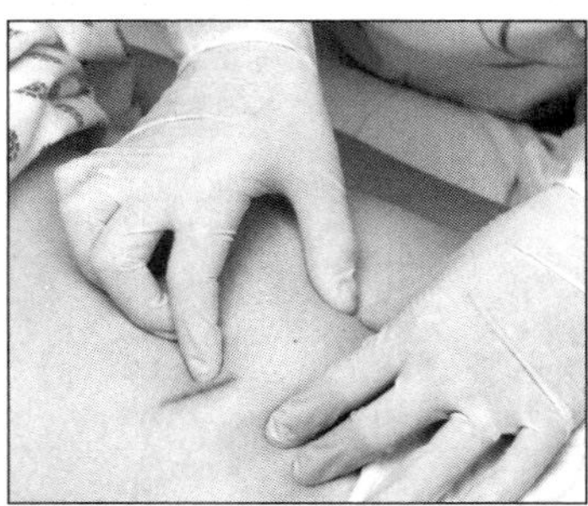

Using an alcohol swab, clean the pump site from the center septum, and work outward beyond the pump's perimeter. Remove and discard your gloves, and put on a mask and sterile gloves. After the alcohol has dried, repeat the same procedure using povidone-iodine swabs.

Place the fenestrated drape supplied in the refill kit over the prepared pump site to create a sterile field. Remove the template (also in the kit), and position it over the pump so it conforms to the shape of the pump (as shown below). The template will help you locate the refill septum.

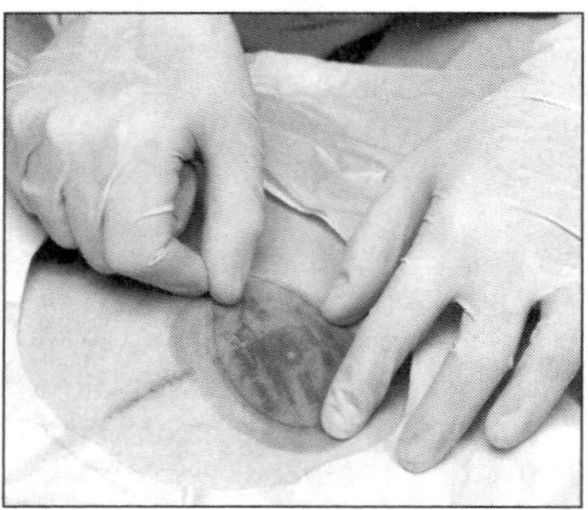

To remove residual medication from the pump, attach the empty syringe barrel from the kit to one end of the stopcock and the 22G needle to the other end (as shown below). Close the stopcock and place this assembly on the sterile field.

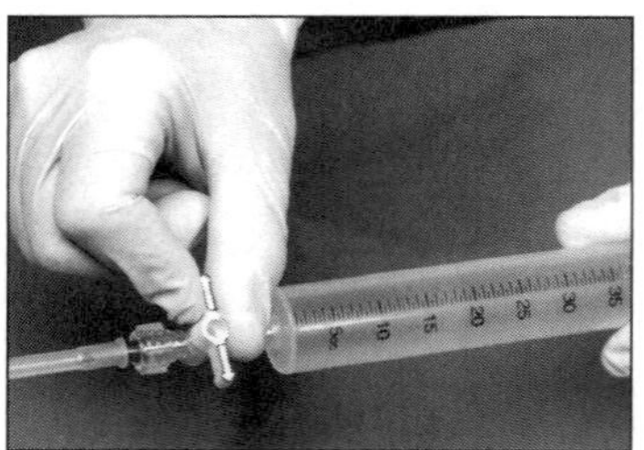

Attach a second 22G needle to the luer-lock connection of the tubing set. Then connect the syringe barrel, stopcock, and needle assembly to the tubing injection port (as shown at the top of the next column).

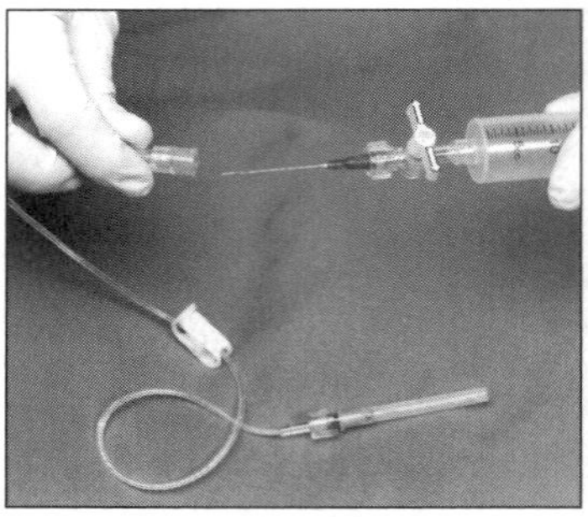

Insert the needle attached to the tubing straight through the template hole and septum into the pump reservoir (as shown below). Be careful not to use the catheter access port located near the pump perimeter. Injecting into it can cause a serious overdose.

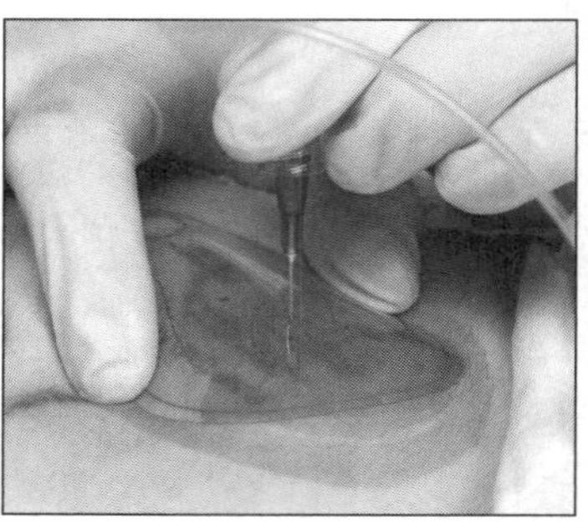

Open the stopcock to let residual medication flow from the pump into the syringe. When the flow stops, turn the stopcock to seal the syringe. Note the amount of liquid in the syringe. The syringe from the kit gives an accurate reading because the scale allows for fluid still in the tubing.

To replace the medication, close the clamp on the extension tubing. Then remove the syringe barrel, stopcock, and needle from the tubing and discard them. Next, attach a needle to the 50-ml syringe containing the refill medication, and insert it into the injection port of the tubing (as shown at the top of the next page).

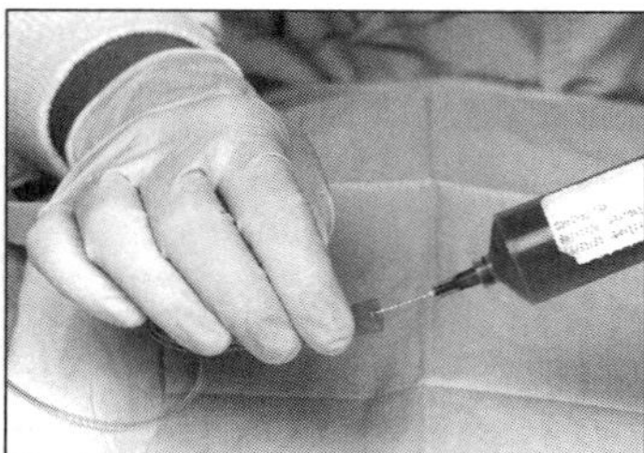

Open the tubing clamp and slowly inject 5 ml of medication into the reservoir (as shown below).

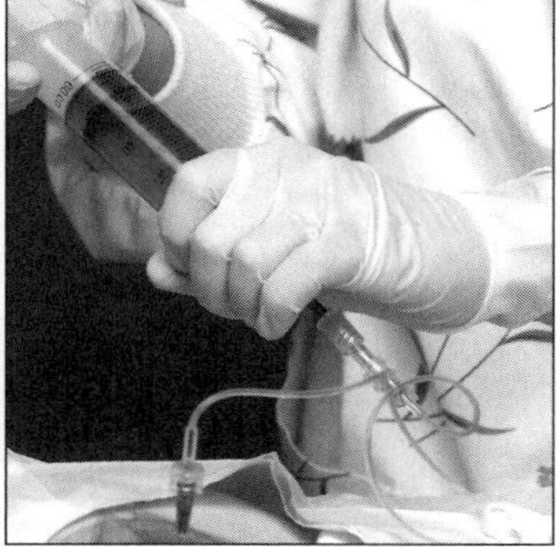

To confirm that the needle is in the reservoir, release pressure on the plunger and allow a small amount of fluid to flow back into the syringe. Don't aspirate fluid from the pump because doing so could cause pump failure. Continue to inject and confirm needle placement at 5-ml increments, until all medication is injected.

While maintaining positive pressure on the syringe plunger, clamp the tubing as close as possible to the needle in the septum. Gently pull the needle out of the septum, and press a sterile gauze pad on the puncture site for 1 minute (as shown at the top of the next column). Discard all needles and sharps in the sharps container.

Remove the template, wash the area with an alcohol pad to remove the povidone-iodine, and allow it to dry.

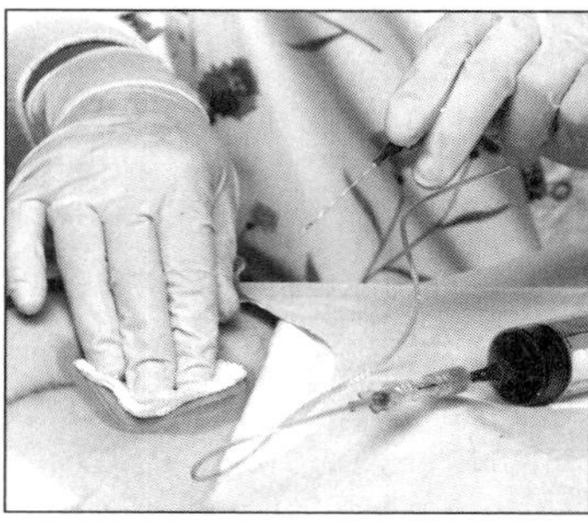

Apply an adhesive bandage or a dressing if needed. Discard all waste in the appropriate container and wash your hands.

Teaching points

- ◆ *Assess the patient's level of understanding about the purpose of the pump, how it works, and how to care for it.*
- ◆ *Evaluate the presence and amount of pump supplies in the patient's home and whether he needs additional materials for appropriate pump care. Coordinate with the patient a convenient time and effective method to have the pump refilled.*
- ◆ *Teach the patient about the type of medication being infused through the pump, expected actions, adverse effects, and potentiating effects.*
- ◆ *Observe the patient's technique for pump care. Reinstruct as needed.*

Special considerations

Not all patients are candidates for implanted infusion pumps. Ideally, the patient with a pump will be ambulatory and able to care for himself. Because the patient probably won't be homebound, Medicare won't reimburse for home care and you'll spend little time with patients who have implanted pumps. Even so, you need to know how to handle this high-tech need should it arise.

Administering chemotherapy

Chemotherapy administered in the home is becoming more common, not only for hospice-certified agencies but also for federally certified ones. Administering chemotherapeutic drugs requires additional training and skills besides those you need for giving other drugs.

Giving chemotherapy in the home is particularly challenging because the usual processes nurses learn and the support nurses have in acute care settings are different. The role of the home care nurse administering chemotherapy is highly autonomous. Home care agencies will have specific qualifications for staff expected to administer chemotherapy in the home.

Rarely will home care nurses be expected to prepare or mix chemotherapy solutions. The agency's pharmacy or contracted home infusion company will prepare and deliver all chemotherapeutic medications to the patient's home. The pharmacy or home infusion company also will provide hazardous material spill kits in case the drug leaks or spills.

Chemotherapy can be provided by several routes. The most common is I.V. All chemotherapy administered in the home must be infused through a volumetric infusion pump. If giving a bolus injection of a chemotherapeutic agent, the correct process is to use a side port of a running I.V.

Equipment and preparation

The equipment needed to administer chemotherapy to a homebound patient is as follows: ◆ chemotherapeutic medications ◆ prescribed compatible infusion fluids ◆ compatible I.V. infusion tubing sets ◆ prescribed antiemetic medication ◆ sterile normal saline solution ◆ 10-100 U/ml heparin solution ◆ other specific catheter flush solution per manufacturer protocols ◆ I.V. infusion pump ◆ 5- and 10-ml syringes for flushing ◆ 5-ml syringes with 23G needles ◆ extravasation antidote for the chemotherapeutic agent ◆ hot and cold compresses as ordered for extravasation ◆ blood sampling supplies, if required ◆ topical antimicrobial pads (povidone-iodine and alcohol) ◆ specially designed chemotherapy gloves or doubled clean disposable gloves ◆ sterile gloves (if needed to access a CV access line) ◆ personal protective equipment, including goggles, gown, mask ◆ spill kits (water-resistant, nonpermeable, long-sleeved gown with cuffs and back closure; shoe covers; two pairs of gloves for double gloving; goggles; mask; disposable dustpan; plastic scraper for collecting broken glass; plastic-backed or absorbable towels; container of desiccant powder or granules to absorb wet contents; two disposable sponges; puncture-proof, leakproof container labeled "biohazard waste"; container of 70% alcohol for cleaning the spill area) ◆ biohazard "chemo bucket" ◆ sharps container ◆ plastic trash bags ◆ hand-washing supplies.

To prepare to administer a course of chemotherapy for a home care patient, you'll need to do the following:

◆ Review your agency's procedure.

◆ Review cardiopulmonary resuscitation, shock, transfusion reaction, and medication reaction policies.

◆ Consult with the doctor for medication orders for pain control and nausea.

◆ Be prepared to tell the patient where to purchase wigs, scarfs, or hats.

◆ Consult with the doctor for fluid intake needs and an opinion about whether the patient would benefit from a psychiatric nursing evaluation for depression or changes in mood and affect.

◆ Consult with the doctor regarding the use of stool softeners for associated constipation.

◆ Monitor the CBC, platelet count, liver function tests, cardiac studies, urine creatinine clearance, and serum electrolyte levels. Notify the doctor of any abnormal or unsafe laboratory values.

Implementation

Begin the visit with a review of the chemotherapeutic agent you'll be giving. Explain its possible adverse effects to the patient, including hair loss, nausea, vomiting, loss of appetite, mouth sores, constipation, diarrhea, and skin and hemopoietic changes. Tell the patient that these effects last only as long as the chemotherapy does. Afterward, the body will recover, unpleasant effects will disappear, and lost hair will regrow.

Obtain a signed informed consent before beginning the infusion.

Explain the procedure, and help the patient to a comfortable position that exposes the I.V. infusion catheter site. Review with the patient any allergies he may have, specifically to medications.

Draw any required samples for ordered laboratory studies. Collect the blood either through venipuncture or through a venous, peripheral, or implanted access device. Follow proper procedure to flush any lines used for blood sampling after drawing the sample. Discard all used equipment properly.

Ideally, the patient should take an antiemetic, if ordered, at least 60 minutes before the start of chemotherapy.

If the patient doesn't have a venous, peripheral, or implanted access device, insert a peripheral catheter following standard precautions. Keep in mind that some drugs are contraindicated by the peripheral route, especially continuous infusion of vesicants.

Wash your hands and put on goggles and clean gloves. Taking the chemotherapeutic medication, carefully open the compatible I.V. tubing, spike the bag or bottle, and prime the tubing. Access the infusion site and disinfect it with the topical antimicrobial pad. Attach the primed tubing to the access site. Turn on the pump or controller and regulate the infusion.

Observe the infusion and site for several minutes to evaluate for signs of extravasation. If you suspect it, react quickly to offset its effects. (See *Responding to chemotherapy extravasation,* page 394.)

If the chemotherapy infuses without incident or evidence of extravasation, discontinue the medication when it has completed infusing. Discard all used sharps in the sharps container. All chemotherapy materials, including bags and tubing, must be discarded in a leakproof container ("chemo bucket").

Flush the infusion site according to protocol. Clean up and provide for patient comfort. Remove your goggles, mask, and gloves, and wash your hands.

If the chemotherapy agent spills, go immediately to your spill kit. Apply the identified contents to the spill, wait for it to solidify, and then clean up according to the manufacturer's instructions.

Teaching points

◆ Review the resources available for obtaining wigs, scarves, and so on. Reassure the patient that hair loss is temporary and that the hair will regrow when the medication is stopped.

Responding to chemotherapy extravasation

If your patient develops swelling at and above the chemotherapy I.V. site as well as discomfort, burning, pain, and blanching, he may be experiencing extravasation. To avoid extensive tissue damage, you'll have to act fast. Do the following:

◆ Stop infusing the chemotherapeutic drug at once.

◆ Leave the needle or catheter in place.

◆ Aspirate any residual drug from the I.V. tubing or the catheter and infiltration site.

◆ Instill the prescribed antidote specific to the chemotherapy agent administered.

◆ Remove the needle if it has clotted, and inject the prescribed antidote subcutaneously, clockwise, into the infiltrated site. Use a new 25G needle with each injection.

◆ Apply a sterile occlusive dressing.

◆ Elevate the extremity.

◆ Apply hot or cold compresses as prescribed by the doctor or warranted by the chemotherapy agent.

◆ *Instruct the patient to eat small, frequent meals that are high in protein.*

◆ *Suggest that the patient increase dietary fiber to help alleviate constipation.*

◆ *Instruct the patient to increase fluid intake to 2 to 3 qt (2 to 3 L) for cystitis.*

◆ *Teach the patient about bleeding precautions, including not using a straight razor. Advise the patient to take care around the home to avoid accidental cuts and bruises.*

◆ *Urge the patient to maintain good personal hygiene and to take other steps to prevent infection. For example, hand washing is crucial to prevent infections. Also tell the patient to avoid crowds and people known to be sick. Make sure the patient knows how to care for I.V. catheters and other sources of infection.*

◆ *Teach the patient and caregivers about the signs and symptoms of infection. Urge them to report infections promptly.*

◆ *Tell the patient to use a soft toothbrush or swab toothettes frequently to minimize the risk of oral mucosal breakdown. Teach him to rinse his mouth frequently with normal saline solution or baking soda and water. Advise against using commercial mouthwashes because they contain alcohol, which can damage mucosa.*

◆ *Instruct the patient to take the prescribed antiemetic at least 1 hour before the scheduled chemotherapeutic dose, around the clock, or before meals.*

◆ *Instruct the patient and home caregivers about the proper handling of chemotherapeutic drugs, the patient's body waste materials, and contaminated linens or other home items. Tell them to wear gloves when handling these items. Contaminated linens should be placed in a pillowcase and laundered separately from other household items. The pillowcase, with the linens inside, should be run through the wash cycle twice.*

◆ *Describe signs and symptoms that should be reported to you or the doctor.*

Special considerations

Before you can (or should) work with chemotherapeutic agents, you'll need special training in how to handle them safely and reduce your exposure to them.

If a chemotherapeutic agent contacts your skin, wash the area thoroughly with soap and water (don't use a germicidal agent). If it splashes in your eye, flood the eye with water or an isotonic eyewash for at least 5 minutes. Hold the eyelid open while performing the eyewash. See a doctor as soon as possible to evaluate any damage.

Do not place food or drinks in the same refrigerator as chemotherapeutic drugs.

When working with patients on chemotherapy, take precautions when handling their body fluids. Wear disposable latex surgical gloves. Empty waste products into the commode, close to the water, to reduce splashing. Close the lid and flush two to three times.

Instruct the patient or home caregivers to make arrangements with either a hospital or private biohazard disposal company for pickup and proper disposal of contaminated wastes.

Administering patient-controlled analgesia

In patient-controlled analgesia (PCA), the patient controls the administration of an analgesic by pressing a button on the delivery pump. The analgesic, usually morphine or a morphine derivative, is delivered only when the patient needs it. PCA can be delivered I.V. or S.C.

PCA devices are built with a patient lock-out mechanism; the mechanism prevents the patient from accidentally overdosing by imposing a lock-out time between doses. The time between doses varies among devices. Even if the patient continues to push the dose button, no analgesic will be delivered.

Two major types of PCA pumps are available. The first is similar to a portable infusion pump. It's an electronically operated, battery back-up system. The pump has a long cord with a button that's similar to a call-button. When the patient pushes the button, the pump delivers a dose of medicine (unless it's still in a lock-out period).

The second type of device is disposable and mechanically operated. It contains an infuser and a unit worn like a wristwatch. A dose of the medication is administered from a collapsible chamber when the patient pushes a button.

As home care becomes more prevalent, pump manufacturers continue to develop new and more efficient units specifically for home use. In fact, PCA pumps are being seen more often in the home care environment, specifically for patients with terminal cancer, painful chronic diseases, and postoperative trauma.

Your role when caring for a home-bound patient with a PCA pump includes:

- ◆ monitoring the effectiveness of the medication
- ◆ assessing the site of the infusion
- ◆ evaluating the amount of medication used
- ◆ instructing the patient and home caregivers on the actions, adverse effects, and potentiating effects of the infused medication.

The PCA pump is usually started while the patient is still in an acute care facility. This is to ensure the patient's tolerance of the medication as well as ongoing monitoring of the patient's respiratory status.

Candidates for PCA include patients who are mentally alert and able to understand and comply with instruc-

Advantages of PCA

Patient-controlled analgesia (PCA) has several advantages, including:
◆ reduced need for intramuscular or subcutaneous injections
◆ pain relief tailored to each patient's size and pain tolerance level
◆ personal control over pain
◆ increased ability to sleep at night with minimal daytime drowsiness
◆ overall lower use of narcotics compared with patients not on PCA
◆ improved patient compliance with overall medical regimen, including such pain-inducing activities as deep breathing, coughing, and frequent position changes.

tions and procedures and who have no history of allergy to the analgesic. Less likely candidates for PCA therapy include those with end-stage respiratory disease, a psychiatric disorder, or a history of drug abuse and those on long-term sedative or tranquilizer therapy. For appropriate candidates, PCA has a number of advantages over traditional pain control. (See *Advantages of PCA*.)

Equipment and preparation

When you receive a referral to care for a patient with PCA, prepare yourself by determining:
◆ the type of analgesic being infused
◆ the frequency of patient dosing
◆ the amount of medication in the pump when the patient is discharged from the acute care facility
◆ the type of pump used
◆ the best way to make additional medication available to the patient
◆ the prescribed lock-out mechanism
◆ the reason the patient is on PCA
◆ the most appropriate education materials to assist with pain control
◆ the site for PCA infusion (I.V. or S.C.).

The home care agency needs to confirm with the doctor the following orders:
◆ loading dose (if applicable)
◆ lock-out mechanism
◆ maintenance dose
◆ amount of analgesic the patient will receive when the pump is activated (bolus dose)
◆ maximum amount the patient can receive within a specific time.

As needed, contact either the agency's pharmacy or another home infusion company to order a pump and infusion supplies to be delivered directly to the patient's home. Also gather the following equipment: ◆ pump-specific I.V. tubing ◆ infusion site dressing supplies ◆ vial of 10-100 U/ml heparin solution ◆ vial of sterile normal saline solution for infusion ◆ 3-, 5-, 10-, and 20-ml syringes ◆ assortment of 20G, 22G, and 25G needles with ⅝", 1", and 1½" lengths ◆ standard precaution supplies, including gloves and gown ◆ hand-washing supplies.

Implementation

When you arrive at the patient's home, assemble all necessary equipment and wash your hands. Measure the patient's vital signs, especially respiratory rate and breath sounds. Use a pain assessment scale to rate the patient's level of pain.

Review the pump, the amount of infusion available in the cartridge, and the integrity of the electrical outlet and battery back-up system. Also review the frequency of patient dosing. (If the patient is keeping a log, review the log.) Assess the reasons why or when the patient will dose.

Examine the infusion site for integrity, signs and symptoms of infection, and the need for a dressing change.

If the cartridge on the PCA pump needs to be changed, follow these steps:

Begin by preparing the new syringe or cartridge, attaching pump-specific tubing to the medication, and priming the tubing. Turn off the pump and clamp the infusion tubing. Remove the tubing from the patient's infusion site. Flush the infusion site, if indicated, with a compatible flush solution. Change the infusion site dressing if indicated.

Remove the used cartridge or syringe from the infusion pump, and discard it in an appropriate plastic container. Attach the new cartridge or syringe in the pump, and attach the new infusion tubing to the patient's access site. Turn on the pump and allow the patient to provide a dose of the medication when needed.

Remove and discard all used disposable items. Discard sharps in the sharps container. Evaluate the integrity of the pump and the patient's response to dosing.

Teaching points

◆ *The patient and home caregivers must be instructed in:*
– pump operation
– how to administer a dose
– when to administer a dose (Ideally, doses should be potent enough to relieve acute pain, but not enough to cause drowsiness.)
– what to do in the event of a power or pump failure
– how to change the cartridge or syringe
– how to check the access site for signs of infection or infiltration
– what to do if the patient continues to have pain throughout the dosing and lock-out periods
– what to do for pain if the infusion site infiltrates or the line comes out or becomes kinked or torn
– emergency procedures in the event of respiratory failure.

Special considerations

Respiratory depression is a primary complication of PCA. Patients receiving PCA for a terminal illness might have an advanced directive prepared, explaining what they want done in the event of respiratory failure. Obtain a copy of this directive, and place it in the patient's home care chart.

If the power fails, make sure the patient or a caregiver has access numbers for emergency 24-hour assistance. If ordered, the patient may also have a supply of analgesic patches to use in case of mechanical failure.

Provide ongoing assessment of the medication's effectiveness and the patient's overall health. A patient receiving PCA for pain after a traumatic event will eventually be weaned from the pump. As his condition improves, pain subsides and the need for ongoing home care nursing will end. Patients in the terminal stages of a disease will likely be receiving PCA until they die. It is with these patients that the home care nurse's compassion, understanding, and instruction will be most crucial.

◆ RESPIRATORY PROCEDURES

The type of respiratory care a home care patient requires ranges from simple oxygen administration to complete ventilator support. Nurses who provide this care must be skilled in assessing oxygenation and respiratory status, signs and symptoms of hypoxemia, types of ventilatory equipment, and emergency respiratory resuscitation procedures.

Home ventilatory support

Patients who have experienced a debilitating illness or disease and are unable to maintain their own airway or respirations are candidates for home ventilatory support.

Mechanical ventilation moves oxygenated air in and out of the lungs. The actual ventilator might successfully provide oxygenated air to the patient being ventilated; however, effective gas exchange within the alveoli is not assured.

The homebound patient requiring mechanical ventilation poses a variety of challenges to the nurse and other caregivers. Ventilator management and airway support are necessary for successful care of the patient requiring home ventilation.

The decision to send a patient on mechanical ventilation home from an acute care or extended care facility is not an easy one to make. A variety of reasons might influence a family to decide to care for the patient at home. These can include social, financial, and personal reasons.

Equipment and preparation

Contact the home medical or respiratory therapy company to determine the best time to deliver the prescribed ventilator and back-up system. The following should be delivered to the patient's home: ◆ ventilator ◆ ventilator circuits and filters ◆ heated humidifier or cascade ◆ condensation drainage bags ◆ external 12-volt battery with power cord ◆ manual self-inflating resuscitation bag ◆ oxygen source (concentrator, tank) ◆ oxygen connecting tubing ◆ pressure-compensated oxygen flowmeter ◆ air compressor (optional) ◆ other home durable medical equipment: hospital bed, communication aids, equipment to aid with bowel and bladder management, wheelchair.

Implementation

Review the patient care manual outlining home management of a ventilator-dependent patient. Review the ventilator-specific manufacturer's instructions regarding the safe function and use of the ventilator.

Prepare other necessary respiratory support equipment, such as artificial airways; tracheostomy supplies; suction equipment; standard precaution supplies, including gown, gloves, mask, goggles; and hand-washing supplies. Also, review your agency's policies and procedures for caring for a patient receiving mechanical ventilation.

The patient will probably be transported home in an ambulance. Upon arrival, the ventilator will need to be set up to deliver the prescribed amount of oxygen at the ordered rate. The medical or respiratory therapy company will review with the patient and caregivers the type of ventilator the patient is on, including the controls, alarms, settings, oxygen connections, and fluid reservoirs.

When you arrive at the patient's home, begin your visit by performing a physical assessment, which should include blood pressure, pulse and respiratory rates, breath sounds, and oxygen saturation.

Also assess for complications of immobility secondary to ventilator dependence, such as skin breakdown, infection, fluid and electrolyte imbalance, malnutrition, and depression.

Review the most recent plan of care to ensure that all orders are being implemented correctly. Assess the home caregiver's comments and observations related to the patient, such as observing the patient experiencing shortness of breath, color change, excessive mucus production, fever greater than 100° F (37.7° C), and equipment concerns.

Assess and evaluate the home caregiver's ability to manage the ventilator and the need for additional teaching. Questions related to the care of the ventilator and other equipment are usually answered by the medical or respiratory therapy company. While you are in the patient's home, contact the company with any questions that require immediate answers.

Also perform a safety check of all equipment. (See *Performing a ventilator safety check*.) Study the ventilator and assess for:

◆ breath rate

◆ tidal volume that the ventilator is giving the patient

◆ low-pressure alarm limit setting; when the pressure falls below the set rate, an alarm will sound (for example, a low-pressure alarm sounds when the ventilator tubing becomes disconnected from the patient or "pinched off")

◆ high-pressure alarm limit setting; when the pressure rises above the set rate, an alarm will sound (for example, a high-pressure alarm sounds if the patient has a mucus plug inhibiting the ventilator's ability to deliver oxygen)

◆ patient's pressures by observing low and high limits as the patient breathes (For more information on alarms, see chapter 13.)

◆ fraction of inspired oxygen (FIO_2) or the amount of prescribed oxygen being delivered; approximate range is between 24% and 40% (FIO_2 greater than 40% is rarely used in home care.)

◆ positive end-expiratory pressure (called PEEP), if used (rarely in home care).

Performing a ventilator safety check

If you care for a patient who's on a ventilator, check to make sure the equipment is safe. Include the following steps:

◆ Drain all tubing of water; consider excess water contaminated, and dispose of it properly.

◆ Make sure tubing is routed to prevent excess water from draining into the patient's airway or back into the humidifier or ventilator.

◆ Inspect the circuits for wear and cracks.

◆ Check all connections for tightness.

◆ Inspect all equipment for proper function and wear, including battery level and operational hours of the ventilator.

◆ Confirm that the equipment is cleaned and changed as ordered or according to the manufacturer's recommendations.

Inform the local power company and emergency medical service that the homebound patient is being mechanically ventilated. They will place the patient on a priority service listing in case a power outage or disaster occurs. Instruct caregivers in how to use emergency back-up ventilator equipment, such as a manual resuscitation bag.

Continue to provide needed airway management and instruction, including suctioning, tracheostomy care, and chest physiotherapy if ordered.

When you complete your visit, document the following:

◆ patient tolerance of ventilator support

◆ patient's cardiopulmonary status

◆ instructions, interventions, and procedures performed

◆ ventilator settings or any changes in findings, such as mode, breath rate, high- and low-pressure alarm limit settings, patient's high and low pressure readings, and FIO_2

◆ other services' involvement in the patient's care, such as respiratory therapy, home health aides, and social services

◆ response of home caregiver to instructions given

◆ home caregiver's questions or concerns about home environment, equipment, resources, or psychosocial needs.

Teaching points

◆ *Instruct the home caregiver to post phone numbers by the telephone for the medical or respiratory therapy company, doctor, local power or electric company, local emergency medical service, and home health agency.*

◆ *The home caregiver must be able to use alternative ventilatory support systems. Review the use of the manual ventilator, and have the caregiver practice providing ventilations to the patient under supervision.*

Special considerations

Expect to make daily visits to the mechanically ventilated home patient for at least the first week. The amount of information the home caregiver needs to learn and be comfortable with can be overwhelming, and the family will need support.

Patients who can breathe on their own occasionally may have a ventilator with a setting called "continuous positive airway pressure" or CPAP. Continuous positive pressure ventilators exert a positive pressure on the airway, causing inspiration while increasing tidal volume. The inspiratory cycles on the positive pressure ventilators may vary in volume, pressure, or time. CPAP works only for patients who are able to breathe spontaneously.

Administering BiPAP

Patients who have other respiratory conditions — such as nocturnal hypoxemia caused by sleep apnea or respiratory fatigue caused by chronic obstructive pulmonary disease — may benefit from the bi-positive airway pressure (BiPAP) ventilator (one form of a CPAP ventilator).

The BiPAP ventilator is designed to provide mask-applied ventilation in the home. It delivers two different levels of positive airway pressure. The system spontaneously cycles between a preset level of inspiratory positive airway pressure (called IPAP) and expiratory positive airway pressure (called EPAP). Through these two levels of pressure, apneic and nonapneic periods can be controlled.

The BiPAP system offers ventilatory support without committing patients to the lifestyle changes associated with a tracheostomy. However, it is noncontinuous and intended to augment the patient's normal breathing pattern. This system must not be used as a life-support ventilation system because it cannot provide the total ventilatory requirements needed by a ventilator-dependent patient.

Equipment and preparation

The medical or respiratory therapy company is responsible for setting up the machine, adjusting settings, and instructing the patient and home caregivers in the operation of equipment and procedural care.

The equipment needed to place a patient on a BiPAP ventilator includes: ◆ BiPAP ventilator ◆ patient circuit ◆ nasal mask and head strap.

Implementation

Explain the procedure to the patient and help him to a comfortable position. Wash your hands and put on gloves.

Assess the patient's cardiopulmonary status, including vital signs, skin color, use of accessory muscles for ventilation, paradoxical movement of the chest wall, breath sounds, oxygen saturation, and pertinent laboratory values.

Assemble all of the equipment in a convenient work area, and place the BiPAP ventilator on a level surface, close to where the patient rests or sleeps. Plug the machine into a standard three-prong home outlet.

Connect one end of the tubing to the airflow outlet port on the front of the BiPAP ventilator. Connect the other end of the tubing to the end of the mask.

Place the mask over the patient's nose. It should extend from the end of the nasal bone to just below the nares. Make sure the mask rests above the patient's upper lip to prevent air leaks and reduce discomfort.

Turn the ventilator on. The ON/OFF switch will light up.

Attach the head strap to the mask, and adjust it until you eliminate all air leaks. Avoid overtightening, which would be uncomfortable for the patient and might cause air leaks by distorting the mask cushion. If possible, have the patient move his head to confirm the mask's seal during normal range of motion.

Check that all connections are secure and then assess the prescribed BiPAP settings. (See *Understanding BiPAP settings,* page 402.)

Assess the patient's comfort level. Observe for the development of ear discomfort or conjunctivitis. Notify the doctor as needed. Consult with the medical or respiratory therapy company and the doctor to add humidification if the patient complains of nasal dryness.

Clean and replace the equipment. Wipe off all ventilator surfaces with a clean, damp cloth. When not in use, place the mask and tubing in a plastic bag to keep them free from dust.

Document the procedure and the patient's tolerance, the patient's cardiopulmonary status, the BiPAP ventilator settings (BiPAP mode, FIO_2, IPAP/EPAP control, and number of breaths per minute), and the response of the patient and home caregiver to instructions. Also describe the patient's or home caregiver's ability to operate the equipment, the condition of supplies, and the need for more to be delivered.

Teaching points

◆ *Teach the patient relaxation techniques to help overcome the anxiety and fear he may experience when using this mask.*

◆ *Teach the patient and caregiver to assess the skin around and under the mask to help prevent skin breakdown.*

Special considerations

Watch for signs of pneumothorax, gastric distention, decreased cardiac output, and a drop in blood pressure.

Reassess the mask from time to time to make sure it still fits snugly.

Understanding BiPAP settings

Although you won't need to set up the patient's bi-positive airway pressure (BiPAP) ventilator, you will need to make sure the settings match the doctor's orders. Make sure you understand the following settings.

Inspiratory positive airway pressure (IPAP) control

- Sets prescribed pressure support level
- Ranges from 4 to 20 cm H_2O
- Active in all modes except continuous positive airway pressure (CPAP)

Expiratory positive airway pressure (EPAP) control

- Sets prescribed positive end-expiratory pressure (PEEP) level
- Ranges from 4 to 20 cm H_2O
- Active in all modes

Breaths per minute (BPM) control

- Sets the number of BPM
- Ranges from 4 to 30 BPM
- Active in the spontaneous/timed and timed modes.

Pressure support modes

- In spontaneous (S) mode, the unit cycles between IPAP and EPAP in response to the patient's rate.
- In spontaneous/timed (S/T) mode, the unit cycles as in the spontaneous mode but, if the patient fails to breathe, it will respond to the BPM control setting.
- In timed (T) mode, the unit cycles between the IPAP and EPAP levels based solely on the set BPM and IPAP time controls.
- CPAP mode allows the system to be used for CPAP delivery.

◆ DIALYSIS

Once viewed as a procedure requiring acute care, or at least outpatient care, renal dialysis is becoming more commonplace in the home environment. The patient on renal dialysis will need either a catheter in the peritoneal cavity (for peritoneal dialysis) or an arteriovenous shunt created in one of his limbs (for hemodialysis). Once the catheter or shunt is inserted and functional, the patient is ready for home dialysis.

The patient who needs peritoneal dialysis at home will be on continuous ambulatory peritoneal dialysis (CAPD). To receive this type of dialysis, the patient will need to have a permanent catheter, such as a Tenckhoff, surgically sutured in place. The external portion of the catheter exits from the middle of his abdomen. Typically, this patient has cardiovascular instability, vascular access problems that limit creation of an arteriovenous shunt, fluid overload, or an electrolyte imbalance.

The patient who needs hemodialysis through an arteriovenous shunt typically has acute reversible renal failure or acute poisoning or needs long-term treatment for chronic end-stage renal disease.

An arteriovenous shunt consists of two segments of tubing joined in the shape of a U. The shunt diverts blood from an artery to a vein. Inserted surgically, the shunt is usually located in the forearm (near the wrist) or, rarely, in the ankle. (See *Hemodialysis access sites*, pages 404 and 405.)

Equipment and preparation

The equipment and preparation you'll need for dialysis depend on the type of procedure you'll be administering.

CAPD

To care for a patient receiving CAPD, gather the following equipment: ◆ prescribed amount of dialysate (usually in 2-L bags) ◆ basin of warm water ◆ 42″ (1-m) connective tubing with drain clamp ◆ three face masks ◆ six to eight packages of sterile 4″ × 4″ gauze pads ◆ povidone-iodine pads and solution ◆ adhesive tape ◆ sterile basin ◆ alcohol pads and solution ◆ sterile gloves ◆ belt or pouch ◆ two sterile water-resistant drapes (one fenestrated) ◆ assortment of syringes and specimen containers.

Hemodialysis

To administer hemodialysis to the home patient, you'll need to be an expert in accessing the shunt, supporting the patient, and caring for the shunt after dialysis. Review your agency's policy for home hemodialysis before making the visit.

When preparing to administer hemodialysis in the home, gather the following equipment: ◆ hemodialysis machine with appropriate dialyzer ◆ I.V. solution, administration sets, tubing, and related equipment ◆ dialysate ◆ vial of 10-100 U/ml heparin solution ◆ 3-ml syringes with ⅝″ and 1″ needles ◆ 4″ × 4″ gauze pads ◆ sterile cotton-tipped applicators ◆ sterile drape ◆ alcohol pads ◆ sterile gloves ◆ two sterile shunt adapters ◆ sterile Teflon connector ◆ two bulldog clamps ◆ two 10-ml syringes ◆ vial of normal saline solution ◆ four strips of adhesive tape ◆ hand-washing supplies ◆ sharps container ◆ two hemostats ◆ elastic gauze bandage.

Usually, the dialysate is delivered directly to the home. Review the agency's procedure for peritoneal dialysis, and prepare patient-education materials.

Implementation

The implementation you provide differs depending on the type of dialysis the patient needs.

CAPD

Explain the procedure to the patient, and provide patient-education materials. While the patient is reviewing the materials, check the dialysate against the doctor's order. Assess and observe the solution; don't use it if it's cloudy. As needed, run warm water over the dialysate bags to bring them to body temperature. Don't place the bags in a conventional or microwave oven.

Weigh the patient. Then help him to a comfortable position that exposes the catheter. Arrange your equipment nearby and wash your hands. Put on gloves and a mask.

Open the protective cover from the dialysate. Gently squeeze the bag to check for any leaks. Insert the connective tubing into the dialysate. Open the drain clamp to prime the tubing. Then close the clamp.

Prepare a sterile field next to the patient. Saturate four pairs of sterile gauze pads with povidone-iodine solution in the basin. Place the alcohol container next to the basin.

Put on a clean mask and provide one for the patient. Remove the dressing covering the peritoneal catheter and discard it. Avoid touching the catheter or the skin. Check the skin at the catheter site for signs of infection, such as drainage, swelling, and redness.

Hemodialysis access sites

Hemodialysis requires vascular access. The site and type of access may vary, depending on the expected duration of dialysis, the surgeon's preference, and the patient's condition.

Subclavian vein catheterization
Using the Seldinger technique, the doctor or surgeon inserts an introducer needle into the subclavian vein. He then inserts a guide wire through the introducer needle and removes the needle. Using the guide wire, he then threads a 5″ to 12″ plastic or Teflon catheter (with a Y hub) into the patient's vein (as shown below).

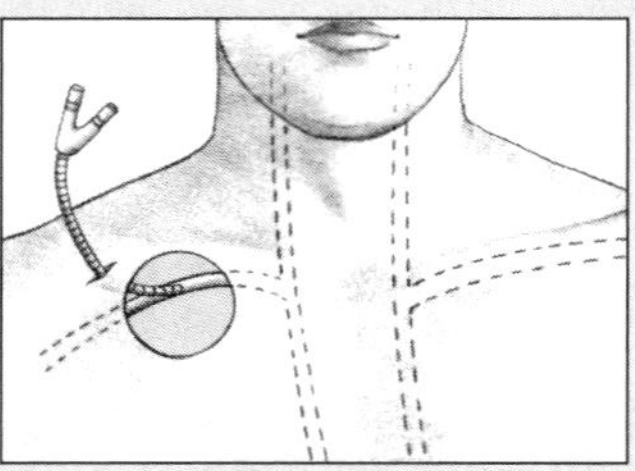

Femoral vein catheterization
Using the Seldinger technique, the doctor or surgeon inserts an introducer needle into the left or right femoral vein. He then inserts a guide wire through the introducer needle and removes the needle. Using the guidewire, he then threads a 5″ to 12″ plastic or Teflon catheter with a Y hub or two catheters, one for inflow and another placed about ½″ (1.3 cm) distal to the first for outflow (as shown above right).

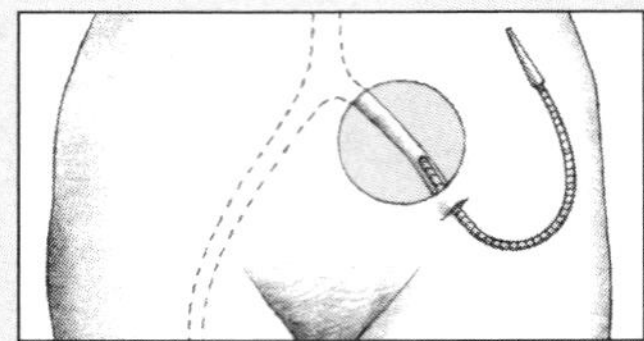

Arteriovenous fistula
To create a fistula, the surgeon makes an incision in the patient's wrist or lower forearm and then a small incision in the side of an artery and another in the side of a vein. He sutures the edges of these incisions together to make a common opening 3 to 7 mm long (as shown below).

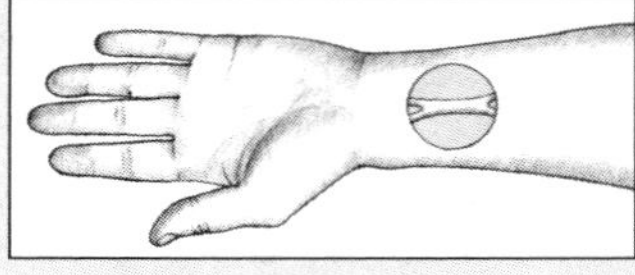

Arteriovenous shunt
To create a shunt, the surgeon makes an incision in the patient's wrist, lower forearm, or (rarely) ankle. He then inserts a 6″ to 10″ transparent Silastic cannula into an artery and another into a vein. Finally, he tunnels the cannulas out through stab wounds and joins them with a piece of Teflon tubing (as shown below).

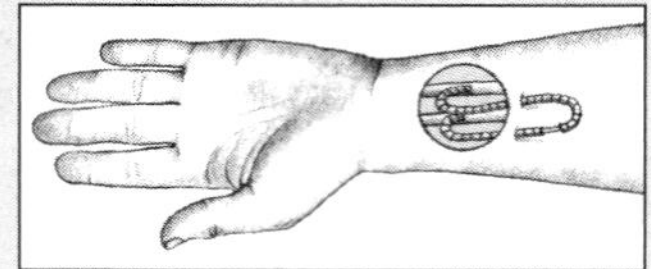

Hemodialysis access sites *(continued)*

Arteriovenous graft
To create a graft, the surgeon makes an incision in the patient's forearm, upper arm, or thigh. He then tunnels a natural or synthetic graft under the skin and sutures the distal end to an artery and the proximal end to a vein (as shown).

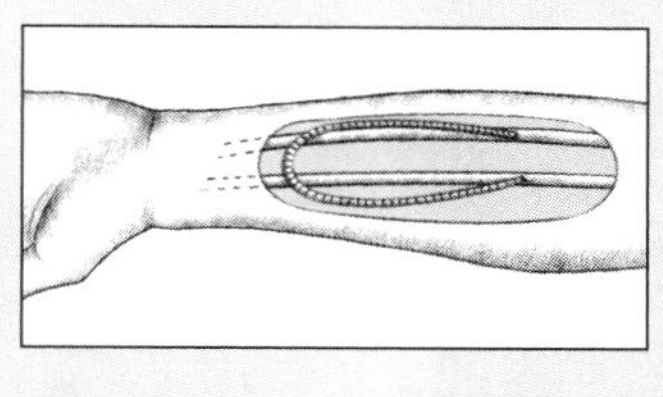

Remove your gloves, use a nonwater hand cleaner, and put on sterile gloves. Wrap one gauze pad saturated with povidone-iodine around the distal end of the catheter, and leave it in place for 5 minutes. Clean the catheter and insertion site with the other saturated gauze pad; begin at the insertion site and work outward, in a circular motion. After using the third saturated gauze pad, place the fenestrated drape around the base of the catheter.

Remove the pad from the tip of the catheter and remove the catheter cap. Attach the connective tubing from the dialysate container to the catheter. Tightly secure the luer-lock connector.

Open the drain clamp on the dialysate container to allow the solution to enter the peritoneal cavity by gravity over 5 to 10 minutes. Leave a small amount of fluid in the bag. Close the drain clamp.

Fold the bag and secure it with a belt or pouch. Clean up all your equipment. Discard disposable items and provide for patient comfort. Remove your mask and gloves and wash your hands.

After the ordered wait or "dwell" time (usually 4 to 6 hours), unfold the bag, open the clamp, and allow the peritoneal fluid to drain back into the bag by gravity.

When drainage is complete, attach a new bag of dialysate, as prescribed, or disconnect the infusion. To disconnect the infusion, wash your hands and put on a mask. Provide a mask for the patient. Clamp the dialysate tubing.

Set up a sterile field, and saturate 4″ × 4″ gauze pads with povidone-iodine solution. Remove the catheter dressing and begin cleaning outward from the site in a circular motion.

Clean the catheter tubing with another saturated sponge for about 1 minute. Disconnect the dialysate tubing and apply the catheter cap. Apply a dressing over the catheter site using sterile technique.

Remove all equipment and discard used supplies. Remove the mask from the patient and provide for his comfort. Remove your mask and gloves, and wash your hands.

Hemodialysis

Explain the procedure to the patient and provide patient-education materials. While the patient is reviewing the materials, check the dialysis machine, dialyzer, and solution. Prepare the machine according to manufacturer's instructions. Follow strict aseptic technique to prevent accidental introduction of bacteria into the patient's bloodstream. Check all of the alarms on the machine.

Weigh the patient. Then help him to a comfortable position that exposes the shunt site. Arrange your equipment nearby and wash your hands. Put on gloves and a mask.

Prepare a sterile field and place the limb with the shunt on it. Remove the clamps from the elastic gauze bandage, and gently remove the bandage from the shunt. Carefully remove the gauze dressing covering the shunt.

Assess the arterial and venous exit sites for signs of infection, including redness, swelling, tenderness, or drainage. Check the blood flow through the shunt by inspecting the color of the blood and comparing the warmth of the shunt with the surrounding skin. The blood in a shunt should be bright red and should feel as warm as the surrounding skin. Using a stethoscope, auscultate the shunt between the arterial and venous access sites. A bruit confirms normal blood flow. Palpate the shunt for a thrill. This also confirms normal blood flow.

Saturate several sterile gauze pads and cotton-tipped applicators with povidone-iodine solution. Put on a pair of sterile gloves.

Select a saturated gauze sponge and start cleaning the skin at one of the exit sites. Wipe away from the site to remove bacteria and reduce the chance of contaminating the shunt. Use the saturated cotton-tipped applicators to remove any crusted material from the exit sites. Encrustation provides a medium for bacterial growth. Clean the other exit site in the same manner.

Clean the remainder of the skin that's covered by the gauze bandage. Apply antimicrobial ointment to the exit sites, if ordered, to help prevent infection.

Assemble the shunt adapters according to the manufacturer's directions. Clean the arterial and venous shunt connection with povidone-iodine–saturated gauze pads. Use a separate pad for each tube, and wipe in one direction, from the insertion site to the connection site. Allow the tubing to air-dry. Remove your gloves, wash your hands, and put on another pair of sterile gloves.

Clamp the arterial side of the shunt with a bulldog clamp to prevent blood from flowing through it. Clamp the venous side to prevent leakage when the shunt is opened.

Open the shunt by separating its sides with your fingers. Expose both sides of the shunt. Inspect the Teflon connector on one side of the shunt to see if it's damaged or bent.

Attach a shunt adapter and 10-ml syringe filled with about 8 ml of normal saline solution to the side of the shunt containing the Teflon connector. Attach a new Teflon connector to the other side of the shunt with the second adapter. Attach the second 10-ml syringe filled with 8 ml of normal saline solution to the same side.

Flush the shunt's arterial tubing by releasing the clamp and gently aspirating it with the normal saline–filled syringe. Then slowly flush the tubing. Repeat the procedure on the venous side of the shunt.

Secure the shunt to the adapter connection with adhesive tape. This prevents accidental separation during treatment.

Connect the arterial and venous lines to the adapters, and secure the connections with tape. Tape each line to the patient's arm to prevent unnecessary strain on the shunt during treatment.

Turn on the machine and begin dialysis. Remove and discard used items in the appropriate containers. Provide for patient comfort. Remove your gloves and wash your hands.

When dialysis is finished, wash your hands and put on sterile gloves. Remove the tape from the connection site of the arterial lines. Clamp the arterial cannula with a bulldog clamp. Then disconnect the lines.

The blood in the machine's arterial line will continue to flow toward the dialyzer, followed by a column of air. Just before the blood reaches the point where the normal saline solution enters the line, clamp it with a hemostat.

Unclamp the normal saline solution, and allow a small amount to flow through the line. Then reclamp it and unclamp the hemostat on the machine line. Just before the last volume of blood enters the patient, clamp the venous cannula with a bulldog clamp and the machine's venous line with a hemostat.

Remove the tape from the connection site of the venous lines. Disconnect the lines. Reconnect the shunt cannula. Remove the older of the two Teflon connectors and discard it. Connect the shunt and remove the bulldog clamps.

Secure the shunt connection with tape to prevent accidental disconnection. Clean the shunt with povidone-iodine–soaked gauze pads followed by alcohol pads. Evaluate the shunt for blood flow.

Apply a dressing to the shunt, and wrap it securely with an elastic gauze bandage. Attach the bulldog clamps to the outside dressing.

Immediately after hemodialysis, measure the patient's weight, vital signs, and mental status.

Teaching points

- *Teach the patient and home caregivers to use sterile technique throughout the CAPD procedure. Sterile technique is especially important for cleaning and dressing changes, to prevent complications such as peritonitis.*
- *Instruct the patient and caregivers about the signs and symptoms of peritonitis, including fever, abdominal pain, and tenderness. Tell them to contact you if any of these signs appears. Signs of an infected catheter site include redness, drainage, swelling, and local tenderness. These signs should also be reported immediately.*
- *Teach the patient to measure daily weights and record them. Teach him to examine his limbs for fluid retention.*
- *Show the patient how to care for the hemodialysis access site, including keeping the incision clean and dry to prevent infection. Remind him to clean the site daily until it's completely healed and the sutures are removed.*
- *Instruct the patient to notify you if the hemodialysis site is painful, begins to swell, is red, or has drainage. Teach him how to use a stethoscope to auscultate for a bruit and how to palpate for a thrill.*
- *Explain that once the hemodialysis site heals, he can use the arm freely. In fact, exercise is beneficial because it helps stimulate vein enlargement. Remind the patient to permit no treatments or procedures on the arm with the shunt, including blood pressure monitoring, venipuncture, or I.V. catheterization.*
- *Urge the patient to avoid putting excess pressure or weight on the arm, sleeping on it, wearing constrictive clothing, or lifting heavy objects with it. He should avoid getting the shunt wet for several hours after dialysis.*
- *Inform the patient that an exercise beneficial for the affected arm is squeezing a small rubber ball or other soft object for about 15 minutes.*
- *Tell the patient to clearly post the telephone number of the dialysis center.*

Special considerations

If CAPD inflow and outflow slows or stops, check the tubing for kinks. Try raising the solution or repositioning the patient to increase the inflow rate. Repositioning the patient or gently applying manual pressure to the lateral aspects of the patient's abdomen helps increase outflow drainage.

The most common complication of CAPD is peritonitis. Although it can be treated, peritonitis can permanently scar the peritoneal membrane, decreasing permeability and reducing the efficiency of dialysis. Excessive fluid loss may result from a concentrated dialysate, improper or inaccurate monitoring of inflow and outflow, or inadequate oral fluid intake.

If you find the patient's blood dark purple or black when you inspect the shunt, and the shunt's temperature is lower than the surrounding skin, the shunt is clotted. Don't use it. Instead, contact the doctor, and prepare the patient to go to an acute care facility to have it repaired or replaced.

In hemodialysis, bacterial contaminants in the dialysate can cause fever. Rapid fluid removal and electrolyte changes during the procedure can cause early dialysis disequilibrium syndrome. Signs and symptoms of this syndrome include headache, nausea, vomiting, restlessness, muscle cramps, backache, and seizures.

Excessive removal of fluid can cause hypovolemia and hypotension. Cardiac arrhythmias can occur from electrolyte and pH changes in the blood after hemodialysis.

Some complications of hemodialysis can be fatal. Air embolism can result if the dialyzer retains air, if tubing connections become loose, or if the normal saline solution container empties.

Hemolysis can result from obstructed flow of the dialysate concentrate or from incorrect setting of the alarm limits. Symptoms include chest pain, dyspnea, cherry-red blood, arrhythmias, acute decrease in hematocrit, and hyperkalemia.

Hyperthermia can result if the dialysate becomes overheated. Exsanguination can result from separations of the blood lines or rupture of the blood lines or dialyzer membrane.

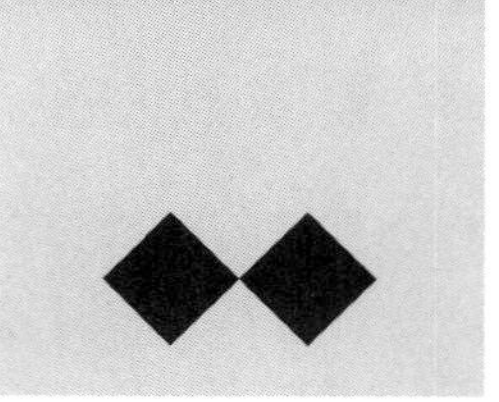

CHAPTER 13

Troubleshooting equipment problems

No matter how carefully and accurately you deliver nursing care, you're bound to have equipment problems now and then. Especially in the home, you'll need to be ready to handle equipment glitches on your own and teach patients and their caregivers how to do the same. This chapter offers some valuable pointers to help you solve equipment problems quickly and get on with the business of patient care.

Managing intravenous (I.V.) access devices requires periodic monitoring and diligence on your part and that of a competent, trained caregiver in the patient's home. You and the caregiver will need to be able to identify high-risk situations and potential problems and correct them promptly. Failing to do so can be dangerous for the patient.

The complications most commonly seen in the home include primarily local complications, such as phlebitis, dislodgment, infiltration, occlusion, and hematoma. Less common, systemic complications include circulatory overload, allergic reaction, and systemic infection. You can minimize or prevent complications by using proper insertion techniques, carefully monitoring the patient, checking the condition of all tubing and other equipment, and scheduling routine site rotations. Thoroughly training the patient or caregiver in aseptic technique and troubleshooting for complications will influence your outcome more than any other factor. (See *Correcting common I.V. catheter problems,* pages 410 and 411.)

◆ PERIPHERAL I.V. THERAPY

Although peripheral I.V. usage in the home provides many benefits, there may be complications associated with the venipuncture, the infusion, the medication being administered, or the equipment. The complication may be local (such as phlebitis) or systemic (such as septicemia). Some complications may begin locally and become systemic, such as an infection at the venipuncture site that progresses to septicemia.

◆ CENTRAL VENOUS THERAPY

If your home care patient has a central venous catheter, patient teaching will form a crucial part of your nursing role. Using manufacturer-supplied materials and your own preparation, teach the patient and home caregiver the following:

- ◆ the reason for central venous therapy
- ◆ catheter placement
- ◆ clean and sterile techniques

(Text continues on page 412.)

Correcting common I.V. catheter problems

The following chart describes how to recognize and manage some common problems with I.V. catheters.

Problem and possible causes	Patient interventions
Medication or flush solution won't infuse ◆ Closed clamp ◆ Displaced or kinked catheter ◆ Thrombus	◆ Check infusion system and clamps. ◆ Straighten any catheter kinks. ◆ Call nurse if actions don't correct problem. ◆ Never force a flush that won't infuse with gentle pressure. *Also, for central catheter:* ◆ Change body position; cough and breathe deeply.
Unable to draw blood ◆ Closed clamp ◆ Displaced or kinked catheter ◆ Thrombus ◆ Catheter movement against vessel wall with negative pressure	◆ Change position of extremity. ◆ Straighten any catheter kinks. ◆ Call nurse if actions don't correct problem. *Also, for central catheter:* ◆ Change body position; cough and breathe deeply.
Fluid leaking at site ◆ Displaced or torn catheter ◆ Lymph fluid leaking from subcutaneous tract	◆ Stop infusion and call nurse.
Catheter dislodgment ◆ Swelling or leaking at insertion site ◆ Catheter backing out of vein	◆ Stop infusion and contact nurse. *Also, for peripheral catheter:* ◆ Remove catheter and apply pressure to site.

Nursing interventions

◆ Attempt to aspirate a clot, if visible; don't force the clot.
◆ Attempt procedures listed under patient interventions.
◆ Try to withdraw blood; flush gently with sterile saline solution.
Also, for peripheral catheter:
◆ Remove catheter that won't flush with gentle pressure; insert new peripheral catheter per agency protocol.
Also, for central catheter:
◆ If catheter placement is ensured with a blood return, contact doctor for an order to use a thrombolytic flush (if agency protocol permits).
◆ If blood return is not obtained, use of lumen may need to be stopped until X-ray confirmation can occur.
◆ If other lumens are available and placement is ensured with a blood return, other lumens can be used.
◆ Tape the malfunctioning lumen so patient or caregiver will not use it.

◆ Check infusion system and clamps.
◆ Remove dressing and examine external portion of catheter.
Also, for peripheral catheter:
◆ Monitor closely for signs of infiltration.
◆ Remove catheter; insert new peripheral catheter per agency protocol.
Also, for central catheter:
◆ Attempt to draw blood from another lumen if it's a multilumen catheter.
◆ Instruct patient or caregiver not to use malfunctioning lumen (identify with tape).
◆ If unable to obtain blood from any lumen, call doctor for an X-ray order; tell patient not to use catheter.

◆ Change dressing and observe site for redness.
◆ Notify doctor.
◆ Prepare for a catheter change, if necessary.

◆ Reinsert new peripheral or central device per agency policy and resume infusion.
◆ Secure catheter.

- drug administration procedures
- maintenance procedures, such as routine flushing; changing dressings, solution, tubing, and injection cap; blood sampling; inspecting the catheter for tears (especially tunneled catheters); and inspecting the site for phlebitis or infiltration
- how to correct complications and equipment problems
- how to dispose of used equipment
- resources for problem solving.

You'll also need to be able to troubleshoot problems as they arise, and teach your patient and his caregivers how to do so as well.

◆ INFUSION CONTROL DEVICES

Monitor infusion control devices — such as pumps and controllers — very carefully. You can avoid several common infusion pump problems by following this advice and teaching your patients to do the same.

- Before you attach an I.V. filter or infuse blood, check the manufacturer's recommendations. Not all pumps are designed for these purposes.
- Follow the manufacturer's instructions precisely when you connect the tubing to the pump.
- Be sure to flush *all* air out of the tubing before connecting it to the patient; this lowers the risk of air embolism.
- To avoid fluid overload, always clamp the tubing before opening the pump door.
- Double-check the flow rate. The control setting may not be accurate. Monitor the flow rate over a specific time span, then adjust the flow as needed.
- Avoid turning the pump on and off excessively. This can clog the catheter.

Also teach patients and caregivers the basic functions and management of alarms. Above all, never disarm an alarm; the patient could suffer injury. Instead, investigate and fix nuisance alarms and other common problems, such as those listed below. (See *Responding to problems with infusion control devices*.)

◆ I.V. FLOW RATES

When an infusion stops, assess the I.V. setup systematically to look for the reason. In your assessment, include the insertion site, tubing, filter, clamps, air vents, and fluid level. (See *Correcting I.V. flow rate deviations,* pages 414 and 415.)

Checking the site

Check for infiltration or phlebitis, which may slow or stop the flow rate.

Checking patency

Evaluate the I.V. device for patency, which may be affected by several factors:

- If the patient's limb is flexed or lying directly on the I.V. site, increased blood pressure may stop the flow. Reposition the limb as needed.
- The tip of the needle may lie against the vein wall or a venous valve. Lift up or pull back the venipuncture device to reestablish the I.V. flow.
- If the patient's arm is wrapped with tape, a tourniquet effect may reduce the flow rate. Taping the I.V. site too tightly can cause the same problem. Release or remove the tape, then reapply it.
- Smaller venipuncture devices may kink or fold, impeding I.V. flow. Pull the device back to reestablish flow.
- Local edema or poor tissue perfusion from disease can block venous flow. Move the I.V. line to an unaffected site.
- Infusion of incompatible fluids or medications may cause precipitation, which can block the tubing and

Responding to problems with infusion control devices

When the alarm on an infusion control device goes off, check for the following problems and intervene as appropriate.

Problem	Intervention
Air in the line	While setting up, make sure all air is out of the line, including air trapped in Y-injection sites. Also, check that the connections are secure and the container is filled properly. Withdraw any air from a piggyback port with a syringe or an air-eliminating filter.
Infusion completed	Reset the pump as ordered or discontinue the infusion and shut off the pump.
Empty container	Check for adequate fluid levels in the I.V. container, and have another container available before the last one runs out. Teach the patient and caregiver to change the I.V. container using aseptic technique.
Low battery	Battery life varies; keep the machine plugged in on AC power as much as possible, especially while the patient is in bed. If the alarm goes off, plug in the machine immediately or power may be lost. Review manufacturer information to determine battery life.
Occlusion	Check that all clamps are open, look for kinked tubing, and check the patency of the venipuncture device.
Rate change	Check that the infusion control device displays the ordered rate. The patient or a family member may have tampered with the controls.
Open door	The door should be closed; it may not shut if the device isn't set up properly (for example, if the cassette isn't inserted all the way).
Malfunction	A mechanical failure usually must be handled by the manufacturer. Disconnect the infusion control device. Label it clearly with a sign that says "BROKEN" and return it to the manufacturer. Replace the infusion device.

Correcting I.V. flow rate deviations

Problem and possible causes	Interventions
Flow rate too fast	
Clamp manipulated by patient or family member	Instruct the patient and family to use the clamp appropriately.
Tubing disconnected from catheter	Use only luer-lock connections.
Change in patient position	Use an infusion pump or a controller to ensure the correct flow rate. Restart I.V. infusion as appropriate.
Bevel against vein wall (positional cannulation)	Manipulate the venipuncture device, and place a 2″ × 2″ gauze pad under or over the catheter hub to change the angle. Reset the flow clamp at the desired rate. If necessary, remove and reinsert the venipuncture device.
Flow clamp drifting from patient movement	Place tape below the clamp.
Flow rate too slow	
Venous spasm after insertion	Apply warm soaks over site.
Venous obstruction from bending arm	Replace I.V. or secure so obstruction doesn't occur.
Pressure change (from decreased fluid in bottle)	Readjust the flow rate.
Elevated blood pressure	Readjust the flow rate. Use an infusion pump or a controller to ensure correct rate.
Change in solution viscosity from drug added	Readjust the flow rate.
I.V. container too low or patient's arm or leg too high	Hang the container higher or remind the client to keep his arm below heart level.
Bevel against vein wall (positional cannulation)	Withdraw the catheter slightly, or place a folded 2″ × 2″ gauze pad over or under the catheter hub to change the angle.
Excess tubing dangling below insertion site	Replace the tubing with a shorter piece. Secure it so the patient can be mobile.

Correcting I.V. flow rate deviations *(continued)*

Problem and possible causes	Interventions
Flow rate too slow *(continued)*	
Infiltration or clotted venipuncture device.	Remove the venipuncture device in use, and insert a new venipuncture device.
Kinked tubing	Check the tubing over its entire length and unkink it.
Clogged filter	Remove the filter and replace it with a new one.
Tubing compressed at clamped area	Massage or milk the tubing by pinching and wrapping it around a pencil four or five times. Then quickly pull the pencil out of the coiled tubing.

venipuncture device, and may even expose the patient to a life-threatening embolism. Always check the compatibility of medications and I.V. solutions before administering them. Replace the venipuncture device if it is occluded.

Checking the filter

Start by making sure the in-line filter is the right size and type. I.V. fluids usually go through a 0.22- or 0.45-micron filter that eliminates air and microorganisms. Don't use single-use filters for in-line filtration. Rather, use them only for drawing up or administering a bolus dose. If the drug solution was particulate filtered at the pharmacy, you may not need an in-line filter.

Remember, if you use the wrong size or type of filter, the solution may not pass through it. For example, drugs such as amphotericin B and lymphocyte immune globulin contain molecules too large to pass through a 0.22-micron filter; they'd rapidly block the filter and stop the I.V. flow. If necessary, replace the filter.

Likewise, if you use a filter longer than recommended, it may become blocked by minute particles and microorganisms. Not only will the I.V. flow stop, but the patient may become exposed to bacterial toxins and sepsis. The interval between filter changes usually ranges from 24 to 48 hours, depending on the manufacturer's instructions. Change the filter, if necessary.

Checking clamps

Make sure that the flow clamps are open. Check all clamps, including the roller clamp and any clamps on secondary sets, such as a slide clamp on a filter (a roller clamp may also become jammed if the roller is pushed up too far).

Checking tubing

Look to see if the tubing is kinked or if the patient is lying on it. Also, check whether the tubing remains crimped where a clamp was tightened around it. If so, gently squeeze the area between your fingers to encourage it to round back out to its original shape.

Checking air vents

If you're using an evacuated glass container, be sure it has an air vent to make the solution flow. Insert one, as necessary. With a volume control set, an air vent is usually located at the top of the calibrated changer. If the solution stops flowing, check the patency of this vent (by following manufacturer instructions) and the position of the vent clamp.

Checking fluid levels

Tell the patient or a caregiver to watch the fluid level in the I.V. container, and to replace it as instructed when it's empty. Remind the patient that a cold solution could cause a venous spasm, thus decreasing the flow rate. Applying warm compresses may relieve it and help increase the flow rate. Tell them to make sure subsequent solutions are the right temperature. Finally, check that the spike at the end of the administration set has been pushed far enough into the container to allow the solution to flow.

If you can't identify the problem with this series of checks, the I.V. line should be removed and restarted at a different site. (See *Troubleshooting I.V. devices and pumps*.) Document the episode in the patient's chart.

◆ VENTILATORS

Always follow the doctor's orders for ventilator settings, and don't reset the controls unless you have an order to do so. Post a sign that displays the prescribed settings.

Tell the patient and a caregiver to check the ventilator throughout the day and before bedtime. Print out a checklist for the patient or caregiver to use when checking the ventilator at bedtime. It should include these items:

- ◆ Settings are correct.
- ◆ Alarm lights are turned on.
- ◆ Machine is functioning.
- ◆ Humidifier is filled.
- ◆ Connections are secure.
- ◆ Tube isn't kinked or filled with water.

Also teach the caregiver to do the following:

- ◆ Position the ventilator close to the patient, with enough slack so the patient can move his head without disconnecting the tubing.
- ◆ Keep the ventilator out of reach of children. Consider a childproof covering over the controls if necessary.
- ◆ Don't use an extension cord on the ventilator.
- ◆ Make sure you have extra supplies on hand, such as a tracheostomy tube, manual resuscitator with tracheostomy adapter, oxygen, suctioning equipment, and a backup power source.
- ◆ Keep the manufacturer's manual and troubleshooting guide near the ventilator.
- ◆ Clean the equipment according to manufacturer recommendations.
- ◆ Respond promptly to ventilator alarms. (See *Responding to ventilator alarms*, page 418.)

CRITICAL DECISIONS

Troubleshooting I.V. devices and pumps

Use the following decision tree to help you intervene appropriately when you encounter problems with I.V. devices and pumps. At each step, reevaluate the status of the problem. If the problem is solved, there is no need to proceed further through the decision tree

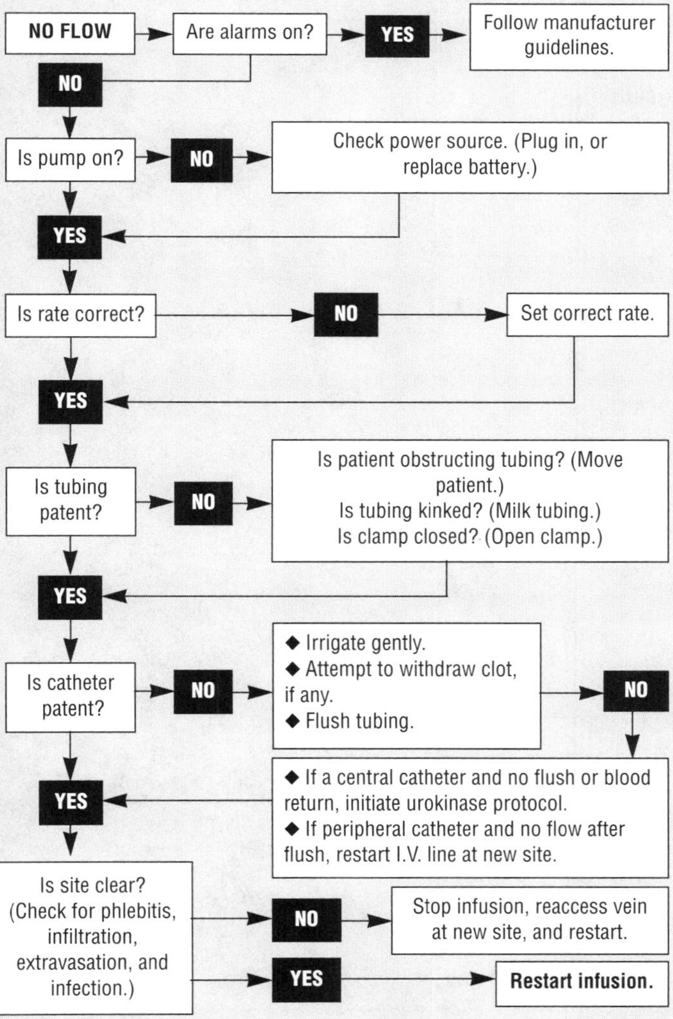

NO FLOW → Are alarms on?
- **YES** → Follow manufacturer guidelines.
- **NO** → Is pump on?

Is pump on?
- **NO** → Check power source. (Plug in, or replace battery.) → YES
- **YES** → Is rate correct?

Is rate correct?
- **NO** → Set correct rate. → YES
- **YES** → Is tubing patent?

Is tubing patent?
- **NO** → Is patient obstructing tubing? (Move patient.) Is tubing kinked? (Milk tubing.) Is clamp closed? (Open clamp.) → YES
- **YES** → Is catheter patent?

Is catheter patent?
- **NO** → ◆ Irrigate gently. ◆ Attempt to withdraw clot, if any. ◆ Flush tubing. → **NO** → ◆ If a central catheter and no flush or blood return, initiate urokinase protocol. ◆ If peripheral catheter and no flow after flush, restart I.V. line at new site. → YES
- **YES** → Is site clear?

Is site clear? (Check for phlebitis, infiltration, extravasation, and infection.)
- **NO** → Stop infusion, reaccess vein at new site, and restart.
- **YES** → **Restart infusion.**

Responding to ventilator alarms

Signal and possible causes	Interventions
Low-pressure alarm	
◆ Tube disconnected from ventilator	◆ Reconnect tube to ventilator.
◆ Endotracheal tube displaced above vocal cords or tracheostomy tube extubated	◆ Check tube placement and reposition if needed. If extubation or displacement has occurred, instruct caregiver to ventilate the patient manually and call the doctor immediately.
◆ Low cuff pressure (from an underinflated or ruptured cuff or a leak in the cuff or one-way valve)	◆ Listen for a whooshing sound around the tube, indicating an air leak. If you hear one, check cuff pressure. If you can't maintain pressure, call the doctor; he may need to insert a new tube.
◆ Ventilator malfunction	◆ Disconnect patient from ventilator and ventilate him manually if necessary. Use a backup ventilator or call the equipment supplier.
◆ Leak in ventilator circuitry (from loose connection or hole in tubing, loss of temperature-sensitive device, or cracked humidification jar)	◆ Make sure all connections are intact. Check for holes or leaks in the tubing and replace if necessary. Check the humidification jar and replace if cracked.
High-pressure alarm	
◆ Increased airway pressure or decreased lung compliance caused by worsening disease	◆ Auscultate the lungs for evidence of increasing lung consolidation or wheezing. Call the doctor if indicated.
◆ Secretions in airway	◆ Look for secretions in the airway. To remove them, suction the patient or have him cough.
◆ Condensate in large-bore tubing	◆ Check tubing for condensate and remove any fluid.
◆ Chest wall resistance	◆ Reposition the patient if it improves chest expansion.
◆ Failure of high-pressure relief valve	◆ Call equipment supplier and have faulty equipment replaced.
◆ Signs of respiratory distress	◆ Remove the patient from the ventilator and ventilate him manually. Call the equipment supplier, doctor, or both, as appropriate.

Dealing with concentrator problems

Problem and possible causes	Interventions
Alarm on, concentrator not running ◆ Not plugged in ◆ No power	◆ Check plug. ◆ Check power source.
No alarm, concentrator not running ◆ Dead battery ◆ Not plugged in	◆ Replace battery. ◆ Plug in.
Unit running but has little or no flow ◆ Flow meter got bumped. ◆ Flow meter dirty and occluded ◆ Tubing or cannula kinked or not attached ◆ Humidifier not properly attached	◆ Reset or replace flow meter. ◆ Unwind or replace tubing. ◆ Check all tubing connections. ◆ Remove, clean, and reattach humidifier. ◆ Unscrew and rescrew humidifier to be sure threaded properly.

◆ OXYGEN

If your patient needs home oxygen therapy, he'll receive either an oxygen concentrator, an oxygen tank, or a liquid oxygen system. No matter which equipment he receives, however, be sure to verify that it's been set up properly and works as expected. If you detect anything abnormal about oxygen equipment, report it to the equipment supplier right away.

Also teach patients the following important points to help them avoid potentially disastrous problems with oxygen equipment:

◆ Use oxygen only in well ventilated areas.

◆ Don't store oxygen equipment in small spaces, such as a closet or car.

◆ Don't permit oil, grease, aerosol sprays, cosmetics, or other flammable material to come in contact with oxygen equipment.

◆ Don't allow children to tamper with or operate the oxygen system.

◆ Don't drop the unit or place it where it could easily be knocked over.

◆ Avoid storing oxygen equipment near a heat source, such as a radiator, portable heater, fireplace, or oven. Keep the equipment at least 5 feet from an open flame.

◆ Always secure oxygen tanks upright in a cart, stand, or other safe location.

◆ Post "oxygen in use" signs.

◆ Obtain a fire extinguisher and smoke alarm.

◆ If a concentrator doesn't seem to be working properly, consider which factors could be causing the problem. (See *Dealing with concentrator problems*.)

◆ PORTABLE SUCTION

Portable suction machines create the air pressure needed to suction mucus and other secretions from the patient's mouth, nose, and trachea. To help avoid problems, set up the system according to the manufacturer's instructions.

The most common problem with suction equipment is a lack of suction. Usually the reason is a lack of power, an occluded suction catheter, or improper use of the control valve. To solve this problem, check the power source, clean the suction catheter or replace it, and review the instructions for using the control valve. Also teach the patient or caregiver how to assess the system and troubleshoot this problem.

◆ FEEDING TUBES

The most common problems with feeding tubes include obstruction or clogging, dislodgment, aspiration of gastric contents, nasal or pharyngeal irritation or necrosis, and such adverse reactions as vomiting, bloating, diarrhea, or cramps. (See *Managing tube feeding problems.*)

◆ HOSPITAL BEDS

Three kinds of hospital beds are available: manual, semi-electric, and fully electric. Manual beds are adjusted by hand cranks at the foot or side of the bed. Electric beds let patients elevate the head or feet without physical effort. They may have manual adjustments for height or be fully electric.

Regardless of the type of hospital bed your patient has, bed rails are essential to keep him from falling out of bed. They're also useful as hand holds when the patient repositions himself in bed. Universal bed rails work with almost any hospital bed.

The most common problem with hospital beds is nonfunctioning controls. The problem may result from a lack of power, either from the bed not being properly plugged in, or having the controls disconnected. If this happens, check the power source and the plug, and reconnect it if necessary. Check that cords are intact and not frayed. Report any malfunction to the equipment supplier for replacement.

◆ WHEELCHAIRS

Wheelchairs are classified as standard (nonmotorized), motorized, and ultralight (for very active patients). Many optional pieces of equipment are available, such as handrims, brakes, arm rests, and leg rests. Wheelchairs should be fitted to the patient's needs by the equipment supplier.

The most common problem encountered with wheelchairs is an inability to move or difficulty steering. If this occurs, first check that the wheel brake isn't on. If it is, release it. If the chair remains difficult to steer or move, call the supplier for a functional assessment.

◆ HYDRAULIC LIFTS

A hydraulic lift is designed to provide a safe way to lift or move a patient with little effort. A variety of slings and accessories is available. Usually, you pump a handle to lift the patient and turn a control knob to lower the patient. Brakes are provided for added safety. Even so, only trained personnel should use these devices.

A common problem with hydraulic lifts is that the patient isn't seated securely and safely in the lift, which raises the risk that he could fall out. This can result from improper ad-

Managing tube feeding problems

Problems	Interventions
Tube obstruction or clogging	◆ Flush the tube with warm water. If necessary, replace the tube. ◆ Flush the tube with 20 to 30 ml of water every 6 to 8 hours, before and after completing formula infusion (or when temporarily stopped), and before and after administering medications.
Aspiration of gastric secretions	◆ Discontinue feeding immediately. ◆ Perform tracheal suction of aspirated contents if possible. ◆ Notify the doctor. Prophylactic antibiotics and chest physiotherapy may be ordered. ◆ Check tube placement before feeding to prevent complications.
Nasal or pharyngeal irritation or necrosis	◆ Change the tube's position. If necessary, replace the tube. ◆ Provide frequent oral hygiene using mouthwash or lemon-glycerin swabs. Use petroleum jelly on cracked lips.
Vomiting, bloating, diarrhea, or cramps	◆ Reduce the flow rate. ◆ As ordered, administer metoclopramide to increase GI motility. ◆ Warm the formula. ◆ For 30 minutes after feeding, position the patient on his right side with his head elevated to facilitate gastric emptying. ◆ Notify the doctor. He may reduce the amount of formula being given during each feeding.
Dislodgment	◆ Secure the tube appropriately and check placement by aspirating for gastric contents before each feeding, if appropriate. Teach the patient or caregiver how to measure the external portion of the tube each day. Tell them to report any change in length. ◆ If you have any doubt about tube placement (especially with small-bore tubes, such as #8 French or smaller), delay the feeding until you can confirm placement with an X-ray.

justment of the chains or straps. The chains or straps should be readjusted according to the manufacturer's guidelines.

If the lift doesn't work, possibly because of an oil leak from the lift cylinder, contact the equipment supplier for service or a replacement.

◆ PRODUCT DEFECT REPORTING

To help safeguard the public from hazardous devices, the Food and Drug Administration created the Medical Products Reporting Program to encourage all health care personnel to report problems with medical devices. In fact, it's mandatory to report any device that causes serious injury or death. You should report even poor product design, poor packaging, or inadequate or hard-to-understand instructions. Consult your supervisor to find out how your agency reports equipment problems.

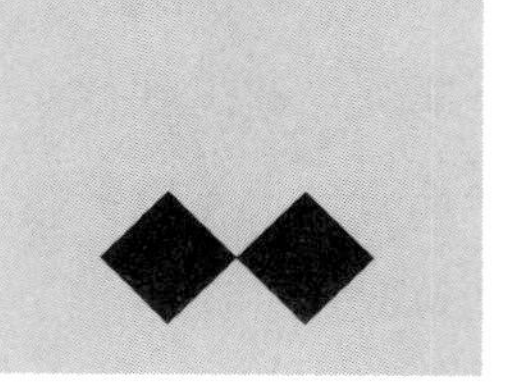

CHAPTER 14

Handling special situations

When you work as a nurse in the home care setting, you quickly learn to expect the unexpected. No matter what kind of nursing care you think you'll be delivering in a patient's home, you may find yourself facing a situation well outside the realm of your initial assignment.

These special situations might involve a patient who's confused or who abuses drugs or other substances. You may be exposed to circumstances that make you suspect abuse or neglect. You may find yourself dealing with a patient who's depressed or suicidal. Or you may arrive at a patient's home only to find that he has died.

Naturally, you'll need to know your agency's policies and your state's laws for dealing with these and all unusual situations. Just as important, however, is knowing how to assess patients carefully and respond appropriately — both professionally and personally — to these trying circumstances. This chapter offers help.

◆ CONFUSION

In its simplest form, confusion is a disorder of orientation to person, place, or time. Everyone becomes confused to varying degrees in varying circumstances. For some, it happens during periods of great stress, grief, or exhaustion. For others, it happens when first awakening. Also, many patients are confused when recovering from anesthesia.

The key to determining when confusion presents a significant problem is in its severity and duration. Nurses are often the first to notice the sometimes subtle signs of confusion, in many cases when addressing an unrelated health problem. Always be alert for confusion and disorientation, especially in elderly patients.

Assessing the problem

If your patient doesn't offer evidence that quickly demonstrates his orientation to person, place, and time, assess the possibility of confusion while performing your systems review and health history interview. Tell him that you'll be asking some questions about his past and present mental and physical health. Assure him that all your questions are simply part of a general assessment to help plan his care.

Confidentiality and privacy are key factors in promoting an atmosphere of open communication needed to take a thorough history. However, if you must conduct this conversation with other people in the room, make sure you talk directly to the patient, and the patient talks directly back to you. The overly helpful wife who answers every question for her husband may not be doing so just because she's

Assessing orientation

To determine whether your patient is oriented to person, place, and time, perform the following assessment.

Person

Ask the person's full name. If other people are in the room, ask him to tell you their names. If no one else is in the room, ask if he has children and what their names are.

Remember that a degree of forgetfulness doesn't necessarily indicate confusion ("I always get my grandsons mixed up and call them by each others' names."). And remember to take your patient's personal characteristics into account when deciding on appropriate questions. For example, a child old enough to talk may not know his parents' names other than to call them "Daddy" or "Mommy."

Place

Ask the person where he is. Keep in mind that an elderly person who seemed confused in an acute care setting may quickly reorient to familiar surroundings. In fact, a home health agency may receive an acute care referral for a "confused" patient who seems well-oriented at home. Even so, it's worth doing a little gentle probing.

If the patient says that he's "home," ask him for more details about where his home is. Ask where he was just before he came home; you may discover that the patient didn't know where he was. Sometimes you'll find that a confused patient believes he was somewhere vastly different, perhaps even for bizarre purposes ("I was in a jail with guards who hurt me."). Document the patient's response and reassess it periodically.

Time

Orientation to time tends to diminish first in unsettling circumstances, and it can be easy to reestablish. Ask the patient to tell you the complete date, the time of day, how old he is, and when significant events occurred. Distant memory may be intact even if the patient is confused about more recent happenings. It's harder to assess a child's concept of time; in fact, to a young child, events may happen either "now" or "not now."

overbearing. It may represent learned behavior unwittingly developed to compensate for her husband's increasing forgetfulness and confusion. Be polite but firm in your efforts to speak directly with the patient.

You should be able to assess your patient's orientation to person, place, and time fairly easily by using a simple set of questions. (See *Assessing orientation*.)

In addition to obvious disturbances in orientation to person, time, and place, confusion can be demonstrated by other behaviors. The patient's hygiene or appearance may be inappropriate or even bizarre. The patient may become agitated during the interview or a treatment, out of keeping with the nature of the interaction. It may stem from fear, misunderstanding, or feeling threatened by a situation the patient perceives as outside of his control. Assess the patient for errors in logic, delusions, flight of ideas, the inability to complete a thought or sentence, and other such manifestations of confusion that can indicate underlying pathology.

Taking action

A patient's confusion can make it difficult to establish a plan of care that you feel confident will be carried out in your absence. To help ensure implementation, make sure the patient has a competent caregiver in the home, or arrange to have a friend or family member visit.

To assess your patient's ability to follow through with the plan of care, ask him such questions as:

- "What would you do if your medicine was nearly gone?"
- "What would you eat if the Meals on Wheels truck couldn't get through the snow?"
- "What would you do if you smelled smoke in the house?"

Use a teaching technique that assesses understanding, such as asking for return demonstrations of changing a dressing. Another effective method (which also can be fun) is to ask the patient to pretend he's the nurse and you are the patient. Have him explain the procedure or information to you.

If you suspect that your patient is confused, consult with his doctor and refer him for evaluation and treatment as necessary. Incorporate any new orders or treatments into the plan of care. Also remember to take action in the patient's home to offset the dangers created by his confusion.

First, take steps to keep the patient safe. By planning ahead, you can reduce the likelihood that family members or caregivers will want to use chemical or physical restraints to keep the patient safe. For example, work together with caregivers to detect and defuse potential fire hazards for a patient who might forget to turn off a stove, including installing smoke and carbon monoxide detectors.

Second, take precautions against falls and other accidents. For example, suggest that caregivers lock up the patient's car keys or, if necessary, disable the patient's car so he can't drive. Consider adding and using side rails on the patient's bed. Suggest that caregivers use a baby monitor so they can hear if the patient needs help. And have them install door locks that the patient can't open but a caregiver easily can in case of fire or other emergency. (For more information, see "Dementia" in chapter 7.)

◆ SUBSTANCE ABUSE

Be aware that the home care population includes known and secret substance abusers. Substances can range from glue to alcohol to heroin, and the abuse and its implications vary with each patient's situation. If the patient is a substance abuser, your care may be directly related to the abuse or not related at all. Even so, be vigilant. If the patient uses a venous access device to administer drugs, for example, he could risk contamination at the site.

In some cases, a family member is an abuser. If so, be aware of drugs prescribed for the patient, whether they're possible targets of abuse, how and where they're stored, and whether the patient receives them as planned.

Assessing the problem

When you deliver care in a patient's home, you can assess potential substance abuse more easily than you can in an acute care setting. To be effective, however, you'll need to shed preconceived notions about substance abusers, and avoid judgmental attitudes. Remember that addictions are disease entities in themselves. A patient's alcoholism may have a genetic link; dependence on or increased tolerance of a drug may result from prescribed therapy, as in pain control.

Of course, you'll want to assess for medication problems that don't involve abuse as well, including adverse reactions, interactions, allergies, and so on. Clearly, you'll need to be familiar with the indications for use, usual dosage, expected effects, contraindications, adverse reactions, and symptoms of toxicity for any drug prescribed for your patient.

Also make sure the patient understands what he's taking, why he's taking it, how much he should take, and how and when he should take it. On each visit with the patient, assess for both desirable and undesirable effects of medications, using subjective and objective assessment data.

Taking action

If you identify a possible drug overdose in the home, you may need to take emergency action. The patient's condition and agency policy will dictate that course of action. You may need to call an ambulance, the doctor, or a supervising nurse. You may also need to notify the patient's insurer to ensure coverage. In many instances, you'll need to take all of these actions and document them appropriately. Once the situation has been successfully resolved, follow up with the patient and his family and caregivers to help avoid another overdose.

Always consider the possibility of intentional overdose. Assess the patient's state of mind, history of depression and past suicide attempts, prognosis, degree of pain, difficulties in interpersonal relationships, and financial situation in considering whether the overdose may have been a suicide attempt. If you have suspicions, ask the patient outright and, if necessary, arrange a referral for evaluation and follow-up as needed.

Dealing with a substance-abusing patient in the home setting can present a variety of problems and issues for the home health care staff. Be aware that in order to serve their addictions, some substance abusers may become skilled in distorting facts, outright lying, storehousing drugs, manipulation, theft, and other coping strategies that few nurses would be skilled at recognizing or handling.

Dealing with these situations requires direct, honest, and open communication among the home health agency, the referring hospital, the infusion company or pharmacist, and the doctor to work out a plan for conditionally accepting these patients for home care services. Naturally, this communication can only occur when the patient gives written consent to have this information shared. Use of written, signed agreements with the patient can be very helpful in avoiding future problems. When such open communication can't be arranged in advance, the home health agency may choose not to accept the referral.

Three procedures can help in dealing with substance-abusing patients at home. The first is predischarge planning for the care of I.V. substance abusers who need infusion care at home. This step helps in assessing whether the patient is an appropriate subject for home care and lays the ground rules for cooperation. (See *I.V. therapy for the known substance abuser*.)

The second is to have the patient sign a special type of informed consent. In it the patient promises to follow his plan of care, take responsibility for the infusions, avoid using or selling drugs during the treatment,

I.V. therapy for the known substance abuser

If you'll be charged with administering home I.V. therapy to a patient known to abuse drugs, you or someone at your agency will need to perform a predischarge assessment before the patient leaves the acute care facility and within 72 hours of the start of I.V. therapy. Your evaluation must demonstrate that:

- ◆ Agency personnel will be safe in and around the patient's home.
- ◆ The patient has a permanent home and isn't facing eviction.
- ◆ The home has running water, a refrigerator, and a telephone.
- ◆ The patient has agreed not to sell or use drugs at home during therapy.
- ◆ The patient has money for food and other necessities.
- ◆ The patient has agreed to undergo mental health treatment for his addiction.
- ◆ The patient or an identified caregiver can learn to administer the infusion.
- ◆ The patient has agreed to sign a release of information permitting communication with caregivers.
- ◆ The patient has agreed to sign a contract stating that he'll follow your care plan.
- ◆ The patient has agreed to be available for scheduled visits.
- ◆ The patient has a doctor available for medical follow-up and consultation with staff.
- ◆ The patient has adequate vascular access for the therapy.

and avoid using the access site for anything but his prescribed medications.

The third is a letter sent from your agency to the patient's doctor. In it the agency should explain the situation and provide a copy of the patient's informed consent.

◆ SUSPECTED NEGLECT OR ABUSE

Few situations are more heartrending than suspecting that a patient or family member is being neglected or abused. But you must face even this trying situation with professionalism and responsibility.

Keep in mind that abuse can be physical, emotional, or sexual. Neglect refers to a failure of the caretaker to provide for the needs of the person in question. Also be aware of possible exploitation, in which someone uses a child or other helpless person for personal or financial gain.

Assessing the problem

If you suspect neglect or abuse, gather more information during your assessments. And look for signs to corroborate your suspicions. (*See Common signs of neglect and abuse*, page 428.)

If the patient is an adult, ask questions that he can answer simply — for example, "Does anyone hurt you?" "Does this person hit, slap, or kick you?" Remember that the patient may never have been asked such questions before and may be anxious about answering truthfully. Don't force the issue. He may need time to develop trust in your relationship, or he may choose to confide in someone else.

Also ask questions such as those listed above when the suspected vic-

Common signs of neglect and abuse

If your assessment reveals any of the following signs, consider neglect or abuse as a possible cause and investigate further.

Neglect
- Failure to thrive in infants
- Malnutrition
- Dehydration
- Poor personal hygiene
- Inadequate clothing
- Severe diaper rash
- Injuries from falls
- Failure of wounds to heal
- Periodontal disease
- Infestations, such as scabies, lice, or maggots in a wound

Abuse
- Recurrent injuries
- Multiple injuries or fractures in various stages of healing
- Unexplained bruises, abrasions, burns, bites, damaged or missing teeth, strap or rope marks
- Head injuries or bald spots from pulling hair out
- Bleeding from body orifices
- Genital trauma
- Sexually transmitted diseases in children
- Pregnancy in young girls or those with physical or mental handicaps
- Verbalized accounts of being beaten, slapped, kicked, or involved in sexual activities
- Precocious sexual behaviors
- Exposure to inappropriately harsh discipline
- Exposure to verbal abuse and belittlement
- Extreme fear or anxiety

Additional signs
- Mistrust of others
- Blunted or flat affect
- Depression or mood changes
- Social withdrawal
- Lack of appropriate peer relationships
- Sudden school difficulties, such as poor grades, truancy, or fighting with peers
- Nonspecific headaches, stomachaches, or eating or sleeping problems
- Clinging behavior directed toward health care providers
- Aggressive speech or behavior toward adults
- Abusive behavior toward younger children and pets
- Use of drugs or alcohol
- Runaway behavior

tim is a child. Remember, though, that if the victim is a very young child or an infant, the person you'll be questioning could be the abuser.

Frank discussion with the person being abused may be impossible if the abuser insists on being present during every interaction, or if one parent is afraid to speak against the other. If you're concerned about possible abuse, you may need to create situations in which you can ask the appropriate questions of the appropriate person, without interference.

Bear in mind that your role isn't to investigate but to report your suspicions of abuse or neglect. Don't underestimate the potential danger to the person who chooses to admit that he's being abused.

Be vigilant in identifying and reporting suspected physical, mental, or emotional abuse. In fact, you may tell patients up front, in your initial interview, that home health agency staff are considered "mandated reporters" and are bound to report suspected abuse.

Keep in mind that a family known to be abusive in the past is at higher risk of repeating those behaviors when a new baby or person is added to the household, when the abuser returns to the household, and during times of increased stress or financial pressures.

If you interview prenatal or postpartum patients being followed with home visits, include questions about experiences the expectant or new parents had with their own parents. Further assessment should include the parents' knowledge of infant growth and development, their expectations of behaviors, and their concept of discipline.

As appropriate, suggest local resources, such as play groups, parent support groups, resources for single parents, toll-free confidential parents' assistance phone lines, and so on.

A home health agency may receive a referral for the express purpose of reuniting a child or other victim with an abuser. This may take the form of supervised visits during which the nurse evaluates a parent's ability to care for and interact with her baby appropriately. It may be observation of the interaction between an adult son and his elderly father as the son gives a bedbath. Regardless of the situation, remain objective and report the slightest concerns.

Taking action

If you suspect neglect, keep in mind that a person you consider neglectful in caring for a child or elderly person may be that way because of inadequate knowledge or resources, resentment of a situation beyond his control, or even simple fatigue. Be aware of the potential for neglect in even the most dedicated caregiver. Strive to prevent it by assisting the caregiver in gaining the knowledge, resources, and respite needed to provide optimal care to the patient.

No matter what the reasons behind them, signs of neglect warrant a conference with the doctor to report your findings, as required by law and agency protocol. Use common sense when deciding on the best way to handle the situation. In cases of neglect, sometimes simple interventions provide the best way to remedy the problem.

If you receive a referral to teach or care for a patient already known to be neglected or abused, look for ways to manage the situation to the patient's benefit. For example, say you're called to treat a patient with a pressure ulcer that was allowed to develop by a tired daughter-in-law who works, cares for her own children, manages the household, and cares for her mother-in-law as well. Situations such as this one can be successfully managed, but they take some initiative and suggestions for improvement on your part. They also require periodic follow-up and reevaluation.

Working with victims of abuse, neglect, or exploitation takes an emotional toll on all staff members, novice and experienced alike. Your home health agency should ensure that all staff have appropriate orientation and training, that supervisors know about sensitive situations, and that staff members have opportunities to vent their emotions and be supported in their efforts to cope with the challenging situations facing them.

Supervisors should also be aware that some staff themselves may have been victimized in their private lives, and may have trouble separating their own issues from those of the case at hand. Not all nurses can be effective with such patients. The supervisor is responsible to ensure that the nurse-patient relationship is a therapeutic one.

Cases of abuse, neglect, and exploitation are more likely to lead into the courtroom than most other situations you'll encounter. Because agency records may be subpoenaed for cases in which an abuser is being prosecuted or parental rights being terminated, your documentation must be accurate, objective, complete, and specific to the patient.

If you receive a call from someone identifying himself as an attorney and requesting your documentation, however, refer the person to your supervisor. The supervisor probably will respond with something like, "Because of the confidential nature of our records and services, I can't confirm whether or not we provide services to that person. Our legal counsel will call you back."

In extreme situations, news of abuse and abusers may appear in the media. Find out your agency's policy about speaking with the press. Be prepared to give a noncommittal response to anyone who expresses interest in your comments on a case or a patient.

◆ DEPRESSION

Statistics in the United States suggest that depression affects as many as 20% of women and 10% of men at least once in their lives. Whether organic, seasonal, genetically linked, chemically induced, or situational in nature, the symptoms can be frightening and even immobilizing or life-threatening to the person experiencing them. In addition, the person can be drastically misunderstood by family, friends, and caregivers.

Assessing the problem

Depression encompasses a broad range of symptoms presenting in varying degrees with each patient. Assess it carefully and thoughtfully. The patient may not recognize his symptoms as depression and may even resist the suggestion that he could be depressed. (For more information, see "Mentally ill patient" in chapter 5.)

Instead of labeling the disorder, question the patient about specific symptoms. He may deny being depressed but admit to difficulty with concentration, irritability, and low energy. Family members may play a key role by offering their perceptions of the patient's mood and daily functioning. Don't consider family perceptions to the exclusion of the patient's, however. (See *Warning signs of depression*.)

When assessing for depression, specifically ask if the patient has any of the following symptoms:

- ◆ depressed mood most of the day
- ◆ diminished interest or pleasure in activities once enjoyed
- ◆ decreased attention to activities of daily living
- ◆ decreased or increased appetite
- ◆ insomnia or hypersomnia
- ◆ decreased energy
- ◆ decreased concentration or indecisiveness
- ◆ decreased motivation
- ◆ feelings of hopelessness, helplessness, worthlessness, or guilt
- ◆ recurrent thoughts of death, with or without suicidal ideation
- ◆ psychotic symptoms (paranoia, suspiciousness, hallucinations)
- ◆ increased anxiety
- ◆ increased somatic complaints
- ◆ cognitive changes.

If the patient has some or all of these symptoms, notify his doctor. Beware that it can take as long as 4 to 6 weeks for a patient to show a response to antidepressant medication. Keep his doctor informed of his progress.

Also assess for a personal or family history of depression and previous psychiatric treatment. Specifically assess any suicide risk.

Altered sleep is one of the most common complaints of depression. Evaluate whether the patient has trouble falling asleep (initial insomnia), wakes frequently during the night (middle insomnia), or wakes early in the morning (early morning awakening). He may need a sleep aid until he starts to respond to treatment for depression.

Also assess nutritional status. Monitor the patient's recovery from physical illness. Depressed people tend to produce increased cortisone levels, which can suppress the immune system and interfere with recovery.

Depression is most common among elderly patients and most likely to be misconstrued in this population. Be alert for increased somatic complaints, cognitive changes, and increased anxiety in addition to the classic symptoms of depression. Don't assume that a patient's symptoms of depression are a normal part of aging.

Of course, no one is immune to depression, including children and teens. They, too, tend to have atypical symptoms. They often present with lowered self-esteem, anger, increased accidents, behavioral problems, or poor school performance — depending largely on developmental stage.

Look closely at family dynamics and current stressors, but don't assume that a functional home can protect a child from depression. Use the same assessment skills with this population as you would with adults. Evaluate typical and atypical symptoms of depression, suicidal ideation, physical illness, social and academic functioning, laboratory findings, and family dynamics.

Because a depressed person has a limited ability to concentrate, teach him and his family carefully and repeatedly about depression and its treatment. Offer written material whenever possible.

Keep in mind that depression can result from endocrine disorders, tumors, adverse effects of medications, nutritional deficiencies, multiple sclerosis, organic brain disorders, and other pathophysiologic factors, some of which, once identified, can be remedied. Diseases found more commonly in elderly people, such as

Warning signs of depression

Look for these subtle and sometimes not-so-subtle signs that your home care patient may be depressed:

- dulled affect
- tearfulness
- feeling hopeless, powerless, worthless, guilty
- difficulty concentrating or making decisions
- dulled sense of pain or pleasure
- decrease in physical or sexual activity
- social withdrawal
- irritability or anger
- anxiety
- recurrent thoughts of death
- suicidal threats or acts.

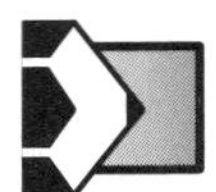

TEACHING POINTS

Living with depression

If your patient has been diagnosed with clinical depression, you can help him and his family by offering the following information:

◆ Teach the patient and family about depression and its symptoms.

◆ Advise the patient not to make major life decisions until the depression has subsided.

◆ Explain that antidepressant medications help ease the patient's symptoms, but that his mood may not lift for 10 to 28 days. It may take up to 8 weeks for the full effect to occur and for the symptoms to subside.

◆ Provide detailed teaching on the proper use of antidepressants. Include a review of their adverse effects and necessary precautions.

◆ Tell the family that depressed patients tend to be forgetful. Encourage the family to remind the patient about the length of time needed for antidepressants to work. Doing so will help to provide hope and stimulate memory.

◆ Explain that adverse effects common to antidepressants — such as dizziness, drowsiness, and hypotension — usually subside after the first few weeks.

◆ Instruct the patient to use extreme caution when working around machinery, driving a car, and crossing streets because of possible drowsiness and decreased reflexes.

◆ Instruct the patient not to drink alcohol because it can interfere with antidepressants.

◆ Explain that taking the full dose at night may reduce adverse effects experienced during the day.

◆ Tell the patient that, if he misses a dose of medication, he should try to take it within the next 3 hours. If more than 3 hours pass, he should skip that day's dose and take the next day's dose as scheduled.

◆ Tell the patient not to double up on doses.

◆ Warn the patient not to stop taking an antidepressant suddenly. Instead, tell him to call his doctor first.

Alzheimer's disease, disabling arthritis, or Parkinson's disease, can result in depression as well.

Taking action

When caring for a patient with depression, promote his safety, facilitate effective coping, and help build self-esteem. Specific interventions include the following:

◆ Teach the patient and his family that depression is an illness and not a weakness. The patient needs support and understanding. Teach them the biological symptoms of depression and the cognitive and psychosocial changes. (See *Living with depression*.)

◆ Ask the patient in a nonjudgmental way if he has thoughts of death or suicide. If so, this signals an immediate need for consultation and evaluation.

◆ Assess losses and how the patient deals with them, including social and cultural factors that may affect how the patient coped with them.

◆ Assess effective and maladaptive coping techniques used by the patient, and emphasize the positive results when he uses healthy techniques.

◆ Include the patient in establishing a realistic plan of care. Doing so tells him you value his opinion and sets the stage for later reinforcement and encouragement of his success when he makes progress — which can bolster his self-esteem and diminish feelings of worthlessness and powerlessness.

◆ Establish patient-centered objectives, and incorporate them into your written plan of care. Establish a rapport with the patient and an unconditional relationship (although you must tell him that you'll have to respond to any threats of self-harm).

◆ Acknowledge the physical pain, emotional stress, financial difficulties, tragic losses, and other situations that the patient may be experiencing. Be positive, empathetic, and encouraging without minimizing the perceived impact of these circumstances.

◆ Assist the patient in identifying stressors, associated emotional responses, and adaptive coping skills. This process will help him gain insight and an increased sense of control. Rehearsing new behaviors in a safe setting can increase self-confidence and self-esteem as well.

◆ Institute measures to ensure relaxation before sleep, such as relaxation techniques and avoidance of stimulants and depressants before bedtime.

◆ If the patient is too immobilized by depression to attend to activities of daily living, such as personal hygiene and grooming, he'll need help in these areas and encouragement to take part as much as possible until he can do so without help.

◆ Establish a simple routine for the patient. This helps establish structure and decreases feelings of helplessness and hopelessness that come with the inability to make decisions.

◆ Listen to the patient when he's ready to discuss his feelings and painful topics. This helps diminish feelings of isolation and aids in recovery. Encourage the patient to verbalize his feelings, including anger, resentment, and fear. This can decrease the need to act feelings out in inappropriate ways.

◆ Encourage the patient to discuss irrational thoughts about himself or others. This helps to put perspective on irrational thinking.

◆ Encouraging independence and practicing techniques of assertiveness and communication can also enhance the patient's progress toward improved self-esteem.

◆ Administer pharmacologic and other treatments as ordered.

◆ Encourage the patient to keep a journal to help dissipate negative energy that goes into feeling worthless, powerless, or hopeless.

◆ SUICIDE

The risk of suicide in a depressed patient is very real. Depression may contribute to as many as 75% of all completed suicides and is one of the strongest risk factors for attempted and completed suicides.

Your agency should have policies and procedures for identification, treatment, and referral of potentially suicidal patients. All staff, including receptionists who might take a phone call threatening suicide, should be oriented to these procedures. (See *Responding to the suicidal patient*, page 434.)

Responding to the suicidal patient

Any time a patient expresses verbal or nonverbal signs of possible suicide, assume that he's asking for help. Help prevent the suicide and find ongoing help for the patient. To do so, follow these guidelines or your agency's policy:

◆ Tell the patient that you and other professionals are concerned for his well-being and safety.

◆ Contact your agency supervisor to ask about any medical or legal protocols you need to follow. Also notify other agency staff of the increased risk.

◆ Contact the patient's doctor to develop a plan for referring the patient or intervening in the current crisis, possibly by arranging transport to a psychiatric facility.

◆ As appropriate, tell the patient's family what's happening.

◆ Document your findings and your conversations with the patient's doctor. Notify team members of any changes in the patient's care.

◆ Ask a social worker and mental health specialist for assistance in making appropriate referrals.

◆ Request a care conference so you can develop a long-term plan for the patient.

If the patient attempts suicide, follow these guidelines or your agency's policy:

◆ Call 911 immediately.

◆ Start cardiopulmonary resuscitation to try to revive the person.

◆ Ask someone to call your agency, or make the call yourself as soon as possible, to tell your supervisor about the situation.

◆ Unless your supervisor does it, call the patient's doctor and arrange for whatever assistance you need.

◆ Stay with the patient until the ambulance arrives.

◆ Do your best to comfort and support the family.

◆ Request a care conference so you can plan additional interventions or referrals for the patient, the family, and staff affected by the crisis.

Assessing the problem

Assess all depressed patients for self-destructive or suicidal tendencies. Remember that healthy, adventurous people may intentionally take death-defying risks, especially during their youth. Risks taken by self-destructive patients, in contrast, are not death-defying, but death-seeking.

Not all depressed patients want to die, but a higher percentage of them commit suicide than patients with other diagnoses. In *subintentional suicide*, a person has no conscious intention of dying but engages in self-destructive acts that could easily prove fatal.

National statistics suggest that white women are three times as likely to attempt suicide but white men are four times as likely to succeed at killing themselves. The person who attempts suicide typically is under age 19 or over age 45. About 25% of successful suicides in the United States are committed by people over age 55, and the risk increases exponentially with age.

Most people who attempt suicide have a history of previous suicide attempts and have been under psychiatric care during the previous year. They may also suffer from chronic, painful, or disabling diseases; be divorced, widowed, or separated; live alone in an urban area; or be unemployed or have suffered a recent and significant loss of income.

Chemically dependent and schizophrenic patients also present a high suicide risk. Suicidal schizophrenics may become agitated instead of depressed. Voices may tell them to kill themselves. Alarmingly, some schizophrenics exhibit only vague warning signs before taking their lives. A patient who has lost touch with reality may cut or mutilate body parts to focus on physical pain, which may be less overwhelming than emotional distress. Such behavior may indicate a borderline personality disorder.

Assessing suicidal ideation involves specifically asking the patient whether he has thoughts of suicide and whether he has a plan for suicide. Some patients have what's called *passive suicidal ideation,* meaning that they have no plan or intent, but they do wish to be dead. Assessment is still necessary to determine if they would ever do anything to hasten death. Don't worry that asking questions about suicide will make a patient begin thinking about it.

Taking action

As with the depressed patient, first report your concerns about potential suicide risk to the patient's doctor for further medical evaluation and referral to a counselor or psychiatric practitioner. Any indication of suicidal ideation, regardless of how passive, should be assessed and taken seriously. In addition, teach paraprofessionals to be on the lookout for warning signs of mental illness and suicide.

Emergency interventions

If you determine that a patient has a plan for committing suicide, regard the situation as a crisis requiring immediate action. Start by ensuring the safest possible environment for him. Dispose of anything that may pose a danger to him.

If the patient is willing to contract with you to avoid attempting suicide, do so, and arrange for a psychiatric evaluation. A contract for safety involves either a verbal or written promise not to act on suicidal impulses.

Give the patient the phone number of a crisis line in case he has trouble distracting himself from suicidal impulses. If the patient isn't willing to contract with you, notify your agency, then stay with him and protect him until the psychiatric evaluation can take place or relief is provided.

Patients at risk for suicide can be successfully treated through psychotherapy, medication, group support, and other treatment. Although these procedures are outside the realm of practice for most home health nurses, you can help many suicidal patients simply by telling them that treatments exist. Sharing this information helps to convey hope for the future, without downplaying the severity of the patient's despair.

Most of all, help the patient see that he isn't alone. Help him see that even if he has no significant others in his personal life, caring and competent professionals are dedicated to seeing him through this low point.

If possible, also encourage the patient to engage in physical activity to help release tension. Whether it involves a hobby that requires physical effort or a motor activity, such as walking, swimming, or gardening, these activities can provide a real sense of release and relief in addition to a sense of accomplishment.

If a patient does attempt suicide, especially if he succeeds, everyone involved will be deeply affected. Your home health agency probably has a plan to help involved staff deal with grief, a sense of failure and guilt, and other normal responses to such a tragedy.

◆ DEATH OF A PATIENT AT HOME

Occasionally, a patient may die unexpectedly at home, either from natural or suspicious causes. In an unexpected death, suicide, or possible homicide in the home care setting, legal procedures take precedence over medical ones; don't disturb the death scene until you're cleared to do so by officials. More often, however, you'll deal with terminally ill patients who choose to die at home in a hospice environment.

Elements of hospice

For the dying patient and his family, home health care provides support and assistance to prepare for death and the dying process. Many home care agencies have a Medicare-certified hospice component or a special program for meeting the needs of dying patients, their families, and significant others.

When caring for a dying patient at home, focus on the objectives and priorities of the hospice concept. For example, direct your care at easing the patient's symptoms and keeping him comfortable — not attempting to improve his condition or prolong his life. Direct much of your efforts at addressing the emotional and spiritual needs of the patient and his family. Safeguard the patient's dignity; help all involved to prepare for the death, express their grief and fears, and participate as fully as possible in the process.

Assisting with death

When dealing with a dying patient and his family, the home care team fills a supportive role, realizing that even though this is an opportunity for the patient to plan and "put things in order," it also is a most difficult and painful time for the family. It requires emotional strength and sensitivity on your part, and it requires you to strictly follow the basic standards of hospice care, including these important goals:

- ◆ alleviating pain and other symptoms
- ◆ promoting comfort and maximizing the quality of remaining life
- ◆ promoting functional autonomy based on the interdependence of the patient and his caregivers
- ◆ facilitating communication between the patient, caregivers, and family
- ◆ helping to adapt the home setting to ensure patient safety and facilitate caregiving
- ◆ educating the patient and family regarding care techniques
- ◆ identifying patient and family needs and developing strategies and interventions to fulfill those needs
- ◆ providing care in a holistic manner, including attention to the physical, psychological, spiritual, and interpersonal needs of the patient
- ◆ providing supportive coping techniques and guidance in developing alternatives
- ◆ coordinating other members of the interdisciplinary team
- ◆ establishing mechanisms to ensure quality care and services, and ongoing monitoring of care plans
- ◆ providing information on resources available in meeting patient and family needs

Warning signs of impending death

To help your patient's family prepare for his impending death, consider giving them a list of signs that commonly precede death, so they can be prepared. Emphasize that not all of these signs appear at once; some may not appear at all. However, each sign reflects the body's progression into the final stage of life.

- The person's arms and legs may become cool to the touch as blood circulation slows down.
- The underside of the body may become darker in color, also as a result of slowed circulation.
- The person will gradually spend more and more time sleeping. At times, he may be difficult to rouse. This is the result of a change in the body's metabolism.
- The person may become increasingly confused about time, place, and the identities of familiar people. This too results from altered metabolism.
- Oral secretions may collect in the back of the throat and produce what some people call a "death rattle." It results from a decrease in fluid intake and the person's inability to cough up normal saliva production.
- Hearing and visual ability may decrease slightly.
- The person may become restless, pull at bed linens, and have visions of people and things that don't exist. These signs result from decreased oxygen circulation to the brain and a change in the body's metabolism.
- The person will have a decreased need for food and fluids.
- During sleep, the person's breathing pattern may become irregular. You may notice periods up to 30 seconds long in which the person doesn't take a breath.
- The person may enter a coma, a state much like a deep sleep, and may no longer respond to you.
- The person may lose control of urinary function and bowel movements, but usually not until death is imminent.

- providing care based on the concepts of case management.

In most agencies, as the patient's primary nurse, you are responsible for making sure the doctor knows about the patient's desire to die at home. Discuss with the doctor the patient's prognosis, advance directives, and the need for a do-not-resuscitate (DNR) order in the home. If appropriate, encourage the patient to prepare advance directives. (See chapter 3 for more information.) Also confirm that the doctor will sign the patient's death certificate after you confirm that he has no signs of life, depending on the requirements of your state's nurse practice act.

Keep the DNR order and the advance directives in the patient's home in an accessible location. Give the patient's family a list of signs and symptoms that warn of approaching death. (See *Warning signs of impending death*.) Tell the family to call your agency at any hour. Suggest that the family keep a list by the phone of people they want to call after the patient's death, along with the numbers of the funeral home, doctor, and medical examiner or coroner, as required by state law.

Review the patient's plans with the patient, family, and caregivers at least every 30 days to reconfirm that they still reflect the patient's wishes. Document his wishes in the clinical record. The DNR order is also recertified every 30 days. To ensure continuity and continued support, make sure your agency supervisor knows about the patient's impending death and any special circumstances involved.

When the patient dies, you may need to make a home visit to confirm that he has no life signs. Document your findings in the clinical record and, if the family requests it, notify the patient's doctor or covering doctor that you need a signature on the death certificate. Also consider removing any temporary tubes and cleaning the body, if necessary. Follow standard precautions.

Remember that many family members take comfort in helping with this last service for their loved one or doing it themselves. Respect their wish to help. When the family is ready, consider offering to call the funeral home for them. As much as you can, offer to help the family with whatever support and comfort measures are indicated. Also help them arrange for relatives or friends to provide ongoing support.

If for some reason the medical examiner's office or the police come to the home, stay there to answer questions. By remaining with the family until all notifications are completed and ongoing support systems are in place, you can help the family through the initial shock that accompanies any death. It can also allow you to help bring closure — for yourself — to one of the most intimate and emotionally challenging of all nurse-patient relationships.

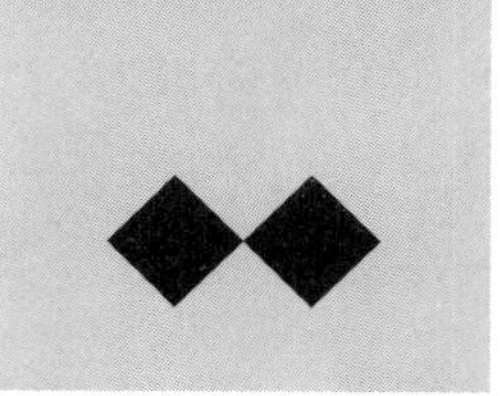

CHAPTER 15

Documenting your care

As you've seen throughout this book, home health nurses need a host of highly developed clinical, personal, and management skills. In addition, though, remember that clear and accurate documentation is the administrative piece that makes the whole home health system run.

Like acute care facilities, rehabilitation centers, and nursing homes, home health agencies are regulated by state and federal laws and governing bodies. Without accurate and complete documentation for each patient, these authorities may refuse to license, accredit, or reimburse your agency.

In no other health care setting are you as responsible for ensuring the fiscal well-being of your employer as you are in the home health setting. In fact, your agency's success or failure is closely linked with your knowledge of reimbursement guidelines and your ability and willingness to document clearly, completely, and appropriately. In this chapter, you'll find important information to help you hone your documentation skills.

◆ REQUIRED DOCUMENTATION

Every home health agency has its own standards, requirements, and forms to be used when documenting a patient's care. Naturally, you'll want to be familiar with your agency's requirements and follow them to the best of your ability.

In a general sense, however, you'll find that all agencies and payers require certain types of documentation, even if they use different forms to report the information. The areas in which you'll need to ensure documentation typically include the referral for home care, assessment (including the Outcome and Assessment Information Set), plan of care, medical update, progress notes, patient or caregiver teaching, recertification, discharge summary, and telephone orders.

Keep in mind that, if your agency is reimbursed by Medicare, you'll need to provide at least some of your documentation on specific forms using particular reimbursement codes.

Referral for home care

Before you begin caring for a patient in his home, your agency will receive information about that patient on a referral or intake form. (See *Referral for home care*, pages 440 and 441.) Either you or someone in your agency will use this form to make sure the patient is eligible for home care — and the agency can provide the services he needs — before taking the new case.

To meet Medicare's criteria for home care reimbursement, the patient will need to meet all of the following conditions:

Referral for home care

Also called an intake form, this form is used to document the patient's needs when you begin your evaluation of a new patient. Use the form below as a guide.

ELECTION BENEFIT PERIOD (1) 2 3 4

Date of Referral: 040198 Branch ______ Chart#: 0001234 H __

Info Taken By: Jane Smith, RN Admit Date: 040298

Patient's Name: John Dough

Address: 11 Second St.

City: Hometown State: PA Zip: 10981

Phone: 881-555-2931 Date of Birth: 050229

Primary Caregiver Name & #: Sarah Dough 881-555-2931

Insurance Name: Medicare Ins.#: 123-45-6789A

Is this a managed care policy (HMO): NO

Primary Dx: (Code 873.50) Open wound Foot/Complications (Onset) Date: 060197

(Code 250.03) Type I IDDM uncontrolled (Exac.) Date: 060197

(Code 443.89) Periph Vascular Disease (Exac.) Date: 060197

Procedures: (Code 86.28) Debridement Wound (Onset) Date: 060197

Referral Source: Dr's office Phone: 000-00-0000

Physician Name & Phone #: (UPIN 22222) Dr. Goodman

Phone: 881-555-6900

Physician Address: Dr's Medical Center, Hometown, PA 10981

Hospital N/A Admit N/A Discharge N/A

Functional Limitations: Pain Management, Pain, ambulation dysfunction

ORDERS/SERVICES (specify amount, frequency and duration):

SN: 5-7 visits/wk x 9 wks for assessment and wound care (L) foot: saline wet to dry drsg

AI: 3-5 visits/wk x 9 wks for assistance with ADLs and personal care

PT, OT, ST: PT 1-3 visits/wk x 9 wks to assess mobility and safety, and develop home exercise program.

MSW: 1-2 visits x 1 mo. for financial assessment and long term planning

Spiritual Coordinator: N/A Counselor: N/A

Volunteer: N/A

Other Services Provided: N/A

Goals: Wound healing without complications.

Equipment: walker and dressing supplies

Company & Phone #: Best Med Equip. Co 881-260-1026

Safety Measures: Correct use of supportive devices Nutritional Req 1800 cal ADA diet

FUNCTIONAL LIMITATIONS: (Circle Applicable)

(1) Amputation
2 Bowel/Bladder
3 Contracture
4 Hearing
5 Paralysis
(6) Endurance
(7) Ambulation
8 Speech
9 Legally Blind
A Dyspnea With Minimal Exer
B Other

ACTIVITIES PERMITTED: (Circle Applicable)

1. Complete Bedrest
2. Bedrest BRP
3. Up as Tolerated
(4) Transfer Bed/Chair
5. Partial Wgt Bearing
6. Independent at Home
7. Crutches
8. Cane
A. Wheelchair
(B) Walker
C. No Restriction
D. Other—specify

Referral for home care *(continued)*

Accessibility to bath Y - (N) Shower Y - (N) Bathroom (Y) - N Exit (Y) - N
Mental Status: (Circle) (Oriented) Comatose (Forgetful) Depressed Disoriented Lethargic Agitated Other
Allergies: *NKA*
• Hospice Appropriate Meds • Med company: *N/A*
MEDICATIONS: *Humulin N 24 units SC q am* — *changed*
Tylenol 325-1000 mg q4h prn pain po — *unchanged*
Darvocet N 100 one tab q4h prn pain po — *new*
MOM 30 cc qhs prn po — *unchanged*
Living Will Yes ____ No *x* Obtained ____ Family to mail to office ____
Guardian, POA, or Responsible Person: *wife*
Address & Phone Number: *same*
Other Family Members: *N/A*
ETOH: *0* Drug Use: ____ Smoker *X* *1-2 ppd x 25 yrs*
HISTORY: *Chronic peripheral vascular disease with periodic open wounds of feet and legs. Seen by Dr. in office 040198 and new wound of (L) foot debrided.*
Social History (place of birth, education, jobs, retirement, etc.): *WWII veteran retired (x 8 yrs) construction worker*

ADMISSION NOTES: VS: T *99°* AP *88* RR *22* BP *150/82*
Lungs: *diminished bilat. at bases* Extremities: *R foot WNL, L foot pale, DP and PT pulses +.*
Wgt: *155 lb.* Recent wgt loss/gain of *denies*
Admission Narrative: *Patient independent in Insulin administration and instructed in Insulin dosage change with good understanding. Wound of L ankle-outer malleolar area = 4 cm x 5 cm x 1 cm deep; open with beefy red appearance, wound edges pink, moderate amount serosanguineous drainage present. Wound care performed by RN per care plan. Pain controlled with Darvocet prn.*
Psychosocial Issues *Wife refuses to be involved with wound care at all.*
Environmental Concerns *Cluttered home, 2 dogs and 1 cat in house*
Are there any cultural or spiritual customs or beliefs of which we should be aware before providing Hospice services? *N/A*

Funeral Home: *N/A* Contact made YES ____ NO ____
DIRECTIONS: *1 block before intersection of Main St, on Second St.*

Agency Representative
Signature: *Jane Smith, RN* Date: *040298*

- ◆ He must be confined to his home.
- ◆ He must need skilled services.
- ◆ He must need those services on an intermittent basis.
- ◆ The care he needs must be reasonable and medically necessary.
- ◆ He must be under the care of a doctor.

Assessment

When you first begin caring for the patient in his home, you'll need to complete a thorough and specific assessment. Chart the information on your agency's assessment form.

Be sure to assess the patient's

- ◆ nutritional status
- ◆ home environment in relation to safety and supportive services and groups such as family, neighbors, and community
- ◆ knowledge of his disease or current condition, prognosis, and treatment plan
- ◆ potential for complying with the treatment plan.

Outcomes and Assessment Information Set

The proposed "Conditions of Participation for Home Health Agencies" requires that Medicare-certified agencies complete a comprehensive assessment of home care patients using a standardized data set called the Outcome and Assessment Information Set (OASIS). Many home health agencies already use OASIS in their documentation. In the near future, many more will follow.

OASIS was developed specifically to measure outcomes for adults who receive home care. (See *Outcome and Assessment Information Set,* pages 443 through 456.) Using this instrument, you'll collect data to measure changes in your patient's health status over time. Typically, you'll need to collect OASIS data when a patient starts home care, at the 60-day recertification point, and when the patient is discharged or transferred to another health care facility, such as a hospital or subacute care facility.

The OASIS data set includes more than 80 topics, including sociodemographic data, physiologic data, functional data, service utilization information, and mental, behavioral, and emotional data. However, keep in mind that OASIS is not a comprehensive assessment tool. Plus, it's not suitable for use with pediatric or maternal patients.

Plan of care

Once you've assessed the patient thoroughly, prepare a comprehensive plan of care for him. As in any health care setting, the nursing process forms the basis for your plan of care. However, more than you would in an acute care environment, you'll need to prepare your plan of care in cooperation with the patient and his caregivers. Remember that they may be providing much of the patient's care. Adjust your interventions, patient goals, and teaching accordingly.

Some agencies use a home health certification and plan of care form — which is required for Medicare reimbursement — as their official plan of care for Medicare patients. This form is also called form 485. (See *Home health certification and plan of care*, pages 457 and 458.) Other agencies use a multidisciplinary, integrated plan of care. (See *Interdisciplinary plan of care*, page 459.)

Whichever form you use, make sure you provide accurate, appropriate documentation. To document effectively on your plan of care, follow these suggestions:

- ◆ Keep a copy of the plan of care in the patient's home for easy reference by the patient and his family.
- ◆ Make sure the plan is comprehensive by including more than the patient's physiologic problems. Also include information about the home environment, needed resources, and the emotional states and attitudes of the patient, family, and caregiver.
- ◆ Document physical changes needed in the patient's home for him to receive proper care. Also document how you helped the family find the resources to implement them.

(Text continues on page 456.)

Outcome and Assessment Information Set

Medicare Home Health Care Quality Assurance and Improvement Demonstration Outcome and Assessment Information Set (OASIS-B)

OASIS Items to be Used at Specific Time Points

Start of Care (or Resumption of Care Following Inpatient Facility Stay): 1-69
Follow-Up: 1, 4, 9-11, 13, 16-26, 29-71
Discharge (not to inpatient facility): 1, 4, 9-11, 13, 16-26, 29-74, 78-79
Transfer to Inpatient Facility (with or without agency discharge): 1, 70-72, 75-79
Death at Home: 1, 79
Note: For items 51-67, please note special instructions at the beginning of the section.

CLINICAL RECORD ITEMS

a. (M0010) Agency ID: 269387HC

b. (M0020) Patient ID Number: SM962

c. (M0030) Start of Care Date: 02/10/1998 (month day year)

d. (M0040) Patient's Last Name: ANDERSON

e. (M0050) Patient State of Residence: PA

f. (M0060) Patient Zip Code: 26911

g. (M0063) Medicare Number: (including suffix if any) 128451941 3
☐ NA- No Medicare

h. (M0066) Birth Date: 01/11/1911 (month day year)

i. (M0080) Discipline of Person Completing Assessment:
☒ 1-RN ☐ 2-LPN ☐ 3-PT
☐ 4-SLP/ST ☐ 5-OT ☐ 6-MSW

j. (M0090) Date Assessment Information Recorded: 02/10/1998 (month day year)

DEMOGRAPHICS AND PATIENT HISTORY

1. (M0100) This Assessment is Currently Being Completed for the Following Reason:
   - ☒ 1-Start of care
   - ☐ 2-Resumption of care (after inpatient stay)
   - ☐ 3-Discharge from agency-not to an inpatient facility [Go to M0150]
   - ☐ 4-Transferred to an inpatient facility-discharged from agency [Go to M0830]
   - ☐ 5-Transferred to an inpatient facility-not discharged from agency [Go to M0830]
   - ☐ 6-Died at home [Go to M0906]
   - ☐ 7-Recertification reassessment (follow-up) [Go to M0150]
   - ☐ 8-Other follow-up [Go to M0150]

2. (M0130) Gender:
   - ☐ 1-Male
   - ☒ 2-Female

3. (M0140) Race/Ethnicity (as identified by patient):
   - ☒ 1-White, non-Hispanic
   - ☐ 2-Black, African-American
   - ☐ 3-Hispanic
   - ☐ 4-Asian, Pacific Islander
   - ☐ 5-American Indian, Eskimo, Aleut
   - ☐ 6-Other
   - ☐ UK-Unknown

(continued)

Outcome and Assessment Information Set *(continued)*

4. (M0150) Current payment sources for home care: (Mark all that apply.)
   - ☐ 0-None: no charge for current services
   - ☒ 1-Medicare (traditional fee-for-service)
   - ☐ 2-Medicare (HMO/managed care)
   - ☐ 3-Medicaid (traditional fee-for-service)
   - ☐ 4-Medicaid (HMO/managed care)
   - ☐ 5-Workers' compensation
   - ☐ 6-Title programs (e.g., Title III, V, or XX)
   - ☐ 7-Other government (e.g., CHAMPUS, VA, etc.) ____________
   - ☒ 8-Private insurance
   - ☐ 9-Private HMO/managed care
   - ☐ 10-Self-pay
   - ☐ 11-Other (specify)
   - ☐ UK-Unknown

5. (M0160) Financial factors limiting the ability of the patient/family to meet basic health needs: (Mark all that apply.)
   - ☐ 0-None
   - ☐ 1-Unable to afford medicine or medical supplies
   - ☐ 2-Unable to afford medical expenses that are not covered by insurance/Medicare (e.g., copayments)
   - ☐ 3-Unable to afford rent/utility bills
   - ☐ 4-Unable to afford food
   - ☒ 5-Other (specify) *Has PACE*

6. (M0170) From which of the following inpatient facilities was the patient discharged <u>during the past 14 days?</u> (Mark all that apply.)
   - ☒ 1-Hospital
   - ☐ 2-Rehabilitation facility
   - ☐ 3-Nursing home
   - ☐ 4-Other (specify)
   - ☐ NA-Patient was not discharged from an inpatient facility [If NA, go to M0200]

7. (M0180) Inpatient discharge date (most recent): *02* / *10* / *1998*
   month / day / year
   - ☐ UK-Unknown

8. (M0190) Inpatient diagnoses and three-digit ICD code categories <u>for only those conditions treated during an inpatient facility stay within the last 14 days</u> (no surgical or V-codes):

Inpatient facility diagnosis	ICD
a. *Heart failure*	(*4 2 8*)
b. *Sacral decubitus*	(*7 0 7*)

9. (M0200) Medical or treatment regimen change within past 14 days: Has this patient experienced a change in medical or treatment regimen (e.g., medication, treatment, or service change due to new or additional diagnosis, etc.) within the last 14 days?
   - ☐ 0-No [If no, go to M0220]
   - ☒ 1-Yes

10. (M0210) List the patient's medical diagnoses and three-digit ICD code categories for those conditions requiring changed medical or treatment regimen (no surgical or V-codes):

Changed medical regimen diagnosis	ICD
a. *Heart failure*	(*4 2 8*)
b. *Sacral decubitus*	(*7 0 7*)
c. ____________	(_ _ _)
d. ____________	(_ _ _)

11. (M0220) Conditions prior to medical or treatment regimen change or inpatient stay within past 14 days: If this patient experienced an inpatient facility discharge or change in medical or treatment regimen within the past 14 days, indicate any conditions that existed prior to the inpatient stay or change in medical or treatment regimen. (Mark all that apply.)
   - ☐ 1-Urinary incontinence
   - ☒ 2-Indwelling/suprapubic catheter
   - ☐ 3-Intractable pain
   - ☐ 4-Impaired decision-making
   - ☐ 5-Disruptive or socially inappropriate behavior
   - ☐ 6-Memory loss to the extent that supervision required
   - ☐ 7-None of the above
   - ☐ NA-No inpatient facility discharge and no change in medical or treatment regimen in past 14 days
   - ☐ UK-Unknown

Outcome and Assessment Information Set *(continued)*

12. (M0230/M0240) Diagnoses and Severity Index: List each medical diagnosis or problem for which the patient is receiving home care and ICD code category (no surgical or V-codes), and rate them using the following severity index. (Choose one value that represents the most severe rating appropriate for each diagnosis.)

0-Asymptomatic, no treatment needed at this time
1-Symptoms well controlled with current therapy
2-Symptoms controlled with difficulty, affecting daily functioning; patient needs ongoing monitoring
3-Symptoms poorly controlled, patient needs further adjustment in treatment and dose monitoring
4-Symptoms poorly controlled, history of rehospitalizations

Primary diagnosis	ICD	Severity rating	Date of onset
a. *Stage 3 sacral decubitus*	(*7 0 7*)	☐ 0 ☐ 1 ☒ 2 ☐ 3 ☐ 4	*1/21/98*
Other diagnosis	**ICD**	**Severity rating**	
b. *Heart failure*	(*4 2 8*)	☐ 0 ☐ 1 ☒ 2 ☐ 3 ☐ 4	*1/21/98*
c. *urinary retention*	(*7 8 8*)	☐ 0 ☒ 1 ☐ 2 ☐ 3 ☐ 4	*1/24/98*
d. ______	(_ _ _)	☐ 0 ☐ 1 ☐ 2 ☐ 3 ☐ 4	______
e. ______	(_ _ _)	☐ 0 ☐ 1 ☐ 2 ☐ 3 ☐ 4	______
f. ______	(_ _ _)	☐ 0 ☐ 1 ☐ 2 ☐ 3 ☐ 4	______

Surgical procedure ______ Code ______ Date ______

13. (M0250) Therapies the patient receives at home: (Mark all that apply.)

☐ 1 - Intravenous or infusion therapy (excludes TPN)
☐ 2 - Enteral nutrition (nasogastric, gastrostomy, jejunostomy, or any other artificial entry into the alimentary canal)
☒ 4 - None of the above

14. (M0260) Overall prognosis: BEST description of patient's overall prognosis for recovery from this episode of illness

☐ 0 - Poor: little or no recovery is expected and/or further decline is imminent
☒ 1 - Good/Fair: partial to full recovery is expected
☐ UK - Unknown

15. (M0270) Rehabilitative prognosis: BEST description of patient's prognosis for functional status

☒ 0 - Guarded: minimal improvement in functional status is expected; decline is possible
☐ 1 - Good: marked improvement in functional status is expected
☐ UK - Unknown

16. (M0280) Life expectancy: (Physician documentation is not required.)

☒ 0 - Life expectancy is greater than 6 months
☐ 1 - Life expectancy is 6 months or fewer

17. (M0290) High risk factors characterizing this patient: (Mark all that apply.)

☒ 1 - Heavy smoking
☐ 2 - Obesity
☐ 3 - Alcohol dependency
☐ 4 - Drug dependency
☐ 5 - None of the above
☐ UK - Unknown

LIVING ARRANGEMENTS

18. (M0300) Current residence:

☒ 1 - Patient's owned or rented residence (house, apartment, or mobile home owned or rented by patient/couple/significant other)
☐ 2 - Family member's residence
☐ 3 - Boarding home or rented room
☐ 4 - Board and care or assisted living facility
☐ 5 - Other (specify)

19. (M0310) Structural barriers in the patient's environment limiting independent mobility: (Mark all that apply.)

☐ 0 - None
☒ 1 - Stairs inside home that must be used by the patient (e.g., to get to toileting, sleeping, eating areas)
☐ 2 - Stairs inside the home that are used optionally (e.g., to get to laundry facilities)
☒ 3 - Stairs leading from inside house to outside
☐ 4 - Narrow or obstructed doorways

(continued)

Outcome and Assessment Information Set *(continued)*

20. (M0320) Safety hazards found in the patient's current place of residence: (Mark all that apply.)

☐ 0 - None
☐ 1 - Inadequate floor, roof, or windows
☐ 2 - Inadequate lighting
☐ 3 - Unsafe gas/electric appliance
☐ 4 - Inadequate heating
☐ 5 - Inadequate cooling
☒ 6 - Lack of fire safety devices
☐ 7 - Unsafe floor coverings
☐ 8 - Inadequate stair railings
☐ 9 - Improperly stored hazardous materials
☐ 10 - Lead-based paint
☐ 11 - Other (specify)

21. (M0330) Sanitation hazards found in the patient's current place of residence: (Mark all that apply.)

☒ 0 - None
☐ 1 - No running water
☐ 2 - Contaminated water
☐ 3 - No toileting facilities
☐ 4 - Outdoor toileting facilities only
☐ 5 - Inadequate sewage disposal
☐ 6 - Inadequate/improper food storage
☐ 7 - No food refrigeration
☐ 8 - No cooking facilities
☐ 9 - Insects/rodents present
☐ 10 - No scheduled trash pickup
☐ 11 - Cluttered/soiled living area
☐ 12 - Other (specify)

22. (M0340) Patient lives with: (Mark all that apply.)

☐ 1 - Lives alone
☒ 2 - With spouse or significant other
☐ 3 - With other family member
☐ 4 - With a friend
☐ 5 - With paid help (other than home care agency staff)
☐ 6 - With other than above

SUPPORTIVE ASSISTANCE

23. (M0350) Assisting person(s) other than home care agency staff: (Mark all that apply.)

☐ 1 - Relatives, friends, or neighbors living outside the home
☒ 2 - Person residing in the home (excluding paid help)
☐ 3 - Paid help
☐ 4 - None of the above (If none of the above, go to M0390)
☐ UK - Unknown (If unknown, go to M0390)

24. (M0360) Primary caregiver taking lead responsibility for providing or managing the patient's care, providing the most frequent assistance, etc. (other than home care agency staff):

☐ 0 - No one person (If no one person, go to M0390)
☒ 1 - Spouse or significant other
☐ 2 - Daughter or son
☐ 3 - Other family member
☐ 4 - Friend or neighbor or community or church member
☐ 5 - Paid help
☐ UK - Unknown (If unknown, go to M0390)

25. (M0370) How often does the patient receive assistance from the primary caregiver?

☒ 1 - Several times during day and night
☐ 2 - Several times during day
☐ 3 - Once daily
☐ 4 - Three or more times per week
☐ 5 - One to two times per week
☐ 6 - Less often than weekly
☐ UK - Unknown

26. (M0380) Type of primary caregiver assistance: (Mark all that apply.)

☒ 1 - ADL assistance (bathing, dressing, toileting, bowel/bladder, eating/feeding)
☒ 2 - IADL assistance (meds, meals, housekeeping, laundry, telephone, shopping, finances)
☐ 3 - Environmental support (housing, home maintenance)
☒ 4 - Psychosocial support (socialization, companionship, recreation)
☒ 5 - Advocates or facilitates patient's participation in appropriate medical care
☐ 6 - Financial agent, power of attorney, or conservator of finance
☐ 7 - Health care agent, conservator of person, or medical power of attorney
☐ UK - Unknown

SENSORY STATUS

27. (M0390) Vision with corrective lenses if the patient usually wears them:

☒ 0 - Normal vision: sees adequately in most situations; can see medication labels, newsprint
☐ 1 - Partially impaired: cannot see medication labels or newsprint, but can see obstacles in path and the surrounding layout; can count fingers at arm's length
☐ 2 - Severely impaired: cannot locate objects without hearing or touching them OR patient nonresponsive

Outcome and Assessment Information Set *(continued)*

28. (M0400) Hearing and ability to understand spoken language in patient's own language (with hearing aids if the patient usually uses them):

- ☒ 0 - No observable impairment; able to hear and understand complex or detailed instructions and extended or abstract conversation
- ☐ 1 - With minimal difficulty, able to hear and understand most multi-step instructions and ordinary conversation; may need occasional repetition, extra time, or louder voice
- ☐ 2 - Has moderate difficulty hearing and understanding simple, one-step instructions and brief conversation; needs frequent prompting or assistance
- ☐ 3 - Has severe difficulty hearing and understanding simple greetings and short comments; requires multiple repetitions, restatements, demonstrations, additional time
- ☐ 4 - Unable to hear and understand familiar words or common expressions consistently OR patient nonresponsive

29. (M0410) Speech and oral (verbal) expression of language (in patient's own language):

- ☒ 0 - Expresses complex ideas, feelings, and needs clearly, completely, and easily in all situations with no observable impairment
- ☐ 1 - Minimal difficulty in expressing ideas and needs (may take extra time, makes occasional errors in word choice, grammar or speech intelligibility; needs minimal prompting or assistance)
- ☐ 2 - Expresses simple ideas or needs with moderate difficulty (needs prompting or assistance, errors in word choice, organization or speech intelligibility); speaks in phrases or short sentences
- ☐ 3 - Has severe difficulty expressing basic ideas or needs and requires maximal assistance or guessing by listener; speech limited to single words or short phrases
- ☐ 4 - Unable to express basic needs even with maximal prompting or assistance but is not comatose or unresponsive (e.g., speech is nonsensical or unintelligible)
- ☐ 5 - Patient nonresponsive or unable to speak

30. (M0420) Frequency of pain interfering with patient's activity or movement:

- ☐ 0 - Patient has no pain or pain does not interfere with activity or movement
- ☐ 1 - Less often than daily
- ☒ 2 - Daily, but not constantly
- ☐ 3 - All of the time

31. (M0430) Intractable pain: Is the patient experiencing pain that is not easily relieved, occurs at least daily, and affects his sleep, appetite, physical or emotional energy, concentration, personal relationships, emotions, or ability or desire to perform physical activity?

- ☒ 0 - No
- ☐ 1 - Yes

INTEGUMENTARY STATUS

32. (M0440) Does patient have a skin lesion or an open wound (excluding "ostomies")?

- ☐ 0 - No (If no, go to M0490)
- ☒ 1 - Yes

33. (M0450) Does patient have a pressure ulcer?

- ☐ 0 - No (If no, got to M0468)
- ☒ 1 - Yes

33a. (M0450) Current number of pressure ulcers at each stage: (Circle one response for each stage.)

Pressure ulcer stages

a) Stage 1: Nonblanchable erythema of intact skin; heralding of skin ulceration. In darker skin, warmth, edema, hardness, or discolored skin may be indicators.

Number of pressure ulcers

0	1	2	3	4 or more

b) Stage 2: Partial thickness skin loss involving epidermis and/or dermis. The ulcer is superficial and presents clinically as an abrasion, blister, or shallow crater.

Number of pressure ulcers

0	1	2	3	4 or more

c) Stage 3: Full-thickness skin loss involving damage or necrosis of subcutaneous tissue that may extend down to, but not through, underlying fascia. The ulcer presents clinically as a deep crater with or without undermining of adjacent tissue.

Number of pressure ulcers

0	(1)	2	3	4 or more

d) Stage 4: Full-thickness skin loss with extensive destruction, tissue, necrosis, or damage to muscle, bone, or supporting structures (e.g., tendon, joint capsule, etc.)

Number of pressure ulcers

0	1	2	3	4 or more

e) In addition to the above, is there at least one pressure ulcer that cannot be observed due to the presence of eschar or a nonremovable dressing, including casts?

☒ 0 - No ☐ 1 - Yes

(continued)

Outcome and Assessment Information Set *(continued)*

33b. (M0460) Stage of most problematic (observable) pressure ulcer:

- ☐ 1 - Stage 1
- ☐ 2 - Stage 2
- ☒ 3 - Stage 3
- ☐ 4 - Stage 4
- ☐ NA - No observable pressure ulcer

33c. (M0464) Status of most problematic (observable) pressure ulcer:

- ☐ 1 - Fully granulating
- ☐ 2 - Early/partial granulation
- ☒ 3 - Not healing
- ☐ NA - No observable pressure ulcer

34. (M0468) Does this patient have a stasis ulcer?

- ☒ 0 - No (If no, go to M0482)
- ☐ 1 - Yes

34a. (M0470) Current number of observable stasis ulcer(s):

- ☐ 0 - Zero
- ☐ 1 - One
- ☐ 2 - Two
- ☐ 3 - Three
- ☐ 4 - Four or more

34b. (M0474) Does this patient have at least one stasis ulcer that cannot be observed due to the presence of a nonremovable dressing?

- ☐ 0 - No
- ☐ 1 - Yes

34c. (M0475) Status of most problematic (observable) stasis ulcer:

- ☐ 1 - Fully granulating
- ☐ 2 - Early/partial granulation
- ☐ 3 - Not healing
- ☐ NA - No observable stasis ulcer

35. (M0482) Does this patient have a surgical wound?

- ☒ 0 - No (If no, go to M0490)
- ☐ 1 - Yes

35a. (M0484) Current number of (observable) surgical wounds: (If a wound is partially closed but has more than one opening, consider each opening as a separate wound.)

- ☐ 0 - Zero
- ☐ 1 - One
- ☐ 2 - Two
- ☐ 3 - Three
- ☐ 4 - Four or more

35b. (M0486) Does this patient have at least one surgical wound that cannot be observed due to the presence of a nonremovable dressing?

- ☐ 0 - No
- ☐ 1 - Yes

35c. (M0488) Status of most problematic (observable) surgical wound:

- ☐ 1- Fully granulating
- ☐ 2 - Early/partial granulation
- ☐ 3 - Not healing
- ☐ NA - No observable surgical wound

RESPIRATORY STATUS

36. (M0490) When is the patient dyspneic or noticeably short of breath?

- ☐ 0 - Never; patient is not short of breath
- ☒ 1 - When walking more than 20 feet, climbing stairs
- ☐ 2 - With moderate exertion (e.g., while dressing, using commode, or bedpan, walking distances less than 20 feet)
- ☐ 3 - With minimal exertion (e.g., while eating, talking, or performing other ADLs) or with agitation
- ☐ 4 - At rest (during day or night)

37. (M0500) Respiratory treatments utilized at home: (Mark all that apply.)

- ☐ 1 - Oxygen (intermittent or continuous)
- ☐ 2 - Ventilator (continually or at night)
- ☐ 3 - Continuous positive airway pressure
- ☒ 4 - None of the above

ELIMINATION STATUS

38. (M0510) Has this patient been treated for a urinary tract infection in the past 14 days?

- ☒ 0 - No
- ☐ 1 - Yes
- ☐ NA - Patient on prophylactic treatment
- ☐ UK - Unknown

39. (M0520) Urinary incontinence or urinary catheter presence:

- ☐ 0 - No incontinence or catheter (includes anuria or ostomy for urinary drainage) (If no, go to M0540)
- ☐ 1 - Patient is incontinent
- ☒ 2 - Patient requires a urinary catheter (i.e., external, indwelling, intermittent, suprapubic) (Go to M0540)

40. (M0530) When does urinary incontinence occur?

- ☐ 0 - Timed voiding defers incontinence
- ☐ 1 - During the night only
- ☐ 2 - During the day and night

Outcome and Assessment Information Set *(continued)*

41. (M0540) Bowel incontinence frequency:

- ☒ 0 - Very rarely or never has bowel incontinence
- ☐ 1 - Less than once weekly
- ☐ 2 - One to three times weekly
- ☐ 3 - Four to six times weekly
- ☐ 4 - On a daily basis
- ☐ 5 - More often than once daily
- ☐ NA - Patient has ostomy for bowel elimination
- ☐ UK - Unknown

42. (M0550) Ostomy for bowel elimination: Does this patient have an ostomy for bowel elimination that (within the last 14 days): a) was related to an inpatient facility stay, or b) necessitated a change in medical or treatment regimen?

- ☒ 0 - Patient does not have an ostomy for bowel elimination
- ☐ 1 - Patient's ostomy was not related to an inpatient stay and did not necessitate change in medical or treatment regimen
- ☐ 2 - Ostomy was related to an inpatient stay or did necessitate change in medical or treatment regimen

NEURO/EMOTIONAL/BEHAVIOR STATUS

43. (M0560) Cognitive functioning: (patient's current level of alertness, orientation, comprehension, concentration, and immediate memory for simple commands)

- ☒ 0 - Alert/oriented, able to focus and shift attention, comprehends and recalls task directions independently
- ☐ 1 - Requires prompting (cuing, repetition, reminders) only under stressful or unfamiliar conditions
- ☐ 2 - Requires assistance and some direction in specific situations (e.g., on all tasks involving shifting of attention), or consistently requires low stimulus environment due to distractibility
- ☐ 3 - Requires considerable assistance in routine situations; is not alert and oriented or is unable to shift attention and recall directions more than half the time
- ☐ 4 - Totally dependent due to disturbances such as constant disorientation, coma, persistent vegetative state, or delirium

44. (M0570) When confused (reported or observed):

- ☒ 0 - Never
- ☐ 1 - In new or complex situations only
- ☐ 2 - On awakening or at night only
- ☐ 3 - During the day and evening, but not constantly
- ☐ 4 - Constantly
- ☐ NA - Patient nonresponsive

45. (M0580) When anxious (reported or observed):

- ☐ 0 - None of the time
- ☐ 1 - Less often than daily
- ☒ 2 - Daily, but not constantly
- ☐ 3 - All of the time
- ☐ NA - Patient nonresponsive

46. (M0590) Depressive feelings reported or observed in patient: (Mark all that apply.)

- ☐ 1 - Depressed mood (e.g., feeling sad, tearful)
- ☐ 2 - Sense of failure or self-reproach
- ☒ 3 - Hopelessness
- ☐ 4 - Recurrent thoughts of death
- ☐ 5 - Thoughts of suicide
- ☐ 6 - None of the above feelings observed or reported

47. (M0600) Patient behaviors (reported or observed): (Mark all that apply.)

- ☐ 1 - Indecisiveness, lack of concentration
- ☐ 2 - Diminished interest in most activities
- ☐ 3 - Sleep disturbances
- ☐ 4 - Recent change in appetite or weight
- ☐ 5 - Agitation
- ☐ 6 - A suicide attempt
- ☒ 7 - None of the above behaviors observed or reported

48. (M0610) Behaviors demonstrated at least once a week (reported or observed): (Mark all that apply.)

- ☐ 1 - Memory deficit: failure to recognize familiar persons/places, inability to recall events of past 24 hours, significant memory loss so that supervision is required
- ☐ 2 - Impaired decision-making: failure to perform usual ADLs or IADLs, inability to appropriately stop activities jeopardizes safety through actions
- ☐ 3 - Verbal disruption: yelling, threatening, excessive profanity, sexual references, etc.
- ☐ 4 - Physical aggression: aggressive or combative to self and others (e.g., hits self, throws objects, punches, performs dangerous maneuvers with wheelchair or other objects)
- ☐ 5 - Disruptive, infantile, or socially inappropriate behavior (excludes verbal actions)
- ☐ 6 - Delusional, hallucinatory, or paranoid behavior
- ☒ 7 - None of the above behaviors demonstrated

(continued)

Outcome and Assessment Information Set *(continued)*

49. (M0620) Frequency of behavior problems (reported or observed) (e.g., wandering episodes, self-abuse, verbal disruption, physical aggression, etc.):

☒ 0 - Never
☐ 1 - Less than once a month
☐ 2 - Once a month
☐ 3 - Several times each month
☐ 4 - Several times a week
☐ 5 - At least daily

50. (M0630) Is this patient receiving psychiatric nursing services at home provided by a qualified psychiatric nurse?

☒ 0 - No
☐ 1 - Yes

ADL/IADLs

For Questions 51 to 67, complete the "current" column for all patients. For these same items, complete the "prior" column at start of care or resumption of care; mark the level that corresponds to the patient's condition 14 days prior to the start of care. In all cases, record what the patient is able to do.

51. (M0640) Grooming: Ability to tend to personal hygiene needs (i.e., washing face and hands, hair care, shaving or makeup, teeth or denture care, fingernail care):

Prior	Current	
☒	☐	0 - Able to groom self unaided, with or without the use of assistive devices or adapted methods
☐	☐	1 - Grooming utensils must be placed within reach before able to complete grooming activities
☐	☒	2 - Someone must assist the patient to groom self
☐	☐	3 - Depends entirely upon someone else for grooming needs
☐		UK - Unknown

52. (M0650) Ability to dress upper body (with or without dressing aids), including pullovers, undergarments, front-opening shirts and blouses, managing zippers, buttons, and snaps:

Prior	Current	
☒	☐	0 - Able to get clothes out of closets and drawers, put them on, and remove them from the upper body without assistance
☐	☐	1 - Able to dress upper body without assistance if clothing is laid out or handed to the patient
☐	☒	2 - Someone must help put on upper body clothing
☐	☐	3 - Depends entirely upon another person to dress the upper body
☐		UK - Unknown

53. (M0660) Ability to dress lower body (with or without dressing aids), including slacks, undergarments, socks or nylons, shoes:

Prior	Current	
☒	☐	0 - Able to obtain, put on, and remove clothing and shoes without assistance
☐	☐	1 - Able to dress lower body without assistance if clothing and shoes are laid out or handed to patient
☐	☒	2 - Someone must help put on undergarments, slacks, socks or nylons, and shoes
☐	☐	3 - Depends entirely upon another person to dress lower body
☐		UK - Unknown

Outcome and Assessment Information Set *(continued)*

54. (M0670) Bathing: Ability to wash entire body; excludes grooming (washing face and hands only):

Prior	Current	
☐	☐	0 - Able to bathe self in shower or tub independently
☒	☐	1 - With the use of devices, able to bathe self in shower or tub independently
☐	☐	2 - Able to bathe in shower or tub with the assistance of another person: (a) for intermittent supervision or encouragement or reminders OR (b) to get in and out of the shower or tub OR (c) for washing difficult-to-reach areas
☐	☒	3 - Participates in bathing self in shower or tub, but requires presence of another person throughout the bath for assistance or supervision
☐	☐	4 - Unable to use the shower or tub and is bathed in bed or bedside chair
☐	☐	5 - Unable to effectively participate in bathing and is totally bathed by another person
☐		UK - Unknown

55. (M0680) Toileting: Ability to get to and from the toilet or bedside commode:

Prior	Current	
☒	☒	0 - Able to get to and from the toilet independently with or without a device
☐	☐	1 - When reminded, assisted, or supervised by another person, able to get to and from the toilet
☐	☐	2 - Unable to get to and from the toilet but is able to use a bedside commode (with or without assistance)
☐	☐	3 - Unable to get to and from the toilet or bedside commode but is able to use a bedpan/urinal independently
☐	☐	4 - Totally dependent in toileting
☐		UK - Unknown

56. (M0690) Transferring: Ability to move from bed to chair, on and off toilet or commode, into and out of tub or shower, and ability to turn and position self in bed if patient is bedfast:

Prior	Current	
☐	☐	0 - Able to transfer independently
☒	☐	1 - Transfers with minimal human assistance or with use of an assistive device
☐	☒	2 - Unable to transfer self but able to bear weight and pivot during the transfer process
☐	☐	3 - Unable to transfer self and unable to bear weight or pivot when transferred by another person
☐	☐	4 - Bedfast, unable to transfer but able to turn and position self in bed
☐	☐	5 - Bedfast, unable to transfer and unable to turn and position self
☐		UK - Unknown

57. (M0700) Ambulation/Locomotion: Ability to walk safely, once in a standing position, or use a wheelchair, once in a seated position, on a variety of surfaces:

Prior	Current	
☒	☐	0 - Able to walk independently on even and uneven surfaces and climb stairs with or without railings (i.e., needs no human assistance or assistive device)
☐	☒	1 - Requires use of a device (e.g., cane, walker) to walk alone or requires human supervision or assistance to negotiate stairs or steps or uneven surfaces
☐	☐	2 - Able to walk only with the supervision of assistance of another person at all times
☐	☐	3 - Chairfast, unable to ambulate but able to wheel self independently
☐	☐	4 - Chairfast, unable to ambulate and unable to wheel self
☐	☐	5 - Bedfast, unable to ambulate or be up in a chair
☐		UK - Unknown

(continued)

Outcome and Assessment Information Set *(continued)*

58. (M0710) Feeding or eating: Ability to feed self meals and snacks: (*Note:* This refers only to the process of eating, chewing, and swallowing, not preparing the food to be eaten.)

Prior Current

- ☒ ☒ 0 - Able to feed self independently
- ☐ ☐ 1 - Able to feed self independently but requires:
  (a) meal set-up OR
  (b) intermittent assistance or supervision from another person; OR
  (c) a liquid, pureed, or ground meat diet
- ☐ ☐ 2 - Unable to feed self and must be assisted or supervised throughout the meal/snack
- ☐ ☐ 3 - Able to take in nutrients orally and receives supplemental nutrients through a nasogastric tube or gastrostomy
- ☐ ☐ 4 - Unable to take in nutrients orally and is fed nutrients through a nasogastric tube or gastrostomy
- ☐ ☐ 5 - Unable to take in nutrients orally or by tube feeding
- ☐ UK - Unknown

59. (M0720) Planning and preparing light meals (e.g., cereal, sandwich) or reheat delivered meals:

Prior Current

- ☐ ☐ 0 - (a) Able to independently plan and prepare all light meals for self or reheat delivered meals; OR
  (b) Is physically, cognitively, and mentally able to prepare light meals on a regular basis but has not routinely performed light meal preparation in the past (i.e., prior to this home care admission)
- ☒ ☐ 1 - Unable to prepare light meals on a regular basis due to physical, cognitive, or mental limitations
- ☐ ☒ 2 - Unable to prepare any light meals or reheat any delivered meals
- ☐ UK - Unknown

60. (M0730) Transportation: physical and mental ability to safely use a car, taxi, or public transportation (bus, train, subway):

Prior Current

- ☐ ☐ 0 - Able to independently drive a regular or adapted car, OR uses a regular or handicap-accessible public bus
- ☒ ☐ 1 - Able to ride in a car only when driven by another person; OR able to use a bus or handicap van only when assisted or accompanied by another person
- ☐ ☒ 2 - Unable to ride in a car, taxi, bus, or van, and requires transportation by ambulance
- ☐ UK - Unknown

61. (M0740) Laundry: Ability to do own laundry—to carry laundry to and from washing machine, to use washer and dryer, to wash small items by hand:

Prior Current

- ☐ ☐ 0 - (a) Able to take care of all laundry tasks independently; OR
  (b) Physically, cognitively, and mentally able to do laundry and access facilities, but has not routinely performed laundry tasks in the past (i.e., prior to this home care admission)
- ☒ ☐ 1 - Able to do only light laundry, such as minor hand wash or light washer loads; due to physical, cognitive, or mental limitations, needs assistance with heavy laundry such as carrying large loads of laundry
- ☐ ☒ 2 - Unable to do any laundry due to physical limitation or needs continual supervision and assistance due to cognitive or mental limitation
- ☐ UK - Unknown

Outcome and Assessment Information Set *(continued)*

62. (M0750) Housekeeping: Ability to safely and effectively perform light housekeeping and heavier cleaning tasks:

Prior	Current	
☐	☐	0 - (a) Able to independently perform all housekeeping tasks; OR (b) Physically, cognitively, and mentally able to perform all housekeeping tasks but has not routinely participated in housekeeping tasks in the past (i.e., prior to this home care admission)
☐	☐	1 - Able to perform only light housekeeping (e.g., dusting, wiping kitchen counters) tasks independently
☐	☐	2 - Able to perform housekeeping tasks with intermittent assistance or supervision from another person
☐	☐	3 - Unable to consistently perform any housekeeping tasks unless assisted by another person throughout the process
☒	☒	4 - Unable to effectively participate in any housekeeping tasks
☐		UK - Unknown

63. (M0760) Shopping: Ability to plan for, select, and purchase items in a store and to carry them home or arrange delivery:

Prior	Current	
☐	☐	0 - (a) Able to plan for shopping needs and independently perform shopping tasks, including carrying packages; OR (b) Physically, cognitively, and mentally able to take care of shopping, but has not done shopping in the past (i.e., prior to this home care admission)
☐	☐	1 - Able to go shopping, but needs some assistance: (a) By self is able to do only light shopping and carry small packages, but needs someone to do occasional major shopping; OR (b) Unable to go shopping alone, but can go with someone to assist
☒	☐	2 - Unable to go shopping, but is able to identify items needed, place orders, and arrange home delivery
☐	☒	3 - Needs someone to do all shopping and errands
☐		UK - Unknown

64. (M0770) Ability to use telephone: Ability to answer the phone, dial numbers, and effectively use the telephone to communicate:

Prior	Current	
☒	☒	0 - Able to dial numbers and answer calls appropriately and as desired
☐	☐	1 - Able to use a specially adapted telephone (i.e., large numbers on the dial, teletype phone for the deaf) and call essential numbers
☐	☐	2 - Able to answer the telephone and carry on a normal conversation but has difficulty placing calls
☐	☐	3 - Able to answer the telephone only some of the time or is able to carry on only a limited conversation
☐	☐	4 - Unable to answer the telephone at all but can listen if assisted with equipment
☐	☐	5 - Totally unable to use the telephone
☐	☐	NA - Patient does not have a telephone
☐		UK - Unknown

MEDICATIONS

65. (M0780) Management of oral medications: Patient's ability to prepare and take all prescribed oral medications reliably and safely, including administration of the correct dosage at the appropriate times/intervals; excludes injectable and IV medications: (*Note:* This refers to ability, not compliance or willingness.)

Prior	Current	
☐	☐	0 - Able to independently take the correct oral medication(s) and proper dosage(s) at the correct times
☒	☒	1 - Able to take medication(s) at the correct time if: (a) individual dosages are prepared in advance by another person; OR (b) given daily reminders; OR someone develops a drug diary or chart
☐	☐	2 - Unable to take medication unless administered by someone else
☐	☐	NA - No oral medications prescribed
☐		UK - Unknown

(continued)

Outcome and Assessment Information Set *(continued)*

66. (M0790) Management of inhalant/mist medications: Patient's ability to prepare and take all prescribed inhalants/mist medications (nebulizers, metered dose devices) reliably and safely, including administration of the correct dosage at the appropriate times/intervals; excludes all other forms of medication (oral tablets, injectable and I.V. medications):

Prior Current

☐ ☐ 0 - Able to independently take the correct medication and proper dosage at the correct times
☐ ☐ 1 - Able to take medication at the correct times if:
(a) individual dosages are prepared in advance by another person; OR
(b) given daily reminders.
☐ ☐ 2 - Unable to take medication unless administered by someone else
☒ ☒ NA - No inhalants/mist medications prescribed
☐ UK - Unknown

67. (M0800) Management of injectable medications: Patient's ability to prepare and take all prescribed injectable medications reliably and safely, including administration of correct dosages at appropriate times/intervals; excludes I.V. medications:

Prior Current

☐ ☐ 0 - Able to independently take the correct medication and proper dosage at the correct times
☐ ☐ 1 - Able to take injectable medication at the correct times if:
(a) individual syringes are prepared in advance by another person, OR
(b) given daily reminders
☐ ☐ 2 - Unable to take injectable medications unless administered by someone else
☒ ☒ NA - No injectable medications prescribed
☐ UK - Unknown

EQUIPMENT MANAGEMENT

68. (M0810) Patient management of equipment (includes only oxygen, I.V./infusion therapy, enteral/parenteral nutrition equipment or supplies): Patient's ability to set up, monitor and change equipment reliably and safely, to add appropriate fluids or medication, and to clean/store/dispose of equipment or supplies using proper technique: (*Note:* This refers to ability, not compliance or willingness.)

☐ 0 - Patient manages all tasks related to equipment completely independently.
☐ 1 - If someone else sets up equipment (i.e., fills portable oxygen tank, provides patient with prepared solutions), patient is able to manage all other aspects of equipment.
☐ 2 - Patient requires considerable assistance from another person to manage equipment, but completes portions of the task independently.
☐ 3 - Patient is only able to monitor equipment (e.g., liter flow, fluid in bag) and must call someone else to manage the equipment.
☐ 4 - Patient is completely dependent on someone else to manage all equipment.
☒ NA - No equipment of this type used in care (If NA, go to M0830).

69. (M0820) Caregiver management of equipment (includes only oxygen, I.V./infusion equipment, enteral/parenteral nutrition, ventilator therapy equipment or supplies): Caregiver's ability to set up, monitor, and change equipment reliably and safely, to add appropriate fluids or medication, and to clean/store/dispose of equipment or supplies using proper technique: (*Note:* This refers to ability, not compliance or willingness.)

☐ 0 - Caregiver manages all tasks related to equipment completely independently.
☐ 1 - If someone else sets up equipment, caregiver is able to manage all other aspects.
☐ 2 - Caregiver requires considerable assistance from another person to manage equipment, but independently completes significant portions of task.
☐ 3 - Caregiver is only able to complete small portions of task (e.g., administer nebulizer treatment, clean/store/dispose of equipment or supplies).
☐ 4 - Caregiver is completely dependent on someone else to manage all equipment.
☐ NA - No caregiver
☐ UK - Unknown

Outcome and Assessment Information Set *(continued)*

EMERGENT CARE

70. (M0830) Emergent care: Since the last time OASIS data were collected, has the patient utilized any of the following services for emergent care (other than home care agency services)? (Mark all that apply.)

☐ 0 - No emergent care services (If no emergent care and patient discharged, go to M0855)
☐ 1 - Hospital emergency room (includes 23-hour holding)
☐ 2 - Doctor's office emergency visit/house call
☐ 3 - Outpatient department/clinic emergency (includes urgicenter sites)
☐ UK - Unknown

71. (M0840) Emergent care reason: For what reason(s) did the patient/family seek emergent care? (Mark all that apply.)

☐ 1 - Improper medication administration, medication adverse effects, toxicity, anaphylaxis
☐ 2 - Nausea, dehydration, malnutrition, constipation, impaction
☐ 3 - Injury caused by fall or accident at home
☐ 4 - Respiratory problems (e.g., shortness of breath, tracheobronchial obstruction, respiratory infection)
☐ 5 - Wound infection, deteriorating wound status, new lesion/ulcer
☐ 6 - Cardiac problems (e.g., fluid overload, exacerbation of heart failure, chest pain)
☐ 7 - Hypoglycemia/hyperglycemia, diabetes out of control
☐ 8 - GI bleeding, obstruction
☐ 9 - Other than above reasons
☐ UK - Reason unknown

DATA ITEMS COLLECTED AT INPATIENT FACILITY ADMISSION OR AGENCY DISCHARGE ONLY

72. (M0855) To which inpatient facility has the patient been admitted?

☐ 1 - Hospital (Go to M0890)
☐ 2 - Rehabilitation facility (Go to M0903)
☐ 3 - Nursing home (Go to M0900)
☐ 4 - Hospice (Go to M0903)
☐ NA - No inpatient facility admission

73. (M0870) Discharge disposition: Where is the patient after discharge from your agency? (Choose only one answer.)

☐ 1 - Patient remained in the community (not in hospital, nursing home, or rehab facility)
☐ 2 - Patient transferred to a noninstitutional hospice (Go to M0903)
☐ 3 - Unknown because patient moved to a geographic location not served by this agency (Go to M0903)
☐ UK - Other Unknown (Go to M0903)

74. (M0880) After discharge, does the patient receive health, personal, or support services or assistance? (Mark all that apply.)

☐ 1 - No assistance or services received
☐ 2 - Yes, assistance or services provided by family or friends
☐ 3 - Yes, assistance or services provided by other community resources (e.g., Meals-on-Wheels, home health services, homemaker assistance, transportation assistance, assisted living, board and care)

(Go to M0903)

75. (M0890) IF the patient was admitted to an acute care hospital, for what reason was he/she admitted?

☐ 1 - Hospitalization for emergent (unscheduled) care
☐ 2 - Hospitalization for urgent (scheduled within 24 hours of admission) care
☐ 3 - Hospitalization for elective (scheduled more than 24 hours before admission) care
☐ UK - Unknown

(continued)

Outcome and Assessment Information Set *(continued)*

76. (M0895) Reason for hospitalization: (Mark all that apply.)

- ☐ 1 - Improper medication administration, medication side effects, toxicity, anaphylaxis
- ☐ 2 - Injury caused by fall or accident at home
- ☐ 3 - Respiratory problems (shortness of breath, infection, obstruction)
- ☐ 4 - Wound or tube site infection, deteriorating wound status, new lesion/ulcer
- ☐ 5 - Hypoglycemia/hyperglycemia, diabetes out of control
- ☐ 6 - GI bleeding, obstruction
- ☐ 7 - Exacerbation of heart failure, fluid overload, heart failure
- ☐ 8 - Myocardial infarction, stroke
- ☐ 9 - Chemotherapy
- ☐ 10 - Scheduled surgical procedure
- ☐ 11 - Urinary tract infection
- ☐ 12 - I.V. catheter-related infection
- ☐ 13 - Deep vein thrombosis, pulmonary embolus
- ☐ 14 - Uncontrolled pain
- ☐ 15 - Psychotic episode
- ☐ 16 - Other than above reasons

(Go to M0903)

77. (M0900) For what reason(s) was the patient admitted to a nursing home? (Mark all that apply.)

- ☐ 1 - Therapy services
- ☐ 2 - Respite care
- ☐ 3 - Hospice care
- ☐ 4 - Permanent placement
- ☐ 5 - Unsafe for care at home
- ☐ 6 - Other
- ☐ UK - Unknown

78. (M0903) Date of last (most recent) home visit:

_ _/_ _/_ _ _ _
month day year

79. (M0906) Discharge/transfer/death date: Enter the date of the discharge, transfer, or death (at home) of the patient.

_ _/_ _/_ _ _ _
month day year

☐ UK - Unknown

◆ Describe the primary caregiver, including whether or not he lives with the patient, their relationship, his age and physical ability, and his willingness to help the patient.

◆ Show in your documentation how you made the most of the patient's strengths and resources. Strengths include support systems, good health habits, coping behaviors, a safe and healthful environment, and financial security. Resources include the doctor, pharmacy, other health team members, and medical equipment supplier.

◆ If the patient is housebound, make sure you document that fact and the reasons behind it. Remember that Medicare requires patients to be housebound to qualify for reimbursement of skilled services at home. Some commercial insurers don't require the patient to be housebound.

◆ Make sure your documentation reflects consistent adherence to the plan of care by all caregivers. Have caregivers document that they demonstrated the procedures used for the care they provided.

◆ Keep the patient's plan of care updated. Note changes in the patient's condition or the care you think he needs. Document that you reported these changes to the doctor. Medicare, Medicaid, and certain third-party payers won't reimburse skilled services not reported to the doctor.

Remember that your plan of care provides the most direct legal evidence of your nursing judgment. If you outline a plan of care and then deviate from it without documenting a good reason for doing so, a court may decide that you strayed from a reasonable standard of care. So be sure to update your plan of care rou-

Home health certification and plan of care

Known as form 485, the form below includes space for assessing functional abilities and documenting plan of care. This information is required for Medicare reimbursement.

1. Patient's HI Claim No. 000491615 5
2. Start of Care Date 040298
3. Certification Period From: 040298 To: 060298

4. Medical Record No. 541234
5. Provider No. 0412

6. Patient's Name and Address
John Dough
11 Second Street
Hometown, PA 10981

7. Provider's Name, Address, and Telephone Number
Very Good Home Care
Health Rd
Hometown, PA 10981

8. Date of Birth 05 02 29
9. Sex ☒ M ☐ F

10. Medications: Dose/Frequency/Route (N)ew (C)hanged
Humulin N 24u sc qam (C)
Tylenol 325 mg=1000 mg q 4h prn pain
Darvocet N 100 one tab q4h prn pain PO (N)
Mom 30 cc qhs prn PO

11. IDC-9-CM	Principal Diagnosis	Date
813.50	Open Wound Foot	040198
12. ICD-9-CM	**Surgical Procedure**	**Date**
86.28	Debridement Wound	040198
13. ICD-9-CM	**Other Pertinent Diagnoses**	**Date**
250.03	Type I IDDM uncontrolled	040198
443.89	Peripheral Vascular Disease	040198

14. DME and Supplies: Walker Wound care Supplies
15. Safety Measures: Correct use of supportive devices

16. Nutritional requirements 1800 cal ADA diet
17. Allergies: NKA

18. a. Functional Limitations
1 ☒ Amputation
2 ☐ Bowel/Bladder (Incontinence)
3 ☐ Contracture
4 ☐ Hearing
5 ☐ Paralysis
6 ☒ Endurance
7 ☒ Ambulation
8 ☐ Speech
9 ☐ Legally Blind
A ☐ Dyspnea with Minimal Exertion
B ☐ Other

18. b Activities Permitted
1 ☐ Complete Bedrest
2 ☐ Bedrest BRP
3 ☐ Up as Tolerated
4 ☒ Transfer Bed/Chair
5 ☐ Exercises Prescribed
6 ☐ Partial Weight Bearing
7 ☐ Independent At Home
8 ☐ Crutches
9 ☐ Cane
A ☐ Wheelchair
B ☒ Walker
C ☐ No Restrictions
D ☐ Other (Specify)

19. Mental Status
1 ☒ Oriented
2 ☐ Comatose
3 ☒ Forgetful
4 ☐ Depressed
5 ☐ Disoriented
6 ☐ Lethargic
7 ☐ Agitated
8 ☐ Other

20. Prognosis:
1 ☐ Poor
2 ☒ Guarded
3 ☐ Fair
4 ☐ Good
5 ☐ Excellent

21. Orders for Discipline and Treatments (Specify Amount/Frequency/Duration)

SN: Observe/assess: cardiopulmonary, respiratory, musculoskeletal, gastrointestinal, and circulatory systems function. Assess: nutritional intake and dietary compliance related to wound healing; skin integrity and peripheral pulses; diabetic home management; and home safety. Instruct patient/caregiver in: diabetic management; signs/symptoms of wound infection; wound care; home safety; and emergency measures. SN to provide: wound care, until patient is independent: daily wound care to Ⓛ ankle area = cleanse area with saline and apply wet to dry saline dressing. SN visits: 5-7/wk x 3 wks; 2-4/wk x 3 wks; 1-3/wk x 3 wks

(continued)

Home health certification and plan of care *(continued)*

22. Goals/Rehabilitation Potential/Discharge Plans

SN: GOALS: wound healing without infection or further complications, compliance with diabetic home management. Rehab potential to achieve goals: fair. D/C plan: to family/self when care is independent.

23. Nurse's Signature and Date of Verbal SOC Where Applicable

Jane Smith, RN 040198

25. Date HHA Received Signed POT

041298

24. Physician's Name and Address

Dr. Goodman
Dr's Medical Center
Hometown, PA 10981

26. I certify/recertify that this patient is confined to his/her home and needs intermittent skilled nursing care, physical therapy and/or speech therapy or continues to need occupational therapy. The patient is under my care, and I have authorized the services on this plan of care and will periodically review the plan.

27. Attending Physician's Signature and Date Signed

M. Goodman, M.D. 040298

28. Anyone who misrepresents, falsifies, or conceals essential information required for payment of Federal funds may be subject to fine, imprisonment, or civil penalty under applicable Federal laws.

FORM HCFA-485-(C-4) (0-94) (Print Aligned) PROVIDER

tinely so it accurately reflects your clinical judgment about the care your patient requires to meet his changing needs.

Medical update

Whenever you update your plan of care, do so on a form accepted by your agency. To continue providing skilled nursing care to a patient at home, you are required to submit the information that the insurer requests on any approved agency form. You are not required to submit the Medical Update and Patient Information form (also known as form 486) unless Medicare requests it. (See *Medical update and patient information*, page 460.)

If you do complete form 486 for Medicare patients, use the following treatment codes to describe skilled nursing care delivered to the patient: (Don't use these codes on form 485, described earlier, or when care is provided by the patient or another caregiver living in the home.)

- A1: Skilled observation and assessment (including vital signs, response to medications, etc.)
- A2: Indwelling urinary catheter insertion
- A3: Bladder instillation
- A4: Open wound care/dressing
- A5: Decubitus care (partial tissue loss with signs of infection or full tissue loss, etc.)
- A6: Venipuncture
- A7: Restorative nursing
- A8: Postcataract care
- A9: Bowel or bladder training
- A10: Chest physiotherapy (percussion and postural drainage)
- A11: Administration of vitamin B_{12}

Interdisciplinary plan of care

The plan of care is individualized for each patient. An example of this form is shown below.

Patient name: John Dough
Primary nurse: Jane Smith, RN
Init. cert. period: 040298-060298
Recert. period #1: ________
Recert. period #2: ________

PROBLEM	GOAL	APPROACH	INITIAL CERT.	RECERT. #1	RECERT. #2
A1 A25 A27 A32	stabilization Independence Independence Wound healing without infection	daily assessment	GOAL MET? Y N INIT:______	GOAL MET? Y N INIT:______	GOAL MET? Y N INIT:______
A25 Teach diabetic care	Competent home management of diabetes	use written handouts, teach only one area at a time	GOAL MET? Y N INIT:______	GOAL MET? Y N INIT:______	GOAL MET? Y N INIT:______
A4	Wound healing without infection	Aseptic wound care technique with daily to frequent reassessment by nurse	GOAL MET? Y N INIT:______	GOAL MET? Y N INIT:______	GOAL MET? Y N INIT:______

Intervention codes
(please circle all that apply)

A1. Skilled observation
A2. Indwelling urinary catheter insertion
A3. Bladder instillation
A4. Irrigation care (wd. dsg.)
A5. Irrigation decub. care–meds.
A6. Venipuncture
A7. Restorative nursing
A8. Postcataract care
A9. Bowel/Bladder training
A10. Chest physiotherapy (incl. postural drainage)
A11. Administer vit. B_{12}
A12. Prepare/Administer insulin
A13. Administer other I.M./S.C.
A14. Administer I.V.
A15. Teach ostomy care
A16. Teach nasogastric feeding
A17. Reposition nasogastric feeding tube
A18. Teach gastrostomy
A19. Teach parenteral nutrition
A20. Teach care of trach
A21. Administer care of trach
A22. Teach inhalation Rx
A23. Administer inhalation Rx
A24. Teach administration of injections
A25. Teach diabetic care
A26. Disimpaction/enema
A27. Other
Foot care (diabetic)
Teach diet
Teach disease process
Teach use of O_2
Instruct Rx: Medication
A28. Wound care/dsg - closed
A29. Decubitus care - simple
A30. Teach care of indwelling catheter
A31. Management and evaluation of patient care plan
A32. Teaching and training (other)

A12: Administration of insulin
A13: Administration of other I.M. or subcutaneous medications
A14: Administration of I.V. clysis
A15: Teaching ostomy or ileostomy conduit care
A16: Teaching nasogastric feeding
A17: Reinsertion of nasogastric feeding tube
A18: Teaching gastrostomy feeding
A19: Teaching parenteral nutrition
A20: Teaching care of tracheostomy
A21: Administration of tracheostomy care

Medical update and patient information

When requested by Medicare, you will have to complete form 486, shown below. This form provides Medicare with information to support the need for skilled nursing care.

Department of Health and Human Services
Health Care Financing Administration

Form Approved
OMB No. 0938-0357

MEDICAL UPDATE AND PATIENT INFORMATION

1. Patient's HI Claim No. 000491615
2. SOC Date 060291
3. Certification Period From: 040298 To: 060298
4. Medical Record No. 541234
5. Provider No. 0412
6. Patient's Name and Address John Dough, 11 Second St., Hometown, PA
7. Provider's Name Very Good Home Care
8. Medicare Covered: ☒ Y ☐ N
9. Date Physician Last Saw Patient: 060191
10. Date Last Contacted Physician: 040298
11. Is the Patient Receiving Care in an 1861 (J)(1) Skilled Nursing Facility or Equivalent? ☐ Y ☒ N ☐ Do Not Know
12. ☒ Certification ☐ Recertification ☐ Modified
13. Dates of Last Inpatient Stay: Admission N/A Discharge N/A
14. Type of Facility: N/A
15. Updated information: New Orders/Treatments/Clinical Facts/Summary from Each Discipline

SN: 041098: Dr. contacted to report temp = 101° orally, increased amt. thick, tan, foul smelling drainage. Pt. started on Cephalexin 500 mg BID po x 10 days, increase wound care to BID and increase SN visits for wound care to 12-14 x 3 wks.

PT: 040198: verbal order received to increase patient to ambulation with straight cane. Continue strengthening home exercise program.

SN: 040898: Decrease wound care to daily. Decrease SN visits to 5-7 x 7 wks.

16. Functional Limitations (Expand From 485 and Level of ADL) Reason Homebound/Prior Functional Status FL: Ambulation, endurance, open, draining wound. RH: unable to ambulate more than 15 ft. before becoming exhausted. PFS: Independent ambulation.
17. Supplementary Plan of Care on File from Physician Other than Referring Physician: ☐ Y ☒ N (If Yes, Please Specify Giving Goals/Rehab. Potential/Discharge Plan)
18. Unusual Home/Social Environment Cluttered home with narrow hallways
19. Indicate Any Time When the Home Health Agency Made a Visit and Patient was Not Home and Reason Why if Ascertainable N/A
20. Specify Any Known Medical and/or Non-Medical Reason the Patient Regularly Leaves Home and Frequency of Occurrence Dr's office visits as needed.
21. Nurse or Therapist Completing or Reviewing Form Jane Smith, RN

Date (Mo., Day, Yr.) 043098

HCFA-486 (C3) (02-94) (Print Aligned) PROVIDER

A22: Teaching inhalation treatment
A23: Administration of inhalation treatment
A24: Teaching administration of injection
A25: Teaching diabetic care
A26: Disimpaction and follow-up enema
A27: Other treatments not listed above but ordered by doctor
A28: Wound care/dressing (closed incision or suture line)
A29: Decubitus care (other than A5)
A30: Teaching care of any indwelling catheter
A31: Management and evaluation of patient plan of care
A32: Teaching and training of other skilled nursing services ordered by the doctor.

Progress notes

In the home setting, as in the acute care setting, progress notes provide a place to document both the patient's condition and significant events that occur while he's under your care. (See *The progress note,* page 462.)

You'll need to write a progress note each time you see a patient. Make sure it provides a chronological accounting of at least the following:

◆ any changes in the patient's condition
◆ skilled nursing interventions performed related to the plan of care
◆ the patient's responses to services provided
◆ any event or incident in the home that would affect the treatment plan
◆ the patient's vital signs
◆ what you taught the patient and caregiver, including what written instructional materials and brochures you gave them.

When writing your progress notes, follow these general guidelines:

◆ Write legibly in black ink.
◆ Avoid spelling and grammatical errors.
◆ Date (day, month, year) and sign each entry you make in the record.
◆ Avoid addendums.
◆ Provide a heading for each entry because many members of the health care team use the progress notes.
◆ Use flow sheets and checklists to record vital signs, intake and output measurements, and nutritional data. Encourage the patient or caregiver to fill out these forms when appropriate.
◆ Complete your progress note within 24 hours of providing care and file it in the medical record within 7 days. Remember that Medicare certification reviews can occur without notice, and charts can be audited at any time. Therefore, all your documentation must be filed appropriately.

Patient and caregiver teaching

Whenever you care for a patient at home, you'll need to teach as many procedures as possible to the patient and his at-home caregivers. In addition, you'll need to document that you've done so on the appropriate form. (See *Patient-teaching certification,* pages 463 and 464.)

Although teaching patients and caregivers to perform some skilled services probably will reduce the frequency of your visits to the patient's home, you'll still need to visit to assess the caregivers' abilities, track the patient's progress, and revise the plan of care. Remember that a skilled service remains skilled even if you teach it to a patient or caregiver.

If you do your best to teach a skill or procedure to a patient or his caregiver and you determine that they're unable or unwilling to learn it, document that fact clearly in the patient's record. In this situation, Medicare is obliged to continue reimbursing for nursing care for as long as it remains reasonable and necessary. Depend-

The progress note

Progress notes describe — in chronological order — patient problems and needs, nursing observations, reassessments, and interventions. A sample appears below.

☐ PHONE REPORT ☐ COORDINATION NOTE ☒ CLINICAL NOTE CONTINUATION

Patient Name *John Dough* ID# *162329M* Date *041098*

T=101° P=100 R=28 BP=160/94. Patient unaware of fever but complaining of increased pain at wound site. Darvocet is controlling pain but patient taking it q 4 hr. while awake. Wound of (L) ankle = 4 cm x 4.5 cm x 1 cm deep. Open area appears pink with increased amounts of thick, tan drainage. Wound is foul smelling. Dr's office contacted and patient to start on Cephalexin PO. SN to increase visits for BID wound care. Pt denies other complaints. Glucometer FBS = 160 this am. Lungs with diminished breath sounds at bases. Appetite good, bowels regular - had BM today. Began instruction to patient on Cephalexin dose, schedule, and side effects. Patient appears quite anxious about wound condition. Explanation of signs, symptoms, and treatment of wound infection reinforced. Pt. able to repeat most explanations. Support offered. SN to return for pm wound care today and patient should have begun antibiotic therapy by then.

Jane Smith, RN

SERVICE BY (SIGNATURE) TITLE

ing on the patient's condition and needs, he may be approved for a limited time or indefinitely.

Remember, however, that Medicare will not reimburse your continued efforts to teach the same material to patients or caregivers unable or unwilling to learn it. After a reasonable period, if it becomes apparent to you that your teaching is fruitless, then it ceases to qualify for Medicare's definition of skilled service.

Obtaining recertification

To ensure continued home health services for patients who need them, you'll have to prove that the patient still requires home care. Here's how it works.

Medicare and many managed care plans certify an initial 62-day period during which your agency can receive reimbursement for the patient's home care. When that period is over, the insurer may certify an additional 62-

Patient-teaching certification

The model patient-teaching form below shows what was taught to a home-care patient with an I.V. line in place. This type of form will help you document your teaching sessions clearly and completely.

PATIENT-TEACHING CHECKLIST/CERTIFICATION OF INSTRUCTION

PATIENT NAME: *John Dough*
CAREGIVER: *self*
TYPE OF THERAPY: *wound care*
DATE: *040298*

CONTENT (Check all that apply; fill in blanks as indicated.)

1. ☒ Reason for Therapy *Open wound*
2. Drug/Solution
   - ☐ Dose
   - ☐ Schedule
   - ☐ Label Accuracy
   - ☐ Storage
   - ☐ Container Integrity
3. Aseptic Technique
   - ☒ Hand Washing
   - ☐ Prepping Caps/Connections
   - ☐ Tubing/Cap/Needle
   - ☐ Needleless Adaptor Changes
4. Access Device Maintenance
   Type/Name ______________
   - ☐ Device/Site Inspection
   - ☐ Site Care/Dsg. Changes
   - ☐ Catheter Clamping
   - ☐ Maintaining Patency
     - ☐ Saline Flushing
     - ☐ Heparin Locking
     - ☐ Fdg. Tube Declogging
     - ☐ Self-Insertion of Device
5. Drug Preparation
   - ☐ Premixed Containers
   - ☐ Compounding
   - ☐ Patient Additives
   - ☐ Piggyback Lipids
6. Method of Administration
   - ☐ Gravity
   - ☐ Pump (name) ______________
   - ☐ Continuous ☐ Intermittent
   - ☐ Cycle/Taper
7. Administration Technique
   - ☐ Pump Rate/Calibration
   - ☐ Priming Tubing
   - ☐ Filter
   - ☐ Filling Syringe
   - ☐ Loading Pump
   - ☐ Access Device Hookup/Disconnect
8. Potential Complications/Adverse Effects
   - ☐ Patient Drug Information Sheet Reviewed
   - ☐ Pump Alarms/Trouble-shooting
   - ☐ Phlebitis/Infiltration
   - ☐ Clotting/Dislodgment
   - ☒ Infection
   - ☐ Air Embolus
   - ☐ Breakage/Cracking
   - ☐ Electrolyte Imbalance
   - ☐ Fluid Balance
   - ☐ Glucose Intolerance
   - ☐ Aspiration
   - ☐ N/V/D/Cramping
   - ☐ Other: ______________
9. Self-Monitoring
   - ☐ Weight
   - ☒ Temperature
   - ☐ P ☐ BP
   - ☐ Urine S & A
   - ☐ Fingersticks
   - ☐ Other: ______________
10. Supply Handling/Disposal
    - ☐ Disposal of Sharps/Supplies
    - ☐ Narcotics
    - ☐ Cleaning Pump
    - ☐ Changing Batteries
    - ☐ Blood/Fluid Precautions
    - ☐ Chemo/Spill Precautions
11. Information Given to Patient Re:
    - ☐ Pharmacy Counseling
    - ☒ Advance Directives
    - ☐ Inventory Checks ______________
    - ☐ Deliveries ______________
    - ☒ 24-Hour On-Call Staff
    - ☐ Reimbursement ______________
    - ☐ Service Complaints ______________
12. Safety/Disaster Plan
    - ☐ Backup Pump Batteries ______________
    - ☐ Emergency Room Use ______________
    - ☐ Electrical ______________
    - ☐ Disaster ______________
    - ☐ Other: ______________
13. Written Instructions
    - ☐ Yes ☐ No
    If No, Why ______________

(continued)

Patient-teaching certification *(continued)*

Patient and/or caregiver demonstrates and/or verbalizes competency to perform home infusion therapy.

COMMENTS: *Patient instructed in signs and symptoms of wound infection with good understanding. Patient able to demonstrate adequate hand-washing technique and he will check his temperature each evening and record result.*

Theory/Skill Reviewed/Return Demonstration Completed:

Jane Smith, RN — *040298*

Signature of RN Educator — Date

CERTIFICATION OF INSTRUCTION

I agree that I have been instructed as described above and understand that the above functions will be performed in the home by myself and/or caregiver, outside a hospital or medically supervised environment.

John Dough — *040298*

Patient/Caregiver Signature — Date

day period based on your written demonstration (and the doctor's agreement) that the patient needs continued care. The second 62-day period and every one after that are called recertification periods.

Naturally, your documentation requesting recertification must clearly support the patient's need for continued care within the insurer's guidelines. A clinical summary of care must be compiled and sent to the patient's doctor and then to the insurer. For Medicare, you'll also need to prepare a new certification and plan of care form (form 485, illustrated on pages 457 and 458) for the recertification period and get it to your agency and Medicare before the current certification period expires. Make sure it includes all updated data as amended by verbal order since the start of care.

When recording the primary diagnosis, make sure it reflects the patient's current needs, not the original reason for home care. Here's an example: Your patient had a primary diagnosis of cerebrovascular accident (CVA) at the start of care. The nursing needs directly related to his CVA have been accomplished, but he developed a pressure ulcer that needs wound care and skilled nursing assessment.

If you'll be visiting during the recertification period primarily to deal with the patient's wound, you'll need to change the original primary diagnosis to something like "open wound" instead of CVA. You may still want to include the CVA as a secondary, supporting diagnosis.

The clinical summary that you include with the new certification and plan of care form must include a summary of all disciplines represented on the patient's care team, including the home health aide. Include all services needed, along with their updated treatments and goals, and the frequency and duration of visits. Also make sure you include what's already been accomplished in addition to realistic goals for continued treatment.

Once you've completed form 485, review the new orders with the patient's doctor and sign the "verbal order for start of care" line. This signature serves as a valid verbal order to continue home care services until the original document is signed by the doctor.

As explained earlier, you're not required to submit Medicare's Medical Update and Patient Information form (form 486, illustrated on page 460) for recertification unless Medicare requests it.

Discharge summary

When the patient no longer needs or is eligible for home health care, you'll have to prepare a discharge summary for the doctor's approval. Use the form provided by your agency for recording your discharge summary. (See *Discharge summary,* page 466.)

When preparing a discharge summary, be sure to include these topics:

- services provided
- patient's clinical and psychosocial condition at discharge
- recommendations for further care
- patient's response to and comprehension of the patient-teaching plan
- outcomes attained.

Telephone orders

Typically, a doctor's order to change some aspect of your home care will come to you by way of the telephone. Either you or the doctor may initiate this conversation for a wide variety of reasons. No matter who originated it or how it came about, it's your job to immediately document any orders received. You'll need to use the appropriate verbal order form and send it to the doctor for a signature. (See *Documenting telephone orders,* page 467.)

Make sure your verbal order form includes the following information:

- patient's complete name
- patient's medical record number (check agency policy)
- date and time the order was received
- complete name, title, and signature of person who received the order
- complete name of doctor who gave the order
- place for doctor's signature
- complete contents of order as it was given.

Keep a copy of your signed verbal order in the patient's record until the original copy with the doctor's signature is returned to the office. The original order must be placed in the patient's medical record within 10 days.

In addition to writing up the verbal order, document in the patient's record the reason it was initiated. Describe the circumstances that prompted your conversation with the patient's doctor as well as the doctor's reason for giving the order. Be sure to communicate the order to everyone on the patient's health team who needs to know it.

Clearly, taking orders from the doctor won't be the only time you use the telephone to accomplish a goal for your home health patient. Even if you simply update the doctor on the patient's condition (a legal requirement), you'll want to document the conversation. Likewise, if you talk with another member of the patient's health-care team, you'll want to record the

Discharge summary

Discharge Summary

CODE 01
Admission Date 040298
Discharge Date 053098
Medical Record No.: 541234

Name: John Dough
Address: 11 Second St., Hometown, PA 10981
Phone No.: 881-555-2931
Primary Diagnosis: Open wound - (L) foot
Physician: Dr. Goodman
Date of Birth: 050229

Services Provided: ☒ Nursing ☐ Occupational Therapy ☐ Speech Therapy
☐ Aide ☒ Physical Therapy ☐ Social Work
☐ Other ______

Reason for Discharge:
☒ Condition Improved ☐ Died in Hospital
☐ Self/Family Choice ☐ Referred to Hospital
☐ Moved Out of Area ☐ Placed in Long-Term Institution
☐ Referred to Another Agency ☐ Referred, Not Admitted
☐ Died at Home ☐ Other ______

Physician Notified of Closure: ☒ Yes ☐ No Date: 053098
Family Notified: ☒ Yes ☐ No Date: 053098

Able to verbalize knowledge of the etiology, signs and symptoms, and sequelae/complications of health problem(s).
Patient: ☐ Yes ☒ Partially ☐ No
Family/Caregiver: ☒ Yes ☐ Partially ☐ No

Able to demonstrate knowledge and skills related to the treatment and management of health problem(s).
Patient: ☐ Yes ☒ Partially ☐ No
Family/Caregiver: ☐ Yes ☒ Partially ☐ No

Patient Status:
The patient's condition is: ☐ Stable ☐ Unstable ☒ Improving
☐ Declining ☐ Other ______

ADL STATUS: ☒ Improving ☐ Unchanged ☐ Declining

	Dependent	Partially Independent	Independent
Bathing			X
Dressing			X
Toileting			X
Transferring			X
Feeding			X
Ambulation		X	
Activity Tolerance	(poor)	(fair) [circled]	(good)

Functional Outcomes:	From	To
Knowledge	poor	fair
Skill	fair	good
Psychosocial	poor	fair
Health Status	poor	fair

SUPPORT SYSTEMS: ☒ Family ☐ Caregiver ☐ Friends
☐ Community Resources ☒ Patient uses support systems appropriately
☐ Support systems inadequate ☐ Patient uses support systems ineffectively
☐ Other ______

COMMENTS: ______

Documenting telephone orders

As a home health nurse, you'll rely heavily on orders given by your patients' doctors over the telephone. Your agency must follow guidelines mandated by the Health Care Financing Administration for taking and documenting these orders. Here's an example of a form used by one agency to fulfill these documentation requirements. The doctor must sign the order within 48 hours.

Facility name		Address	
Very Good Home Care		Health Rd, Hometown, PA	
Last name	**First name**	**Attending doctor**	**Admission no.**
Dough	John	Dr. Goodman	N/A

Date ordered	Date discontinued	ORDERS
041098		Start cephalexin 500 mg BID po.
		Increase wound care to BID
		Increase SN visits to 12-14/wk x 3 wks

Signature of nurse receiving order	Time	Signature of doctor	Date
Jane Smith, RN	1400	M. Goodman, MD	041198

contents of the conversation.

At times, you may find it necessary to instruct patients or family members and even implement care over the phone. Or you may need to follow up by phone to verify a patient's condition or his understanding and retention of something you taught him earlier.

Interdisciplinary and interagency telephone communication is essential to case management, coordination, problem solving, and discharge planning. Your agency may use a particular form to document telephone communication, or you may record it in the clinical note. Either way, be sure to include:

- ◆ date and time of contact
- ◆ name and title of person with whom you spoke
- ◆ reason the call was made and by whom
- ◆ content of the conversation
- ◆ outcome of the conversation and any agreements made by the two parties
- ◆ any actions you need to take
- ◆ your signature and title.

◆ DOCUMENTING COMMUNITY REFERRALS

Whether or not your patient needs continued skilled care at home, you'll want to think about community resources that can help maintain and promote his health and well-being. As you know, state public health departments offer many preventive programs and resources free of charge. Classes on such topics as cardiopulmonary resuscitation, smoking cessation, hypertension management, and cooking and disease management for diabetics are available in most communities.

Also consider making referrals for emotional support services through local community health agencies. Specific support groups may be available for people with the patient's disease or disability. Keep abreast of such services so you can educate your patients about them

Mobile health units may provide an additional community resource for patients. Mobile units usually provide assessment and screening services, such as blood pressure screening, glucose monitoring, or cholesterol measurement. Mobile units may be sponsored by hospitals, service organizations, managed health care plans or, occasionally, pharmaceutical companies.

Whenever you make a referral for community services, be sure to document your actions and the reasons why you made the referral.

◆ HOME HEALTH AIDES

Home health aide services are similar to those provided by nursing assistants in acute and long-term care settings. Home health aides provide hands-on personal care to the patient or services needed to maintain the patient's health or facilitate his medical treatment. Aides also provide respite to family members. Remember that Medicare will reimburse only for care provided by a certified level III home health aide.

Because they provide nonskilled services, home health aides can be used to make more frequent visits to your patient's home than you can make. Even so, you'll need to carefully record in your clinical notes the patient's level of independence, mental status, preferences, and available support.

If the aide visits the patient's home four or five times weekly, your notes will need to document the patient's inability to perform self-care activities, the absence of a caregiver, or the complex nature of the physical care he requires. Be sure to follow general principles of good documentation throughout. (See *Principles of documentation.*)

If the patient's condition improves or worsens, the frequency of the home health aide's visits — or the activities performed during visits — can be changed during the certification period. It's up to you to justify the change to the patient, family, aide, doctor, and agency. Carefully document the need for a change in your notes.

You're also responsible for developing the aide's plan of care and supervising her activities in the patient's home. Most agencies use a standard care plan or duty assignment sheet for this purpose that can be adapted to fit each patient's needs. On this document, you must itemize every activity the aide is permitted to provide. You may find it most convenient to use a checklist of services. Simply indicate the services to be performed and when the aide should perform them.

To maintain state licensure and certification from Medicare and the Joint Commission on Accreditation of Healthcare Organizations, your agency must require the home health aide to follow the patient's plan of care and to complete a separate home health aide note or entry in the patient's clinical record for every visit. If the aide visits more than once in a day, the record should reflect more than one visit. Each entry should contain a record of the care provided and the length of the visit, including in and out times.

Principles of documentation

Use this round-up of documentation principles to make sure your documentation is complete.

◆ Use only agency-approved abbreviations and symbols.

◆ State clearly why the patient is homebound. If he leaves home for doctor appointments or other medical care, make sure your documentation reinforces his continuing homebound status.

◆ If the patient receives skilled nursing and makes doctor visits on the same day, document the reason for each visit, for example, "During skilled nursing visit, assessment revealed respiratory rate 32 and labored, blood pressure 190/120, heart rate 124 and irregular. Doctor notified and patient directed to go to doctor's office."

◆ Document only pertinent medical information. Avoid unrelated details, such as what the patient was wearing or what a family member said. Keep statements brief, concise, consistent, and specific.

◆ Establish the patient's continuing need for care. Medicare will question the need for home visits if your documentation says, "The patient is improving" and indicates no further assessment of ongoing needs.

◆ Avoid using terms like "stable" and "chronic" because they can cause Medicare to question the need for skilled care.

◆ Record objective rather than subjective data. For example, record specific wound dimensions instead of writing "Wound healing nicely."

◆ Document specific skilled care provided and how it relates to the diagnosis and plan of care. The level of care must be greater than that which a layperson could provide.

◆ Chart all verbal and written instructions, return demonstrations, verbalization of learning, and any resistance to learning.

◆ Justify the need to repeat instructions. For example, state "Patient newly diagnosed with IDDM and recent CVA is having difficulty manipulating syringe and understanding how to self-inject insulin."

◆ Refer to the plan of care and the patient's progress toward outcomes identified in the plan.

◆ Document how home care is helping the patient achieve goals, and outline steps you're taking to decrease the frequency of visits as goals are met.

◆ Record changes in the patient's condition that require continued skilled care or doctor contact.

◆ When possible and helpful, use pictures, diagrams, measurements, and even video to accurately and effectively represent your patient's condition.

◆ Include all doctor calls and verbal orders in your documentation. Identify the day, time, and reason for the doctor call, and indicate any orders received.

◆ Treat the home health care chart as a legal document. Do not erase entries or use correction fluid. Follow specific agency guidelines for correcting errors.

(continued)

Principles of documentation *(continued)*

- To help prevent the patient from feeling neglected, limit the time you spend charting in the home. When possible, take time to complete your charting while the patient sleeps or is otherwise occupied.
- Involve the patient in his own care and documentation as much as possible. Let him see what you wrote about his care; then let him make additional comments that you can add.
- If the patient has a medical emergency while you are with him, accompany him to the hospital or emergency unit and stay until another caregiver takes over. Notify your supervisor, who will arrange coverage for your other patients, if necessary. Record all assessments and interventions performed until you're relieved. Note the date and the time of transfer and the name of the caregiver who assumed responsibility.
- If documentation materials were completed and left in the patient's home, collect them at least once a week and take them to your agency.

The Health Care Financing Administration requires that you — the supervising nurse — visit the patient's home personally at least every 2 weeks. Coordinate an on-site meeting that includes you, the home health aide, and the patient so you can all participate in developing the aide's plan of care. Typically, this joint meeting takes place at the aide's first visit, during which you'll verify the aide's ability to perform the required tasks. Then you can leave your written plan of care at the patient's home for later reference by the aide.

Be sure to update the aide about any changes in the patient's condition, changes in the aide's plan of care, revised short- and long-term goals for the patient, and discharge planning for the patient. Document all conversations you have with the home health aide.

Don't forget that you're also responsible for evaluating and documenting the patient's and family's satisfaction with care provided by the aide. You can gather this information during your visit, when the aide isn't present.

◆ COMPUTERIZED DOCUMENTATION

If you're not already, you may soon be using a laptop computer equipped with special software designed for documentation. Like the manual method, computerized medical records provide a detailed account of the patient's clinical status, diagnostic tests, treatments, and medical history. Unlike the manual method, computerized records store all the patient's medical data in a single, easily accessible location.

Using a computer to accomplish your documentation can help increase your speed and accuracy, reduce your reliance on recall, and expedite the exchange of data among care providers and third-party payers. By improving legibility, it can reduce the risk of misinterpretation. It can also help to standardize care by providing structures, input formats, and mandatory charting fields for assessments and other notes.

Computer programs are currently available to help you develop the plan of care, formulate goals, monitor patient progress, update medications, and generate visit notes. You enter the information into your computer in the patient's home.

Many agencies have programmed their computer systems to produce exactly the information Medicare wants in the format Medicare wants it. Not only can you complete the certification and plan of care (form 485), but in some agencies you also can fill out agency forms on disk. These include baseline assessment as well as ongoing assessment, safety assessment, medication record, and plans of care. Many times, you can record information with a simple "yes" or "no" keystroke. Some agencies use the computerized systems to augment patient teaching by generating medication and disease information sheets that can be used as teaching tools.

Usually, you'll connect your computer to a central server via a modem when you've finished your daily visits. All your activities and notes for the day will be uploaded to the central computer and, at the same time, new patient information will be downloaded to your laptop so your information is always current and available.

Billing information can also be calculated by some programs and is already in use at some home health agencies. Eventually attending doctors will be able to view their patients' home care via their office computers. At some point in the future, each patient may have a central computerized medical record that follows him throughout life.

The down side

Although computer documentation offers many benefits, it may have some drawbacks as well. For example, relying on a computer may mean fewer opportunities for interaction and communication with coworkers and patients. In addition, patients may be less truthful when providing detailed medical histories if they know the information is going into a computer.

Also, many of the questions you'll need to answer about your patient's needs and responses to treatment can't be standardized into a checklist. They're too individualized and based on circumstances specific to each patient.

Sometimes computerized records raise legal concerns as well. The most pressing concerns involve issues of patient privacy and confidentiality. With traditional records, information is restricted simply by keeping the chart in the office and locking the doors. In contrast, it may be possible to access computer records at any terminal or laptop unit in the system, even at a patient's home.

What's more, E-mail and faxes can easily end up in the wrong hands. In fact, if you need to transmit information about a patient by E-mail or fax, consider blacking out or leaving out information that could be used by an unauthorized person to identify the patient.

Various state laws protect the privacy of a patient's medical records. In addition, some state nurse practice acts impose an ethical duty to guard each patient's privacy. However, no one can fully guarantee that unauthorized persons won't gain access to computerized records.

Your liability when working with computer documentation is the same as when working with a manual system. You may be liable for any patient injuries associated with charting errors. To minimize your legal risks:

◆ Make sure your computer files are password-protected to prevent unauthorized people from reading them.

◆ Always double-check the patient information you enter.

◆ Don't divulge your signature code to anyone.

◆ Inform your supervisor if you suspect that someone is using your code.

◆ Date and time all your computer entries.

◆ Know your state's rules and regulations and your agency's policies regarding privileged data, confidentiality, and disclosure.

By faithfully following through on the procedures outlined here and throughout this book, you'll set yourself up for continued success in the expanding field of home health nursing.

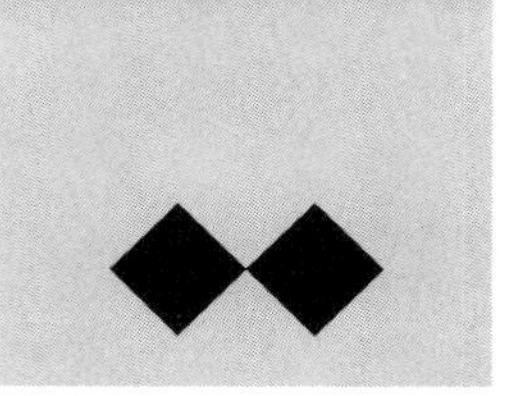

APPENDIX A

NANDA Taxonomy I, Revised

The North American Nursing Diagnosis Association's Taxonomy I, Revised, organized around nine human response patterns, is the currently accepted classification system for nursing diagnoses. The complete taxonomic structure is listed below.

◆ PATTERN 1

Exchanging: A human response pattern involving mutual giving and receiving

1.1.2.1	Altered nutrition: More than body requirements
1.1.2.2	Altered nutrition: Less than body requirements
1.1.2.3	Altered nutrition: Risk for more than body requirements
1.2.1.1	Risk for infection
1.2.2.1	Risk for altered body temperature
1.2.2.2	Hypothermia
1.2.2.3	Hyperthermia
1.2.2.4	Ineffective thermoregulation
1.2.3.1	Dysreflexia
1.3.1.1	Constipation
1.3.1.1.1	Perceived constipation
1.3.1.1.2	Colonic constipation
1.3.1.2	Diarrhea
1.3.1.3	Bowel incontinence
1.3.2	Altered urinary elimination
1.3.2.1.1	Stress incontinence
1.3.2.1.2	Reflex incontinence
1.3.2.1.3	Urge incontinence
1.3.2.1.4	Functional incontinence
1.3.2.1.5	Total incontinence
1.3.2.2	Urinary retention
1.4.1.1	Altered (specify type) tissue perfusion (renal, cerebral, cardiopulmonary, gastrointestinal, peripheral)
1.4.1.2.1	Fluid volume excess
1.4.1.2.2.1	Fluid volume deficit
1.4.1.2.2.2	Risk for fluid volume deficit
1.4.2.1	Decreased cardiac output

1.5.1.1	Impaired gas exchange
1.5.1.2	Ineffective airway clearance
1.5.1.3	Ineffective breathing pattern
1.5.1.3.1	Inability to sustain spontaneous ventilation
1.5.1.3.2	Dysfunctional ventilatory weaning response
1.6.1	Risk for injury
1.6.1.1	Risk for suffocation
1.6.1.2	Risk for poisoning
1.6.1.3	Risk for trauma
1.6.1.4	Risk for aspiration
1.6.1.5	Risk for disuse syndrome
1.6.2	Altered protection
1.6.2.1	Impaired tissue integrity
1.6.2.1.1	Altered oral mucous membrane
1.6.2.1.2.1	Impaired skin integrity
1.6.2.1.2.2	Risk for impaired skin integrity
1.7.1	Decreased adaptive capacity: Intracranial
1.8	Energy field disturbance

◆ PATTERN 2

Communicating: A human response pattern involving sending messages

2.1.1.1	Impaired verbal communication

◆ PATTERN 3

Relating: A human response pattern involving establishing bonds

3.1.1	Impaired social interaction
3.1.2	Social isolation
3.1.3	Risk for loneliness
3.2.1	Altered role performance
3.2.1.1.1	Altered parenting
3.2.1.1.2	Risk for altered parenting
3.2.1.1.2.1	Risk for altered parent/infant/child attachment
3.2.1.2.1	Sexual dysfunction
3.2.2	Altered family processes
3.2.2.1	Caregiver role strain
3.2.2.2	Risk for caregiver role strain
3.2.2.3.1	Altered family process: Alcoholism
3.2.3.1	Parental role conflict
3.3	Altered sexuality patterns

◆ PATTERN 4

Valuing: A human response pattern involving the assigning of relative worth

4.1.1	Spiritual distress (distress of the human spirit)
4.2	Potential for enhanced spiritual well-being

◆ PATTERN 5

Choosing: A human response pattern involving the selection of alternatives

5.1.1.1	Ineffective individual coping
5.1.1.1.1	Impaired adjustment
5.1.1.1.2	Defensive coping
5.1.1.1.3	Ineffective denial
5.1.2.1.1	Ineffective family coping: Disabling
5.1.2.1.2	Ineffective family coping: Compromised
5.1.2.2	Family coping: Potential for growth
5.1.3.1	Potential for enhanced community coping
5.1.3.2	Ineffective community coping
5.2.1	Ineffective management of therapeutic regimen: Individuals
5.2.1.1	Noncompliance (specify)
5.2.2	Ineffective management of therapeutic regimen: Families
5.2.3	Ineffective management of therapeutic regimen: Community
5.2.4	Effective management of therapeutic regimen: Individual
5.3.1.1	Decisional conflict (specify)
5.4	Health-seeking behaviors (specify)

◆ PATTERN 6

Moving: A human response pattern involving activity

6.1.1.1	Impaired physical mobility
6.1.1.1.1	Risk for peripheral neurovascular dysfunction
6.1.1.1.2	Risk for perioperative positioning injury
6.1.1.2	Activity intolerance
6.1.1.2.1	Fatigue
6.1.1.3	Risk for activity intolerance
6.2.1	Sleep pattern disturbance
6.3.1.1	Diversional activity deficit
6.4.1.1	Impaired home maintenance management
6.4.2	Altered health maintenance
6.5.1	Feeding self-care deficit
6.5.1.1	Impaired swallowing
6.5.1.2	Ineffective breast-feeding
6.5.1.2.1	Interrupted breast-feeding
6.5.1.3	Effective breast-feeding
6.5.1.4	Ineffective infant feeding pattern
6.5.2	Bathing or hygiene self-care deficit
6.5.3	Dressing or grooming self-care deficit
6.5.4	Toileting self-care deficit
6.6	Altered growth and development
6.7	Relocation stress syndrome
6.8.1	Risk for disorganized infant behavior
6.8.2	Disorganized infant behavior
6.8.3	Potential for enhanced organized infant behavior

◆ PATTERN 7

Perceiving: A human response pattern involving the reception of information

7.1.1	Body image disturbance
7.1.2	Self-esteem disturbance
7.1.2.1	Chronic low self-esteem
7.1.2.2	Situational low self-esteem
7.1.3	Personal identity disturbance
7.2	Sensory or perceptual alterations (specify — visual, auditory, kinesthetic, gustatory, tactile, olfactory)
7.2.1.1	Unilateral neglect
7.3.1	Hopelessness
7.3.2	Powerlessness

◆ PATTERN 8

Knowing: A human response pattern involving the meaning associated with information

8.1.1	Knowledge deficit (specify)
8.2.1	Impaired environmental interpretation syndrome
8.2.2	Acute confusion
8.2.3	Chronic confusion
8.3	Altered thought processes
8.3.1	Impaired memory

◆ PATTERN 9

Feeling: A human response pattern involving the subjective awareness of information

9.1.1	Pain
9.1.1.1	Chronic pain
9.2.1.1	Dysfunctional grieving
9.2.1.2	Anticipatory grieving
9.2.2	Risk for violence: Self-directed or directed at others
9.2.2.1	Risk for self-mutilation
9.2.3	Post-trauma response
9.2.3.1	Rape-trauma syndrome
9.2.3.1.1	Rape-trauma syndrome: Compound reaction
9.2.3.1.2	Rape-trauma syndrome: Silent reaction
9.3.1	Anxiety
9.3.2	Fear

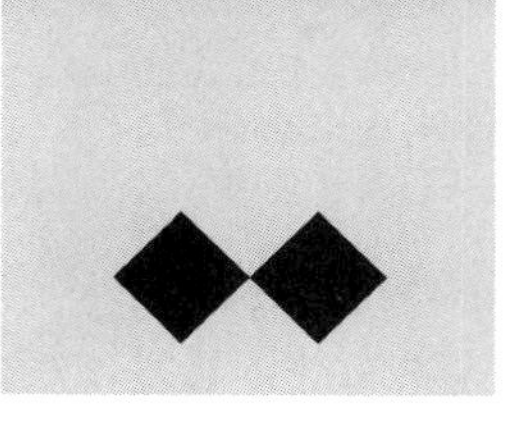

APPENDIX B

Special diets

As a home health care nurse, you're likely to encounter many patients who have special dietary requirements. Some patients may need to eat more high-fiber foods, others may need to reduce their sodium or cholesterol intake, and still others may need to increase or decrease the amount of potassium in their diets.

◆ ADDING FIBER TO YOUR PATIENT'S DIET

Fiber makes up a crucial part of the diet, even though it's completely indigestible. Fiber's benefit is primarily mechanical: It promotes bowel movements, thereby minimizing the risk of constipation, a helpful effect when treating diverticulitis and when administering a drug known to cause constipation. Here are four easy ways to add fiber to your patient's diet.

Whole-grain breads and cereals

For the first few days of a new fiber regimen, have your patient eat one serving daily of whole-grain breads (1 slice), cereal (½ cup), pasta (½ cup), or brown rice (⅓ cup). Examples of whole-grain breads are whole wheat and pumpernickel. Examples of high-fiber cereals are bran or oat flakes and shredded wheat. Have your patient gradually increase the number of servings to four or more daily.

Fresh fruits and vegetables

Begin by suggesting that your patient eat one serving daily of raw or cooked, unpeeled fruit (one medium-sized piece, ½ cup cooked) or unpeeled vegetables (½ cup cooked, 1 cup raw). Have your patient gradually increase the number of servings to four daily. Examples of high-fiber fruits include apples, oranges, and peaches. Some high-fiber vegetables are carrots, corn, and peas.

Dried peas and beans

Begin by suggesting that your patient eat one serving (⅓ cup) a week of peas and beans. Then have him increase the number of servings to at least two a week.

Unprocessed bran

Have your patient add bran to his food, starting with 1 teaspoon daily. Over a 3-week period, have him work up to 2 to 3 tablespoons daily, but not more than 3. Remember to have him drink at least six 8-oz glasses of liquid a day.

A small amount of bran can be beneficial, but too much can irritate the digestive tract, cause gas, interfere with mineral absorption, and even lodge in the intestine.

Note: Crisp, fresh fruits and vegetables, cooked foods with husks, and nuts must be chewed thoroughly so that large particles don't pass whole into the intestine and lodge there, causing problems.

A sample menu

Breakfast
½ grapefruit
Oatmeal with milk and raisins (add bran, if desired)
Bran muffin
8 oz liquid

Lunch
Cabbage slaw
Tuna salad sandwich on whole-wheat bread
Fresh pear with skin
8 oz liquid

Dinner
Vegetable soup
Broiled fish with almond topping
Baked potato with skin
Carrots and peas
Canned crushed pineapple
8 oz liquid

Snack
Dried fruit and nut mix
8 oz liquid

◆ CUTTING DOWN ON SALT

The doctor may recommend reducing your patient's salt intake because too much salt can affect his health. Reducing salt intake isn't hard to do. The following information and suggestions will help your patient get started.

Facts about salt

- Table salt is composed of about 40% sodium.
- Americans consume about 20 times more salt than their bodies need.
- About three-fourths of the salt you consume is already in the foods you eat and drink.
- One teaspoon of salt contains about 2 g (2,000 mg) of sodium.

Tips for reducing salt intake

Have your patient reduce his salt intake to a teaspoon or less daily. This is easy to do if he:

- reads labels on drugs and foods
- puts away his salt shaker or, if he must use salt, uses "light salt," which contains half the sodium of ordinary table salt
- buys fresh meats, fruits, and vegetables instead of canned, processed, and convenience foods

◆ substitutes spices and lemon juice for salt
◆ looks for and avoids sources of hidden sodium — for example, carbonated beverages, nondairy creamers, cookies, and cakes
◆ avoids salty foods, such as bacon, sausage, pretzels, potato chips, mustard, pickles, and some cheeses.

Sodium sources

Canned, prepared, and "fast" foods are loaded with sodium; so are condiments, such as ketchup. Some foods that don't taste salty contain high amounts of sodium. Consider the values below:

Food	Amount of sodium/(mg)
1 can tomato soup	872
1 cup canned spaghetti	1,236
1 hot dog	639
1 cheeseburger	709
1 slice pepperoni pizza	817
1 tbs ketchup	156
1 tsp salt	1,955
1 dill pickle	928
1 cup cornflakes	256
3 oz lean ham	1,128
2½ oz dried chipped beef	3,052

Other high-sodium sources include baking powder, baking soda, barbecue sauce, bouillon cubes, celery salt, chili sauce, cooking wine, garlic salt, onion salt, softened water, and soy sauce.

Surprisingly, sodium is also found in many drugs and other nonfood items, such as alkalizers for indigestion, laxatives, aspirin, cough medicine, mouthwash, and toothpaste.

◆ CUTTING DOWN ON CHOLESTEROL

By reducing his intake of high-cholesterol foods and saturated fats, your patient can help lower his cholesterol level and ensure better health. This means cutting down drastically on eggs, dairy products, and fatty meats and relying instead on poultry, fish, fruits, vegetables, and high-fiber breads.

Use this list as a starting point to teach your patient about his new diet. If he does a lot of home baking, tell him to adjust recipes by using modest amounts of unsaturated oils. Remind your patient to substitute two egg whites when a recipe calls for one whole egg.

Bread and cereals

Have your patient eliminate:

◆ breads containing whole eggs as a major ingredient
◆ egg noodles
◆ pies, cakes, doughnuts, biscuits, high-fat crackers and cookies.

Have your patient substitute:
- ◆ oatmeal, multigrain, and bran cereals; whole-grain and rye bread
- ◆ pasta, rice
- ◆ angel food cake; low-fat cookies, crackers, and home-baked goods.

Eggs and dairy products
Have your patient eliminate:
- ◆ whole milk, 2% milk, imitation milk
- ◆ cream, half and half, most nondairy creamers, whipped toppings
- ◆ whole-milk yogurt and cottage cheese
- ◆ cheese, cream cheese, sour cream, light cream cheese, light sour cream
- ◆ egg yolks
- ◆ ice cream.

Have your patient substitute:
- ◆ skim milk, 1% milk, buttermilk
- ◆ no replacements for creamers and whipped toppings
- ◆ nonfat or low-fat yogurt, low-fat (1% or 2%) cottage cheese
- ◆ cholesterol-free sour cream alternative, such as King Sour
- ◆ egg whites
- ◆ sherbet, frozen tofu.

Fats and oils
Have your patient eliminate:
- ◆ coconut, palm, and palm kernel oils
- ◆ butter, lard, bacon fat
- ◆ dressings made with egg yolks
- ◆ chocolate.

Have your patient substitute:
- ◆ unsaturated vegetable oils (corn, olive, canola, safflower, sesame, soybean, and sunflower)
- ◆ unsaturated margarine and shortening, diet margarine
- ◆ mayonnaise, unsaturated or low-fat salad dressings
- ◆ baking cocoa.

Meat, fish, and poultry
Have your patient eliminate:
- ◆ fatty cuts of beef, lamb, or pork
- ◆ organ meats, spare ribs, cold cuts, sausage, hot dogs, bacon
- ◆ sardines, roe.

Have your patient substitute:
- ◆ lean cuts of beef, lamb, or pork
- ◆ poultry
- ◆ sole, salmon, mackerel.

◆ ADDING OR CUTTING DOWN ON POTASSIUM

If your patient is taking a drug such as furosemide or if he has had severe GI fluid loss from vomiting, diarrhea, or laxative abuse that decreases his potassium level, the doctor may recommend adding potassium to his diet. If your patient has acute or chronic renal failure or hypoaldosteronism or is taking a potassium-sparing diuretic such as spironolactone, he may need to reduce his intake of dietary potassium to prevent the development of hyperkalemia.

How much potassium does your patient need?

Doctors recommend 300 to 400 mg of potassium daily. A potassium deficiency can cause leg cramps, weakness, paralysis, and spasms. Too much potassium, however, can cause heart problems and fatigue.

The following chart lists potassium-rich foods along with their potassium content (the number of milligrams in a 3½-oz serving). Because some of these foods are also high in calories, check with your patient's doctor or dietitian if your patient is on a weight-reduction diet.

Potassium content of common foods

Meats	**mg**
Beef	370
Chicken	411
Lamb	290
Liver	380
Pork	326
Turkey	411
Veal	500
Fish, shellfish	**mg**
Bass	256
Flounder	342
Haddock	348
Halibut	525
Oysters	203
Perch	284
Salmon	421
Sardines, canned	590
Scallops	476
Tuna	301
Fruits	**mg**
Apricots	281
Bananas	370
Dates	648
Figs	152
Nectarines	294
Oranges	200
Peaches	202
Plums	299
Prunes	262
Raisins	355

Vegetables	**mg**
Asparagus	238
Brussel sprouts	295
Cabbage	233
Carrots	341
Endive	294
Lima beans	394
Peppers	213
Potatoes	407
Radishes	322
Spinach	324
Sweet potatoes	300
Juices	**mg**
Orange, fresh	200
Orange, reconstituted	186
Tomato	227
Other foods	**mg**
Gingersnap cookies	462
Graham crackers	384
Ice milk	195
Milk, dry (nonfat solids)	745
Molasses (light)	917
Oatmeal cookies (with raisins)	370
Peanut butter	670
Peanuts	674

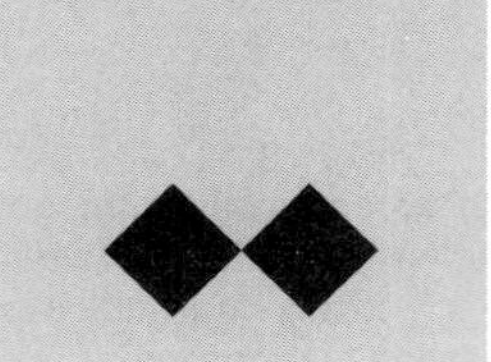

Index

i refers to an illustration; t to a table.

i refers to an illustration; t to a table.

C ◆

i refers to an illustration; t to a table.

D ◆

E ◆

i refers to an illustration; t to a table.

G ◆

H ◆

i refers to an illustration; t to a table.

J ◆

K ◆

L ◆

N ◆

O ◆

i refers to an illustration; t to a table.

i refers to an illustration; t to a table.

T ◆

i refers to an illustration; t to a table.

U ◆

V ◆

WX ◆

Y 

Z ◆

i refers to an illustration; t to a table.

Commonly used abbreviations *(continued from inside front cover)*

LA	left atrium
	long-acting
LAP	left atrial pressure
	leucine aminopeptidase
LBBB	left bundle-branch block
LD	lactate dehydrogenase
	lethal dose
LDL	low-density lipoprotein
LE	lupus erythematosus
LES	lower esophageal sphincter
LH	luteinizing hormone
LLQ	left lower quadrant
LOC	level of consciousness
LR	lactated Ringer's solution
LSB	left scapular border
	left sternal border
LUQ	left upper quadrant
LV	left ventricle
LVEDP	left ventricular end-diastolic pressure
LVET	left ventricular ejection time
LVF	left ventricular failure
m	meter
M	molar (solution)
m^2	square meter
MAO	monoamine oxidase
mcg	microgram
MCH	mean corpuscular hemoglobin
MCHC	mean corpuscular hemoglobin concentration
MCV	mean corpuscular volume
MD	manic depressive
	medical doctor
	muscular dystrophy
mEq	milliequivalent
mg	milligram
mgtt	microdrip or minidrop
MI	mitral insufficiency
	myocardial infarction
	myocardial ischemia
ml	milliliter
µg	microgram
µL	microliter
mm	millimeter
mm^3	cubic millimeter
MMEF	maximal midexpiratory flow
mmol	millimole
MRI	magnetic resonance imaging
MS	mitral sounds
	mitral stenosis
	morphine sulfate
	multiple sclerosis
	musculoskeletal
MUGA	multiple-gated acquisition (scanning)
MVI	multivitamin infusion
MVP	mitral valve prolapse
MVV	maximal voluntary ventilation
Na	sodium
NaCl	sodium chloride
NAHC	National Association for Home Care
NCQA	National Commission on Quality Assurance
ng	nanogram
NG	nasogastric
NIDDM	non-insulin-dependent diabetes mellitus
NKA	no known allergies
NP	nasopharynx
	new patient
	not palpable
NPO	nothing by mouth
NR	nonreactive
	no report
	no respirations
N/R	not remarkable
NS, NSS	normal saline solution (0.9% sodium chloride)
NSAID	nonsteroidal anti-inflammatory drug
O_2	oxygen
OASIS	Outcome and Assessment Information Set
OBQI	outcome-based quality improvement
OD	occupational disease
	oculus dexter (right eye)
	overdose
OS	oculus sinister (left eye)
O_2 sat	oxygen saturation
OSHA	Occupational Safety and Health Administration
OT	occupational therapist
OTC	over-the-counter
OU	oculus uterque (each eye)
oz	ounce
PA	posteroanterior
	pulmonary artery
PAC	premature atrial contraction
PaO_2	partial pressure of arterial oxygen
$PaCO_2$	partial pressure of arterial carbon dioxide
PAP	primary atypical pneumonia
	pulmonary artery pressure
Pap (test)	Papanicolaou test
PAT	paroxysmal atrial tachycardia
PAWP	pulmonary artery wedge pressure
p.c.	after meals
PCA	patient-controlled analgesia
PDA	patent ductus arteriosus
PE	physical examination
	pulmonary embolism
PEEP	positive end-expiratory pressure
PEFR	peak expiratory flow rate
per	by or through
PHO	physician hospital organization
PICC	peripherally inserted central catheter
PID	pelvic inflammatory disease
PKU	phenylketonuria
PMI	point of maximal impulse
PMS	premenstrual syndrome
PND	paroxysmal nocturnal dyspnea
	postnasal drip

D & C	dilatation and curettage
DD	differential diagnosis
	discharge diagnosis
	dry dressing
D & E	dilatation and evacuation
DIC	disseminated intravascular coagulation
dil	dilute
disp	dispense
DJD	degenerative joint disease
DKA	diabetic ketoacidosis
dl	deciliter
DNA	deoxyribonucleic acid
DNR	do not resuscitate
DOA	date of admission
	dead on arrival
DRG	diagnosis-related group
DS	double-strength
DSA	digital subtraction angiography
DTP	diphtheria and tetanus toxoids and pertussis vaccine
DVT	deep vein thrombosis
D_5W	dextrose 5% in water
EBV	Epstein-Barr virus
EC	enteric-coated
ECF	extended care facility
	extracellular fluid
ECG	electrocardiogram
ECHO	echocardiography
ECMO	extracorporeal membrane oxygenator
ECT	electroconvulsive therapy
EDTA	ethylenediamine tetra-acetic acid
EEG	electroencephalogram
EENT	eyes, ears, nose, throat
EF	ejection fraction
ELISA	enzyme-linked immunosorbent assay
elix	elixir
EMG	electromyography
ENG	electronystagmography
EOM	extraocular movement
ER	emergency room
	expiratory reserve
ERCP	endoscopic retrograde cholangiopancreatography
ERV	expiratory reserve volume
ESR	erythrocyte sedimentation rate
ESWL	extracorporeal shock-wave lithotripsy
F	Fahrenheit
FEF	forced expiratory flow
FEV	forced expiratory volume
FFP	fresh frozen plasma
FFS	fee for service
FHR	fetal heart rate
fl, fld	fluid
FRC	functional residual capacity
FSH	follicle-stimulating hormone
FSP	fibrinogen-split products
FT_3	free triiodothyronine
FT_4	free thyroxine
FTA	fluorescent treponemal antibody (test)
FTA-ABS	fluorescent treponemal antibody absorption (test)
FUO	fever of undetermined origin
FVC	forced vital capacity
G	gauge
g, gm	gram
GFR	glomerular filtration rate
GI	gastrointestinal
G6PD	glucose-6-phosphate dehydrogenase
gr	grain
gtt	drop
GU	genitourinary
GVHD	graft-versus-host disease
HAV	hepatitis A virus
Hb	hemoglobin
HBIG	hepatitis B immunoglobulin
HBsAg	hepatitis B surface antigen
HBV	hepatitis B virus
HCA	home care aide
HCFA	Health Care Financing Administration
hCG	human chorionic gonadotropin
HCO_3	bicarbonate
Hct, HCT	hematocrit
HDL	high-density lipoprotein
HF	heart failure
hGH	human growth hormone
HHNS	hyperosmolar hyperglycemic nonketotic syndrome
HIV	human immunodeficiency virus
HLA	human leukocyte antigen
HMO	health maintenance organization
h.s.	at bedtime
HSV	herpes simplex virus
HZV	herpes zoster virus
IA	intra-arterial
	intra-articular
IABP	intra-aortic balloon pump
IC	inspiratory capacity
ICD	International Classification of Diseases
ICP	intracranial pressure
ID	identification
	initial dose
	inside diameter
	intradermal
I & D	incision and drainage
IDDM	insulin-dependent diabetes mellitus
IM	infectious mononucleosis
I.M.	intramuscular
IMV	intermittent mandatory ventilation
IND	investigational new drug
IPPB	intermittent positive-pressure breathing
IRV	inspiratory reserve volume
IU	International Unit
IUD	intrauterine device
I.V.	intravenous
IVH	intravenous hyperalimentation
IVP	intravenous pyelography
JCAHO	Joint Commission on Accreditation of Healthcare Organizations
JVD	jugular vein distention
JVP	jugular venous pressure
kg	kilogram
KUB	kidney-ureter-bladder
KVO	keep vein open
L	liter
	lumbar
	left

(continued inside back cover)